T0293563

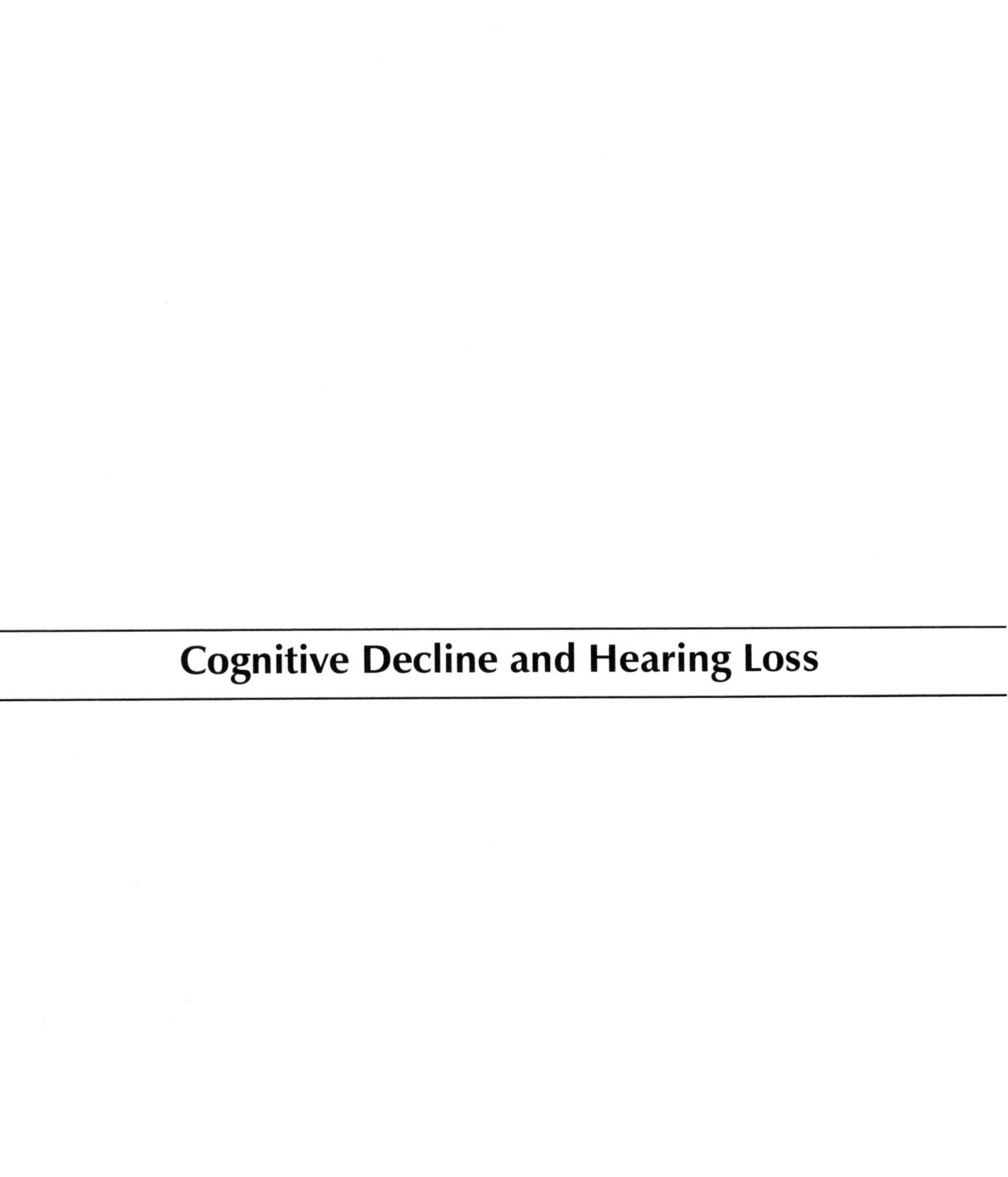

Cognitive Decline and Hearing Loss

Cognitive Decline and Hearing Loss

Editor: Blake Haldeman

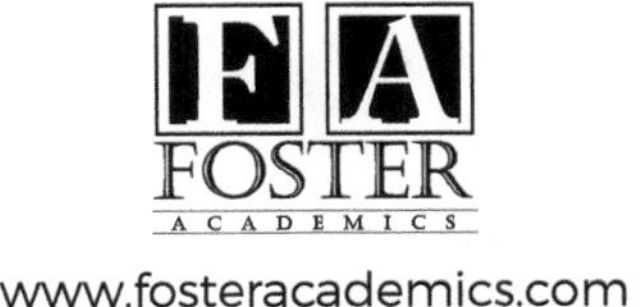

www.fosteracademics.com

www.fosteracademics.com

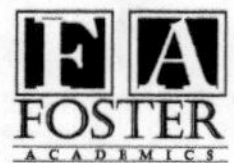

Cataloging-in-Publication Data

Cognitive decline and hearing loss / edited by Blake Haldeman.
p. cm.
Includes bibliographical references and index.
ISBN 978-1-64646-579-8
1. Deafness. 2. Hearing disorders. 3. Nervous system--Diseases.
4. Neurology. I. Haldeman, Blake.
RF290 .H433 2023
617.8--dc23

Foster Academics,
118-35 Queens Blvd., Suite 400,
Forest Hills, NY 11375, USA

ISBN 978-1-64646-579-8 (Hardback)

Contents

Preface

The main aim of this book is to educate learners and enhance their research focus by presenting diverse topics covering this vast field. This is an advanced book which compiles significant studies by distinguished experts in the area of analysis. This book addresses successive solutions to the challenges arising in the area of application, along with it; the book provides scope for future developments.

Cognitive decline refers to a type of condition wherein a person experiences memory loss, slower or diminished thinking skills, or other impairments in mental capabilities. It is a reaction to the slower rate at which the brain functions due to the ageing of neurons. Environmental factors that are not conducive to a person's brain health can contribute to cognitive decline. This condition might range from dementia to mild cognitive impairment. Hearing loss is a partial or whole loss of hearing in one or both ears which can range from minor to profound. Its common causes include ageing, heredity, exposure to loud noise and illness. Hearing loss is independently linked to both incident cognitive impairment and accelerated cognitive decline in community-dwelling older adults. This book aims to understand the clinical perspectives of cognitive decline and hearing loss. It aims to shed light on some of the unexplored aspects of these medical conditions. This book will serve as a reference to a broad spectrum of readers.

It was a great honour to edit this book, though there were challenges, as it involved a lot of communication and networking between me and the editorial team. However, the end result was this all-inclusive book covering diverse themes in the field.

Finally, it is important to acknowledge the efforts of the contributors for their excellent chapters, through which a wide variety of issues have been addressed. I would also like to thank my colleagues for their valuable feedback during the making of this book.

Editor

1

Association of Hearing Acuity and Cognitive Function Among a Low-Income Elderly Population in Rural China

Yi Xu[1†], Yan Li[2†], Dandan Guo[3†], Xin Zhang[3†], Huiying Guo[1], Hui Cao[1], Xin Li[4], Jing Zhang[1], Jun Tu[3,5,6], Jinghua Wang[3,5,6], Xianjia Ning[3,5,6*] and Dong Yang[1*]*

[1] Department of Otorhinolaryngology, Tianjin Medical University General Hospital, Tianjin, China, [2] Department of Anesthesiology, Tianjin Jizhou People's Hospital, Tianjin, China, [3] Department of Neurology, Tianjin Medical University General Hospital, Tianjin, China, [4] Department of Otorhinolaryngology, Beijing Tsinghua Changgung Hospital, School of Clinical Medicine, Tsinghua University, Beijing, China, [5] Laboratory of Epidemiology, Tianjin Neurological Institute, Tianjin, China, [6] Key Laboratory of Post-Neuroinjury Neuro-Repair and Regeneration in Central Nervous System, Tianjin Neurological Institute, Ministry of Education and Tianjin City, Tianjin, China

***Correspondence:**
Dong Yang
entyd@sohu.com
Xianjia Ning
xning@tmu.edu.cn
Xin Li
entlixin@sina.com

†These authors have contributed equally to this work

Hearing loss is a modifiable risk factor for dementia and cognitive decline. However, the association between cognition and hearing acuity at different frequencies is unknown. We aimed to assess the relationships between hearing acuity at different frequencies with global cognitive function and five domains of cognition among a low-income elderly population in northern rural China. A population-based cross-sectional study was conducted to collect basic information from elderly residents aged 60 years and older in rural areas of Tianjin, China from April 2012 to November 2013. Pure tone averages (PTAs) at different frequencies in the ear with better hearing and Mini-Mental State Examination (MMSE) scores were measured, and the relationships between these variables were assessed. A total of 737 residents aged 60 years or more were enrolled in this study, and the prevalence of hearing impairment was 60.7%. After adjusting for sex, age, education, income, smoking, drinking, systolic blood pressure (SBP), total cholesterol (TC), and low-density lipoprotein cholesterol level (LDL-C), MMSE score and immediate recall score were negatively associated with overall PTA (OPTA) at four frequencies (0.5, 1, 2, and 4 kHz), PTA at low frequencies (LPTA; 0.5, 1, and 2 kHz), and PTA at high frequencies (HPTA; 3, 4, and 8 kHz) in the ear with better hearing. Moreover, orientation score was negatively associated with OPTA and LPTA, and the attention and calculation scores were negatively associated with OPTA and HPTA. Each 10-dB increase in OPTA was associated with a MMSE score decrease of 0.464. Each 10-dB increase in LPTA or HPTA was associated with a MMSE score decrease of 0.441 (95% CI: −0.795, −0.086) and 0.351 (95% CI: −0.592, −0.110), respectively. The present study demonstrated significant but weak relationships between OPTA, LPTA, and HPTA with global cognitive function, as defined using MMSE scores; these relationships were independent of age, education, lifestyle factors, and laboratory test values. These results indicated that hearing was associated with cognitive decline among older individuals, who should be screened routinely to identify risk for cognitive decline.

Keywords: cognitive function, hearing loss, pure tone average, low-frequency pure tone average, aging

INTRODUCTION

Cognitive impairment is the leading cause of disability and a global public health priority for aging populations (Wortmann, 2012; GBD 2017 DALYs and HALE Collaborators, 2018). The World Alzheimer Report estimated there were over 50 million people living with dementia globally, and this number was estimated to increase to more than 152 million by 2050 (Wimo et al., 2013). Moreover, most people with dementia live in developing countries, and the number of people living with dementia in China accounts for approximately 25% of total dementia population worldwide, posing a substantial economic and social burden (GBD 2016 Neurology Collaborators, 2019).

Hearing impairment is the third most prevalent chronic condition in older age (Yueh et al., 2003). According to the Global Burden of Disease study, there were 1.4 billion people living with hearing impairment in 2017, and approximately 90% of people with moderate to severe hearing impairment reside in developing countries (GBD 2017 Disease and Injury Incidence and Prevalence Collaborators, 2018). Hearing impairment has also been recognized as the largest potentially modifiable risk factor for dementia and cognitive decline (Livingston et al., 2017; Loughrey et al., 2018). Numerous epidemiological studies have demonstrated hearing impairment at older age was associated with cognitive decline (Lin et al., 2013; Gurgel et al., 2014; Deal et al., 2017; Pabst et al., 2021; Saji et al., 2021). For example, the Health, Aging and Body Composition Study found that hearing impairment at baseline was related to a 24% increased risk of dementia over a 6-year period (Lin et al., 2013). Hearing loss at older age usually impacts high-frequency hearing long before low-frequency hearing (Panza et al., 2015). Thus, it is important to determine whether hearing loss at high frequencies is associated with impaired cognitive function. However, studies exploring significant association between hearing acuity and cognition have used the pure tone average (PTA) threshold at overall or low frequencies (Bush et al., 2015; Golub et al., 2020). To our knowledge, only one cross-sectional study enrolling 307 elderly demonstrated PTA at low frequencies, but not high frequencies, was related to cognitive performance among older individuals (Mukari et al., 2017). The association between PTA at different frequencies and cognitive function is not as well established.

Moreover, socioeconomic inequality is related to the risk of hearing loss (Emmett and Francis, 2015; Ping et al., 2018), and low income is associated with poor auditory function, with approximately 90% residents living in low- and middle-income countries having moderate to profound hearing impairment (Davis and Hoffman, 2019). There is a high burden of hearing impairment in northern China, where the prevalence of hearing impairment is 49.3% among the low-income rural population aged over 45 years (Yang et al., 2021). Only four studies in China have focused on the mediating role of social isolation, cognitive reserve, and leisure activities between self-reported hearing impairment and cognitive decline (Chen and Lu, 2019; Chen and Zhou, 2020; Gao et al., 2020; Chen, 2021). However, the relationship between cognitive performance and PTA at different frequencies as measured using standardized audiometric tests in an older population has not been reported in China, especially in low-income rural areas.

Thus, the aim of this study was to evaluate the relationships between cognitive function and hearing acuity at different frequencies among a low-income elderly population in northern rural China.

MATERIALS AND METHODS

Study Population

This population-based, cross-sectional study recruited older individuals from 18 administrative villages in rural areas of Tianjin, China from April 2012 to November 2013 based on the Tianjin Brain Study (Wang et al., 2014; Hu et al., 2016). Owing to the national health policy, all residents aged 60 years and older visit the health center for free physical examinations annually. From this population, all older residents (≥ 60 years old) with previous diagnosis of total hearing loss (over 120 dB) and blindness (best-corrected distance visual acuity < 3/60 or visual field < 10 central degrees) in the better ear/eye were excluded (Martin, 1986; World Health Organization (WHO), 2020).

The study was approved by the ethics committee at the Tianjin Medical University General Hospital, and written informed consent was obtained from all participants.

Risk Factors and Physical Examinations

This study was conducted through face-to-face interviews by trained researchers. Demographic information (including name, sex, date of birth, income, and educational level), individual medical history (including the presence of hypertension, diabetes mellitus, stroke, and coronary heart disease), and lifestyle factors (including smoking, drinking, and exercise) were collected using a pre-designed questionnaire; data regarding exercise was missing for six individuals. The participants were categorized into three age groups (60–64, 65–69, and ≥ 70 years), three educational groups (0–5, 6–8, and ≥ 9 years), and three groups of annual per capita income (< 300 USD, 300–650 USD, and > 650 USD). Smoking was defined as smoking ≥ 1 cigarette daily for more than 1 year. Drinking was defined as drinking > 50 mL of alcohol at least once per week for more than 6 months.

Body height, weight, waist circumference, systolic blood pressure (SBP), and diastolic blood pressure (DBP) were obtained by local general practitioners with the participant wearing thin clothing. The levels of fasting blood glucose (FBG), total cholesterol (TC), triglycerides (TG), high-density lipoprotein cholesterol (HDL-C), and low-density lipoprotein cholesterol (LDL-C) were tested in the central laboratory of the Tianjin Ji County People's Hospital. Hypertension was defined as a SBP ≥ 140 mm Hg, DBP ≥ 90 mm Hg, the use of antihypertensive drugs, or a history of hypertension. Diabetes was defined as a FBG ≥ 7.0 mmol/L, taking medication for diabetes, or a self-reported history of diabetes. Body mass index (BMI) was calculated as the individual's weight (kg) divided by the square of the individual's height (m^2) and was classified into four categories (low-weight, < 18.5 kg/m^2; normal, 18.5–23.9 kg/m^2; overweight, 24.0–27.9 kg/m^2; and obese, ≥ 28.0 kg/m^2; Zhou, 2002).

Cognitive Impairment

Cognitive function was measured using the Chinese version of the Mini-Mental State Examination (MMSE) owing to its high sensitivity and specificity of screening for cognitive impairment (Li et al., 1989; Canadian Task Force on Preventive Health Care et al., 2016). The diagnostic criteria of cognitive impairment were based on MMSE score according to educational levels. The MMSE is a 30-point scale that assesses five different cognitive domains including orientation, immediate recall, attention and calculation, recall, and language. Cognitive impairment was defined as an MMSE score < 17 points in the illiterate group, < 22 points in the primary school group, and < 26 points in the junior school and above group (Nunes et al., 2010).

Hearing Test

Audiometric assessments in each ear were performed at seven frequencies (0.5, 1, 2, 3, 4, 6, and 8 kHz) in a quiet, soundproof room using the Denmark XETA Audiometer (Xeta EN60645-1 type:3 REF:8-04-12207 GN Otometrics A/S Hoerskaetten 92360 Taastrup DENMARK) and TDH 50P transducer (Telephonics, Huntington, NY). Audiometric thresholds were measured at 5-dB increments in decibels of hearing level (dB HL). Outcome variables reported in this study were overall PTA (OPTA) at four frequencies (0.5, 1, 2, and 4 kHz), PTA at low frequencies (LPTA; 0.5, 1, and 2 kHz), and PTA at high frequencies (HPTA; 3, 4, and 8 kHz) in the ear with better hearing. Hearing impairment was defined as OPTA > 25 dB of the better ear according to the World Health Organization's definition of impairment [World Health Organization (WHO), 1997]. Participants suspected of having hearing impairment were referred to audiologists for final diagnoses.

Statistical Analysis

Continuous variables (age, BMI, waist circumference, SBP, DBP, FBG, TC, TG, LDL-C, HDL-C, and PTA) are described as means and standard deviations. Categorical variables (binary variables: sex, smoking, drinking, physical exercise, hypertension, diabetes, stroke, hearing impairment, and MMSE group; multi-categorical variables: age, education, income, and BMI groups) are presented as numbers with frequencies. The Student *t*-test was used to compare MMSE score differences between binary variables; the ANOVA test was used to compare MMSE score differences between multi-categorical variables. Univariate linear analyses were used to evaluate the relationship between each continuous variable and the MMSE score. Multiple linear regression analyses were used to evaluate the relationship between PTA and MMSE score after adjusting for independent variables that were statistically significant in the univariate analyses. The univariate analysis results are shown as unadjusted β-values and 95% confidence intervals (CIs); the multivariate analysis results are shown as adjusted β-values and 95% CIs after adjusting for covariates.

All statistical analyses were performed with SPSS version 19.0 statistical software (SPSS Inc., Chicago, IL, United States), and a two-sided *P*-value ≤ 0.05 was considered statistically significant.

RESULTS

Demographic Characteristics

A total of 737 residents aged more than 60 years (mean age, 68.95 years) were enrolled in this study, including 324 men (44.0%; mean age, 69.65 years) and 413 women (56.0%; mean age, 68.39 years). In this rural population, the prevalence of hearing impairment was 60.7% overall, 64.2% in men, and 57.9% in women. The mean OPTA of all residents was 30.27 dB HL, with 28.99 dB in LPTA, and 35.44 dB in HPTA. The average education level of the participants was low: 41.7% were illiterate. Moreover, 733 (99.5%) participants had annual per capita incomes of < 650 USD (**Table 1**).

Factors Associated With MMSE Score in the Univariate Analysis

The MMSE score was higher among participants with female sex, older age, high education, high income, smoking, and drinking, compared with other groups (all, $P < 0.001$). Compared with individuals with normal hearing, MMSE score of those with hearing impairment did not approached statistical significance ($P = 0.872$; **Table 2**).

In the linear regression analysis, MMSE score was negatively associated with SBP, TC, and LDL-C (all, $P < 0.05$; **Table 3**).

Association of MMSE Score and Its Domains With PTA in the Univariate Analysis

Linear regression analysis showed that MMSE score and its domains, immediate recall, and attention and calculation, were negatively correlated with OPTA, LPTA, and HPTA (all, $P < 0.05$). Orientation was negatively correlated with OPTA and LPTA in the univariate analysis (**Table 4**).

TABLE 1 | Demographic characteristics and risk factors for all participants by sex group.

Risk factors	Men	Women	Total
Total, *n* (%)	324 (44.0)	413 (56.0)	737 (100.0)
Age group, *n* (%)			
60–64 years	84 (25.9)	133 (32.2)	217 (29.4)
65–69 years	97 (29.9)	130 (31.5)	227 (30.8)
70–74 years	63 (19.4)	77 (18.6)	140 (19.0)
≥ 75 years	80 (24.7)	73 (17.7)	153 (20.8)
Education, *n* (%)			
0–6 years	57 (17.6)	250 (60.5)	307 (41.7)
6–8 years	190 (58.6)	125 (30.3)	315 (42.7)
≥ 9 years	77 (23.8)	38 (9.2)	115 (15.6)
Annual per-capital income			
< 300 USD	262 (80.9)	392 (94.9)	654 (88.7)
300–650 USD	60 (18.5)	19 (4.6)	79 (10.7)
> 650 USD	2 (0.6)	2 (0.5)	4 (0.5)
Smoking, *n* (%)			
No	181 (55.9)	386 (93.5)	567 (76.9)
Yes	143 (44.1)	27 (6.5)	170 (23.1)
Drinking, *n* (%)			
No	194 (59.9)	397 (96.1)	591 (80.2)
Yes	130 (40.1)	16 (3.9)	146 (19.8)
Physical exercise, *n* (%)			
No	231 (72.9)	295 (73.0)	526 (73.0)
Yes	86 (27.1)	109 (27.0)	195 (27.0)
Hypertension, *n* (%)			
No	174 (53.7)	214 (51.8)	388 (52.6)
Yes	150 (46.3)	199 (48.2)	349 (47.4)
Diabetes, *n* (%)			
No	296 (91.4)	361 (87.4)	657 (89.1)
Yes	28 (8.6)	52 (12.6)	80 (10.9)
CHD, *n* (%)			
No	271 (83.6)	330 (79.9)	601 (81.5)
Yes	53 (16.4)	83 (20.1)	136 (18.5)
Stroke, *n* (%)			
No	311 (96.0)	396 (95.9)	707 (95.9)
Yes	13 (4.0)	17 (4.1)	30 (4.1)
Hearing impairment, *n* (%)			
No	116 (35.8)	174 (42.1)	290 (39.3)
Yes	208 (64.2)	239 (57.9)	447 (60.7)
BMI category, *n* (%)			
Low-weight	13 (4.0)	9 (2.2)	22 (3.0)
Normal	150 (46.3)	178 (43.1)	328 (44.5)
Overweight	120 (37.0)	161 (39.0)	281 (38.1)
Obese	41 (12.7)	65 (15.7)	106 (14.4)
MMSE group, *n* (%)			
Non-CI	59 (18.2)	31 (7.5)	90 (12.2)
CI	265 (81.8)	382 (92.5)	647 (87.8)
Age, means (SD)	69.65 (6.45)	68.39 (6.10)	68.95 (6.28)
BMI (kg/m^2), mean (SD)	24.10 (3.31)	24.66 (3.51)	24.42 (3.43)
Waist (cm), mean (SD)	86.90 (9.65)	86.53 (9.22)	86.69 (9.41)
SBP, mean (SD)	5.48 (1.24)	5.55 (1.35)	5.52 (1.30)
DBP, mean (SD)	4.34 (0.86)	4.89 (0.94)	4.65 (0.94)
FBG, mean (SD)	1.19 (0.72)	1.56 (0.90)	1.40 (0.84)
TC, mean (SD)	1.36 (0.43)	1.43 (0.53)	1.40 (0.49)
TG, mean (SD)	2.27 (0.98)	2.74 (1.00)	2.53 (1.02)
HDL-C, mean (SD)	157.85 (23.80)	159.76 (23.83)	158.92 (23.82)
LDL-C, mean (SD)	92.38 (12.28)	91.44 (12.62)	91.85 (12.47)
MMSE score, mean (SD)	22.45 (4.55)	19.18 (5.31)	20.62 (5.24)
OPTA, mean (SD), dB HL	31.30 (10.54)	29.46 (8.59)	30.27 (9.54)
LPTA, mean (SD), dB HL	29.07 (9.44)	28.91 (8.48)	28.99 (8.91)
HPTA, mean (SD), dB HL	38.69 (15.61)	32.87 (11.61)	35.43 (13.81)

SD, standard deviation; CHD, coronary heart disease; BMI, body mass index; MMSE, Mini-Mental state examination; CI: cognitive impairment; SBP, systolic blood pressure; DBP, diastolic blood pressure; FBG, fasting blood glucose; TC, total cholesterol; TG, triglycerides; HDL-C, high-density lipoprotein cholesterol; LDL-C, low-density lipoprotein cholesterol; OPTA, overall pure tone average; LPTA, low-frequency pure tone average; HPTA, high-frequency pure tone average.

TABLE 2 | Differences in mean MMSE score, according to demographic characteristics and risk factors groups.

Characteristics	Mean MMSE	*F/t*	*P*
Sex		9.015	< 0.001
Men	22.45 (4.55)		
Women	19.18 (5.31)		
Age group		21.077	< 0.001
60–64 years	21.64 (4.63)		
65–69 years	21.70 (4.78)		
70–74 years	20.21 (5.28)		
≥ 75 years	17.94 (5.71)		
Education		138.452	< 0.001
0–5 years	17.54 (4.98)		
6–8 years	22.13 (4.38)		
≥ 9 years	24.70 (3.09)		
Annual per-capital income		10.266	< 0.001
< 300 USD	20.31 (5.31)		
300–650 USD	22.95 (3.95)		
> 650 USD	24.50 (3.11)		
Smoking		−4.224	< 0.001
No	20.20 (5.33)		
Yes	22.00 (4.72)		
Drinking		−5.347	< 0.001
No	20.15 (5.30)		
Yes	22.49 (4.58)		
Hypertension		−0.317	0.751
No	20.56 (5.23)		
Yes	20.68 (5.27)		
Diabetes		−0.082	0.935
No	20.61 (5.25)		
Yes	20.66 (5.23)		
CHD		−1.438	0.152
No	20.49 (5.32)		
Yes	21.17 (4.87)		
Stroke		−0.728	0.462
No	20.59 (5.25)		
Yes	21.30 (5.12)		
Hearing impairment		0.162	0.872
No	20.66 (4.91)		
Yes	20.59 (5.45)		

CHD, coronary heart disease.

Association of MMSE Score and Its Domains With PTA in the Multiple Linear Regression Analysis

Mini-Mental State Examination score and immediate recall score were negatively associated with OPTA, LPTA, and HPTA in multiple linear regression analyses after adjusting for sex, age, education, income, smoking, drinking, SBP, TC, and LDL-C (all, $P < 0.05$). Moreover, orientation score was negatively associated with OPTA and LPTA (all, $P < 0.05$), and attention and calculation score were negatively associated with OPTA and HPTA after adjusting for sex, age, education, income, smoking, drinking, SBP, TC, and LDL-C (all, $P < 0.05$; **Table 5**). The R^2 value in linear regression was similar between LPTA and HPTA (adjusted R^2 0.332 vs. 0.334).

DISCUSSION

This study evaluated the associations between peripheral hearing with global cognitive function and five domains of cognition

TABLE 3 | Association of MMSE score with measured parameters in the linear regression analysis.

Characteristics	β (95% CI)	P
SBP	−0.020 (−0.036, −0.004)	0.012
DBP	0.020 (−0.010, 0.050)	0.197
FBG	0.042 (−0.250, 0.333)	0.779
TC	−0.762 (−1.160, −0.363)	< 0.001
TG	−0.211 (−0.663, 0.241)	0.359
HDL-C	−0.635 (−.411, 0.140)	0.108
LDL-C	−0.611 (−0.982, −0.241)	0.001

SBP, systolic blood pressure; DBP, diastolic blood pressure; FBG: fasting blood glucose; TC, total cholesterol; TG, triglycerides; HDL-C, high-density lipoprotein cholesterol; LDL-C, low-density lipoprotein cholesterol.

TABLE 4 | Association of MMSE and its domains with pure tone average in the linear regression analysis.

Parameters	β	SE	95% CI	P
OPTA				
MMSE score	−0.520	0.202	−0.917, −0.124	0.010
Orientation	−0.126	0.057	−0.238, −0.015	0.026
Immediate recall	−0.127	0.035	−0.196, −0.058	< 0.001
Attention and calculation	−0.157	0.068	−0.291, −0.023	0.022
Recall	0.072	0.048	−0.022, 0.166	0.133
Language	−0.087	0.079	−0.242, 0.068	0.269
LPTA				
MMSE score	−0.601	0.216	−1.025, −0.177	0.006
Orientation	−0.157	0.061	−0.276, −0.038	0.010
Immediate recall	−0.129	0.038	−0.203, −0.055	0.001
Attention and calculation	−0.155	0.073	−0.298, −0.011	0.035
Recall	0.089	0.051	−0.011, 0.189	0.082
Language	−0.137	0.084	−0.303, 0.028	0.104
HPTA				
MMSE score	−0.347	0.140	−0.621, −0.073	0.013
Orientation	−0.065	0.039	−0.142, 0.012	0.096
Immediate recall	−0.092	0.024	−0.140, −0.044	< 0.001
Attention and calculation	−0.130	0.047	−0.222, −0.037	0.006
Recall	0.023	0.033	−0.042, 0.088	0.695
Language	−0.034	0.054	−0.141, 0.073	0.532

β, regression coefficient; SE, standard error; CI, confidence interval; OPTA, overall pure tone audiometry; LPTA, low-frequency pure tone average; HPTA, high-frequency pure tone average.

among low-income elderly individuals in northern rural China. The prevalence of hearing impairment was 60.7% in this low-income rural population. LPTA and HPTA were negatively and independently related to MMSE score and its domains; this association was independent of age, education, lifestyle factors, and laboratory test values. In multiple linear regression analysis, both LPTA and HPTA accounted for a minimal proportion variance of MMSE score after adjusting for other covariates. There was a 0.441-point and 0.351-point MMSE score decrease associated with each 10-dB increase in LPTA and HPTA, respectively.

Hearing loss is prevalent among older adults and associated with a high prevalence of cognitive decline, apathy, and poor functional status (Sugawara et al., 2011; Miyake et al., 2020). In the present study, four-frequency PTA in the ear with better hearing was an independent risk factor for global cognitive status (MMSE score) and its domains; these findings are consistent with most previous studies. For instance, a longitudinal community-dwelling study found that hearing loss was related to accelerated cognitive decline and dementia among older adults, and individuals with hearing impairment at baseline was related to a 24% increased risk of dementia after a 6-year follow-up (Lin et al., 2013). Two American epidemiologic studies also found an independent association between cognitive performance and subclinical hearing loss; there was a 0.97-point decrease in the Digit Symbol Substitution Test score associated with a 10-dB increase of the PTA (Golub et al., 2020). Furthermore, a systematic review and meta-analysis demonstrated that hearing impairment was associated with a decline of global cognition, cognitive domains of executive function, and episodic memory, as well as increased risk of incident dementia and cognitive impairment (Loughrey et al., 2018). Other studies found stronger associations between hearing decline and lower episodic memory levels (Maharani et al., 2018b; Guglielmi et al., 2020). As a proxy measurement for episodic memory, immediate recall was strongly associated with worse hearing acuity in present study. Moreover, hearing aids use helps to slow down cognitive decline and improve functional status of older individuals (Maharani et al., 2018a; Sarant et al., 2020). However, a prospective cohort study in four American metropolitan areas demonstrated that vision, but not hearing impairment, was associated with cognitive decline (Lin et al., 2004). Another longitudinal study found that hearing loss did not accelerate cognitive decline over time after adjusting for the non-linear effects of age (Croll et al., 2021). In the present study, PTA was negatively and independently related to MMSE score and its domains independent of age, education, lifestyle factors, and laboratory test values.

Additionally, we found an independent association of both LPTA and HPTA with MMSE score. To our knowledge, only one study has assessed the association between PTA of different frequencies and cognitive performance; this prior study reported that LPTA, but not HPTA, was significantly and independently related to the MMSE score (Mukari et al., 2017). Studies

TABLE 5 | Association of MMSE and its domains with pure tone average in the multiple linear analysis.

Parameters	β (95% CI)		
	OPTA	LPTA	HPTA
MMSE score	−0.464 (−0.798, −0.130)**	−0.441 (−0.795, −0.086)*	−0.351 (−0.592, −0.110)**
Orientation	−0.114 (−0.218, −0.009)*	−0.122 (−0.232, −0.012)*	–
Immediate recall	−0.107 (−0.175, −0.040)**	−0.100 (−0.171, −0.028)**	−0.082 (−0.131, −0.034)**
Attention and calculation	−0.130 (−0.253, −0.007)*	−0.101 (−0.232, 0.029)	−0.121 (−0.210, −0.033)**

$^*P < 0.05$. $^{**}P < 0.01$. Adjusted for sex, age, education, income, smoking, drinking, TC, LDL-C, and SBP.

have consistently confirmed that PTA is highly correlated with speech recognition (Coren and Hakstian, 1994; Vermiglio et al., 2012). In addition, a cross-section study demonstrated that PTA at low frequency exhibited the highest effect on speech recognition threshold compared to PTA at full range and high frequencies (Coren and Hakstian, 1994). High LPTA was more associated with poor speech recognition, which resulted in difficulty in communicating and maintaining interpersonal relationships (Lindenberger and Baltes, 1994; Maharani et al., 2019). These reasons will further cause social isolation, loneliness, and cognitive decline.

Three hypotheses have been proposed to explain the association between hearing and cognitive function (Wayne and Johnsrude, 2015; Uchida et al., 2019). In the cognitive load hypothesis, auditory signals are degraded among individuals with hearing loss (Lavie, 1995). Consequently, greater cognitive resource is required to understand speech, which affects other cognitive tasks and results in cognitive reserve depletion (Tun et al., 2009). Excessive cognitive load in daily life would cause neurodegeneration and structural changes in the brain, which subsequently impairs cognitive function (Martini et al., 2014). In addition, according to the common cause hypothesis, hearing impairment usually occurs simultaneously with cognitive decline at older ages; both hearing impairment and cognitive decline are results of neuropathological cause without direction of causality (Stahl, 2017). Finally, the sensory deprivation hypothesis suggests that sensory impairment, like hearing and vision impairment, could prevent older adults from communicating, resulting in social isolation, loneliness, and poor cognitive status (Rutherford et al., 2018). Some studies have reported the mediating effect of social isolation and loneliness between hearing and cognition (Rutherford et al., 2018; Maharani et al., 2019).

This was a population-based real-world study. Although studies have shown that hearing impairment increases the risk of cognitive decline, the relationship between hearing acuity and cognition remains inconclusive, especially in studies of large-scale low-income people. Moreover, many factors including age, sex, education, income, blood pressure, serum lipids, diabetes, smoking, and drinking can affect cognitive function (Yaffe et al., 2021). In the present study, both LPTA and HPTA accounted for a minimal proportion variance of the MMSE score; this association was independent of age, education, lifestyle factors, and laboratory test values. Moreover, due to earlier hearing loss at high frequencies, it is of great importance to discover and manage hearing loss to reduce risk for cognitive decline on the early stage.

There are several limitations in this study. First, cognitive function was evaluated using MMSE scores rather than a cognitive test battery; therefore, cognitive domain deficit could not be further diagnosed. Second, the speech-in-noise test could better simulate communication environments of daily living. The Mandarin Quick Speech-in-Noise test (M-Quick SIN) is quick and reliable with high clinical feasibility (Zhou et al., 2014) in population-based study. As M-Quick SIN was not established until 2014, it was not included in the present study. In the future, we plan to conduct a study including the speech-in-noise test. Third, the study population was from a low-income, low-education, rural population in northern China, thus its representativeness and generalizability are limited. Fourth, other confounding factors, including APOE4 genotype and diet, are important factors for cognitive decline and were not excluded in this study (Davies et al., 2018; Kivipelto et al., 2018). Fifth, asymmetrical hearing can be detrimental to cognitive function (Brännström et al., 2018) but was not included in the present study. Our follow-up research will further focus on asymmetrical hearing. Last, this was a cross-sectional study, and therefore causal relationships could not be identified.

CONCLUSION

The present study demonstrated significant but weak relationships between OPTA, LPTA, and HPTA with global cognitive function, as defined using MMSE scores, independent of age, education, lifestyle factors, and laboratory test values. These results indicate that hearing was associated with cognitive decline among older individuals, who should be screened routinely to identify risk for cognitive decline.

AUTHOR CONTRIBUTIONS

DY, XL, and XN were involved in the conception and design of the study, data interpretation, and critically reviewed the manuscript. YX, YL, DG, XZ, HG, HC, XL, JZ, JT, and DY were involved in the data collection, case diagnosis, and confirmation for this manuscript. YX, YL, DG, and XZ were involved in the manuscript drafting and revision. JW was involved in the data analysis for this manuscript. All authors contributed to the article and approved the submitted version.

ACKNOWLEDGMENTS

We thank all participants of the Tianjin Brain Study and local medical care professionals for their valuable contributions.

REFERENCES

Brännström, K. J., Karlsson, E., Waechter, S., and Kastberg, T. (2018). Extended high-frequency pure tone hearing thresholds and core executive functions. *Int. J. Audiol.* 57, 639–645. doi: 10.1080/14992027.2018.1475755

Bush, A., Lister, J. J., Lin, F. R., Betz, J., and Edwards, J. D. (2015). Peripheral hearing and cognition: evidence from the staying keen in later life (skill) study. *Ear Hear.* 36, 395–407. doi: 10.1097/aud.0000000000000142

Canadian Task Force on Preventive Health Care, Pottie, K., Rahal, R., Jaramillo, A., Birtwhistle, R., Thombs, B. D., et al. (2016). Recommendations on screening for cognitive impairment in older adults. *CMAJ* 188, 37–46.

Chen, L. (2021). Self-reported hearing difficulty increases 3-year risk of incident cognitive impairment: the role of leisure activities and psychological resilience. *Int. J. Geriatr. Psychiatry.* 36, 1197–1203. doi: 10.1002/gps.5511

Chen, L., and Lu, B. (2019). Cognitive reserve regulates the association between hearing difficulties and incident cognitive impairment evidence from a longitudinal study in China. *Int. Psychogeriatr.* 32, 635–643. doi: 10.1017/S1041610219001662

Chen, L., and Zhou, R. (2020). Does self-reported hearing difficulty decrease older adults' cognitive and physical functioning? The mediating role of social isolation. *Maturitas* 141, 53–58. doi: 10.1016/j.maturitas.2020.06.011

Coren, S., and Hakstian, A. R. (1994). Predicting speech recognition thresholds from pure tone hearing thresholds. *Percept. Mot. Skills* 79, 1003–1008. doi: 10.2466/pms.1994.79.2.1003

Croll, P. H., Vinke, E. J., Armstrong, N. M., Licher, S., Vernooij, M. W., Baatenburg de Jong, R. J., et al. (2021). Hearing loss and cognitive decline in the general population: a prospective cohort study. *J. Neurol.* 268, 860–871. doi: 10.1007/s00415-020-10208-8

Davies, G., Lam, M., Harris, S. E., Trampush, J. W., Luciano, M., Hill, W. D., et al. (2018). Study of 300,486 individuals identifies 148 independent genetic loci influencing general cognitive function. *Nat. Commun.* 9:2098. doi: 10.1038/s41467-018-04362-x

Davis, A. C., and Hoffman, H. J. (2019). Hearing loss: rising prevalence and impact. *Bull. World Health Organ.* 97, 646A–646A. doi: 10.2471/BLT.19.224683

Deal, J. A., Betz, J., Yaffe, K., Harris, T., Purchase-Helzner, E., Satterfield, S., et al. (2017). Hearing impairment and incident dementia and cognitive decline in older adults: the health ABC study. *J. Gerontol. A Biol. Sci. Med. Sci.* 72, 703–709. doi: 10.1093/gerona/glw069

Emmett, S. D., and Francis, H. W. (2015). The socioeconomic impact of hearing loss in U.S. adults. *Otol. Neurotol.* 36, 545–550. doi: 10.1097/mao.0000000000000562

Gao, J., Armstrong, N. M., Deal, J. A., Lin, F. R., and He, P. (2020). Hearing loss and cognitive function among Chinese older adults: the role of participation in leisure activities. *BMC Geriatr* 20:215. doi: 10.1186/s12877-020-01615-7

GBD 2016 Neurology Collaborators (2019). Global, regional, and national burden of neurological disorders, 1990-2016: a systematic analysis for the Global Burden of Disease Study 2016. *Lancet Neurol.* 18, 459–480. doi: 10.1016/S1474-4422(18)30499-X

GBD 2017 DALYs and HALE Collaborators (2018). Global, regional, and national disability-adjusted life-years (DALYs) for 359 diseases and injuries and healthy life expectancy (HALE) for 195 countries and territories, 1990-2017: a systematic analysis for the Global Burden of Disease Study 2017. *Lancet* 392, 1859–1922. doi: 10.1016/S0140-6736(18)32335-3

GBD 2017 Disease and Injury Incidence and Prevalence Collaborators (2018). Global, regional, and national incidence, prevalence, and years lived with disability for 354 diseases and injuries for 195 countries and territories, 1990-2017: a systematic analysis for the Global Burden of Disease Study 2017. *Lancet* 392, 1789–1858. doi: 10.1016/S0140-6736(18)32279-7

Golub, J. S., Brickman, A. M., Ciarleglio, A. J., Schupf, N., and Luchsinger, J. A. (2020). Association of subclinical hearing loss with cognitive performance. *JAMA Otolaryngol. Head Neck Surg.* 146, 57–67. doi: 10.1001/jamaoto.2019.3375

Guglielmi, V., Marra, C., Picciotti, P. M., Masone Iacobucci, G., Giovannini, S., Quaranta, D., et al. (2020). Does hearing loss in the elderly individuals conform to impairment of specific cognitive domains. *J. Geriatr. Psychiatry Neurol.* 33, 231–240. doi: 10.1177/0891988719874117

Gurgel, R. K., Ward, P. D., Schwartz, S., Norton, M. C., Foster, N. L., and Tschanz, J. T. (2014). Relationship of hearing loss and dementia: a prospective, population-based study. *Otol. Neurotol.* 35, 775–781. doi: 10.1097/mao.0000000000000313

Hu, Y., Zhao, L., Zhang, H., Yu, X., Wang, Z., Ye, Z., et al. (2016). Sex differences in the recurrence rate and risk factors for primary giant cell tumors around the knee in China. *Sci. Rep.* 6:28173. doi: 10.1038/srep28173

Kivipelto, M., Mangialasche, F., and Ngandu, T. (2018). Lifestyle interventions to prevent cognitive impairment, dementia and Alzheimer disease. *Nat. Rev. Neurol.* 14, 653–666. doi: 10.1038/s41582-018-0070-3

Lavie, N. (1995). Perceptual load as a necessary condition for selective attention. *J. Exp. Psychol. Hum. Percept. Perform.* 21, 451–468. doi: 10.1037/0096-1523.21.3.451

Li, G., Shen, Y., Chen, C., Li, S., Zhang, W., and Liu, M. (1989). Mini Mental State Examination (MMSE) in different population test study. *Chin. Mental Health J.* 4, 148–151.

Lin, F. R., Yaffe, K., Xia, J., Xue, Q. L., Harris, T. B., Purchase-Helzner, E., et al. (2013). Hearing loss and cognitive decline in older adults. *JAMA Intern. Med.* 173, 293–299. doi: 10.1001/jamainternmed.2013.1868

Lin, M. Y., Gutierrez, P. R., Stone, K. L., Yaffe, K., Ensrud, K. E., Fink, H. A., et al. (2004). Vision impairment and combined vision and hearing impairment predict cognitive and functional decline in older women. *J. Am. Geriatr. Soc.* 52, 1996–2002. doi: 10.1111/j.1532-5415.2004.52554.x

Lindenberger, U., and Baltes, P. B. (1994). Sensory functioning and intelligence in old age: a strong connection. *Psychol. Aging* 9, 339–355. doi: 10.1037/0882-7974.9.3.339

Livingston, G., Sommerlad, A., Orgeta, V., Costafreda, S. G., Huntley, J., Ames, D., et al. (2017). Dementia prevention, intervention, and care. *Lancet* 390, 2673–2734. doi: 10.1016/S0140-6736(17)31363-6

Loughrey, D. G., Kelly, M. E., Kelley, G. A., Brennan, S., and Lawlor, B. A. (2018). Association of age-related hearing loss with cognitive function, cognitive impairment, and dementia: a systematic review and meta-analysis. *JAMA Otolaryngol. Head Neck Surg.* 144, 115–126. doi: 10.1001/jamaoto.2017.2513

Maharani, A., Dawes, P., Nazroo, J., Tampubolon, G., Pendleton, N., and Sense-COG WP1 Group (2018a). Longitudinal relationship between hearing aid use and cognitive function in older Americans. *J. Am. Geriatr. Soc.* 66, 1130–1136. doi: 10.1111/jgs.15363

Maharani, A., Dawes, P., Nazroo, J., Tampubolon, G., Pendleton, N., and Sense-COG WP1 Group (2018b). Visual and hearing impairments are associated with cognitive decline in older people. *Age Ageing* 47, 575–581. doi: 10.1093/ageing/afy061

Maharani, A., Pendleton, N., and Leroi, I. (2019). Hearing impairment, loneliness, social isolation, and cognitive function: longitudinal analysis using English longitudinal study on ageing. *Am. J. Geriatr. Psychiatry* 27, 1348–1356. doi: 10.1016/j.jagp.2019.07.010

Martin, M. C. (1986). Total deafness: the need and possibility for a working definition. *Br. J. Audiol.* 20, 85–88. doi: 10.3109/03005368609079000

Martini, A., Castiglione, A., Bovo, R., Vallesi, A., and Gabelli, C. (2014). Aging, cognitive load, dementia and hearing loss. *Audiol. Neurootol.* 19(Suppl. 1), 2–5. doi: 10.1159/000371593

Miyake, Y., Tanaka, K., Senba, H., Ogawa, S., Suzuki, H., Fujiwara, Y., et al. (2020). Hearing impairment and prevalence of mild cognitive impairment in Japan: baseline data from the Aidai Cohort Study in Yawatahama and Uchiko. *Ear Hear.* 41, 254–258. doi: 10.1097/aud.0000000000000773

Mukari, S., Ishak, W. S., Maamor, N., and Wan Hashim, W. F. (2017). A preliminary study investigating the association between hearing acuity and a screening cognitive tool. *Ann. Otol. Rhinol. Laryngol.* 126, 697–705. doi: 10.1177/0003489417727547

Nunes, B., Silva, R. D., Cruz, V. T., Roriz, J. M., Pais, J., and Silva, M. C. (2010). Prevalence and pattern of cognitive impairment in rural and urban populations from Northern Portugal. *BMC Neurol.* 10:42. doi: 10.1186/1471-2377-10-42

Pabst, A., Bär, J., Röhr, S., Löbner, M., Kleineidam, L., Heser, K., et al. (2021). Do self-reported hearing and visual impairments predict longitudinal dementia in older adults. *J. Am. Geriatr. Soc.* 69, 1519–1528. doi: 10.1111/jgs.17074

Panza, F., Solfrizzi, V., and Logroscino, G. (2015). Age-related hearing impairment-a risk factor and frailty marker for dementia and AD. *Nat. Rev. Neurol.* 11, 166–175. doi: 10.1038/nrneurol.2015.12

Ping, H., Luo, Y., Hu, X., Rui, G., Xu, W., Zheng, X., et al. (2018). Association of socioeconomic status with hearing loss in Chinese working-aged adults: a population-based study. *PLoS One* 13:e0195227. doi: 10.1371/journal.pone.0195227

Rutherford, B. R., Brewster, K., Golub, J. S., Kim, A. H., and Roose, S. P. (2018). Sensation and psychiatry: linking age-related hearing loss to late-life depression and cognitive decline. *Am. J. Psychiatry* 175, 215–224. doi: 10.1176/appi.ajp.2017.17040423

Saji, N., Makizako, H., Suzuki, H., Nakai, Y., Tabira, T., Obuchi, S., et al. (2021). Hearing impairment is associated with cognitive function in community-dwelling older adults: a cross-sectional study. *Arch. Gerontol. Geriatr.* 93:104302. doi: 10.1016/j.archger.2020.104302

Sarant, J., Harris, D., Busby, P., Maruff, P., Schembri, A., Lemke, U., et al. (2020). The effect of hearing aid use on cognition in older adults: can we delay decline or even improve cognitive function. *J. Clin. Med.* 9:254. doi: 10.3390/jcm9010254

Stahl, S. M. (2017). Does treating hearing loss prevent or slow the progress of dementia? Hearing is not all in the ears, but who's listening. *CNS Spectr.* 22, 247–250. doi: 10.1017/s1092852917000268

Sugawara, N., Sasaki, A., Yasui-Furukori, N., Kakehata, S., Umeda, T., Namba, A., et al. (2011). Hearing impairment and cognitive function among a community-dwelling population in Japan. *Ann. Gen. Psychiatry* 10:27. doi: 10.1186/1744-859x-10-27

Tun, P. A., McCoy, S., and Wingfield, A. (2009). Aging, hearing acuity, and the attentional costs of effortful listening. *Psychol. Aging* 24, 761–766. doi: 10.1037/a0014802

Uchida, Y., Sugiura, S., Nishita, Y., Saji, N., Sone, M., and Ueda, H. (2019). Age-related hearing loss and cognitive decline–the potential mechanisms linking the two. *Auris Nasus Larynx* 46, 1–9. doi: 10.1016/j.anl.2018.08.010

Vermiglio, A. J., Soli, S. D., Freed, D. J., and Fisher, L. M. (2012). The relationship between high-frequency pure-tone hearing loss, hearing in noise test (HINT) thresholds, and the articulation index. *J. Am. Acad. Audiol.* 23, 779–788. doi: 10.3766/jaaa.23.10.4

Wang, J., Ning, X., Yang, L., Tu, J., Gu, H., Zhan, C., et al. (2014). Sex differences in trends of incidence and mortality of first-ever stroke in rural Tianjin, China, from 1992 to 2012. *Stroke* 45, 1626–1631. doi: 10.1161/strokeaha.113.003899

Wayne, R. V., and Johnsrude, I. S. (2015). A review of causal mechanisms underlying the link between age-related hearing loss and cognitive decline. *Ageing Res. Rev.* 23(Pt B), 154–166. doi: 10.1016/j.arr.2015.06.002

Wimo, A., Jönsson, L., Bond, J., Prince, M., Winblad, B., and Alzheimer Disease International (2013). The worldwide economic impact of dementia 2010. *Alzheimers Dement.* 9, 1.e–11.e. doi: 10.1016/j.jalz.2012.11.006

World Health Organization (WHO) (1997). *Prevention of Deafness and Hearing Impaired Grades of Hearing Impairment.* Geneva: WHO.

World Health Organization (WHO) (2020). *Blindness and Vision Impairment.* Geneva: WHO.

Wortmann, M. (2012). Dementia: a global health priority–highlights from an ADI and World Health Organization report. *Alzheimers Res. Ther.* 4:40. doi: 10.1186/alzrt143

Yaffe, K., Vittinghoff, E., Hoang, T., Matthews, K., Golden, S. H., and Zeki Al Hazzouri, A. (2021). Cardiovascular risk factors across the life course and cognitive decline: a pooled cohort study. *Neurology* 96, e2212–e2219. doi: 10.1212/WNL.0000000000011747

Yang, D., Liu, J., Yang, Q., Lin, Q., Zhang, X., Wang, M., et al. (2021). Hearing impairment prevalence and risk factors among adults in rural China: a population-based cross-sectional study. *Postgrad. Med.* 133, 369–376. doi: 10.1080/00325481.2020.1855852

Yueh, B., Shapiro, N., MacLean, C. H., and Shekelle, P. G. (2003). Screening and management of adult hearing loss in primary care: scientific review. *JAMA* 289, 1976–1985. doi: 10.1001/jama.289.15.1976

Zhou, B. F. (2002). Effect of body mass index on all-cause mortality and incidence of cardiovascular diseases–report for meta-analysis of prospective studies open optimal cut-off points of body mass index in Chinese adults. *Biomed. Environ. Sci.* 15, 245–252.

Zhou, R., Hua, Z., Wang, S., Jing, C., and Peng, Z. (2014). Scoring formula research and equivalence evaluation of mandarin quick speech-in-noise test materials in mainland China. *Lin chung.Er Bi Yan Hou Ke Za Zhi J. Clin. Otorhinolaryngol.* 28, 1104–1108.

2

Cerebral Representation of Sound Localization using Functional Near-Infrared Spectroscopy

Xuexin Tian[1], Yimeng Liu[1], Zengzhi Guo[2], Jieqing Cai[1], Jie Tang[1,3,4,5], Fei Chen[2]* and Hongzheng Zhang[1,4]**

[1] Department of Otolaryngology Head & Neck Surgery, Zhujiang Hospital, Southern Medical University, Guangzhou, China, [2] Department of Electrical and Electronic Engineering, Southern University of Science and Technology, Shenzhen, China, [3] Department of Physiology, School of Basic Medical Sciences, Southern Medical University, Guangzhou, China, [4] Hearing Research Center, Southern Medical University, Guangzhou, China, [5] Key Laboratory of Mental Health of the Ministry of Education, Southern Medical University, Guangzhou, China

***Correspondence:**
Jie Tang
jietang@smu.edu.cn
Fei Chen
fchen@sustech.edu.cn
Hongzheng Zhang
redtrue@smu.edu.cn

Sound localization is an essential part of auditory processing. However, the cortical representation of identifying the direction of sound sources presented in the sound field using functional near-infrared spectroscopy (fNIRS) is currently unknown. Therefore, in this study, we used fNIRS to investigate the cerebral representation of different sound sources. Twenty-five normal-hearing subjects (aged 26 ± 2.7, male 11, female 14) were included and actively took part in a block design task. The test setup for sound localization was composed of a seven-speaker array spanning a horizontal arc of 180° in front of the participants. Pink noise bursts with two intensity levels (48 dB/58 dB) were randomly applied *via* five loudspeakers (–90°/–30°/–0°/+30°/+90°). Sound localization task performances were collected, and simultaneous signals from auditory processing cortical fields were recorded for analysis by using a support vector machine (SVM). The results showed a classification accuracy of 73.60, 75.60, and 77.40% on average at –90°/0°, 0°/+90°, and –90°/+90° with high intensity, and 70.60, 73.6, and 78.6% with low intensity. The increase of oxyhemoglobin was observed in the bilateral non-primary auditory cortex (AC) and dorsolateral prefrontal cortex (dlPFC). In conclusion, the oxyhemoglobin (oxy-Hb) response showed different neural activity patterns between the lateral and front sources in the AC and dlPFC. Our results may serve as a basic contribution for further research on the use of fNIRS in spatial auditory studies.

Keywords: sound localization, functional near-infrared spectroscopy (fNIRS), spatial hearing, cerebral cortex, auditory cortex (AC), dorsolateral prefrontal cortex (dlPFC)

INTRODUCTION

Auditory perception is one of the most important sensory modalities in creatures. There are multiple types of information presented in sounds. Identifying the source of the sound makes wild animals aware of the danger or its prey and is important in communicative interactions in human society. For decades, auditory neuroscientists have examined the neuronal mechanisms underlying spatial hearing (Middlebrooks and Green, 1991; Skottun, 1998; Grothe et al., 2010). For mammals, the localization and identification of sounds are constructed from the precise relative intensity and timing between the two ears [two binaural cues mostly play roles in the horizontal plane: interaural time difference (ITD) and interaural level difference (ILD)] as well as from patterns of frequencies mapped at the two ears (play roles mostly in the vertical plane) (Middlebrooks and Green, 1991). In addition to the acoustic features, scientists found that the behavioral state of a listener (like task performance and attention) affects neuronal spatial selectivity (Harrington et al., 2008; van der Heijden et al., 2018). Taken together, humans integrate input from the ears and cognitive processes to derive the location of sound sources (Nothwang, 2016; Zhang and Liu, 2019). However, the neural encoding of sound locations and especially the processing of sound sources in the cortex remains a matter of ongoing discussion, and there are still divergent views (Ahveninen et al., 2014).

Electrophysiological research in non-human primates and non-invasive research in humans have provided evidence from a neuroanatomical and functional perspective for acoustic spatial neuron encoding. Regarding the insights into the cortical encoding, evidence for a broader dichotomy between the anterior "what" vs. posterior "where" pathways of the non-primary auditory cortex (AC) aggregates from human neuroimaging studies (Ahveninen et al., 2006; Barrett and Hall, 2006). The dorsal "where" pathway views sound localization as a higher-order sound attribute in higher-level areas including inferior parietal lobule, premotor cortex, dorsolateral prefrontal cortex (dlPFC), and inferior frontal cortex (Rauschecker, 2018; Czoschke et al., 2021). Several published studies have mentioned that the planum temporale (PT) plays an essential role in mediating human horizontal sound localization. Functional MRI (fMRI) research showed that the sound location processing activates the posterior superior temporal gyrus (pSTG) and the inferior parietal cortex (Deouell et al., 2007; van der Zwaag et al., 2011). However, studies demonstrated that goal-oriented sound localization can induce adaptive changes in spectrotemporal tuning in the "dorsal" pathway areas [especially in the primary auditory cortex (PAC)], which can facilitate target detection (Atiani et al., 2009; Lee and Middlebrooks, 2013). fMRI studies reported that the dlPFC might be the source of origin of the top-down modulations that translate sensory representations into task-based representations (Jiang et al., 2018). These findings might suggest that the cortical encoding of sound localization involves recurrent and dynamic processing in PAC and higher-level areas and highlight the need for cortical representation of sound localization in spatial auditory networks.

Besides, there is a contralateral biased tuning of different sound sources with a different degree of bias across the cerebral hemisphere. Non-human primates' measurements demonstrated that cortical spatial tuning is generally broad and predominantly contralateral (Ortiz-Rios et al., 2017). Similar spatial tuning properties have been observed in fMRI studies (Derey et al., 2016; McLaughlin et al., 2016; Higgins et al., 2017). However, inconsistent patterns were reported in human neuroimaging studies. Some electroencephalogram (EEG) and fMRI measures show that the left hemisphere (LH) responds maximally to the contralateral sound source direction and that the right hemisphere (RH) responds more equally to both the contralateral and ipsilateral sounds (Briley et al., 2013; Higgins et al., 2017). Some magnetoencephalography (EMG) studies have shown more activities in RH than LH (Johnson and Hautus, 2010; Salminen et al., 2010). Further measurements using a new image technology are needed to reveal the brain asymmetry in neural sound location encoding.

The development of functional near-infrared spectroscopy (fNIRS) has recently advanced imaging studies in acoustic and audiology, overcoming interference issues in EEG and fMRI. There is an increased oxygen requirement in the brain regions responsible for the specific functions when people are performing the relevant activity. fNIRS is an optical imaging modality that assesses brain hemodynamic responses by its inexpensiveness, safety, non-invasion, and 1–2-cm spatial resolution. This technique is designed to detect changes in the concentration of oxygenated and deoxygenated hemoglobin molecules in the blood (Leon-Carrion and Leon-Dominguez, 2012). Studies have shown that neural activity and the hemodynamic response maintain a linear relationship (Arthurs and Boniface, 2003), and the NIR signal maintains a strong correlation with PET measures of changes in regional cerebral blood flow (rCBF) and the fMRI blood oxygen level-dependent (BOLD) signal (Toronov et al., 2003; Huppert et al., 2006), suggesting that fNIRS is an effective method for assessing cerebral activity. Compared with imaging devices, such as EEG, MEG, and fMRI (Coffey et al., 2016; Dalenberg et al., 2018), fNIRS has no ill-posed inverse problem in EEG and MEG (Helmholtz, 1853) and less interference from the external environment. Whereas the spatial resolution determines anatomical details, the temporal resolution determines the precision in which we can investigate successive neuronal events. With a better spatial resolution than EEG and a similar temporal resolution of fMRI, fNIRS is a relatively good measurement of neuronal activity. In addition, fNIRS is allowable for electrical artifact and ferromagnetic component features, which suggests that fNIRS is a potential tool for the study of auditory perception in special populations.

In fNIRS studies, the existing literature on spatial auditory perception is limited and focuses mainly on speech perception, sound intensity and loudness, and the cross-modal cortex with audiovisual stimulation. For sound intensity, several new fNIRS studies were performed by Chen et al. (2015), Bauernfeind et al. (2018), and Weder et al. (2018, 2020). Those studies found evidence of a linear correlation of the hemodynamic responses with perceived loudness rather than sound intensity in the bilateral superior temporal gyrus (STG). Moreover, no interhemispheric differences are seen in the STG bilaterally. Brain asymmetry was also reported in fNIRS studies. A recent study of dichotic listening suggested that a stronger RH activity in the right prefrontal region can be observed during focused attention tasks (Eskicioglu et al., 2019). However, they neglected the effect of sound source orientation in the cortical representation. This remains the question, what is the cortical representation of a simple spatial sound source detected with fNIRS?

To our knowledge, there are no studies examining the cerebral representation in the prefrontal and auditory cortices during sound localization tasks *via* fNIRS. As fNIRS does not share the issue mentioned in EEG (ill-posed inverse problem) and fMRI (intrinsic noise), it may yield a new understanding of the cerebral cortex-modulated process and brain asymmetry in sound localization. Since localization acuity is higher for broadband than for narrowband sounds and the neural sound location encoding was influenced by the attention of listening (Butler, 1986), here, we presented pink noise bursts with different sound intensities and sources randomly in blocks of a run, allowing participants to attend the sound localization task and avoid speech understanding.

The aims of this study included the following two aspects: (1) does fNIRS detect differences in cortical representations of human attention to different sound source directions between −90°, 0°, and +90°, and if so, (2) are there differences in cortical representations for sound source orientations between −30°, 0°, and +30°? We hypothesized that our spatial stimulus presentation could result in different cerebral representations in both AC and the prefrontal cortex, showing an asymmetric bilateral cortical activation pattern.

MATERIALS AND METHODS

Participants

Twenty-five normal-hearing participants [subject1–subject25 (S1–S25), 11 males and 14 females, all right-handed, all native speakers of Chinese, ages 26.0 ± 2.7 years] took part in this study. This study was approved by the Human Subjects Committee of the Southern Medical University. All individuals were paid an hourly wage for their participation and gave written informed consent prior to the beginning of testing. Otoscopy and acoustic audiometry were conducted with each subject to determine eligibility in this study. Pure tone audiometry showed no significant difference in the hearing thresholds at frequencies 125–8,000 Hz between left (as shown in **Figure 1A**).

Materials and Experiment Paradigm

Apparatus

The sound localization experiments were carried out in a completely darkened anechoic chamber (dimensions L × W × H = 3.3 × 3.5 × 2.5 m^3) in which the apparatus was installed. Seven loudspeakers (Genelec 8010, Genelec Oy, Iisalmi, Finland, matched within 2 dB at 74–20,000 Hz) were positioned in a horizontal arc with a radius of r = 1.46 m at ear level of the subject. The speakers spanned an angle of −90° left to +90° right with a spacing of 30°. Since more sound source directions could increase the test duration and thus cause the subject fatigue, only five of seven loudspeakers (all speakers were real and available) were used for sound presentation in this experiment (Godar and Litovsky, 2010; Zaleski-King et al., 2019). A schematic diagram of the loudspeaker arrangement is shown in **Figure 1E**. The frequency response of each loudspeaker was individually calibrated using our experiment stimuli (seen in **Figure 1B**) in ±1 dB at the subject's head position using an integrating–averaging sound level meter (Xingqiu, HS5670A). Hardware including an eight-channel Yamaha Ro8-D in conjunction with a PC host and software including dante virtual soundcard, dante controller, and MATLAB (MathWorks 2020a, United States) was responsible for stimulus presentation.

Experiment Paradigm and Stimuli

In the behavioral and fNIRS part, the participant was seated facing the front loudspeaker at a distance of approximately 1.46 m and was instructed to calm down and not move their body. A computer monitor placed underneath the front loudspeaker was used as part of the computerized experimental paradigm. A "+" was placed in front of the participant, and the participant was instructed to maintain eye contact with the "+" for the duration of the test. **Figure 1B** shows the experimental paradigm (Moghimi et al., 2012; Weder et al., 2020). At the beginning of the experiment, a preparation time of 10 s was given to the participants. Each 10-s stimulus consists of 77 pink noise bursts each with a duration of 10 ms and with a 120-ms inter-burst gap. The stimuli varied in intensity (low intensity with 48 dB SPL, high intensity with 58 dB SPL) and sound location (loudspeakers 1, 3, 4, 5, 7) (Grieco-Calub and Litovsky, 2010; Weder et al., 2018). In preliminary studies, some researchers used pink noise bursts or broadband noise bursts as a stimulus signal for acoustic source localization (Ching et al., 2005; Grantham et al., 2007; Veugen et al., 2017). The reason for using broadband noise bursts was to activate broad cortical auditory areas. Besides, compared to speech sounds, pink noise is a simpler acoustic stimulus and does not affect the cortical representation of direction recognition due to speech understanding.

During presentation of the sound for 10 s, they were asked to concentrate on the sound location internally without a head movement. Each participant was asked to point to the perceived direction of the sound source at the end of a stimulus. A surveillance camera in the anechoic chamber was used to record the feedback of the subjects. After a 10-s break, the same procedure was repeated. Each of 5 different sound locations * 2 intensity was repeated 10 times and was presented randomly during the localization test. In total, the whole test lasted for approximately 40 min. Feedback was not provided. The subject was unaware that only five of the loudspeakers were used, so that valid responses ranged from 1 to 7. Customized software for stimulus presentation and data collection was written in MATLAB programming language. We used Psychtoolbox in MATLAB to send the trigger for stimulus marking to the NIRS system.

Data Acquisition

During the experiments, task-related cerebral hemodynamic responses were recorded using a multichannel near-infrared spectroscopy (NIRS) imaging system (LIGHTNIRS, Shimadzu Co. Ltd., Kyoto, Japan). The change of oxyhemoglobin [oxy-Hb] and deoxyhemoglobin [deoxy-Hb] and total hemoglobin [total-Hb] was calculated using a modification of the Beer–Lambert law approach. For data recording, we parted all participants' hair and adjusted the signal-to-noise ratio of the NIRS signals using the automatic adjustment function in the measurement software (fNIRS, Shimadzu Co. Ltd., Kyoto, Japan). The signals were digitized at 13.3 Hz, and the 16 optical fiber probes consisting of eight sources (three wavelengths each source, 780, 805, and 830 nm) and eight detectors were attached to the subject's scalp. The probe layout resulted in 20 channels, as

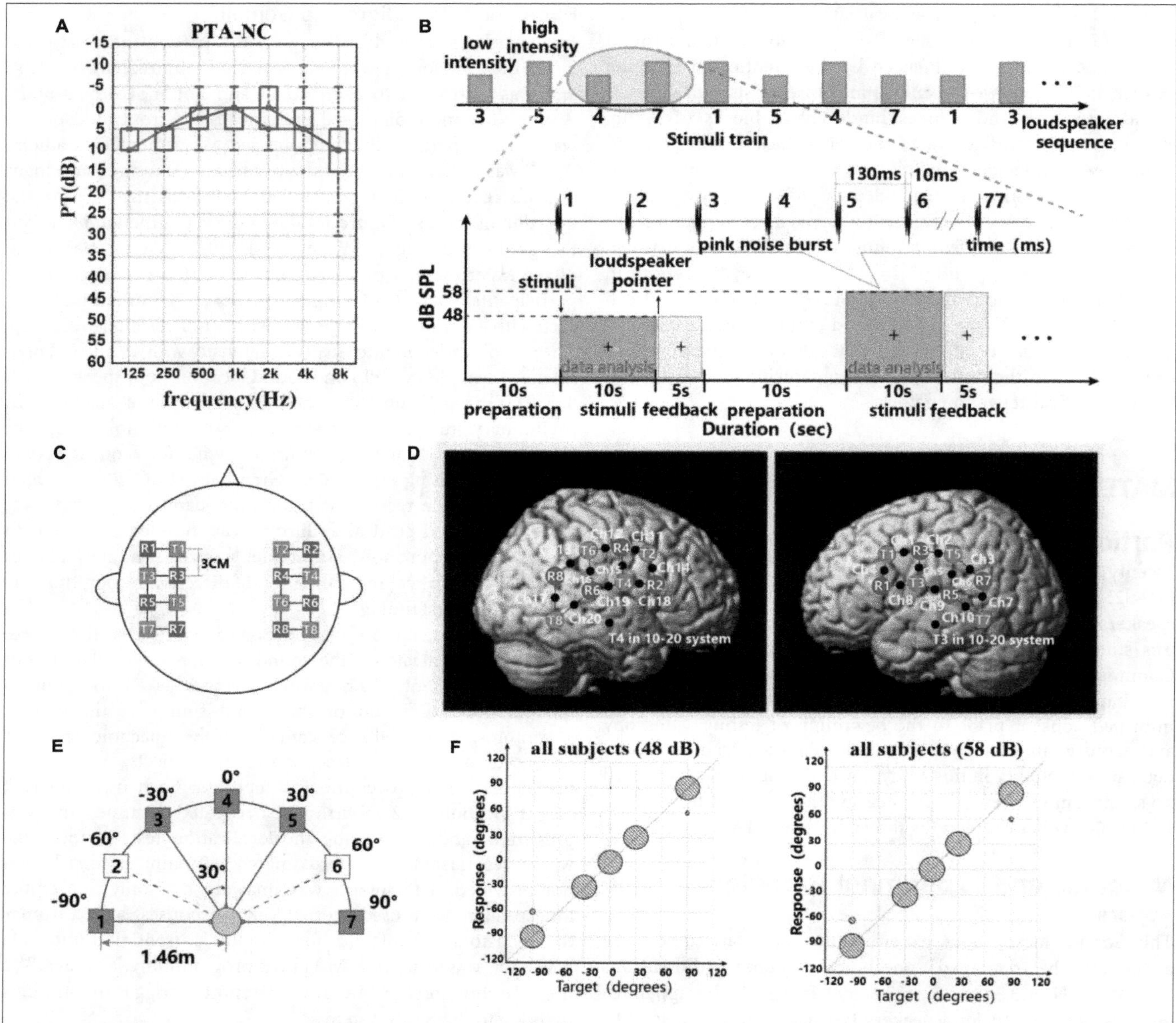

FIGURE 1 | (A) Participants' pure tone threshold information. **(B)** Experimental paradigm and stimulus waveform. Block design used for recording task-related hemodynamic responses: five speakers and two different intensity levels were presented in order randomly. Stimulus waveform representations of pink noise bursts. **(C,D)** Probe layout of the eight sources and eight detectors. **(C)** Placement of the fNIRS optodes (red squares are sources, blue squares are detectors, and black points on lines are channels). **(D)** Optode arrangement in both hemispheres. **(E)** Schematic representation of the seven-loudspeaker system. Loudspeaker 1 and loudspeaker 7 were placed 90° to the left and right of the straight-ahead (0°) position. Loudspeakers 2–6 were placed 30° apart between loudspeakers 1 and 7. Filled symbols indicate "active" loudspeakers; open symbols indicate "dummy" loudspeakers. **(F)** Scatter plots for sound source identification with a five-active-loudspeaker array of all subjects in 48 and 58 dB.

shown in **Figures 1C,D**. Source and detectors were arranged over both hemispheres with 3-cm source-detector separation for maintaining acceptable signal quality and sensing depth (Power et al., 2011). The NIRS optode configuration used in this study followed previous research, which reports the engagement of the pSTG, premotor cortex, and dlPFC in binaural sound cue tuning (McLaughlin et al., 2016).

To allow probabilistic reference to cortical areas underlying the measurement channels and enable the results comparable to results provided by similar fMRI studies. Brain surface MNI (Montreal Neurological Institute) coordinates of channel midpoints were determined and fed into the SPM anatomy toolbox to allocate them to brain areas using a 3D digitizer system (FasTrak, Shimadzu, Japan). The MNI coordinates and anatomical locations of channels and regions of interest (ROIs) are shown in **Table 1** (Eickhoff et al., 2005; Tsuzuki and Dan, 2014).

TABLE 1 | Coordinates and related Brodmann and anatomical areas (based on 25 subjects).

Hem.	ROI	ch	MNI-space			Cortical areas		Proportion
			X	Y	Z	BA		
Left	1	1	−60	3	39	6	Pre-motor and supplementary motor cortex	0.7964
		2	−65	−18	39			0.3576
		5	−66	−6	29			0.6310
		8	−64	6	17			0.5016
	2	3	−68	−39	30	40	Supramarginal gyrus part of Wernicke's area	0.9527
		6	−6	−29	25			0.6075
	3	4	−69	−16	27	9	dlPFC	0.5610
	4	7	−68	−50	7	22	Superior temporal gyrus	0.5290
		10	−71	−39	2			0.5092
	5	9	−68	−16	14	42	Auditory association cortex	0.4658
Right	6	11	62	2	40	6	Pre-motor and supplementary motor cortex	0.8272
		12	67	−18	41			0.3588
		15	68	−5	31			0.7785
		18	67	4	18			0.5342
	7	13	69	−40	31	40	Supramarginal gyrus part of Wernicke's area	0.9968
		16	71	−29	27			0.7037
	8	14	63	14	27	9	dlPFC	0.6111
	9	17	69	4	18	22	Superior temporal gyrus	0.4618
		20	72	−41	1			0.5140
	10	19	71	−17	14	42	Auditory association cortex	0.4969

The table shows 20 channels with MNI space correspondence (x, y, z with SD) and Brodmann areas (BA). The mean MNI coordinates represent the locations of the most likely MNI coordinates for the fNIRS channel projected on the cortical surface.BA, Brodmann area; STG, superior temporal gyrus; dlPFC, dorsolateral prefrontal cortex.

Data Analysis

Behavioristics

Localization performance was determined by calculating the average root-mean-square (RMS) error in degree. For each response, the loudspeaker identified by the subject as delivering the sound was recorded, resulting in a total of 100 speaker location responses for each participant. The error for each response was subsequently converted to degrees and the RMS error for each subject in each listening condition (Zheng et al., 2015). The purpose of calculating subjects' behavioral indicators was to assess subjects' performance in our experimental setting and to maintain subjects' attention during the feedback task. Therefore, we did not set groups.

A non-parametric test was calculated to examine whether there were any statistically significant differences between stimulus levels (48 dB, 58 dB).

Functional Near-Infrared Spectroscopy Data

The fNIRS data analysis procedure consisted of preprocessing, feature extraction, feature selection, and classification stages (for details, see Power et al., 2011; Aydin, 2020). In this study, only the [oxy-Hb] data were used for data analysis, as [oxy-Hb] is a more suitable and robust parameter that has a higher correlation with the fMRI-BOLD response to investigate cortical activity (Plichta et al., 2007). Data preprocessing and analysis were executed in MATLAB (MathWorks, United States) and SPSS (version 26, IBM Corp., United States). We extracted the data preprocessing functions from the open-source toolbox HOMER2 to write the data analysis script and used the MATLAB self-contained toolbox SVM in the classification process. The following steps were executed:

Preprocessing

A common average reference (CAR) spatial filtering approach was used to reduce global influences and task-evoked physiological noise. The mean of all channels was calculated and subtracted from each single channel for each time point (Bauernfeind et al., 2014). To minimize physiological noises such as heartbeat (1–1.5 Hz) and respiration (0.2–0.5 Hz), the signals were low-pass filtered using the Butterworth fourth-order filter at a cutoff frequency of 0.2 Hz. Additionally, a 0.03-Hz high-pass Butterworth filter of order 4 was used to remove baseline drifts (Scholkmann et al., 2014). Then, data were segmented in 10-s windows from the stimulus onset for further processing.

For statistical analyses, the 20 channels were divided into ROIs which limited the need for multiple statistical comparisons and gave a more simplified overview. We combined neighboring channels which hold the same anatomical locations and similar grand average waveform patterns present in the oxy-Hb response, generating 10 ROIs for the whole cortex we covered in total, as shown in **Table 1**. For each ROI, two or four neighboring channels with similar waveform patterns in oxy-Hb were averaged.

Feature Extraction

We used different time windows to extract candidate features since task-related hemodynamic responses appear with a varying delay of 3–8 s (Bauernfeind et al., 2011). The analysis time period was segregated for 14 parts for feature calculation, consisting of a 2-s time window of 2–4, 3–5, 4–6, 5–7, 6–8, 7–9, and 8–10 s; a 3-s time window of 4–7, 5–8, 6–9, and 7–10 s; and a 4-s time window of 4–8, 5–9, and 6–10 s. Then, the temporal features of fNIRS signals [oxy-Hb], including mean, variance, skewness, kurtosis, and slope values, were independently evaluated for all different time windows, 20 channels to create a candidate-feature pool (Noori et al., 2017).

Feature Selection

For each two-class problem, there were a large number of features causing overfitting of a classifier constructed from the training data. In this study, we used the fisher criterion for the feature selection (Power et al., 2011; Moghimi et al., 2012; Hwang et al., 2014). The fisher score based on the Fisher criterion was computed *via*

$$FS_k = \frac{(\mu_{i=1} - \mu_{i=2})^2}{\sigma_{i=1} + \sigma_{i=2}}$$

where μ and σ are the mean and variance, respectively, of the designated class i. The subscript k represents the kth feature element. Since a higher Fisher score signifies larger separability between different classes, the best feature subset was generally constructed by selecting the top *j* feature sets of dimension dim = 1 through dim = 20 we considered.

Classification

We evaluated the performance of each subject and the ability to discriminate between their response of different states using a linear support vector machine (SVM) with the leave-one-out cross-validation (LOOCV) method which was commonly used to classify hemodynamic response (Noori et al., 2017; Hosni et al., 2020). SVM has been applied to binary distinction problems for brain machine interfaces (BMIs) and is also widely used for fNIRS signal analysis. In this study, we used SVM to classify oxy-Hb waveforms into different attention-of-direction trials. LOOCV involves one fold per observation (each observation by itself plays the role of the validation set). The (N-1) observations play the role of the training set, and refitting of the model can be avoided. The classification accuracy and mean percentage of observations correctly classified of the 20 repeated model fittings were then calculated and taken as the result.

RESULTS

This study aimed to examine the cerebral representation in the prefrontal and auditory cortices during sound localization tasks *via* fNIRS. We extracted two sets of fNIRS data for analysis based on behavioral results, used a dichotomous classification method to differentiate the fNIRS signals in different conditions, and presented them in the form of figure legends, which are presented below as part of the results of this experiment.

Localization Performance

To determine the performance of the subject's sound source localization in this experimental setup, we recorded the subject's localization feedback and evaluated it in terms of root mean square error. In addition, we illustrated the specific behavioral performance of all subjects by drawing bubble diagrams.

The RMS results of all participants for different levels are shown in **Table 2.** Normal-hearing subjects had good sound source localization with root mean square errors in the range of 0°–12°. There were 16 subjects with a 0° RMS and nine with a clear bias. Target–response relationships in two sound levels are depicted in **Figure 1F**, illustrating the main behavioral results of the study. Sixteen subjects exhibited perfect performance with an accuracy of 100%; some subjects ($n = 9/25$) failed to identify the sound source at ±90°, with mainly −90° being identified as −60° and +90° as +60°. All subjects except two were 100% accurate for 0° and ±30° discrimination. Specifically, S14 mistook sound source 0° as −30° one time, and S19 mistook sound source 0° as 90° one time. We accepted this error and assumed that the participants could successfully identify sound sources from 0° and ±30°. For stimulus levels, there were no statistically significant differences in RMS results between 48 dB and 58 dB (Wilcoxon signed-rank test, $p = 0.865 > 0.05$).

In conclusion, all participants had good performance in the sound localization task in our experimental apparatus.

TABLE 2 | RMS results of low intensity, high intensity, and all trials.

Subject	RMS (low intensity)	RMS (high intensity)	RMS (all trials)
S1*	0	0	0
S3	6	0	4.24
S11	11.23	11.23	11.23
S14	0	4.24	3
S15	4.24	0	3
S17	6	12.73	9.95
S19	15.30	4.24	11.22
S21	10.39	10.39	10.39
S22	7.35	10.39	8.49
S24	0	4.24	3

**The RMS result of S2, S4, S5, S6, S7, S8, S9, S10, S12, S13, S16, S18, S20, S23, S25 is same as S1.*

Functional Near-Infrared Spectroscopy Results

In this study, to simplify calculation and analysis, we extracted fNIRS data in response to the two questions to be addressed. (1) Does fNIRS detect differences in cortical representations of human attention to different sound source directions between −90°, 0°, and +90°, and if so, (2) are there differences in cortical representations for sound source orientations between −30°, 0°, and +30°?

Cortex Representation of −90°, 0°, and +90° Conditions

The feature values of the relative value change of oxy-Hb of all subjects were calculated using a dichotomous method. The details of the classification are listed below:

For high intensity: (1) −90° versus 0°, (2) 0° versus +90°, (3) −90° versus +90°.

For low intensity: (1) −90° versus 0°, (2) 0° versus +90°, (3) −90° versus +90°.

For the same loudspeaker: (1) high intensity versus low intensity for −90°, (2) high intensity versus low intensity for 0°, and (3) high intensity versus low intensity for +90°.

For ipsilateral and contralateral neural ascending: (1) ipsilateral hemisphere: ROIs of the LH for −90° versus ROIs of the right hemisphere for +90° and (2) contralateral hemisphere: ROIs of the right hemisphere for −90° versus ROIs of the LH for +90.

Lateral and Front Conditions

Table 3 shows the best classification accuracies of each subject for oxy-Hb responses related to six conditions, including stimuli from −90°/0° in 48 dB, 0°/+90° in 48 dB, −90°/+90° in 48 dB, −90°/0° in 58 dB, 0°/+90° in 58 dB, and −90°/+90° in 58 dB. Most of the subjects (n = 18/25, 21/25, 23/25, 21/25, 21/25, 19/25, respectively) showed significantly higher classification accuracies than the marginal classification accuracy of 70%. The mean classification accuracies of the oxy-Hb features were 70.60, 73.60, 78.60, 73.60, 75.60, and 77.40%, respectively. Although the classification accuracies of high intensity were higher than those of low intensity, there was no significant difference

TABLE 3 | Classification accuracies of each participant using an optimal selected feature set for oxy-Hb response (–90°/0°/+90°).

		S1 %	S2 %	S3 %	S4 %	S5 %	S6 %	S7 %	S8 %	S9 %	S10 %	S11 %	S12 %	S13 %
48 dB	–90°/0°	80.00	70.00	70.00	75.00	70.00	60.00	75.00	80.00	70.00	60.00	75.00	65.00	75.00
	0°/+90°	70.00	80.00	65.00	70.00	75.00	75.00	70.00	70.00	70.00	70.00	75.00	60.00	75.00
	–90°/+90°	85.00	70.00	85.00	85.00	85.00	80.00	75.00	65.00	90.00	70.00	70.00	80.00	60.00
58 dB	–90°/0°	65.00	85.00	75.00	65.00	65.00	75.00	65.00	85.00	85.00	70.00	70.00	70.00	70.00
	0°/+90°	65.00	85.00	75.00	65.00	85.00	65.00	75.00	70.00	75.00	75.00	70.00	70.00	85.00
	–90°/+90°	70.00	55.00	75.00	85.00	95.00	85.00	90.00	75.00	65.00	75.00	90.00	65.00	80.00
		S14 %	**S15 %**	**S16 %**	**S17 %**	**S18 %**	**S19 %**	**S20 %**	**S21 %**	**S22 %**	**S23 %**	**S24 %**	**S25 %**	**Mean**
48 dB	–90°/0°	75.00	80.00	65.00	70.00	75.00	70.00	65.00	60.00	75.00	70.00	70.00	65.00	70.60
	0°/+90°	80.00	75.00	65.00	75.00	80.00	85.00	75.00	75.00	90.00	85.00	70.00	60.00	73.60
	–90°/+90°	70.00	80.00	80.00	80.00	70.00	85.00	100.00	70.00	90.00	90.00	80.00	70.00	78.60
58 dB	–90°/0°	75.00	70.00	70.00	70.00	85.00	70.00	80.00	75.00	80.00	80.00	70.00	70.00	73.60
	0°/+90°	85.00	70.00	80.00	85.00	80.00	75.00	75.00	75.00	80.00	90.00	70.00	65.00	75.60
	–90°/+90°	75.00	65.00	65.00	90.00	80.00	85.00	100.00	60.00	95.00	75.00	70.00	70.00	77.40

between sound level conditions (one-way ANOVA: −90°/0°: $p = 0.091 > 0.05$; 0°/+90°: $p = 0.114 > 0.05$; −90°/+90°, $p = 0.694 > 0.05$).

The grand oxy-Hb responses averaged over all subjects are shown in **Figure 2**, with the best feature set of lateral and front classification with optimal analysis time periods. As shown in the figure, the optimal feature set of −90°/0° was ROIs 3, 7, 8, 9, 10 in 5–8 s and ROIs 4 and 5 in 4–8 s, while 0°/+90° was for ROIs 1, 2, 4, 5, 8, and 9 in 5–8 s, indicating that the bilateral non-primary auditory cortex [including Brodmann (BA) 42 auditory-associated cortex, BA22 STG, and BA 40 Wernicke's area] executed more use of oxy-Hb for a lateral sound source. For stimuli from −90°, we observed a steeper increase of oxy-Hb in the bilateral BA22, BA42, and BA40 regions of the right hemisphere. For stimuli from +90°, a significant difference was shown in bilateral BA22 and BA42 and BA42 of the LH.

BA9 and BA6 also showed significant differences in our classification. For stimuli from −90°, steeper activation patterns were found in the bilateral BA9. For stimuli from +90°, a significant difference was shown in BA9 of the right hemisphere and BA6 of the LH.

Oxy-Hb change waveform patterns of stimuli from −90° and +90° are shown in **Figure 3A**. Significant differences were observed in BA6, BA9, BA22, and BA42 of the LH and in BA40 and BA42 of the right hemisphere.

Despite the distinct feature type shown in different ROIs, slope is the most frequently selected feature type during the whole LOOCV steps over all subjects. As the feature set results of the two sound levels were not much different, we only presented the high sound intensity in **Figure 2**. (Low-intensity results are shown in **Supplementary Figure S1**).

Interhemisphere Analysis

In this study, we investigated the difference in spatial tuning between ROIs in the hemisphere ipsilateral and contralateral to the stimulated ear. In comparing the modulation of sound localization cues at the interhemisphere level, the processed signals of symmetrical hemisphere ROIs on stimuli presented from −90° and +90° were then classified using SVM. **Figure 3B** shows the grand-average oxy-Hb response recorded for all subjects with standard errors. Our statistical analysis indicated significant differences in oxy-Hb changes in the contralateral brain region BA40 and ipsilateral brain regions BA42 and BA22 to the stimulated ear. Grand-average oxy-Hb response showed that the waveform from the −90° source reached its peak 2−3 s earlier than that from the +90° source in both BA42 and BA22 ipsilateral to the stimuli. The kurtosis between the two conditions showed a significant difference in BA40 contralateral to the stimuli during the time period of 6–10 s.

Sound Level Conditions

For the sound level, we further calculated the data to clarify whether this influencing factor affects the results in our experimental setup. **Figure 4** shows the grand-average oxy-Hb response recorded between two sound levels (48 and 58 dB) in the −90° sound source for 10 ROIs (the results for 0° and +90° are shown in **Supplementary Figure S2**). The classification accuracies of the oxy-Hb features on each ROI with five feature types were counted. The average classification accuracy of all subjects in each ROI was lower than 70% (50.81 ± 4.63%). As seen in **Figure 4**, the grand average oxy-Hb change showed a similar waveform at the two sound levels, indicating that the cortical representation of high intensity was not much different than that of low intensity.

Cortex Representation of −30°, 0°, and +30° Conditions

To investigate whether there were significant differences in the cortical representation of −30°/0°/30° sound sources, we further calculated the classification accuracy at high and low sound intensities for sound location of −30° and 0°, 0° and 30°, and −30° and 30° using the optimally selected feature set in −90°/0°/+90°.

The classification accuracy statistics for all subjects are shown in **Table 4**. The average accuracy for all six classification questions was below 70%, specifically, 66.60, 68.00, 60.00, 68.60, 65.60, and 63.80% corresponding to −30°/0° (48 dB),

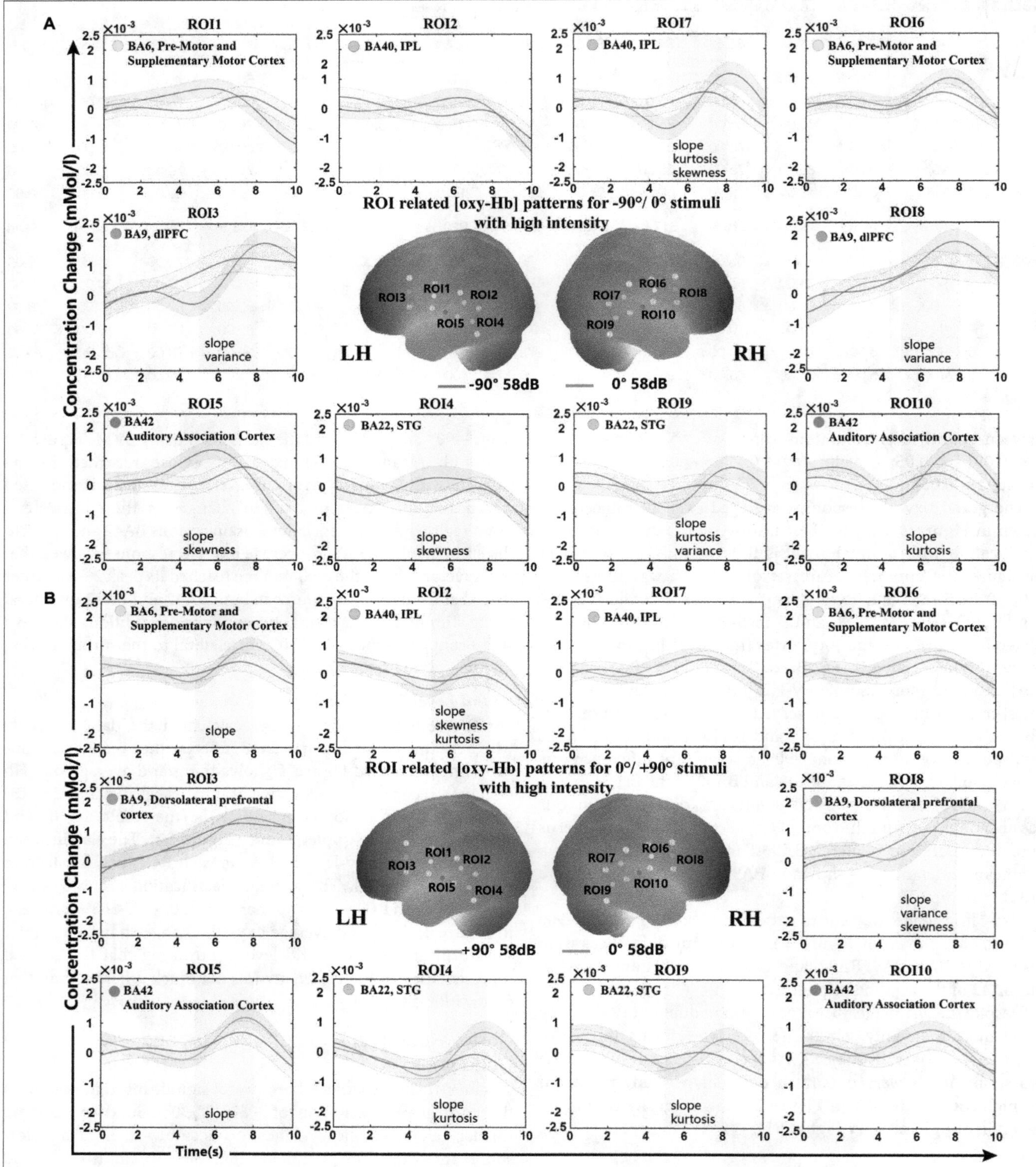

FIGURE 2 | Grand-averaged [oxy-Hb] responses recorded from different locations in high sound intensity (58 dB) for all ROIs and the optimal selected feature set. **(A)** Sound sources from −90° and 0°. **(B)** Sound sources from +90° and 0°. The stimuli were presented at 0 s, and all subjects started concentrating on the sound source. The anatomical location diagram of 10 ROIs is shown in the center of the figure. The lines in blue, red, and green represent the sound sources from −90°/0°/+90°. The selected ROIs with optimal analysis time periods (blue rectangles) and features (shown on the bottom of the blue rectangle) are presented. The shaded regions indicate the standard errors computed across all subjects for the relative condition.

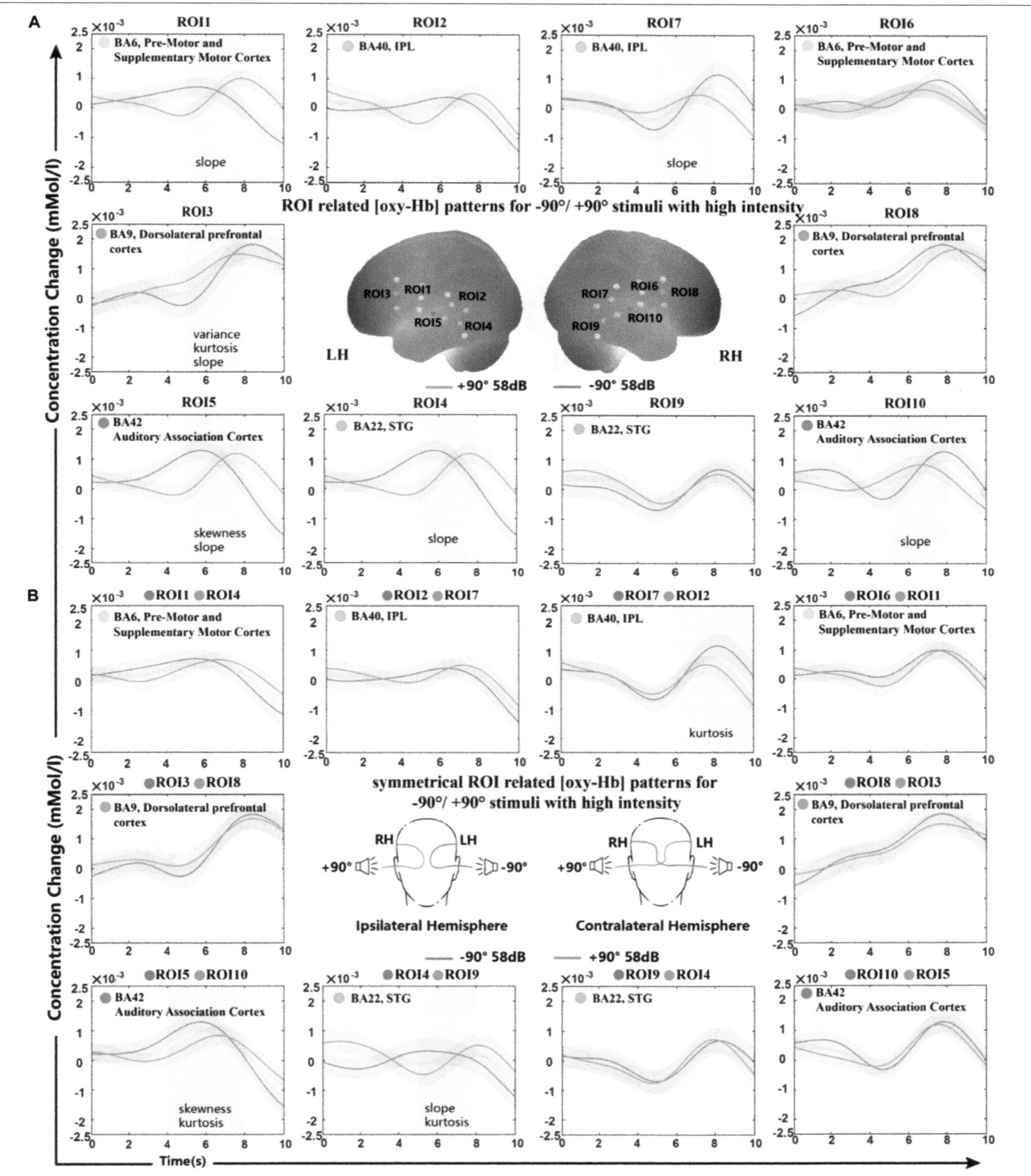

FIGURE 3 | Grand-average oxy-Hb response recorded for −90° and +90° sound sources for all ROIs. **(A)** ROIs in the right and left hemisphere. **(B)** Ipsilateral and contralateral ROI signals of the two conditions. The blue squares on the panel represent time periods in which significant differences in oxy-Hb responses between signals of symmetrical hemisphere ROIs take place. The shaded regions indicate the standard errors computed across all subjects for the relative condition.

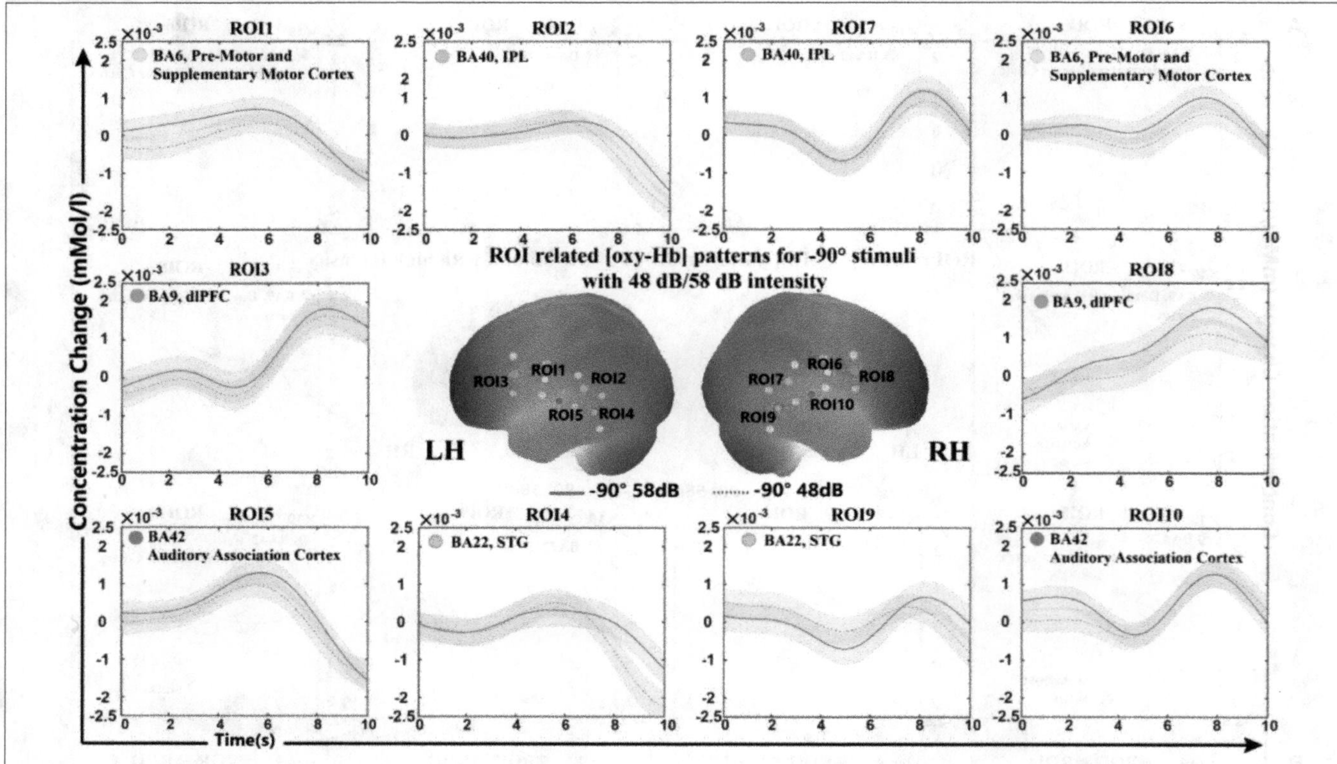

FIGURE 4 | Grand-average oxy-Hb response recorded between different sound levels in the same sound source for 10 ROIs. The blue line in solid and dashed lines on the panel represent oxy-Hb responses between high and low intensities at –90°. The shaded regions indicate the standard errors computed across all subjects for the relative condition.

TABLE 4 | Classification accuracies of each participant using an optimal selected feature set for oxy-Hb response (–30°/0°/+30°).

		S1 %	S2 %	S3 %	S4 %	S5 %	S6 %	S7 %	S8 %	S9 %	S10 %	S11 %	S12 %	S13 %
48 dB	–30°/0°	65.00	70.00	80.00	65.00	80.00	70.00	80.00	60.00	80.00	75.00	60.00	70.00	65.00
	0°/+30°	75.00	60.00	60.00	65.00	35.00	45.00	70.00	70.00	70.00	85.00	60.00	70.00	80.00
	–30°/+30°	65.00	70.00	60.00	60.00	80.00	0.00	70.00	65.00	65.00	65.00	60.00	70.00	60.00
58 dB	–30°/0°	65.00	60.00	65.00	75.00	80.00	75.00	80.00	60.00	65.00	65.00	65.00	60.00	65.00
	0°/+30°	70.00	80.00	50.00	65.00	70.00	65.00	65.00	65.00	55.00	70.00	70.00	70.00	80.00
	–30°/+30°	60.00	65.00	65.00	0.00	65.00	60.00	40.00	60.00	80.00	60.00	80.00	80.00	60.00

		S14 %	S15 %	S16 %	S17 %	S18 %	S19 %	S20 %	S21 %	S22 %	S23 %	S24 %	S25 %	Mean
48 dB	–30°/0°	70.00	65.00	25.00	65.00	40.00	65.00	70.00	70.00	65.00	70.00	70.00	70.00	66.60
	0°/+30°	70.00	90.00	75.00	70.00	65.00	80.00	60.00	65.00	80.00	65.00	65.00	70.00	68.00
	–30°/+30°	65.00	60.00	5.00	70.00	75.00	60.00	50.00	70.00	70.00	80.00	60.00	45.00	60.00
58 dB	–30°/0°	70.00	65.00	70.00	75.00	75.00	65.00	60.00	75.00	70.00	65.00	70.00	75.00	68.60
	0°/+30°	65.00	75.00	70.00	40.00	35.00	85.00	65.00	60.00	70.00	65.00	75.00	60.00	65.60
	–30°/+30°	70.00	80.00	65.00	70.00	65.00	75.00	65.00	65.00	80.00	65.00	60.00	60.00	63.80

0°/+30° (48 dB), −30°/+30° (48 dB), −30°/0° (58 dB), 0°/+30° (58 dB), and −30°/+30° (58 dB), which verified that there were no significant differences in a 30-degrees-of-sound location change on average.

Grand average concentration change data for sound locations of −30°/0° are shown in **Figure 5**. The grand-averaged oxy-Hb showed similar waveforms under the −30° and 0° conditions.

DISCUSSION

This study aimed to investigate what difference the cortical representation was in different sound source localization tasks *via* fNIRS. Differentiation in brain responses related to sound location in 25 subjects was observed. Our experimental evaluation indicated that the lateral and front sound sources revealed different neural activity patterns in the AC and dlPFC.

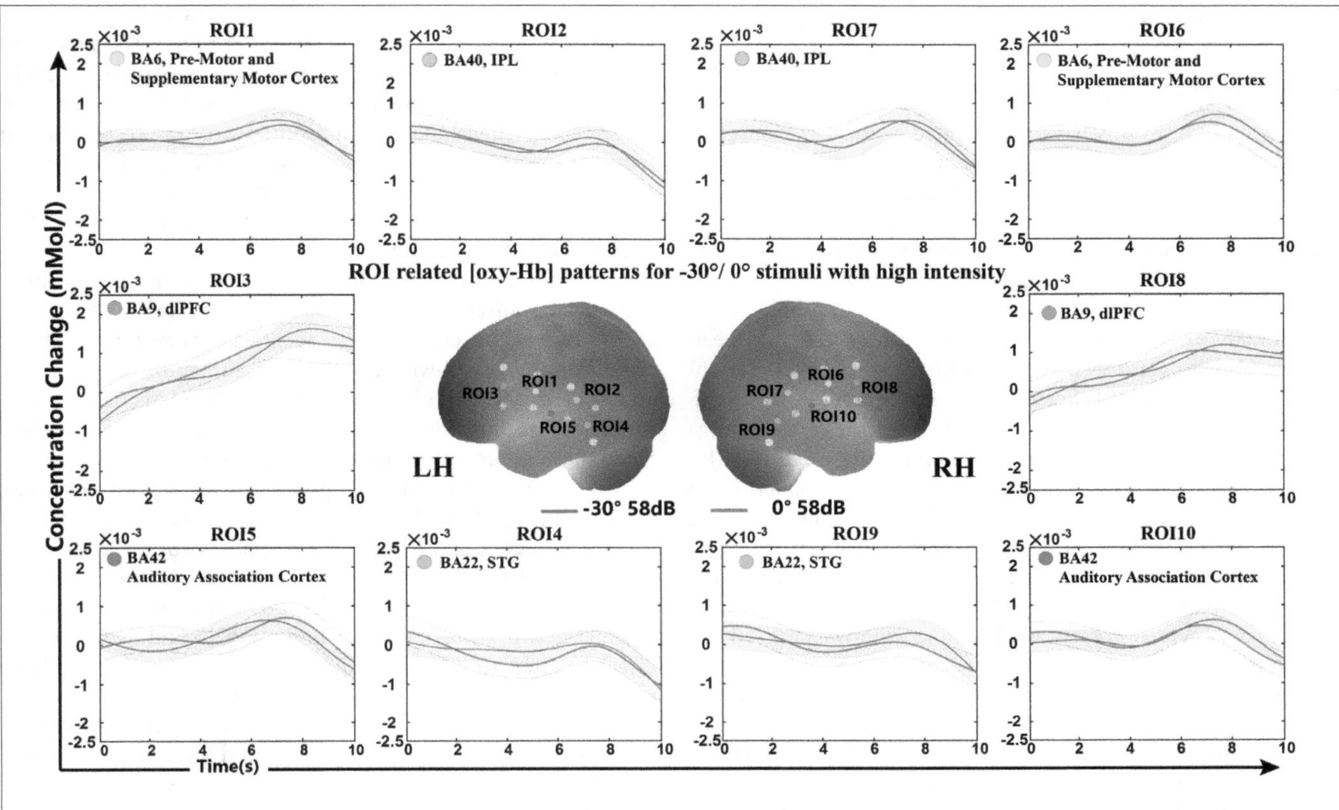

FIGURE 5 | Grand-averaged [oxy-Hb] responses recorded from different locations (–30°/0°) in high sound intensity (58 dB) for all ROIs and the optimally selected feature set.

Many spatial auditory paradigms have proven successful for fMRI and EEG studies (Ebisawa et al., 2011; McLaughlin et al., 2016; van der Heijden et al., 2018). Previous studies using these auditory paradigms identified cortical activation with different sound sources. The block design was generated by referencing the fNIRS and psychophysical experimental methodology. The presented results show a changing amplitude of the oxy-Hb response to the various auditory stimulus sound sources, confirming the feasibility of our experimental design.

Classification Accuracy and Feature Set

Our behavioral data showed that all subjects had 100% accuracy in identifying the 0° source, while some of them had confusion in −90° and +90°. Although the total trial RMS ranged from 0° to 12°, showing the existence of individual variation in psychophysical performance, our interpretation tended to base on the differences in the mental state between individuals. As shown in **Figure 1F**, the subjects show a good performance in our sound localization task.

The SVM classification accuracy pointed to the non-primary auditory cortex, including Wernicke's area and STG, as the structures that showed significant variation in oxy-Hb contribution with different sound sources. The results demonstrated that the fNIRS response to lateral and front sound could be classified with a mean classification accuracy higher than the acceptable practical standard (>70%). As shown in **Figure 5**, both −90° and +90° sound sources brought about a steep slope and revealed an increased oxy-Hb response during 5–8 s over the STG and part of Wernicke's area in the contralateral hemisphere, while signals for sound from the front presented a flat curve. Over all of the feature sets selected from LOOCV, the slope showed statistically higher frequencies selected among five different feature types, which indicated that the growth rate of oxy-Hb in different sound sources may characterize the conditions.

Interestingly, a similar result has been shown over the dlPFC in the hemisphere ipsilateral to stimulus sources. The dlPFC is a region most typically associated with higher-level cognitive functions, including working memory and selective attention (Fehr and Krajbich, 2014; Sturm et al., 2016). A previous study indicated that it is possible to causally influence subjects' choices by making them less likely to express social preferences by disrupting this region. Recently, a high-quality article reviewed and integrated the latest insights from neurophysiological, neuroimaging, and computational modeling studies of mammalian spatial hearing. They proposed that the cortical representation of sound location emerges from recurrent processing taking place in a dynamic, adaptive network of early (primary) and higher-order (posterior-dorsal and dorsolateral prefrontal) auditory regions (van der Heijden et al., 2019). In our research, different neural activities were observed in the dlPFC in both hemispheres between −90°, 0°, and +90°, providing evidence that this region may be involved in the human selection of sound source attention.

Cortical Correlations of Sound Level

Several research groups have investigated cortical responses to auditory stimuli presented with different sound intensities using different recording techniques (Neuner et al., 2014). Researchers have found different sound intensity modulations of cortical responses to binaural stimuli in the middle and lateral primary auditory cortices, and a linear increase in BOLD signals has been shown in fMRI studies (Uppenkamp and Rohl, 2014). Additionally, the volume of the brain-activated area has been confirmed to be positively correlated with the stimulus level (Rohl and Uppenkamp, 2012). Since the signals measured by fNIRS strongly correlate with the fMRI BOLD signal, the same findings were also found in studies that combined the use of fNIRS (Langers et al., 2007; Behler and Uppenkamp, 2016; Bauernfeind et al., 2018; Weder et al., 2020). It has been shown that the channels overlying the supramarginal and caudal STG evoked a phasic response, and the antero-STG and Broca's areas showed a broad tonic pattern, where a significant effect of sound intensity level can be observed in early and late time windows, respectively (Weder et al., 2018).

In a previous study, we were interested in sound localization cues rather than sound intensity because we used different sound levels to reduce the monaural effect and check the conformances of oxy-Hb signal shape in the same sound location. As sound intensities at different levels were applied in previous studies from 0 to 100 dB SPL with a gap of approximately 20–30 dB SPL and an analysis time period from onset to 30 s, the results established before may not have been visible in our studies. The sound intensities presented in this study were 48 and 58 dB. The classification accuracy of the oxyhemoglobin waveforms with different sound intensities is below 70%. We considered that such a small difference between sound levels resulted in a marginal difference in waveforms *via* fNIRS. However, it can be observed from the waveform plots that the average waveform peak at 58 dB is above 48 dB in a tiny degree; we conjecture that if we increase the stimulus sound intensity difference, the significant difference between waveforms of sound level will be observed. This might explain why we did not see differences in the cortex of sound intensity in our study.

Limitation of the Study

fNIRS recordings of auditory stimulation are challenging due to the limitation of time resolution and the limited region we targeted. Since it measures neuronal activity indirectly *via* hemodynamic response, the time resolution reaches the second state, which is a hundred times that in EEG. Previous fMRI studies showed that the initial bilateral transient signal subserved rapid sound detection and that the subsequent lateralized sustained signal subserved detailed sound characterization (Lehmann et al., 2007), which indicated that the time range we analyzed may affect the conclusion we obtained. Moreover, in our study, we used only eight sources and eight detectors fNIRS systems. The cerebral region we covered was limited, and whether there were other region participants in the sound localization activity was unknown. Researchers had applied many stimulus sounds in sound source localization tasks, including pure tones, broadband noise, bandpass noise, and speech sounds. Our study used pink noise in the hope of excluding the effect of speech comprehension on sound source direction recognition in cortical representation. In subsequent studies, we will use speech sound stimuli in complex environments to explore the cortical representation of sound source recognition from the perspective of everyday life applications.

While the best discrimination rate in the same classification among all subjects was 90–95%, the worst was 60–65%. For each subject, the classification accuracies varied in different classifications, as shown in **Table 3** (accuracy of 65% at −90° and 0° and 90% at 0° and +90° at high intensities for S4), suggesting an individual variation in our classification models. Since there are many features that may affect the classification, further development of data preprocessing and algorithms needs to be optimized to make the system more flexible. It has been well documented that [deoxy-Hb] responses appear to be more localized and topographically closer to activated areas (Kaiser et al., 2014). Therefore, we plan to search for an effective channel network that combines both oxy-Hb and deoxy-Hb for discrimination to achieve a high-performance system, perhaps *via* classification methods other than SVM.

Although we observed different oxy-Hb response patterns in the non-primary auditory cortex for sound localization, whether this representation is the fusion of bilateral loudness perception and spatial sound perception is not clear. Recent research has shown that non-primary ACs are the regions involved in many auditory perceptions, including horizontal sound direction changes, movement, intensity-independent distance cues, and separation of multiple sound sources (Ahveninen et al., 2014). It is a main concern to provide an effective experimental paradigm for further investigation in spatial cue encoding and functional specialization. Some scientists pointed that future research needed experimental setups using real-life, complex sounds in ecologically valid listening scenes to gain a better understanding of the full complexity of cortical sound location processing. Since sound source localization is a high-order processing and visual information is involved in an important part of the sound localization activity, a dark room environment was used in this experiment to avoid the extent of visual information input. The inclusion of visual information stimuli and attention to the visual, audiovisual cortex is needed in subsequent studies.

Numerous studies have concentrated on brain function in transmitting and tuning binaural sound localization cues by means of neurophysiological methods, EEG, MEG, and fMRI over the past decade (Zatorre et al., 2004; Krumbholz et al., 2005; Palomaki et al., 2005). In general, our study only investigated the availability of fNIRS on sound localization irrespective of whether ITD and/or ILD were used to produce spatial perception. Although we observed the cortical representation of different spatial origins of sounds, it is not known when distinguishing the location of sound sources to what degree the binaural spatial cue weighs in our recorded fNIRS signals in the revolved cortex. Besides, the sound level to the ipsilateral eardrum would be increased when a sound source is moved from frontal position to lateral position because of the sound scattering characteristics of the head and ear (Liang and Yu, 2020; Liang et al., 2021). Since none of the alternative methods completely eliminates monaural level cues, the available neuroimaging studies of ILD processing all have monaural cues as a potential confound (Ahveninen et al., 2014). Therefore, further comparison and integration of studies are needed to obtain cortical activity representations of separate spatial cues from sound sources.

Outlook

Our study shows that fNIRS is a valid and reliable assessment tool for sound localization task-associated oxygenated blood. However, we know that in real life, sound source localization activities are not just about the directional recognition of simple sounds. Multidirectional speech perception in noisy environments and competing speech sounds are also spatial sound source perceptions. We speculate that future research on spatial acoustic brain function will be devoted to a better understanding of sound source localization processing in real-life complex speech environments.

The application of fNIRS to investigate cross-modal plasticity and speech processing has been of interest in disabled groups like cochlear implantation (CI) users in recent years, from which we have identified the potential of speech development among children early and timely intervened for treatment. As the increasing number of binaural cochlear implant users results in more demands, such as better speech perception in noise and sound localization ability, understanding the cortical representation differences between normal people and guiding and assessing the fitting of bimodal or bilateral CI have been new issues. Due to the previous fNIRS contributions in speech perception, we hold the opinion that the cortical perception of spatial speech sounds will be carried out well off.

We believe that fNIRS holds great potential for growth and application in the clinic, offering new possibilities for the functional organization of the brain in the spatial auditory field.

CONCLUSION

This study presented an experimental paradigm for measuring the cortical representation of sound localization under sound fields *via* fNIRS. We investigated the differences in cortical representations of different sound sources during listening tasks *via* fNIRS. The main waveform patterns of oxy-Hb demonstrated that the front and lateral sound sources extracted different neural activity in non-primary AC and dlPFC.

Taken together, our findings suggested that fNIRS could detect differences in cortical representations of sound source directions from the lateral and the front, providing evidence for the cerebral activation patterns of spatial hearing.

AUTHOR CONTRIBUTIONS

HZ and FC designed the research. XT performed the research and wrote the first draft of the manuscript. XT and ZG analyzed the data. XT, YL, JC, HZ, FC, and JT edited the manuscript. XT, YL, JC, and HZ wrote the manuscript. All authors contributed to the article and approved the submitted version.

ACKNOWLEDGMENTS

The authors would like to thank Xin Zhou and Changhai Ding for assistance with the experimental design, and Mianmian Lin for assistance with data collection.

REFERENCES

Ahveninen, J., Jääskeläinen, I. P., Raij, T., Bonmassar, G., Devore, S., and Hämäläinen, M. (2006). Task-modulated "what" and "where" pathways in human auditory cortex. *Proc. Natl. Acad. Sci. U S A* 103, 14608–14613. doi: 10.1073/pnas.051048 0103

Ahveninen, J., Kopčo, N., and Jääskeläinen, I. P. (2014). Psychophysics and neuronal bases of sound localization in humans. *Hear. Res.* 307, 86–97.

Arthurs, O. J., and Boniface, S. J. (2003). What aspect of the fMRI BOLD signal best reflects the underlying electrophysiology in human somatosensory cortex? *Clin. Neurophys.* 114, 1203–1209. doi: 10.1016/s1388-2457(03)00080-4

Atiani, S., Elhilali, M., David, S. V., Fritz, J. B., and Shamma, S. A. (2009). Task difficulty and performance induce diverse adaptive patterns in gain and shape of primary auditory cortical receptive fields. *Neuron* 61, 467–480. doi: 10.1016/j.neuron.2008.12.027

Aydin, E. A. (2020). Subject-Specific feature selection for near infrared spectroscopy based brain-computer interfaces. *Comput Methods Prog. Biomed.* 195:105535. doi: 10.1016/j.cmpb.2020.10 5535

Barrett, D. J. K., and Hall, D. A. (2006). Response preferences for "what" and "where" in human non-primary auditory cortex. *NeuroImage* 32, 968–977. doi: 10.1016/j.neuroimage.2006.03.050

Bauernfeind, G., Scherer, R., Pfurtscheller, G., and Neuper, C. (2011). Single-trial classification of antagonistic oxyhemoglobin responses during mental arithmetic. *Med. Biol. Eng. Comput.* 49, 979–984. doi: 10.1007/s11517-011-0792-5

Bauernfeind, G., Wriessnegger, S. C., Daly, I., and Muller-Putz, G. R. (2014). Separating heart and brain: on the reduction of physiological noise from multichannel functional near-infrared spectroscopy (fNIRS) signals. *J. Neural. Eng.* 11:056010. doi: 10.1088/1741-2560/11/5/056010

Bauernfeind, G., Wriessnegger, S. C., Haumann, S., and Lenarz, T. (2018). Cortical activation patterns to spatially presented pure tone stimuli with different intensities measured by functional near-infrared spectroscopy. *Human Brain Mapp.* 39, 2710–2724. doi: 10.1002/hbm.24034

Behler, O., and Uppenkamp, S. (2016). The representation of level and loudness in the central auditory system for unilateral stimulation. *NeuroImage* 139, 176–188. doi: 10.1016/j.neuroimage.2016.06.025

Briley, P. M., Kitterick, P. T., and Summerfield, A. Q. (2013). Evidence for opponent process analysis of sound source location in humans. *J. Assoc. Res. Otolaryngol.* 14, 83–101.

Butler, R. A. (1986). The bandwidth effect on monaural and binaural localization. *Hear. Res.* 21, 67–73. doi: 10.1016/0378-5955(86)90047-x

Chen, L. C., Sandmann, P., Thorne, J. D., Herrmann, C. S., and Debener, S. (2015). Association of Concurrent fNIRS and EEG Signatures in Response to Auditory and Visual Stimuli. *Brain Topogr.* 28, 710–725. doi: 10.1007/s10548-015-0424-8

Ching, T. Y., Hill, M., Brew, J., Incerti, P., Priolo, S., Rushbrook, E., et al. (2005). The effect of auditory experience on speech perception, localization, and functional performance of children who use a cochlear implant and a hearing aid in opposite ears. *Int. J. Audiol.* 44, 677–690. doi: 10.1080/0022293050027 1630

Coffey, E. B., Herholz, S. C., Chepesiuk, A. M., Baillet, S., and Zatorre, R. J. (2016).

Cortical contributions to the auditory frequency-following response revealed by MEG. *Nat. Commun.* 7:11070.

Czoschke, S., Fischer, C., Bahador, T., Bledowski, C., and Kaiser, J. (2021). Decoding Concurrent Representations of Pitch and Location in Auditory Working Memory. *J. Neurosci.* 41, 4658–4666. doi: 10.1523/JNEUROSCI.2999-20.2021

Dalenberg, J. R., Hoogeveen, H. R., and Lorist, M. M. (2018). Physiological Measurements:EEG and fMRI, in *Methods in Consumer Research. Exp. Psychol.* 2, 253–277.

Deouell, L. Y., Heller, A. S., Malach, R., D'Esposito, M., and Knight, R. T. (2007). Cerebral responses to change in spatial location of unattended sounds. *Neuron* 55, 985–996. doi: 10.1016/j.neuron.2007.08.019

Derey, K., Valente, G., de Gelder, B., and Formisano, E. (2016). Opponent Coding of Sound Location (Azimuth) in Planum Temporale is Robust to Sound-Level Variations. *Cereb. Cortex* 26, 450–464. doi: 10.1093/cercor/bhv269

Ebisawa, M., Kogure, M., Yano, S.-H., Matsuzaki, S.-I., and Wada, Y. (2011). Estimation of direction of attention using EEG and out-of-head sound localization. *Annu. Intern. Conf. IEEE Eng. Med. Biol. Soc.* 2011, 7417–7420. doi: 10.1109/IEMBS.2011.6091727

Eickhoff, S. B., Stephan, K. E., Mohlberg, H., Grefkes, C., Fink, G. R., Amunts, K., et al. (2005). A new SPM toolbox for combining probabilistic cytoarchitectonic maps and functional imaging data. *Neuroimage* 25, 1325–1335. doi: 10.1016/j.neuroimage.2004.12.034

Eskicioglu, E., Taslica, S., Narin, B., Guducu, C., Oniz, A., and Ozgoren, M. (2019). Brain asymmetry in directing attention during dichotic listening test: An fNIRS study. *Laterality* 24, 377–392. doi: 10.1080/1357650X.2018.1527847

Fehr, E., and Krajbich, I. (2014). Social Preferences and the Brain. *Neuroeconomics* 2014, 193–218.

Godar, S. P., and Litovsky, R. Y. (2010). Experience with bilateral cochlear implants improves sound localization acuity in children. *Otol. Neurotol.* 31, 1287–1292.

Grantham, D. W., Ashmead, D. H., Ricketts, T. A., Labadie, R. F., and Haynes, D. S. (2007). Horizontal-plane localization of noise and speech signals by postlingually deafened adults fitted with bilateral cochlear implants. *Ear. Hear.* 28, 524–541. doi: 10.1097/aud.0b013e31806dc21a

Grieco-Calub, T. M., and Litovsky, R. Y. (2010). Sound localization skills in children who use bilateral cochlear implants and in children with normal acoustic hearing. *Ear. Hear.* 31, 645–656. doi: 10.1097/aud.0b013e3181e50a1d

Grothe, B., Pecka, M., and McAlpine, D. (2010). Mechanisms of sound in mammals. *Physiol. Rev.* 90, 983–1012. doi: 10.1152/physrev.00026.2009

Harrington, I. A., Stecker, G. C., Macpherson, E. A., and Middleb, J. C. (2008). Spatial sensitivity of neurons in the anterior, posterior, and primary fields of cat auditory cortex. *Hear. Res.* 240, 22–41. doi: 10.1016/j.heares.2008.02.004

Helmholtz, H. (1853). Ueber einige Gesetze der Vertheilung elektrischer Ströme in körperlichen Leitern, mit Anwendung auf die thierisch-elektrischen Versuche (Schluss.). *Annal. Physik* 165, 353–377.

Higgins, N. C., McLaughlin, S. A., Rinne, T., and Stecker, G. C. (2017). Evidence for *cue-independent spatial representation in the human auditory cortex during active listening. Proc. Natl. Acad. Sci. U S A* 114, E7602–E7611. doi: 10.1073/pnas.1707522114

Hosni, S. M., Borgheai, S. B., McLinden, J., and Shahriari, Y. (2020). An fNIRS-Based Motor Imagery BCI for ALS: A Subject-Specific Data-Driven Approach. *IEEE Trans. Neural. Syst. Rehabil. Eng.* 28, 3063–3073. doi: 10.1109/TNSRE.2020.3038717

Huppert, T. J., Hoge, R. D., Diamond, S. G., Franceschini, M. A., and Boas, D. A. (2006). A temporal comparison of BOLD, ASL, and NIRS hemodynamic responses to motor stimuli in adult humans. *Neuroimage* 29, 368–382. doi: 10.1016/j.neuroimage.2005.08.065

Hwang, H. J., Lim, J. H., Kim, D. W., and Im, C. H. (2014). Evaluation of various *mental task combinations for near-infrared spectroscopy-based brain-computer interfaces. J. Biomed. Opt.* 19:77005. doi: 10.1117/1.JBO.19.7.077005

Jiang, X., Chevillet, M. A., Rauschecker, J. P., and Riesenhuber, M. (2018). Training Humans to Categorize Monkey Calls: Auditory Feature- and Category-Selective Neural Tuning Changes. *Neuron* 2018:2. doi: 10.1016/j.neuron.2018.03.014

Johnson, B. W., and Hautus, M. J. (2010). Processing of binaural spatial information in human auditory cortex: neuromagnetic responses to interaural timing and level differences. *Neuropsychologia* 48, 2610–2619. doi: 10.1016/j.neuropsychologia.2010.05.008

Kaiser, V., Bauernfeind, G., Kreilinger, A., Kaufmann, T., Kubler, A., Neuper, C., et al. (2014). Cortical effects of user training in a motor imagery based brain-computer interface measured by fNIRS and EEG. *Neuroimage* 85(Pt 1), 432–444. doi: 10.1016/j.neuroimage.2013.04.097

Krumbholz, K., Schonwiesner, M., von Cramon, D. Y., Rubsamen, R., Shah, N. J., Zilles, K., et al. (2005). Representation of interaural temporal information from left and right auditory space in the human planum temporale and inferior parietal lobe. *Cereb Cortex* 15, 317–324. doi: 10.1093/cercor/bhh133

Langers, D. R. M., van Dijk, P., Schoenmaker, E. S., and Backes, W. H. (2007). fMRI activation in relation to sound intensity and loudness. *NeuroImage* 35, 709–718. doi: 10.1016/j.neuroimage.2006.12.013

Lee, C.-C., and Middlebrooks, J. C. (2013). Specialization for sound localization in fields A1, DZ, and PAF of cat auditory cortex. *J. Assoc. Res. Otolaryngol.* 14, 61–82. doi: 10.1007/s10162-012-0357-9

Lehmann, C., Herdener, M., Schneider, P., Federspiel, A., Bach, D. R., Esposito, F., et al. (2007). Dissociated lateralization of transient and sustained blood oxygen level-dependent signal components in human primary auditory cortex. *NeuroImage* 34, 1637–1642. doi: 10.1016/j.neuroimage.2006.11.011

Leon-Carrion, J., and Leon-Dominguez, U. (2012). Functional Near-Infrared Spectroscopy (fNIRS): Principles and Neuroscientific Applications. *Neuroimag. Methods* 2012, 47–74.

Liang, L., and Yu, G. (2020). Binaural speech transmission index with spatialized virtual speaker in near field: Distance and direction dependence. *J. Acoust. Soc. Am.* 148:EL202. doi: 10.1121/10.0001808

Liang, L., Yu, L., Zhao, T., Meng, Q., and Yu, G. (2021). Speech intelligibility for various head orientations of a listener in an automobile using the speech transmission index. *J. Acoust. Soc. Am.* 149:2686. doi: 10.1121/10.0004265

McLaughlin, S. A., Higgins, N. C., and Stecker, G. C. (2016). Tuning to Binaural Cues in Human Auditory Cortex. *J. Assoc. Res. Otolaryngol.* 17, 37–53. doi: 10.1007/s10162-015-0546-4

Middlebrooks, J. C., and Green, D. M. (1991). Sound localization by human listeners. *Annu. Rev. Psychol.* 42, 135–159. doi: 10.1146/annurev.ps.42.020191.001031

Moghimi, S., Kushki, A., Power, S., Guerguerian, A. M., and Chau, T. (2012). Automatic detection of a prefrontal cortical response to emotionally rated music using multi-channel near-infrared spectroscopy. *J. Neural. Eng.* 9:026022. doi: 10.1088/1741-2560/9/2/026022

Neuner, I., Kawohl, W., Arrubla, J., Warbrick, T., Hitz, K., Wyss, C., et al. (2014). Cortical response variation with different sound pressure levels: a combined event-related potentials and FMRI study. *PLoS One* 9:e109216. doi: 10.1371/journal.pone.0109216

Noori, F. M., Naseer, N., Qureshi, N. K., Nazeer, H., and Khan, R. A. (2017). Optimal feature selection from fNIRS signals using genetic algorithms for BCI. *Neurosci. Lett.* 647, 61–66. doi: 10.1016/j.neulet.2017.03.013

Nothwang, H. G. (2016). Evolution of ma*mmalian sound localization circuits: A developmental perspective. Prog. Neurobiol.* 141, 1–24. doi: 10.1016/j.pneurobio.2016.02.003

Ortiz-Rios, M., Azevedo, F. A. C., Kuśmierek, P., Balla, D. Z., Munk, M. H., Keliris, G. A., et al. (2017). Widespread and Opponent fMRI Signals Represent Sound Location in Macaque Auditory Cortex. *Neuron* 2017:4. doi: 10.1016/j.neuron.2017.01.013

Palomaki, K. J., Tiitinen, H., Makinen, V., May, P. J., and Alku, P. (2005). Spatial processing in human auditory cortex: the effects of 3D, ITD, and ILD stimulation techniques. *Brain Res. Cogn. Brain Res.* 24, 364–379. doi: 10.1016/j.cogbrainres.2005.02.013

Plichta, M. M., Herrmann, M. J., Baehne, C. G., Ehlis, A. C., Richter, M. M., Pauli, P., et al. (2007). Event-related functional near-infrared spectroscopy (fNIRS) based on craniocerebral correlations: reproducibility of activation? *Hum. Brain Mapp.* 28, 733–741. doi: 10.1002/hbm.20303

Power, S. D., Kushki, A., and Chau, T. (2011). Towards a system-paced near-infrared spectroscopy brain-computer interface: differentiating prefrontal activity due to mental arithmetic and mental singing from the no-control state. *J. Neural. Eng.* 8:066004. doi: 10.1088/1741-2560/8/6/066004

Rauschecker, J. P. (2018). Where, When, and How: Are they all sensorimotor? Towards a unified view of the dorsal pathway in vision and audition. *Cortex* 98, 262–268. doi: 10.1016/j.cortex.2017.10.020

Rohl, M., and Uppenkamp, S. (2012). Neural coding of sound intensity and loudness in the human auditory system. *J. Assoc. Res. Otolaryngol.* 13, 369–379.

Salminen, N. H., Tiitinen, H., Miettinen, I., Alku, P., and May, P. J. (2010). Asymmetrical representation of auditory space in human cortex. *Brain Res.* 1306, 93–99. doi: 10.1016/j.brainres.2009.09.095

Scholkmann, F., Kleiser, S., Metz, A. J., Zimmermann, R., Mata Pavia, J., Wolf, U., et al. (2014). A review on continuous wave functional near-infrared spectroscopy and imaging instrumentation and methodology. *Neuroimage* 85(Pt 1), 6–27.

Skottun, B. C. (1998). Sound localization and neurons. *Nature* 393:531. doi: 10.1038/31134

Sturm, V. E., Haase, C. M., and Levenson, R. W. (2016). Emotional Dysfunction in Psychopathology and Neuropathology: Neural and Genetic Pathways. *Genom. Circuits Pathways Clin. Neuropsych.* 2016, 345–364. doi: 10.1016/b978-0-12-800105-9.00022-6

Toronov, V., Walker, S., Gupta, R., Choi, J. H., Gratton, E., Hueber, D., et al. (2003). The roles of changes in deoxyhemoglobin concentration and regional cerebral blood volume in the fMRI BOLD signal. *NeuroImage* 19, 1521–1531. doi: 10.1016/s1053-8119(03)00152-6

Tsuzuki, D., and Dan, I. (2014). Spatial registration for functional near-infrared spectroscopy: from channel position on the scalp to cortical location in individual and group analyses. *Neuroimage* 85(Pt 1), 92–103. doi: 10.1016/j.neuroimage.2013.07.025

Uppenkamp, S., and Rohl, M. (2014). Human auditory neuroimaging of intensity and loudness. *Hear. Res.* 307, 65–73. doi: 10.1016/j.heares.2013.08.005

van der Heijden, K., Rauschecker, J. P., de Gelder, B., and Formisano, E. (2019). Cortical mechanisms of spatial hearing. *Nat. Rev. Neurosci.* 20, 609–623. doi: 10.1038/s41583-019-0206-5

van der Heijden, K., Rauschecker, J. P., Formisano, E., Valente, G., and de Gelder, B. (2018). Active Sound Localization Sharpens Spatial Tuning in Human Primary Auditory Cortex. *J. Neurosci.* 38, 8574–8587. doi: 10.1523/JNEUROSCI.0587-18.2018

van der Zwaag, W., Gentile, G., Gruetter, R., Spierer, L., and Clarke, S. (2011). Where sound position influences sound object representations: a 7-T fMRI study. *NeuroImage* 54, 1803–1811. doi: 10.1016/j.neuroimage.2010.10.032

Veugen, L. C. E., Chalupper, J., Mens, L. H. M., Snik, A. F. M., and van Opstal, A. J. (2017). Effect of extreme adaptive frequency compression in bimodal listeners on sound localization and speech perception. *Cochlear Implants Int.* 18, 266–277. doi: 10.1080/14670100.2017.1353762

Weder, S., Shoushtarian, M., Olivares, V., Zhou, X., Innes-Brown, H., and McKay, C. (2020). Cortical fNIRS Responses Can Be Better Explained by Loudness Percept than Sound Intensity. *Ear Hear.* 41, 1187–1195. doi: 10.1097/AUD.0000000000000836

Weder, S., Zhou, X., Shoushtarian, M., Innes-Brown, H., and McKay, C. (2018). Cortical Processing Related to Intensity of a Modulated Noise Stimulus-a Functional Near-Infrared Study. *J. Assoc. Res. Otolaryngol.* 19, 273–286. doi: 10.1007/s10162-018-0661-0

Zaleski-King, A., Goupell, M. J., Barac-Cikoja, D., and Bakke, M. (2019). Bimodal Cochlear Implant Listeners' Ability to Perceive Minimal Audible Angle Differences. *J. Am. Acad. Audiol.* 30, 659–671. doi: 10.3766/jaaa.17012

Zatorre, R. J., Bouffard, M., and Belin, P. (2004). Sensitivity to auditory object features in human temporal neocortex. *J. Neurosci.* 24, 3637–3642. doi: 10.1523/JNEUROSCI.5458-03.2004

Zhang, Y. D., and Liu, W. (2019). A study of auditory localization mechanism based on thought experiments. *Phys. Life Rev.* 31, 206–213. doi: 10.1016/j.plrev.2019.01.005

Zheng, Y., Godar, S. P., and Litovsky, R. Y. (2015). Development of Sound Localization Strategies in Children with Bilateral Cochlear Implants. *PLoS One* 10:e0135790. doi: 10.1371/journal.pone.0135790

3

Serotonin Transporter Defect Disturbs Structure and Function of the Auditory Cortex in Mice

Wenlu Pan[1,2], Jing Pan[3,4], Yan Zhao[1], Hongzheng Zhang[3,4] and Jie Tang[1,3,4,5]**

[1] Department of Physiology, School of Basic Medical Sciences, Southern Medical University, Guangzhou, China, [2] Functional Nucleic Acid Basic and Clinical Research Center, Department of Physiology, School of Basic Medical Sciences, Changsha Medical College, Changsha, China, [3] Department of Otolaryngology Head and Neck Surgery, Zhujiang Hospital, Southern Medical University, Guangzhou, China, [4] Hearing Research Center, Southern Medical University, Guangzhou, China, [5] Key Laboratory of Mental Health of the Ministry of Education, Southern Medical University, Guangzhou, China

***Correspondence:**
Hongzheng Zhang
redtrue@smu.edu.cn
Jie Tang
jietang@smu.edu.cn

Serotonin transporter (SERT) modulates the level of 5-HT and significantly affects the activity of serotonergic neurons in the central nervous system. The manipulation of SERT has lasting neurobiological and behavioral consequences, including developmental dysfunction, depression, and anxiety. Auditory disorders have been widely reported as the adverse events of these mental diseases. It is unclear how SERT impacts neuronal connections/interactions and what mechanism(s) may elicit the disruption of normal neural network functions in auditory cortex. In the present study, we report on the neuronal morphology and function of auditory cortex in SERT knockout (KO) mice. We show that the dendritic length of the fourth layer (L-IV) pyramidal neurons and the second-to-third layer (L-II/III) interneurons were reduced in the auditory cortex of the SERT KO mice. The number and density of dendritic spines of these neurons were significantly less than those of wild-type neurons. Also, the frequency-tonotopic organization of primary auditory cortex was disrupted in SERT KO mice. The auditory neurons of SERT KO mice exhibited border frequency tuning with high-intensity thresholds. These findings indicate that SERT plays a key role in development and functional maintenance of auditory cortical neurons. Auditory function should be examined when SERT is selected as a target in the treatment for psychiatric disorders.

Keywords: serotonin transporter, auditory cortex, dendritic spines, tonotopic map, hearing disorder

INTRODUCTION

Serotonin, one of the most widely spread neurotransmitters in the central nervous system, has been known to play a critical role in brain morphogenesis and functions (Azmitia, 2001; Gaspar et al., 2004). The defects of serotonergic neurons are related to many psychiatric disorders, including depression, anxiety, and autism spectrum disorder (ASD) (Simpson et al., 2011). Acting as a key regulator of serotonergic activity, the serotonin transporter (SERT) is usually selected as the target of antidepressant treatments. SERT represents a potential mediator for anxiety- and depression-related behaviors. However, chronic exposure to selective serotonin reuptake inhibitors (SSRIs) was reported to elicit hearing disorders, such as tinnitus (Kehrle et al., 2015; Pattyn et al., 2016), auditory hallucinations (Kogoj, 2014), and hearing loss (Blazer and Tucci, 2018).

However, how the functions of SERT affect the auditory system remains unclear. Both increases and decreases in serotonin levels during early development have been found to impair the formation and function of the primary somatosensory cortex of rodents (Cases et al., 1996; Persico et al., 2000; Jennings et al., 2006). Pre- and post-natal exposure to the SSRI disturbed the chemoarchitecture of the mouse auditory cortex (AC) and resulted in ASD-like behavior (Simpson et al., 2011). Our previous study found that both SSRI treatment and SERT knockout (KO) did not change the auditory brain responses but abolished the auditory mismatch negativity in adult animals (Pan et al., 2020). These investigations suggest that SERT may affect the auditory functions by manipulating the serotonin level and serotonergic neurons of AC.

In rodents, 2 weeks after birth, layer IV afferent neurons in the primary visual, auditory, and somatosensory cortex are innervated by aggregates of serotonin-containing processes (D'Amato et al., 1987; Blue et al., 1991). At present, the morphological and especially the functional implications of SERT in AC remain unclear. In the present study, we examined the fine dendritic structure of the neurons in primary AC. We found that although expression of SERT is low in the AC, both pyramidal neurons and interneurons in SERT KO mice showed significant reductions in dendritic length, the number, and density of dendritic spines than did wild-type (WT) mice. The electrophysiological features of AC were also impaired by the SERT deficit. These results suggest that SERT plays a key role in development and functional maintenance of AC. This may explain the observed hearing disorders in patients utilizing drugs that target SERT, such as SSRIs, in the treatment for psychiatric disorders.

MATERIALS AND METHODS

All the animal experiments involved in this study were approved by the Institutional Animal Care and Use Committee (IACUC) of Southern Medical University. The principles formulated by the Animal Care Committee of Southern Medical University were followed throughout the experiment.

Subjects

SERT KO mice were derived from the Jackson Laboratory (Stock No. 008,355) and backcrossed with C57BL/6J background mice (Bengel et al., 1998). Polymerase chain reaction (PCR) protocol used for genotyping SERT KO mice has been reported in our previous literature (Pan et al., 2020). Male and female mice aged 2–4 months and weighting 20–26 g were employed in our test. Animals were housed in a room maintained at 22°C (±2°C) and kept on a 12:12 light/dark cycle with lights on at 8:00 a.m.

Immunohistochemistry

In this study, adult C57BL/6J mice were deeply sedated with pentobarbital sodium (50 mg/kg) administered *via* intraperitoneal injection. The mice were perfused intravascularly *via* the left ventricle with phosphate-buffered saline (PBS; pH 7.4), followed by a fixative, viz., 4% (w/v) paraformaldehyde. The mice were decapitated; the brain and cochleae were harvested and fully fixed in 4% paraformaldehyde, at 4°C overnight. Then the brain was sectioned on a freezing microtome to a thickness of 50 μm. The cochleae were washed in PBS, then placed into 10% ethylenediaminetetraacetic acid (EDTA) decalcifying solution, and replaced with fresh decalcifying solution every day for 6–8 days. Decalcification is terminated when the cochleae were transparent and elastic. Then the cochleae were sliced up parallel to the modiolar plane of the cochlea, and thickness of the slices was 10 μm. Brain and cochleae tissue samples were permeabilized in 0.3% Triton X-100 (Gibco, Grand Island, NY, United States) for 1 h and immunoblocked with a solution of 10% goat serum albumin for an additional hour. The specimens were incubated overnight at 4°C with SERT antibody (Millipore, Billerica, MA, United States; cat. no. 2828614) diluted in 10% goat serum albumin. After several washes in PBS, the specimens were then incubated with the Alexa-Fluor-488-conjugated secondary antibody at a concentration of 1:1,000 for 1 h at room temperature. To assign neurons, sections were counterstained for 20 min at room temperature with a fluorescent dye NeuroTrace 530/615 (1:100, Invitrogen, Carlsbad, CA, United States). Samples were then washed with PBS for three times and examined by using a Nikon confocal microscope (Nikon Instruments Inc., Melville, NY, United States).

Golgi Staining

Golgi staining was used to visualize the dendritic branching complexity and spines of the neurons in the mice. Mice were anesthetized with 10% chloral hydrate. The brains were taken after being fully infused with 0.9% saline and 4% paraformaldehyde, successively. Then, the brains were immersed in Golgi-Cox solution (Glaser and Loos, 1981) and stored at room temperature for 2 weeks in the dark. Next, the brains were transferred to a 30% sucrose solution and dehydrated at 4°C for 2–5 days, avoiding light. The brain tissues were completely coated with OCT embedding agent (Tissue-Tek 4583; Sakura Finetek United States, Inc., Torrance, CA, United States). The 100-μm-thick sections were prepared on gelatin-coated slides in a coronal plane parallel to the base and left to air-dry away from light for 2 days before being processed for Golgi–Cox impregnation. The brain slides were put into a special opaque staining box, and Golgi–Cox staining was performed as the literature (Zhang et al., 2009).

Sholl's Analysis

Dendrites in each of the selected neurons were quantitatively analyzed using Sholl's concentric circle method (Sholl, 1953). The neurons were selected from layers IV and II/III in AC using the following criteria: (1) the cell body was in the subregion of interest, (2) the staining of the branches was efficient and complete throughout the length, and (3) the branches were isolated from their neighbors. A series of concentric rings, spaced 20 μm apart, were placed over the neuron and centered on the cell body, and the number of dendrites intersecting each circle in the series of concentric circles was counted blind to the experimental conditions to estimate the total dendritic length, branch points, and dendritic complexity.

Dendritic Spine Density Analysis

Spine analyses were conducted blind to the experimental conditions on coded Golgi impregnated brain sections containing the AC. Spines were examined on dendrites of pyramidal neurons and inter neurons. Briefly, all protruding dendritic spines were counted on per 25-μm dendritic segments. Spine density was expressed as the number of spines per 25 μm. Two to three dendritic segments were analyzed per neuron. Only intact, properly stained, and unbranched dendritic segments were included in the analyses. To acquire images for spine analysis, the dendritic segments were imaged under bright field illumination on a Zeiss Axioimager microscope (Carl Zeiss, Oberkochen, Germany) with a 63× oil immersion objective.

Recording in the Primary Auditory Cortex (AI)

WT and SERT KO mice weighing 20–26 g were anesthetized by pentobarbital sodium (30 mg/kg, i.p.), followed by atropine sulfate (0.25 mg/kg, i.h.) to prevent asphyxia. The level of anesthesia was maintained by additional dosages of sodium pentobarbital (30 mg/kg, i.p.) administered approximately every 40 min throughout the physiological experiments. Under anesthesia, the mouse's head was fixed in a head holder by rigidly clamping on a nail about 1.5 cm long fixed on the surface of the skull vertically with dental cement (Tang et al., 2008; Tang and Suga, 2009).

The scalp, muscles, and soft tissues of the skull were then removed; an opening above the left AC was made using a dental driller; and the dura was gently removed. The anatomical location of AI in AC was marked according to the brain map (bregma −2.7 mm, left/right of the midline 3.5 mm) (Umbricht et al., 2005), and the size of the parietal open window was 0.2 × 0.2 mm^2. The cortex was maintained under artificial cerebrospinal fluid to prevent desiccation. The mouse was placed on a feedback-controlled heating pad to maintain its body temperature at 37°C. All electrophysiological experiments were performed in a soundproof and echo-attenuated chamber.

Microelectrodes with a ~1-μm tip diameter (7–12 MΩ, filled with 3 mol/L of KCl) were used for recordings. At every recording site, the microelectrode was lowered orthogonally into the cortex to depths of 200–375 μm (layers II/III) or 475–600 μm (layers IV/V), where the evoked spikes of a neuron or a small cluster of neurons were collected. After the best frequency (BF) of neurons was found at a recording point once, the electrode was moved toward the rostral or caudal side to the next point 200–300 μm away from the previous recording point, and the same measurement was repeated. Complete examinations were repeated in this way until no response at the two adjacent voice-induced recording sites was observed in any direction.

Pure tones were generated and played with a TDT 3 system (Tucker-Davis Technologies, Alachua, FL, United States) for auditory mapping. A real-time processor (RP2.1) and a program written in RPvdsEx software were used to synthesize the sound signals. Sound intensity was adjusted by an attenuator (PA5). The synthesized sound signal was amplified by an electric driver (ED1) with an open-field speaker (ES1). Before the OpenEx software (sampling rate = 25 kHz) recording, the speakers were calibrated with 1/8- and 1/4-inch microphones (Brüel and Kjaer 4138, 4135, Naerum, Denmark). Neural signals were amplified 10,000× using a digital amplifier (RA16) with a 0.3- to 3-kHz filter and monitored online by a software Brainware (Tucker-Davis Technologies). Frequency–intensity receptive fields (RFs) were reconstructed in detail by presenting pure tones (50-ms duration, 5-ms ramps) of six frequencies (2–32 kHz) at nine sound intensities [0–90 dB sound pressure level (SPL), in 10-dB increments] at a rate of two stimuli per second. The tones were presented in a random, interleaved sequence.

To generate the cortical map, we used Matlab functions to create colored polygons, constructed by connecting a record point and intermediate points between four and six adjacent record points (Bao et al., 2003). The electrode penetration point was located in its center, and each polygon was the BF with responsive neurons at this point. In the topological diagram, the RF of auditory neurons in area AI was continuous, single-peaked, and V-shaped. Moreover, the BF of the neurons in this region was tonotopically organized, with high frequencies in the rostrally and low frequencies in the caudally.

Data Processing and Statistical Analysis

We defined the minimum threshold (MT) and BF to enable neurons to respond to the minimum stimulus sound intensity at the corresponding sound frequency when firing maximum number of spikes at this site. The BF of the cortical region AI was defined as the frequency at the tip of the tuning curve, that is, the sound frequency corresponding to the MT of the neuron at this place. The sharpness of the frequency-tuning curve, defined for all recording sites, was represented by the value Q30 (Tang et al., 2012). Q30 was equal to the BF divided by the bandwidth value of 30 dB above the MT within the frequency–intensity RF range. The larger the Q30, the sharper the tuning curve representing the neurons, and the better the frequency selectivity of the neurons. A customized MatLab program (MathWorks, Natick, MA, United States) was used to analyze and plot tonotopic map of A1. Tonotopic index (TI) was used to evaluate the tonotopic organization by following the methods described in previous studies (Zhang et al., 2001; Bao et al., 2004).

We used SPSS 20 software (IBM, Armonk, NY, United States) to perform statistical analysis. The two-tailed t-tests (for unpaired comparisons) and two-way ANOVA (for multiple-group comparisons) were used to test for significant differences between groups. Statistical significance was defined as $p < 0.05$. GraphPad Prism 7 (GraphPad Software, San Diego, CA, United States) was used for plotting.

RESULTS

By using immunostaining, the expression of SERT in the auditory neural system was examined systematically. As shown in **Figure 1**, no robust SERT expression was detected in the cochlea (spiral ganglion neurons; **Figure 1A**), auditory brainstem (cochlear nuclei, superior olivary complex, and inferior colliculus; **Figures 1B–D**), or auditory thalamus (medial

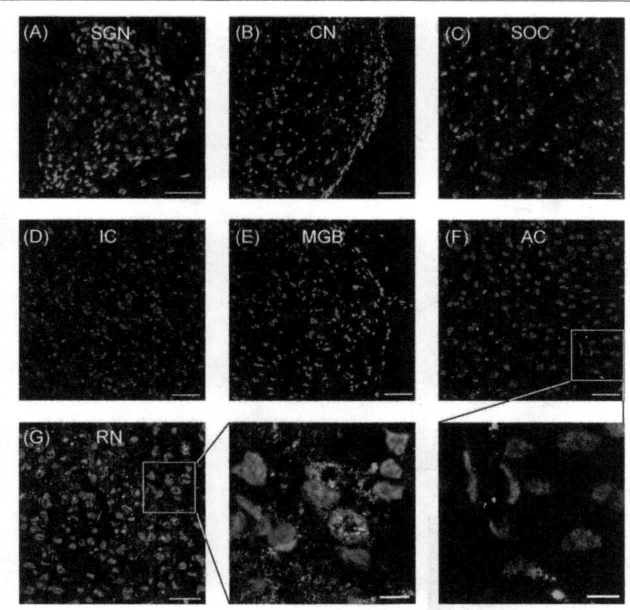

FIGURE 1 | Representative images show the serotonin transporter (SERT) expression in different regions of auditory system. **(A–G)** Confocal images show the SERT (green) expression in the spiral ganglion neurons (SGN), cochlear nuclei (CN), superior olivary complex (SOC), inferior colliculus (IC), medial geniculate body (MGB), auditory cortex (AC), and raphe nuclear complex (RN). Insets are the magnified images of the boxes in **(F,G)**. The soma and nucleus of neurons are colored in red (Nissl) and blue (DAPI), respectively. SERT is colored in green. Scale bars: 50 μm for **(A–G)** and 10 μm for insets.

geniculate body; **Figure 1E**). Hence, we examined the SERT expression in the primary AC. Our data from AC exhibit sporadic spread of SERT immunoreactive puncta, which represents the SERT immunoreactive fibers (**Figure 1F**). However, the SERT immunoreactive puncta was usually detected around the soma of cortical neurons (inset of **Figure 1F**) with a much lower density than the expression in the raphe nuclear complex (**Figure 1G**). This result suggests that AC neurons receive sparse serotonergic projections, if any.

To determine the roles of these serotonergic projections, the morphology of AC neurons from SERT KO mice was examined in comparison with that of WT mice. Our data show that for pyramidal cells in layer IV, the number of intersections and the total length of dendrites were significantly reduced in both apical and basal dendrites of the SERT KO AC neurons (**Figure 2**). Moreover, the reduction of dendrites was also found in layer II/III interneurons of SERT KO AC (**Figures 2F,G**).

Most excitatory synaptic connections occur on dendritic spines. Spines can individually detect the temporal coincidence of pre- and post-synaptic activities and thus serve as basic functional units of neuronal integration (Gray, 1959; Yuste and Denk, 1995; Spacek and Harris, 1998; Arellano et al., 2007). To further determine whether synaptic function at neuronal junctions was altered in SERT KO mice, we looked at the morphologic structure of the dendritic spines of AC neurons. We measured the number and density of total dendritic spines in layer IV pyramidal cells and layer II/III interneurons from the AC of WT and SERT KO mice (**Figure 3A**). In apical dendrites, the total number of dendritic spines of layer IV pyramidal cells was less in SERT KO mice [vs. WT, $F(1,159) = 252.5$, $p < 0.0001$, two-way ANOVA]. Significant reduction was observed at a distance of 25–125 μm from cell bodies (vs. WT, $p < 0.001$, two-tailed t-test; **Figure 3B**). The mean density of apical dendritic spines reduced significantly in SERT KO mice (vs. WT, $p < 0.0001$, two-tailed t-test; **Figure 3E**). The total number of basal dendritic spines of layer IV pyramidal cells was also reduced in SERT KO mice [vs. WT, $F(1,356) = 109.6$, $p < 0.0001$, two-way ANOVA] and significantly reduced at a distance of 25–150 μm from cell bodies (vs. WT, $p < 0.001$, two-tailed t-test; **Figure 3C**). Meanwhile, the mean density of basal dendritic spines reduced significantly in SERT KO mice (vs. WT, $p < 0.0001$, two-tailed t-test; **Figure 3F**). However, the total number of dendritic spines in layer II/III interneurons in SERT KO mice was not significantly different [vs. WT, $F(1,292) = 10.93$, $p = 0.011$, two-way ANOVA]. The density was only found reduced at a distance of 25–75 μm from cell bodies (vs. WT, $p < 0.05$, two-tailed t-tests; **Figure 3D**). The mean density of dendritic spines was also significantly reduced in SERT KO mice (vs. WT, $p < 0.0001$, two-tailed t-test; **Figure 3G**). Together with the results of our Sholl's analysis, these morphological data implied that synaptic transmission between the subcortical and cortical neurons, as well as the neurons within the AC, might be weakened in the auditory system of SERT KO mice. These defects may affect the functions of SERT KO AC neurons.

Electrophysiological experiments were conducted to investigate the functional alteration of auditory neurons in primary AC (AI) of SERT KO mice. Previous studies have found that neurons at different locations within the same layer of AI respond to different frequencies (Kelly and Sally, 1988; Kaas et al., 1999; Zhang et al., 2001; de Villers-Sidani et al., 2007). Therefore, we measured the "frequency-tonotopic map" of neurons in the AI region of cortex. A total 246 sites and 243 sites were recorded from the auditory cortical area of WT and SERT KO mice, respectively. Normally in WT mice, high-frequency sensitive neurons are located in the rostral sites of the AI region, and low-frequency sensitive neurons are located in caudal side (Stiebler et al., 1997).

As shown in the representative data in **Figure 4A**, the BFs of AC neurons were distributed regularly from the rostral to caudal sites, forming a compact and ordered "tonotopic map" in WT mice. However, for AC neurons of SERT KO mice, their frequency selectivity did not show a systematic organization, although the neurons that respond to high frequencies were still mostly located to the rostral side. We further analyzed the frequency range and the total area of the AI region. No statistical difference was found between SERT KO and WT mice ($p > 0.05$, two-tailed t-test; **Figures 4B,C**). The BFs of all recorded sites were plotted against a normalized AC axis (**Figure 4D**). The distribution of BFs was quantified with the TI, which was significantly increased in SERT KO mice ($p < 0.01$, two-tailed t-test). These results showed that a disrupted tonotopic map was found in the AC of SERT KO mice, suggesting that SERT may mainly affect the neuron's tuning property.

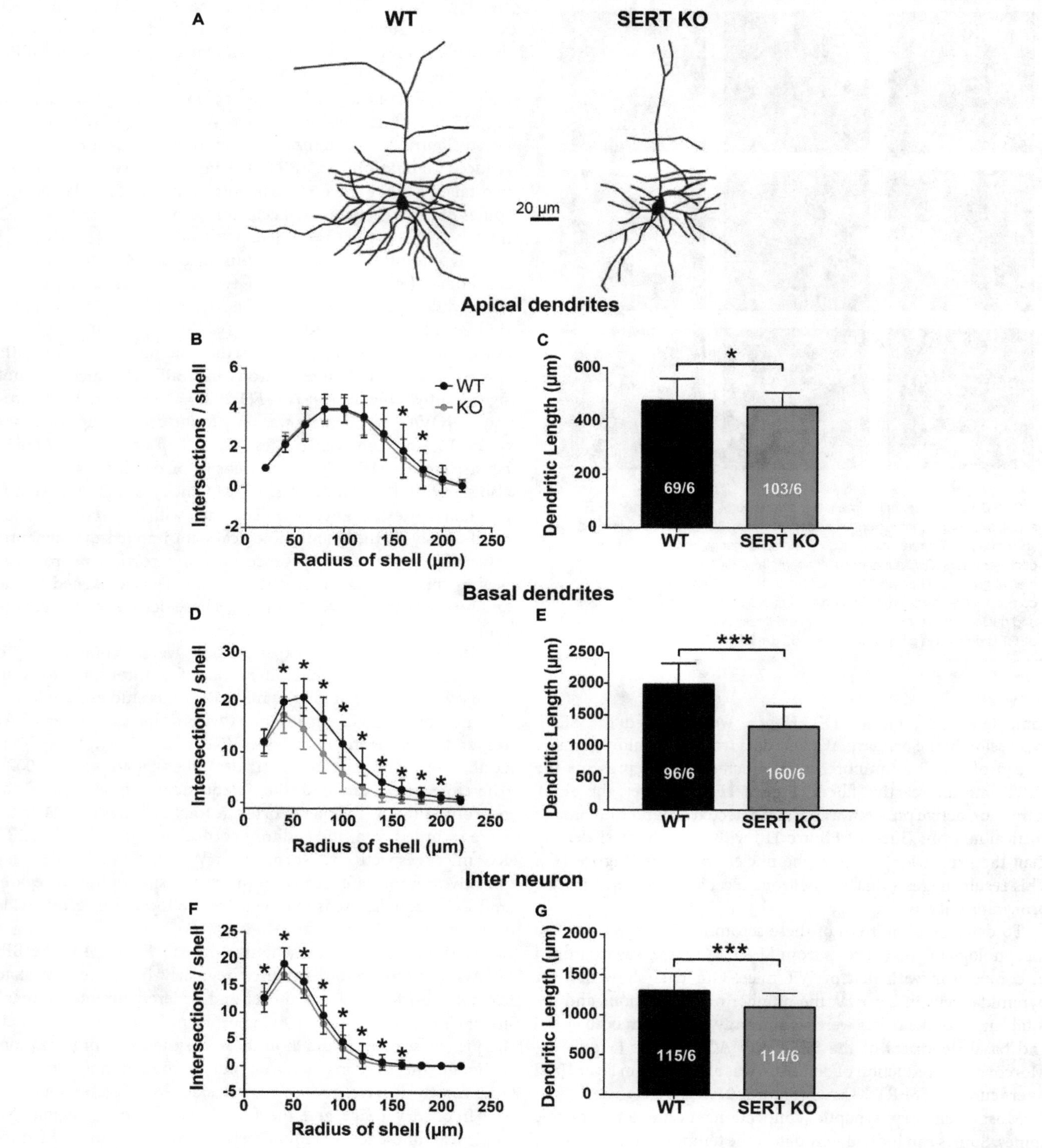

FIGURE 2 | Serotonin transporter (SERT) knockout (KO) degrades the dendrites of layer IV pyramidal neurons and layer II/III interneurons in auditory cortex. **(A)** Representative dendritic morphology of layer IV pyramidal cells in auditory cortex from wild-type (WT) and SERT KO mice. Scale bar: 20 µm. **(B,C)** Comparing the number of intersections and the total length of the apical dendrites of layer IV pyramidal cells in WT mice with SERT KO mice. **(D,E)** Comparing the number of intersections and the total length of the basal dendrites of layer IV pyramidal cells in WT mice with SERT KO mice. **(F,G)** The number of intersections and the total length of the dendrites of layer II/III interneurons were significantly reduced in SERT KO mice, compared with WT mice. The number of intersections of dendrites was measured with 20-µm concentric spheres centered on the soma by Sholl's analysis. The numbers in the column indicate the numbers of neurons/numbers of animals analyzed. Data are presented as means ± SD. * $p < 0.05$; *** $p < 0.001$, Student's *t*-tests and two-way ANOVA.

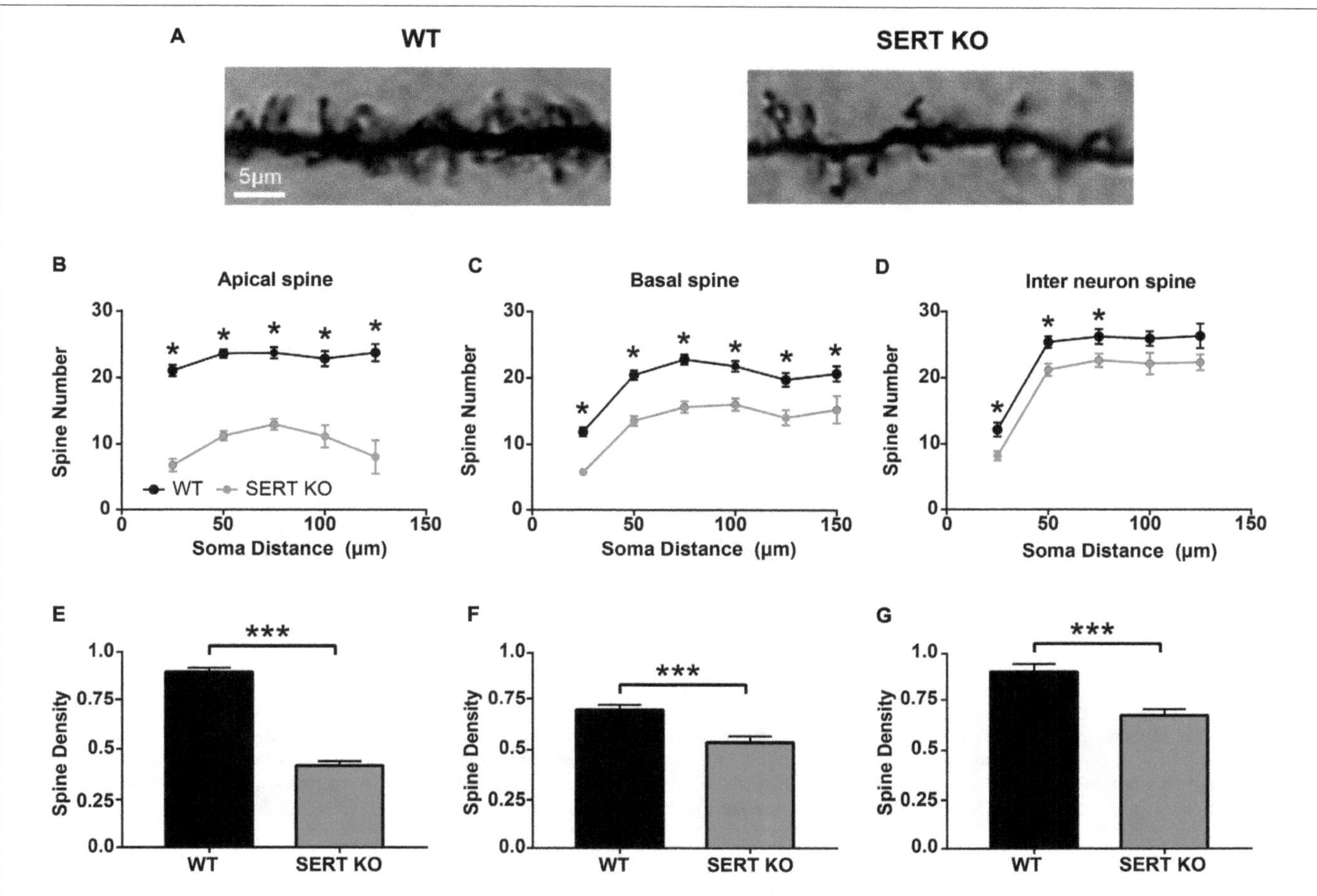

FIGURE 3 | Dendritic spines density decreased in serotonin transporter (SERT) knockout (KO) mice. **(A)** Representative photomicrographs of dendritic spines of basal dendrites in layer IV pyramidal neurons from wild-type (WT) and SERT KO mice. **(B,C)** Comparing the total number of apical and basal dendritic spines at a distance of per 25 μm from the cell body of layer IV pyramidal cells in WT mice with SERT KO mice, respectively. **(D)** Comparing the total number of dendritic spines at a distance of per 25 μm from the cell body of layer II/III interneurons in WT mice with SERT KO mice. **(E–G)** The dendritic spine densities of apical and basal dendrites in layer IV pyramidal neurons and in layer II/III interneurons of the auditory cortex. Data are presented as means ± SD. $n = 6$ for each group. * $p < 0.05$, *** $p < 0.001$, Student's t-test and two-way ANOVA. Scale bar: 5 μm.

We then measured the BF and the MT of AC neurons recorded from SERT KO and WT mice, by which the frequency selectivity and sound sensitivity of neurons were compared. The BFs and MTs of SERT KO and WT neurons were pooled in **Figures 5A,B**, respectively. Interestingly, although no change was found in BFs, the MTs of SERT KO neurons were significantly elevated. The MTs of WT neurons were generally below 40 dB SPL with an average of 27.09 ± 12.81 dB SPL. However, the MTs of SERT KO neurons were significantly higher with an average of 53.85 ± 11.33 dB SPL ($p < 0.0001$, two-tailed t-test; **Figure 5C**). These data suggest that individual neurons in SERT KO mice were significantly less sensitive to sound stimulation.

Auditory neurons respond not only to their most sensitive frequency (i.e., BF) but also to other frequencies of sound. One of the most important functions of auditory neurons is that they can selectively respond to sound within a range of frequencies. In WT mice, individual neurons respond to sound frequencies in addition to the BF at sound levels above MT. These frequency-threshold intensity points formed a "V-shaped" frequency-tuning curve (**Figure 6A**). In SERT KO mice, the frequency-tuning curves of cortical neurons have much wider bandwidth (**Figure 6B**). To evaluate the frequency selectivity of a single neuron, we used "Q30" value to analyze the changes in frequency selectivity of AC neurons. The higher the value of Q30, the sharper the frequency-tuning curve of the neuron, and the better the frequency selectivity. For AC neurons of WT mice, their Q30 values mostly ranged from 1 to 2.5, with an average of 1.78 ± 0.91 (**Figures 6C,D**). But in SERT KO mice, Q30 values of most AC neurons were below 1 (0.65 ± 0.27, mean ± SD; **Figures 6C,D**). This result suggested that AC neurons in SERT KO mice have less selectivity to sound frequency.

DISCUSSION

Our results of immunohistochemical study in the whole auditory system showed that SERT was rarely expressed in the auditory

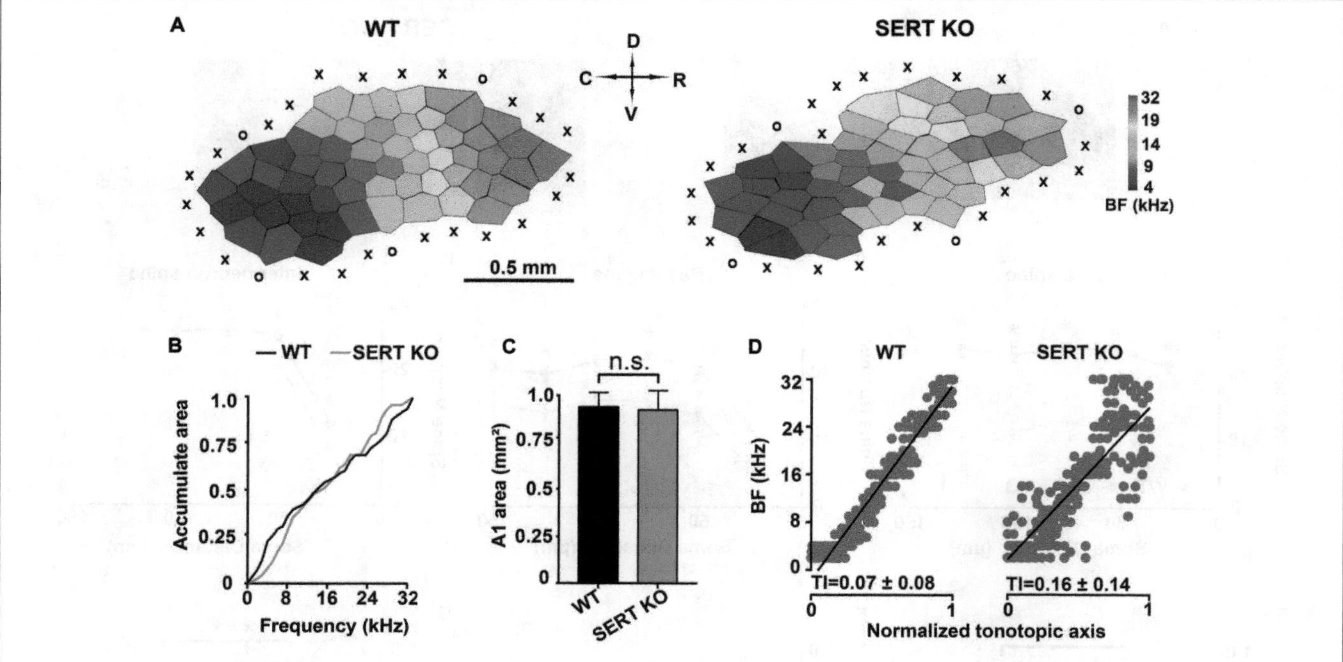

FIGURE 4 | Disturbed tonotopic organization of primary auditory cortex in serotonin transporter (SERT) knockout (KO) mice. **(A)** Representative A1 characteristic-frequency map from a wild-type (WT) mouse (left) and a SERT KO mouse (right). Scale bar: 0.5 mm. X, unresponsive cortical site; O, non-A1 cortical site (see section "Materials and Methods"). **(B)** Plotting accumulated response areas at best frequency for neurons of primary auditory cortex in WT and SERT KO mice. **(C)** The total areas of primary auditory cortex in WT mice and SERT KO mice. **(D)** The best frequencies of all recorded sites in WT and SERT KO mice were plotted against a normalized tonotopic axis. The tonotopic index (TI) represents the increased scatter of best frequencies around the ideal tonotopic axis (black diagonal line) (see section "Materials and Methods"). Data are presented as means ± SD. ns, no statistical difference, $p > 0.05$. Student's t-test.

neurons, including those in the AC, of adult WT mice (**Figure 1**). These data suggest that the morphological and functional defects observed in AC neurons of SERT KO mice may not due to the disruption of serotonergic innervations directly but more likely related to the effects of SERT deficit on cortical circuit development.

FIGURE 5 | Serotonin transporter (SERT) knockout (KO) elevates the threshold of neurons in primary auditory cortex. Pooled data show minimum thresholds at the best frequency of auditory neurons recorded from the A1 region of wild-type (WT) **(A)** and SERT KO mice **(B)**. WT: $n = 6$, recording site = 246. SERT KO: $n = 6$, recording site = 243. **(C)** The average minimum threshold (MT) of neurons in SERT KO mice was significantly higher than that in WT mice. Data are means ± SD. *** $p < 0.001$. Student's t-test.

As the staining results showed, the length of basal dendrites of pyramidal cells was significantly shortened (**Figure 2**), and the number and density of dendritic spines were significantly reduced in SERT KO mice (**Figure 3**), suggesting that the ability of pyramidal cells to receive input information was decreased, which might cause less sensitivity to sound response (**Figure 5**). Moreover, the reduction of the length, the number, and density of dendritic spines in inhibitory interneurons of SERT KO mice suggests that the reduced inhibitory of the interneurons might cause less frequency selectivity of neurons (**Figure 6**). However, deficient SERT may change the neural morphology in different ways in different brain regions. The length of dendrite and the density of dendritic spines were increased in the infralimbic cortex of SERT KO mice. Meanwhile, SERT KO has little effects on the morphology of basolateral amygdala neurons (Wellman et al., 2007). These different results suggest that the morphology of neurons was also specifically determined by their circuits; even the SERT was abolished in the early stage of the development. Interestingly, many evidences have suggested that SERT is expressed not only on serotonin neurons but also on other neurons such glutamatergic neurons during development. The loss of SERT in these neurons may affect the neural circuit in the cortex during development (Chen et al., 2015). This may explain why the morphology of AC neurons was altered by SERT

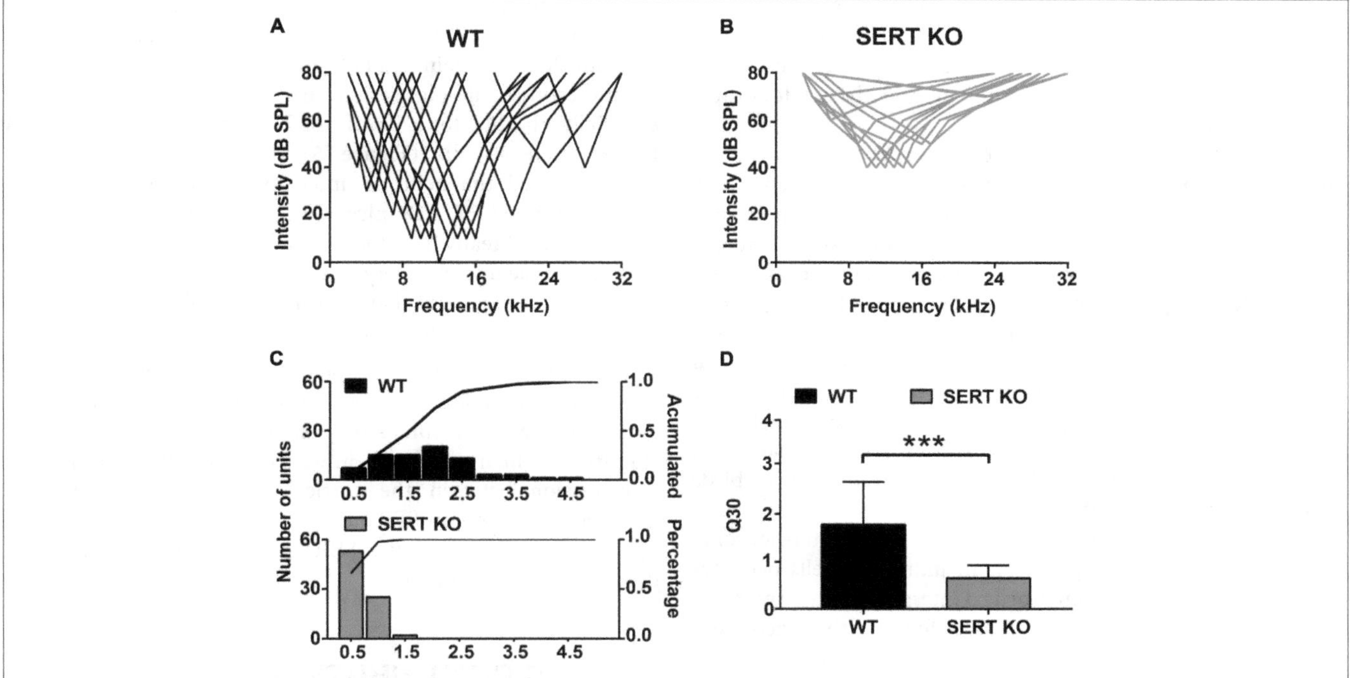

FIGURE 6 | Broader frequency tuning for primary auditory cortical neurons in serotonin transporter (SERT) knockout (KO) mice. Pooled data show the frequency-tuning curves of cortical neurons in wild-type (WT) **(A)** and SERT KO **(B)** AI. **(C)** The distribution of the Q30 values for cortical neurons in WT (top panel) and SERT KO (bottom panel) AI. The lines in the panels represent the cumulative percentage of the Q30 value. **(D)** The mean Q30 value of all auditory neurons recorded from WT mice and SERT KO AI. Data are presented as means ± SD. $n = 6$ for each group. *** $p < 0.001$. Student's *t*-test.

KO, although few direct serotonergic projections were detected in AC of WT animals.

SERT is a target of SSRIs treatments and regulates the activity of serotonergic system (Kalueff et al., 2009). In the present study, we examined the role of SERT function in primary AC by using SERT KO mice. In WT mice, the primary AC formed a compact and ordered "tonotopic map"; the optimal response frequencies from the rostral to caudal side was regularly distributed. But in SERT KO mice, the primary AC formed a distorted tonotopic organization (**Figure 4**). However, in SERT KO mice, the disordered frequency topology did not show a systematic decrease in frequency, although the neurons that respond to high frequencies were still mostly medial to the rostral side, and the neurons that respond to low frequencies were still mostly lateral to the caudal. Next, we further analyzed the total area of the tonotopic map in the AI region and the frequency range of the response to sound (**Figure 4B**). There was no statistical difference between SERT KO mice and WT mice (**Figure 4B**). It suggests that SERT may mainly affect the orderliness of the neuron's frequency response. Similarly, manipulations of rodent brain serotonin levels during early development, through either increases (produced in SERT or monoamine oxidase KO mice) or decreases (produced by parachlorophenylalanine or other treatments), alter the formation of the whisker (barrel) representation in the primary somatosensory cortex and promote aggressive and/or anxiety-related behaviors (Cases et al., 1995, 1996; Persico et al., 2000; Persico et al., 2001; Holmes et al., 2003; Jennings et al., 2006). In our previous study, auditory mismatch negativity response was found abolished by SERT KO, indicating the low ability in frequency discrimination (Pan et al., 2020). This finding was supported by the functional changes of AC observed in the present study. Under the administration of SSRIs, the animal showed anxiety-related and ASD-like behavior (Simpson et al., 2011; Pan et al., 2020). Although the abnormal behavior and auditory function were quite consistent in SERT KO and SSRI-administered animals, the direct evidence is still very limited for us to understand the effects of SSRIs on development and function of cortical circuits. However, the SERT KO mouse model used in the present study is constitutive and global. To investigate the role of SERT and SSRI in the development of ASD and anxiety, a knock-in SERT mouse model, such as SERT Ala56, should be expected in future studies (Siemann et al., 2017).

One of previous findings related to serotonin and early cortical organization found that the primary sensory cortex of mice, especially the layer IV neurons of visual, auditory, and somatosensory cortex, is transiently innervated with dense 5-HT-containing projection (D'Amato et al., 1987; Blue et al., 1991; Bennett-Clarke et al., 1994). Moreover, in early brain development, 5-HT is taken up into glutamatergic thalamocortical terminals (Bennett-Clarke et al., 1996; Lebrand, 1996) and used in combination with the 5-HT 1B receptor on layer IV afferents (Salichon et al., 2001). Serotonin plays a trophic role in brain morphogenesis, including cell proliferation, migration, and differentiation. It is also one of the first neurotransmitters to appear in the central nervous system (Azmitia, 2001; Gaspar et al., 2004). We found that the typical dendritic morphology was shortened (**Figure 2**) and that the density of dendritic spines was lower in SERT KO mice compared with WT mice (**Figure 3**). In SERT KO mice, the deficit of SERT may alter neural morphology and distort tonotopic organization in primary AC.

The structure and arborization of dendrites have a profound impact on the processing of neuronal information because they determine the extent of a neuron's synaptic field. Thousands of spines stud the pyramidal cell's apical and basal dendritic branches, increasing the neuron's receptive surface area and allowing for integration of thousands of excitatory signals to influence the output (Spruston, 2008). Obviously, dendritic spines receive most of the excitatory impulses of a pyramidal cell, consistent with the information processing capacity of the neuron. A cell with spiny processes in homologous nuclei has more spines, the higher level of the subject in the animal series. Thus, as an example in vertebrates, the Purkinje cell of birds shows fewer spines than that of mammals.

Since neural circuits are defined by inter-neuronal communications, output precision in individual cells becomes essential to network function. Cortical interneurons use rhythmic inhibition to create narrow windows for effective excitation, entraining excitatory pyramidal cells to fire certain oscillatory patterns (Beierlein et al., 2000; Uhlhaas and Singer, 2010). Moreover, optogenetic manipulation of specific excitatory and inhibitory circuits directly caused changes in social and cognitive behaviors in mice (Yizhar et al., 2011). Thus, circuits tend to be malleable but vulnerable during post-natal development. Notably, several neurodevelopmental disorders, such as ASD and schizophrenia (SCZ), manifest during this plasticity period (Zoghbi, 2003; Hossein and Folsom, 2009).

Interestingly, in our results, the neuron functions altered; especially, the MT for a BF of SERT KO mice was significantly higher than 40 dB (**Figure 5**). It suggested that absent SERT reduced the neurons' intensity sensitivity to response. Moreover, in SERT KO mice, Q30 values were mostly below 1 (**Figure 6**). Meanwhile, the frequency-tuning curve was dull, and the frequency selectivity of neurons was significantly worse (**Figure 6**). It suggested that neurons in SERT KO mice showed less frequency selectivity to response.

All of these results may be related to shortened typical dendritic morphology of neurons (**Figure 2**) and the lower density of dendritic spines of primary AC in SERT KO mice (**Figure 3**), which may result in weakened synaptic information transmission between the cortical pyramidal cells and the interneurons of AC in SERT KO mice. The altered function of the primary AC suggests that SERT plays a critical role in circuit development and function.

AUTHOR CONTRIBUTIONS

HZ and JT designed the experiments. WP, JP, and YZ performed the experiments. All authors wrote, reviewed, edited, and approved the final manuscript.

REFERENCES

Arellano, J. I., Benavides-Piccione, R., Defelipe, J., and Yuste, R. (2007). Ultrastructure of dendritic spines: correlation between synaptic and spine morphologies. *Front. Neurosci.* 1:131–143. doi: 10.3389/neuro.01.1.1.010.2007

Azmitia, E. C. (2001). Modern views on an ancient chemical: serotonin effects on cell proliferation, maturation, and apoptosis. *Brain Res. Bull.* 56, 413–424. doi: 10.1016/S0361-9230(01)00614-1

Bao, S., Chang, E. F., Davis, J. D., Gobeske, K. T., and Merzenich, M. M. (2003). Progressive degradation and subsequent refinement of acoustic representations in the adult auditory cortex. *J. Neurosci.* 23, 10765–10775. doi: 10.1523/JNEUROSCI.23-34-10765.2003

Bao, S., Chang, E. F., Woods, J., and Merzenich, M. M. (2004). Temporal plasticity in the primary auditory cortex induced by operant perceptual learning. *Nat. Neurosci.* 7, 974–981. doi: 10.1038/nn1293

Beierlein, M., Gibson, J. R., and Connors, B. W. (2000). A network of electrically coupled interneurons drives synchronized inhibition in neocortex. *Nat. Neurosci.* 3, 904–910. doi: 10.1038/78809

Bengel, D., Murphy, D. L., Andrews, A. M., Wichems, C. H., Feltner, D., Heils, A., et al. (1998). Altered brain serotonin homeostasis and locomotor insensitivity to 3,4-methylenedioxymethamphetamine ("Ecstasy") in serotonin transporter-deficient mice. *Mol. Pharmacol.* 53:649. doi: 10.1124/mol.53.4.649

Bennett-Clarke, C. A., Chiaia, N. L., and Rhoades, R. W. (1996). Thalamocortical afferents in rat transiently express high-affinity serotonin uptake sites. *Brain Res.* 733, 301–306. doi: 10.1016/0006-8993(96)00791-3

Bennett-Clarke, C. A., Leslie, M. J., Lane, R. D., and Rhoades, R. W. (1994). Effect of serotonin depletion on vibrissa-related patterns of thalamic afferents in the rat's somatosensory cortex. *J. Neurosci.* 14, 7594–7607. doi: 10.1523/JNEUROSCI.14-12-07594.1994

Blazer, D. G., and Tucci, D. L. (2018). Hearing loss and psychiatric disorders: a review. *Psychol. Med.* 49, 891–897. doi: 10.1017/S0033291718003409

Blue, M. E., Erzurumlu, R. S., and Jhaveri, S. (1991). A comparison of pattern formation by thalamocortical and serotonergic afferents in the rat barrel field cortex. *Cereb. Cortex* 1, 380–389. doi: 10.1093/cercor/1.5.380

Cases, O., Seif, I., Grimsby, J., Gaspar, P., Chen, K., Pournin, S., et al. (1995). Aggressive behavior and altered amounts of brain serotonin and norepinephrine in mice lacking MAOA. *Science* 268, 1763–1766. doi: 10.1126/science.7792602

Cases, O., Vitalis, T., Seif, I., De Maeyer, E., Sotelo, C., and Gaspar, P. (1996). Lack of barrels in the somatosensory cortex of monoamine oxidase a-deficient mice: role of a serotonin excess during the critical period. *Neuron* 16, 297–307. doi: 10.1016/S0896-6273(00)80048-3

Chen, X., Ye, R., Gargus, J. J., Blakely, R. D., Dobrenis, K., and Sze, J. Y. (2015). Disruption of transient serotonin accumulation by non-serotonin-producing neurons impairs cortical map development. *Cell Rep.* 10, 346–358. doi: 10.1016/j.celrep.2014.12.033

D'Amato, R. J., Blue, M. E., Largent, B. L., Lynch, D. R., Ledbetter, D. J., Molliver, M. E., et al. (1987). Ontogeny of the serotonergic projection to rat neocortex: transient expression of a dense innervation to primary sensory areas. *Proc. Natl. Acad. Sci. U.S.A.* 84, 4322–4326. doi: 10.1073/pnas.84.12.4322

de Villers-Sidani, E., Chang, E. F., Bao, S., and Merzenich, M. M. (2007). Critical period window for spectral tuning defined in the primary auditory cortex (A1) in the rat. *J. Neurosci.* 27, 180–189. doi: 10.1523/JNEUROSCI.3227-06.2007

Gaspar, P., Cases, O., and Maroteaux, L. (2004). The developmental role of serotonin: news from mouse molecular genetics. *Nat. Rev. Neurosci.* 4, 1002–1012. doi: 10.1038/nrn1256

Glaser, E. M., and Loos, H. (1981). Analysis of thick brain sections by obverse-reverse computer microscopy: application of a new, high clarity Golgi-Nissl stain. *J. Neurosci. Methods* 4, 117–125. doi: 10.1016/0165-0270(81)90045-5

Gray, E. G. (1959). Electron microscopy of synaptic contacts on dendrite spines of the cerebral cortex. *Nature* 183, 1592–1593. doi: 10.1038/1831592a0

Holmes, A., Yang, R. J., Lesch, K. P., Crawley, J. N., and Murphy, D. L. (2003). Mice lacking the serotonin transporter exhibit 5-HT(1A) receptor-mediated abnormalities in tests for anxiety-like behavior. *Neuropsychopharmacology* 28, 2077–2088. doi: 10.1038/sj.npp.1300266

Hossein, F. S., and Folsom, T. D. (2009). The neurodevelopmental hypothesis of schizophrenia, revisited. *Schizophr. Bull.* 35, 528–548. doi: 10.1093/schbul/sbn187

Jennings, K. A., Loder, M. K., Sheward, W. J., Pei, Q., Deacon, R. M., Benson, M. A., et al. (2006). Increased expression of the 5-HT transporter confers a low-anxiety phenotype linked to decreased 5-HT transmission. *J. Neurosci.* 26, 8955–8964. doi: 10.1523/JNEUROSCI.5356-05.2006

Kaas, J. H., Hackett, T. A., and Tramo, M. J. (1999). Auditory processing in primate cerebral cortex. *Curr. Opin. Neurobiol.* 9, 164–170. doi: 10.1016/S0959-4388(99)80022-1

Kalueff, A. V., Olivier, J., Nonkes, L., and Homberg, J. R. (2009). Conserved role for the serotonin transporter gene in rat and mouse neurobehavioral endophenotypes. *Neurosci. Biobehav. Rev.* 34, 373–386. doi: 10.1016/j.neubiorev.2009.08.003

Kehrle, H. M., Sampaio, A., Granjeiro, R. C., Oliveira, T., and Oliveira, C. A. C. P. (2015). Tinnitus annoyance in normal-hearing individuals: correlation with depression and anxiety. *Anna. Otol. Rhinol. Laryngol.* 125, 185–194. doi: 10.1177/0003489415606445

Kelly, J. B., and Sally, S. L. (1988). Organization of auditory cortex in the albino rat: binaural response properties. *J. Neurophysiol.* 59, 1756–1769. doi: 10.1152/jn.1988.59.6.1756

Kogoj, A. (2014). Selective serotonin reuptake inhibitors-induced delirium: a case review. *Psychiatr. Danub.* 26, 277–280.

Lebrand, C. (1996). Transient uptake and storage of serotonin in developing thalamic neurons. *Neuron* 17, 823–835. doi: 10.1016/S0896-6273(00)80215-9

Pan, W., Lyu, K., Zhang, H., Li, C., and Tang, J. (2020). Attenuation of auditory mismatch negativity in serotonin transporter knockout mice with anxiety-related behaviors. *Behav. Brain Res.* 379:112387. doi: 10.1016/j.bbr.2019.112387

Pattyn, T., Van Den Eede, F., Vanneste, S., Cassiers, L., Veltman, D. J., Van De Heyning, P., et al. (2016). Tinnitus and anxiety disorders: a review. *Hear. Res.* 333, 255–265. doi: 10.1016/j.heares.2015.08.014

Persico, A. M., Ltamura, C. A., Calia, E., Puglisi-Allegra, S., Ventura, R., Lucchese, F., et al. (2000). Serotonin depletion and barrel cortex development: impact of growth impairment vs. serotonin effects on thalamocortical endings. *Cereb. Cortex* 10, 181–191. doi: 10.1093/cercor/10.2.181

Persico, A. M., Mengual, E., Moessner, R., Hall, S. F., Revay, R. S., Sora, I., et al. (2001). Barrel pattern formation requires serotonin uptake by thalamocortical afferents, and not vesicular monoamine release. *J. Neurosci.* 21, 6862–6873. doi: 10.1523/JNEUROSCI.21-17-06862.2001

Salichon, N., Gaspar, P., Upton, A. L., Picaud, S., Hanoun, N., Hamon, M., et al. (2001). Excessive activation of serotonin (5-HT) 1B receptors disrupts the formation of sensory maps in monoamine oxidase A and 5-HT transporter knock-out mice. *J. Neurosci.* 21, 884–896. doi: 10.1523/JNEUROSCI.21-03-00884.2001

Sholl, D. A. (1953). Dendnitic organization in the neurons of the visual and motor cortices of the cat. *J. Anat.* 87, 387–406. doi: 10.1038/171387a0

Siemann, J. K., Muller, C. L., Forsberg, C. G., Blakely, R. D., Veenstra-VanderWeele, J., and Wallace, M. T. (2017). An autism-associated serotonin transporter variant disrupts multisensory processing. *Transl. Psychiatry* 7:e1067. doi: 10.1038/tp.2017.17

Simpson, K. J., Weaver, K. J., de Villers-Sidani, E., Lu, J. Y. F., Cai, Z., Pang, Y., et al. (2011). Perinatal antidepressant exposure alters cortical network function in rodents. *Proc. Natl. Acad. Sci. U.S.A.* 108, 18465–18470.

Spacek, J., and Harris, K. M. (1998). Three-dimensional organization of cell adhesion junctions at synapses and dendritic spines in area CA1 of the rat hippocampus. *J. Comp. Neurol.* 393, 58–68.

Spruston, N. (2008). Pyramidal neurons: dendritic structure and synaptic integration. *Nat. Rev. Neurosci.* 9, 206–221. doi: 10.1038/nrn2286

Stiebler, I., Neulist, R., Fichtel, I., and Ehret, G. (1997). The auditory cortex of the house mouse: left-right differences, tonotopic organization and quantitative analysis of frequency representation. *J. Compar. Physiol. A* 181, 559–571.

Tang, J., and Suga, N. (2009). Corticocortical interactions between and within three cortical auditory areas specialized for time-domain signal processing. *J. Neurosci.* 29, 7230–7237.

Tang, J., Xiao, Z. J., and Shen, J. X. (2008). Delayed inhibition creates amplitude tuning of mouse inferior collicular neurons. *Neuroreport* 19, 1445–1449.

Tang, J., Yang, W., and Suga, N. (2012). Modulation of thalamic auditory neurons by the primary auditory cortex. *J. Neurophysiol.* 108, 935–942.

Uhlhaas, P. J., and Singer, W. (2010). Abnormal neural oscillations and synchrony in schizophrenia. *Nat. Rev. Neurosci.* 11, 100–113.

Umbricht, D., Vyssotki, D., Latanov, A., Nitsch, R., and Lipp, H. P. (2005). Deviance-related electrophysiological activity in mice: is there mismatch negativity in mice? *Clin. Neurophysiol.* 116, 353–363.

Wellman, C. L., Izquierdo, A., Garrett, J. E., Martin, K. P., Carroll, J., Millstein, R., et al. (2007). Impaired stress-coping and fear extinction and abnormal corticolimbic morphology in serotonin transporter knock-out mice. *J. Neurosci.* 27, 684–691.

Yizhar, O., Fenno, L. E., Prigge, M., Schneider, F., Davidson, T. J., O'Shea, D. J., et al. (2011). Neocortical excitation/inhibition balance in information processing and social dysfunction. *Nature* 477, 171–178.

Yuste, R., and Denk, W. (1995). Dendritic spines as basic units of synaptic integration. *Nature* 375, 682–684. doi: 10.1038/375682a0

Zhang, L., Wang, B., Zhang, L., Wang, J., Zhang, M., Cui, M., et al. (2009). A modified Golgi-Cox staining method for study the structure and morphology of neurons in the striatum. *Chin. J. Neuroanat.* 25, 343–347.

Zhang, L. I., Bao, S., and Merzenich, M. M. (2001). Persistent and specific influences of early acoustic environments on primary auditory cortex. *Nat. Neurosci.* 4, 1123–1130. doi: 10.1038/nn745

Zoghbi, H. Y. (2003). Postnatal neurodevelopmental disorders: meeting at the synapse? *Science* 302, 826–830. doi: 10.1126/science.1089071

4

Acute Recreational Noise-Induced Cochlear Synaptic Dysfunction in Humans with Normal Hearing

Qixuan Wang[1,2,3†], Lu Yang[1,4†], Minfei Qian[1,2,3†], Yingying Hong[1,4], Xueling Wang[1,2,3,5], Zhiwu Huang[1,2,3,4] and Hao Wu[1,2,3*]*

Department of Otolaryngology-Head and Neck Surgery, Ninth People's Hospital, Shanghai Jiao Tong University School of Medicine, Shanghai, China, [2] Ear Institute, Shanghai Jiao Tong University School of Medicine, Shanghai, China, Shanghai Key Laboratory of Translational Medicine on Ear and Nose Diseases, Shanghai, China, [4] Hearing and Speech Center, Ninth People's Hospital, Shanghai Jiao Tong University School of Medicine, Shanghai, China, [5] Biobank, Ninth People's Hospital, Shanghai Jiao Tong University School of Medicine, Shanghai, China

***Correspondence:**
Zhiwu Huang
huangzw86@126.com
Hao Wu
wuhao@shsmu.edu.cn

†These authors have contributed equally to this work and share first authorship

Objectives: The objective of the study was to identify the acute high-intensity recreational noise-induced effects on auditory function, especially the cochlear synaptopathy-related audiological metrics, in humans with normal hearing.

Methods: This prospective cohort study enrolled 32 young adults (14 males and 18 females); the mean age was 24.1 ± 2.4 years (ranging from 20 to 29). All participants with normal hearing (audiometric thresholds ≤25 dB HL at frequencies of 0.25, 0.5, 1, 2, 3, 4, 6, and 8 kHz for both ears) had already decided to participate in the outdoor music festival. Participants were asked to measure the noise exposure dose and complete auditory examinations, including the air-conduction pure-tone audiometry (PTA), distortion product otoacoustic emission (DPOAE), contralateral suppression (CS) on transient evoked otoacoustic emission (TEOAE), auditory brainstem response (ABR) test and Mandarin Hearing in Noise Test (MHINT), at baseline and 1 day and 14 days after music festival noise exposure.

Results: The mean time of attending the music festival was 7.34 ± 0.63 h (ranging from 6.4 to 9.5), the mean time-weighted average (TWA) of noise exposure dose was 93.2 ± 2.39 dB(A) (ranging from 87.9 to 97.7). At neither 1 day nor 14 days post exposure, there were no statistically significant effects on PTA thresholds, DPOAE amplitudes, CS on TEOAEs, or MHINT signal-to-noise ratios (SNRs) of acute outdoor music festival noise exposure, regardless of sex. While the ABR wave I amplitudes significantly decreased at 1 day after exposure and recovered at 14 days after exposure, the exposed/unexposed ABR wave I amplitude ratio was significantly correlated with MHINT SNR change at 1 day after exposure, although it was not correlated with the noise exposure dose.

Conclusion: In young adults with normal hearing, we found the self-compared decrement of ABR wave I amplitudes at 1 day post acute recreational noise exposure at high intensity, which also contributes to the change in speech perceptual ability in noisy backgrounds. This study indicated that auditory electrophysiological metric changes might be a more sensitive and efficient indicator of noise-induced cochlear synaptic dysfunction in humans. More attention should be paid to the recreational noise-induced cochlear synaptopathy and auditory perceptual disorder.

Keywords: noise-induced hearing loss, acute recreational noise exposure, hidden hearing loss, cochlear synaptopathy, auditory brainstem response, speech recognition in noise

INTRODUCTION

According to the United States Centers for Disease Control and Prevention, 14% of adults aged 20–69 years have hearing loss (Hoffman et al., 2017). Noise exposure is the most common environmental factor causing hearing loss in adults; noise-induced hearing loss (NIHL) may occur even due to daily noise exposure, such as loud music at concerts (Eichwald et al., 2018), portable media players and earphones (le Clercq et al., 2018), and public transport (Yao et al., 2017). There have been many concerns about the trend of increasing incidence of NIHL since noise exposure is unexpectedly pervasive in modern life, especially in younger populations (Murphy et al., 2018).

A recent mouse study demonstrated that even moderate noise exposure that induces a "temporary" hearing threshold shift (TTS) could result in permanent loss of ribbon synapses accompanied with abnormal suprathreshold auditory brainstem response (ABR), which was known as the cochlear synaptopathy (Kujawa and Liberman, 2009). Several studies further indicated that the cochlear synaptopathy might be the primary cause of hearing difficulties in individuals with normal hearing thresholds, which has been referred to as "hidden hearing loss" (HHL) (Kujawa and Liberman, 2009; Mehraei et al., 2016; Lobarinas et al., 2017). Recent surveys reported that approximately 12–15% of the population with normal hearing thresholds might have the HHL (Kohrman et al., 2020), which also contribute to tinnitus (Schaette and McAlpine, 2011; Gu et al., 2012) and age-related hearing loss (Sergeyenko et al., 2013; Fernandez et al., 2015; Liberman et al., 2015). However, it remains unknown whether daily loud recreational noise exposure could induce the irreversible HHL. Although many studies have made efforts in the identification of the noise-induced HHL-related auditory function changes in humans, this topic remains controversial, mainly due to the difficulty in controlling of the noise exposure and self-comparison data before and after noise exposure.

Most noise-induced HHL studies are based on retrospective design, and conclusions of which are inconsistent. A number of studies have suggested that individuals with experiences of loud noise exposure have greater difficulties in complex listening tasks under noisy background environments (Liberman et al., 2016) and decreased suprathreshold stimulating peak I amplitudes of ABR and electrocochleogram (Stamper and Johnson, 2015; Liberman et al., 2016), despite the normal audiological thresholds. In contrast, some studies failed to associate the noise exposure experience with audiological electrophysiology or perception measures in humans (Prendergast et al., 2017a,b).

To date, there are still very few prospective studies on recreational noise-induced HHL. The only self-comparison evidence from 26 young adults with normal hearing found no permanent auditory function changes after the recreational noise exposure, suggesting little risk of HHL (Grinn et al., 2017). However, in that study, recreational events included movie, bar music, concert, and dance at noise exposure level of mean 92.7 ± 7.7 dB(A) (ranging from 73.1 to 104.2) for 3.3 ± 0.9 h (ranging 1.5–4.5 h). It is still unknown whether louder recreational events would cause the cochlear synaptopathy or HHL in consistent with animal studies.

Outdoor music festivals, which include multiple concerts and often last for several hours, have recently become increasingly popular and should be a considerable source of recreational noise exposure. A recent study including 51 young adults observed the TTS after an outdoor music festival lasting 4.5 h at approximately 100 dB(A) noise exposure (Kraaijenga et al., 2018). Here, we conducted a prospective cohort study including 32 normal-hearing young adults who participated in the outdoor music festival with personal sound level measurements, in order to identify whether the acute recreational noise exposure at high intensity would contribute to cochlear synaptopathy or auditory perceptual disorder.

MATERIALS AND METHODS

Subjects

We recruited volunteers from young adults who had already decided to participate in the outdoor music festival in eastern China. There were 47 healthy participants aged 20–29 years initially recruited, and 32 (14 males and 18 females, sex was self-reported) with normal hearing were included based on the following criteria: (1) no family history of hearing loss, no history of otological injuries or diseases, no history of occupational noise exposure, and no history of outdoor music festival noise exposure within 2 months before participation in this study; (2) both ears show normal external ear canal and tympanic membrane with otoscope, type A tympanogram with 226 Hz probe tone, and air-conduction pure tone audiometric thresholds ≤25 dB HL at frequencies of 0.25, 0.5, 1, 2, 3, 4, 6, and 8 kHz; and (3) have enough language ability for the mandarin Chinese speech recognition test.

Procedure

Subjects were requested to complete the basic information collection (including age, previous visits of music festival/concert/night club, earphone use, and self-reported hearing difficulty) and baseline auditory function examinations within 1 week before participation in the outdoor music festival.

Participants with self-reported tinnitus were asked to complete the mandarin Tinnitus Handicap Inventory (THI) (Meng et al., 2012). The noise exposure dose during the festival was measured for each subject. Follow-up auditory function examinations were performed at 1 day post exposure (follow-up 1) and 14 days post exposure (follow-up 2) of the outdoor music festival. The noise exposure dose received by each subject during the outdoor music festival was measured using a personal sound exposure meter (ASV 5910 type, Hangzhou Aihua, China). Subjects were requested to wear the instrument on their shoulders (near the auricle level), and the duration of festival visits, time-weighted average (TWA), and the C-weighted peak level (L_{Cpeak}) of the noise exposure from the beginning to the end of attendance of the music festival were recorded.

Figure 1 shows the flowchart of this cohort study. All protocols and procedures were approved by the ethics committee of the Ninth People's Hospital affiliated with Shanghai Jiao Tong University School of Medicine. All participants signed written informed consent forms and were informed that participation can be withdrawn at any time. Subjects were offered a 600 (China Yuan) stipend after completion of the study.

Auditory Function Examinations

Auditory function examinations at unexposed baseline and follow-up included the air-conduction pure-tone audiometry (PTA), distortion product otoacoustic emissions (DPOAEs), and contralateral suppression (CS) on transient evoked otoacoustic emissions (TEOAEs), the ABR test and the Mandarin Hearing in Noise Test (MHINT), which were performed by certified audiological technicians in a soundproof and electromagnetic shielding booth [background noise level <25 dB(A)].

Pure-tone audiometry at frequencies of 0.25, 0.5, 1, 2, 3, 4, 6, and 8 kHz in both ears was performed using an audiometer (Madsen Astera, GN Otometrics, Denmark) with inserted earphones in accordance with the regulations of ISO 8253-1:2010.

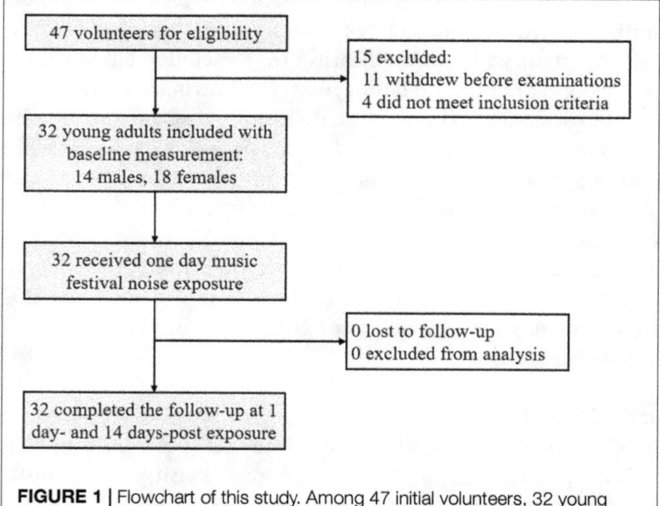

FIGURE 1 | Flowchart of this study. Among 47 initial volunteers, 32 young participants with normal hearing were enrolled and completed this two-stage follow-up study.

Distortion product otoacoustic emission tests were performed using a cochlear emission analyzer (Capella, GN Otometrics, Denmark), which were considered valid when the emission amplitude exceeded the noise by at least 3 dB. DPOAEs were elicited by two tones [L_1 = 65 dB sound pressure level (SPL), L_2 = 55 dB SPL]; the determined f_2/f_1 ratio was equal to 1.22, and the $2f_1–f_2$ cubic distortion product (DP1) component for each pair of stimuli was recorded at frequencies of 1, 2, 3, 4, 6, and 8 kHz. The probe fitting check and the two-tone adjustments were performed before each measurement session.

Contralateral suppression on TEOAEs is a reliable measure to monitor the medial olivocochlear (MOC) efferent reflex status over time (Stuart and Cobb, 2015). In this study, TEOAEs were evoked with 60 dB peak equivalent SPL (peSPL) linear click stimuli at a rate of 19.3/s with and without a contralateral 50 dB SL white noise suppressor (delivered by the audiometer and insert earphone) without probe removal. The intensity of this suppressor stimulus was well below the threshold of the stapedial muscle reflex for all the subjects. Responses were averaged to 2,080 sweeps, and the stimulus stability was at least 90%. Suppression was calculated by subtracting the TEOAE amplitude with contralateral stimulation from those without contralateral stimulation. The frequency bands measured were centered at frequencies of 1, 2, 3, 4, and 5 kHz, and all frequencies were averaged.

Auditory brainstem response tests were performed using SmartEP (Intellegent Hearing System, United States). The recording electrode was placed on the high forehead, the reference electrode was placed on the mastoid, and the grounding electrode was placed on the low forehead. Electrode impedance was less than 5 kΩ. Stimuli were presented using 100-μs clicks at 90 dB normal hearing level (nHL) with alternating polarity at a rate of 11.1/s via insert earphones (ER-3C, Etymotic Research, United States). Waveforms were collected, passed through a bandpass filter from 100 to 3,000 Hz, and averaged across 1,024 stimulus presentations. Two replications of each waveform were obtained, and the peak amplitude of wave I was calculated according to a previous study (Stamper and Johnson, 2015).

We used MHINT (Wong et al., 2007) consisting of 12 lists, each containing 20 sentences, and each sentence contained 10 Chinese characters. The BLIMP software (version 1.3, House Ear Institute, United States) was used to present the sentences at various signal-to-noise ratio (SNR) controls via a personal computer and headphones (HD200, Sennheiser, Germany). The test followed an adaptive procedure as previously described (Zhang et al., 2010). During the test, the ipsilateral white noise level was fixed at 65 dB(A), and the first sentence was presented at 0 dB SNR; the conventional rule required that the entire sentence be repeated accurately. SNR was finally calculated at the presentation level necessary for a listener to recognize the sentence materials correctly 50% of the time.

Statistical Analysis

Data analysis was performed using IBM SPSS software (version 24.0, SPSS Inc., United States) and Prism (version 8.0, GraphPad Software, United States). Continuous variables are presented as the mean ± SD, and categorical variables are presented as percentages [n (%)]. The normality of continuous variables was assessed by the Kolmogorov–Smirnov test. Characteristics, MHINT SNRs and ABR wave I amplitudes at baseline between males and females were compared using unpaired t-tests or χ^2 tests. Differences in PTA thresholds, DPOAE amplitudes, and CS on TEOAEs between males and females were analyzed using the two-way repeated measures ANOVA with sexes and frequencies as dependent variables. Differences in PTA thresholds, DPOAE amplitudes, and CS on TEOAEs between the baseline, follow-up 1, and follow-up 2 groups were analyzed using the two-way repeated measures ANOVA with noise exposure and frequencies as dependent variables. MHINT SNRs and ABR wave I amplitudes between baseline, follow-up 1, and follow-up 2 groups were analyzed using the two-way repeated measures ANOVA with noise exposure and sexes as dependent variables. Pearson correlation analysis was used to screen the significant association between the TWA and auditory function changes; then correlations of the TWA, exposed/unexposed ABR wave I amplitudes ratio, and MHINT SNR changes were determined using linear regression analysis. A two-tailed $P < 0.05$ was considered statistically significant.

RESULTS

Characteristics of Subjects

A total of 32 participants aged 20–29 years [14 males (43.8%), 18 females (56.2%), mean age: 24.1 ± 2.4 years] who completed this study were included in the analyses. The distributions of characteristics at baseline (age, previous visits of music festival/concert/night club, earphone use, and self-reported hearing difficulty) and during the outdoor music festival (duration of festival visit and TWA of noise exposure) were not significantly different between males and females, while the mean L_{Cpeak} of females was slightly higher than that of males (shown in **Table 1**). We noticed that nine participants (three males and six females) experienced at least one self-reported tinnitus, but none of them was indeed troubled from tinnitus according to THI scores. Among all the participants, the mean duration of festival visits was 7.34 ± 0.63 h (ranging from 6.4 to 9.5), the mean TWA was 93.2 ± 2.39 dB(A) (ranging from 87.9 to 97.7), and the mean L_{Cpeak} was 135.4 ± 4.1 dB (ranging from 129.9 to 139.6). None of the participants used hearing protective devices such as earplugs during the festival visit.

Although all the participants showed normal hearing at baseline with PTA thresholds ≤25 dB HL, females showed a lower PTA threshold at a 1-kHz frequency for both the left ear (**Figure 2A**, $P = 0.003$) and the right ear (**Figure 2B**, $P = 0.021$) and a higher DPOAE DP1 amplitude at a 2-kHz frequency for the left ear (**Figure 2D**, $P = 0.011$) than males. We did not observe significant differences in DPOAE DP1 amplitudes for the right ear ($P = 0.058$), CS on TEOAEs (see **Table 2**) for both left ($P = 0.841$) and right ($P = 0.608$) ears, MHINT SNRs (see **Figure 2E**) for both left ($P = 0.999$) and right ($P = 0.916$) ears, or ABR wave I peak amplitudes (see **Figure 2F**) for both left ($P = 0.999$) and right ($P = 0.197$) ears between males and females.

TABLE 1 | Participant characteristics at baseline and during the music festival.

Characteristics	Males (n = 14)	Females (n = 18)	t/χ^2	P
Age, mean (SD)	25 (2.9)	23 (1.7)	1.888	0.069
Previous visits to music festivals/concerts/nightclubs			4.092	0.129
≤once/year, n (%)	5 (35.7)	2 (11.1)		
≥2 times/year, n (%)	7 (50)	15 (83.3)		
≥2 times/month, n (%)	2 (14.3)	1 (5.6)		
Tinnitus history			0.552	0.759
Almost never, n (%)	11 (78.6)	12 (66.7)		
Yes, spontaneously, n (%)	2 (14.3)	4 (22.2)		
Yes, after exposure to noise, n (%)	1 (7.1)	2 (11.1)		
Previous use of personal earphones			1.169	0.557
Almost never, n (%)	2 (14.3)	5 (27.8)		
0–2 h/day, n (%)	8 (57.1)	10 (55.6)		
2–5 h/day, n (%)	4 (28.6)	3 (16.7)		
Previous use of earplugs			0.803	0.370
Almost never, n (%)	14 (100)	17 (94.4)		
Yes, n (%)	0 (0)	1 (5.6)		
Self-reported hearing difficulty			3.418	0.181
Almost never, n (%)	5 (35.7)	2 (11.1)		
Yes, only amid noise, n (%)	6 (42.9)	13 (72.2)		
Yes, in daily life, n (%)	3 (21.3)	3 (16.7)		
During festival				
Duration of visit, mean (SD), hours	7.2 (0.9)	7.4 (0.4)	−0.750	0.463
TWA, mean (SD), dB(A)	93.8 (1.6)	93.4 (1.8)	0.769	0.448
L_{Cpeak}, mean (SD), dB	136.7 (4.0)	133.8 (3.7)	−2.074	0.047

SD, standard deviation; TWA, time-weighted average. There were no statistically significant differences in most characteristics except for the L_{Cpeak} between male and female participants. Analyses were performed by the unpaired t-test or χ^2 test.

Auditory Function Changes Caused by Outdoor Music Festivals

Overall, in this study, PTA thresholds (total: $P = 0.699$ for left ear, $P = 0.591$ for right ear; males: $P = 0.775$ for left ear, $P = 0.509$ for right ear; females: $P = 0.816$ for left ear, $P = 0.931$ for right ear; see **Figure 3**), DPOAE DP1 amplitudes (total: $P = 0.955$ for left ear, $P = 0.997$ for right ear; males: $P = 0.947$ for left ear, $P = 0.984$ for right ear; females: $P = 0.974$ for left ear, $P = 0.997$ for right ear; see **Figure 4**), CS on TEOAEs (total: $P = 0.936$ for left ear, $P = 0.560$ for right ear; males: $P = 0.248$ for left ear, $P = 0.161$ for right ear; females: $P = 0.333$ for left ear, $P = 0.576$ for right ear; see **Table 2**), and MHINT SNRs (total: $P = 0.999$ for left ear, $P = 0.999$ for right ear; males: $P = 0.999$ for left ear, $P = 0.583$ for right ear; females: $P = 0.859$ for left ear, $P = 0.598$ for right ear; see **Figure 5**) at 1 day or 14 days after the outdoor music festival noise exposure were comparable with those at unexposed baseline for both ears, despite sex.

Notably, we observed that the peak amplitudes of ABR wave I significantly decreased at 1 day after exposure (**Figure 6A** for left ear, **Figure 6B** for right ear), with a recovery at 14 days after exposure among all the participants (both

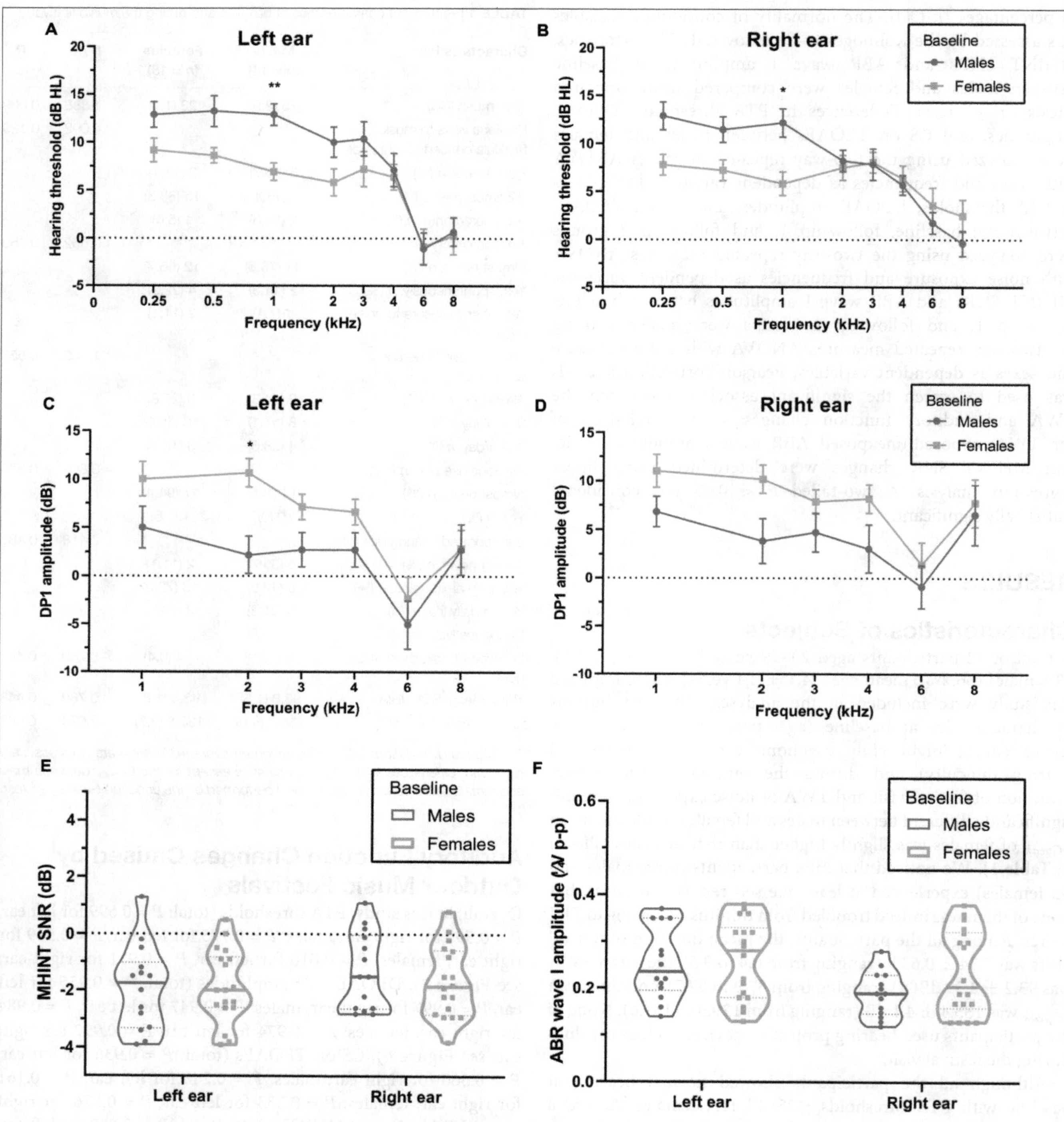

FIGURE 2 | Comparison of auditory function between males and females at baseline. Females (pink) show a lower pure-tone audiometry (PTA) threshold at a 1 kHz frequency than males (blue) for the left ear **(A)** and the right ear **(B)**. Females show higher distortion product otoacoustic emission (DPOAE) amplitudes at a 1 kHz frequency than males for the left ear **(C)** but not the right ear **(D)**, analyses were performed by the two-way repeated measures ANOVA. There were no statistically significant differences in signal-to-noise ratios (SNRs) of Mandarin Hearing in Noise Test (MHINT) **(E)** and auditory brainstem response (ABR) wave I amplitudes **(F)** between males and females for either ear, analyses were performed by the unpaired *t*-test. **P* < 0.05, ***P* < 0.01.

P-values < 0.001). For females, the peak amplitudes at 1 day after exposure were significantly lower than baseline for both the left ear (*P* < 0.001) and the right ear (*P* = 0.008). For males, the decrement of peak amplitudes 1 day after exposure was significantly different from baseline only for the left ear (*P* = 0.002) but not the right ear

TABLE 2 | Effects of noise exposure on contralateral suppression (CS) on transient evoked otoacoustic emissions (TEOAEs).

CS on TEOAEs (dB)	Males (n = 14)						Females (n = 18)					
	Left ear			Right ear			Left ear			Right ear		
	Before	1 day post	14 days post	Before	1 day post	14 days post	Before	1 day post	14 days post	Before	1 day post	14 days post
1 kHz	1.10 (3.22)	1.84 (2.26)	1.11 (3.41)	2.09 (1.99)	2.22 (2.27)	2.31 (2.54)	2.43 (2.36)	1.35 (2.79)	2.06 (2.66)	2.82 (2.74)	2.00 (2.29)	2.38 (2.19)
2 kHz	1.21 (3.22)	1.33 (2.76)	1.68 (2.97)	1.41 (2.28)	1.52 (1.57)	2.15 (2.43)	2.57 (2.75)	1.85 (2.16)	2.03 (2.87)	2.99 (3.14)	2.37 (2.26)	2.67 (3.04)
3 kHz	1.86 (2.33)	1.34 (1.74)	1.14 (2.58)	1.40 (2.49)	1.24 (3.28)	1.11 (1.98)	1.68 (3.02)	0.73 (1.79)	1.57 (1.77)	2.26 (2.55)	2.24 (2.48)	2.68 (2.10)
4 kHz	1.21 (2.56)	1.64 (2.81)	1.19 (2.14)	1.01 (2.15)	1.11 (1.76)	1.85 (1.65)	1.73 (1.33)	1.10 (1.70)	1.43 (1.45)	1.38 (2.16)	1.13 (1.81)	1.24 (1.53)
5 kHz	1.15 (2.18)	0.87 (1.73)	1.04 (1.99)	0.54 (1.29)	1.00 (1.71)	0.14 (1.6)	0.64 (2.16)	0.74 (1.86)	0.85 (2.05)	1.11 (2.81)	0.80 (2.78)	1.47 (1.85)
All	1.99 (2.31)	1.91 (1.69)	1.63 (2.69)	1.86 (1.82)	1.91 (0.95)	2.05 (1.49)	2.16 (1.97)	1.34 (1.79)	2.24 (1.86)	2.45 (2.49)	1.82 (1.95)	2.77 (1.65)

There are no statistically significant differences in CS on TEOAEs over 1–5 kHz frequencies and average value between males and females at baseline (before noise exposure) for the left ear (P = 0.841) and right ear (P = 0.608). There are no statistically significant differences in CS on TEOAEs over 1–5 kHz frequencies and average value of males (P = 0.248 for left ear, P = 0.161 for right ear) or females (P = 0.333 for left ear, P = 0.576 for left ear) between the baseline, 1 day and 14 days post the outdoor music festival noise exposure. Analyses were performed by the two-way repeated measures ANOVA.

(P = 0.055). The mean ABR waveforms are shown in **Supplementary Figure 1**.

Relationship Between Noise Exposure Dose and Auditory Function

To further explore the association between the acute outdoor music festival noise exposure dose and auditory function changes, we performed Pearson correlation analysis but did not observe any statistically significant correlation (see **Supplementary Figure 2**). However, only the normalized exposed/unexposed ABR wave I amplitude changes (ratio of amplitude at 1 day post exposure to amplitude at baseline) seems to show a decreasing tendency with higher noise exposure doses for both ears (**Figure 7A** for the left ear, P = 0.14; **Figure 7B** for the right ear, P = 0.35). Correlation analyses were also performed to explore the relationship between several auditory function changes in this study. We found that the exposed/unexposed ABR wave I amplitude ratio was significantly associated with MHINT SNR changes at 1 day after the outdoor music festival noise exposure (see **Figure 7C** for the left ear, P = 0.010; **Figure 7D** for the right ear, P = 0.021), although it was not significantly correlated with the noise exposure dose (see **Figure 7E** for the left ear, P = 0.92; **Figure 7F** for the right ear, P = 0.75).

DISCUSSION

In this study, to identify whether acute high-level recreational noise exposure would induce HHL or other audiological impairments in humans, we followed up on the temporary and sustained changes in auditory function in 32 normal-hearing young adults who attended the outdoor music festival. To our knowledge, this is the first prospective cohort study that identified that the auditory electrophysiological indicator of suprathreshold stimulating ABR wave I amplitude decreased transiently with subsequent recovery after acute loud recreational noise exposure, without other significant auditory functional changes in humans. In addition, we found that the ABR wave I amplitude changed in relation to speech recognition ability in noisy environments after noise exposure, although the correlations between auditory function changes and noise exposure dose were not significant.

In consideration of the sex differences in auditory characteristics and susceptibility to NIHL (Wang et al., 2021), we compared auditory function between males and females at baseline. Generally, consistent with previous studies (Delhez et al., 2020), females showed a slightly better PTA threshold and DPOAE amplitude (see **Figure 2**) than males at baseline, which would not affect the efficiency of conclusion in this study, since we analyzed the auditory function changes not only in participants overall but also in males and females separately.

Acute Recreational Noise-Induced Auditory Effects Depend on Exposure Doses

Numerous recent studies have indicated that long-term exposure to high-intensity recreational and professional music potentially increases the risk of hearing loss (Schink et al., 2014; Pouryaghoub et al., 2017; le Clercq et al., 2018). Several previous studies that had well-quantified exposure doses demonstrated that short-term music exposure at high intensity has the potential to induce a TTS. According to a randomized clinical trial in Amsterdam to assess the effectiveness of earplugs in preventing TTSs following music exposure, 22 of 52 ears (42%) among the normal-hearing adult volunteers who experienced unprotected outdoor music exposure [TWA approximately 100 dB(A) during the festival] showed a TTS over frequencies of 3 and 4 kHz and a significant decrement in DPOAE amplitude over frequencies of 2–8 kHz (Ramakers et al., 2016). Le Prell et al. (2012) described the effects of carefully controlled 4-h digital audio player use for three different music listening levels [at 93–95, 98–100, and 100–102 dB(A)] on audiometric threshold changes of 33 normal-hearing young adult college students. The largest TTS

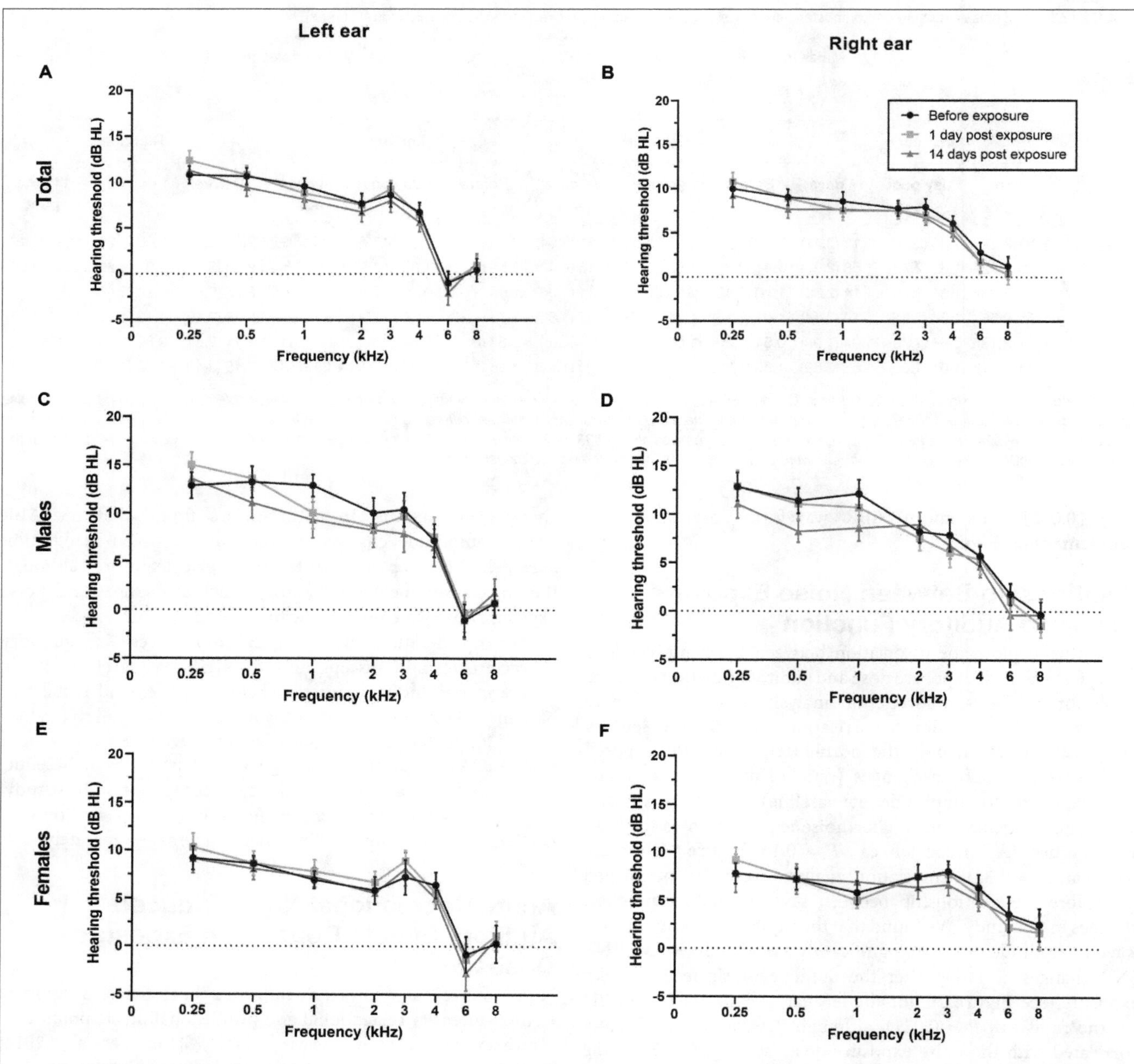

FIGURE 3 | Effects of noise exposure on PTA. There were no statistically significant differences in the PTA hearing thresholds of either ear at frequencies of 0.25–8 kHz in the overall sample **(A,B)**, in males specifically **(C,D)**, or in females specifically **(E,F)** among baseline (black), 1 day after outdoor music festival noise exposure (orange) and 14 days (blue) after exposure. Analyses were performed by the two-way repeated measures ANOVA.

was observed at a 4-kHz frequency (averaged 6.3 ± 3.9 dB, ranging from 0 to 13 dB) 15 min after higher levels of sound exposure, which almost recovered completely within the first 4 h after exposure. In contrast, in another study on young participants with a normal hearing threshold, there were no statistically significant correlations between noise exposure and changes in audiometric threshold or DPOAE amplitude either the day after the loud event [based on noise exposure level of 92.7 ± 7.7 dB(A), range 73.1−104.2 dB(A) for 3.3 ± 0.9 h (range 1.5−4.5 h)] or 1 week later (Grinn et al., 2017).

In our study, the sound exposure dose during the outdoor music festival was measured for each individual, and the dose of TWA was averaged 93.2 ± 2.39 dB(A), ranging from 87.9 to 97.7 dB(A). Our results of TWA were comparable with the noise exposure measurements at a Norwegian outdoor music festival (Tronstad and Gelderblom, 2016) and outdistanced the limit dose of daily noise exposure in most countries and the World Health Organization's recommendations (Neitzel and Fligor, 2019). Since the effect on auditory function are associated with the duration and intensity of sound exposure (Peng et al., 2007;

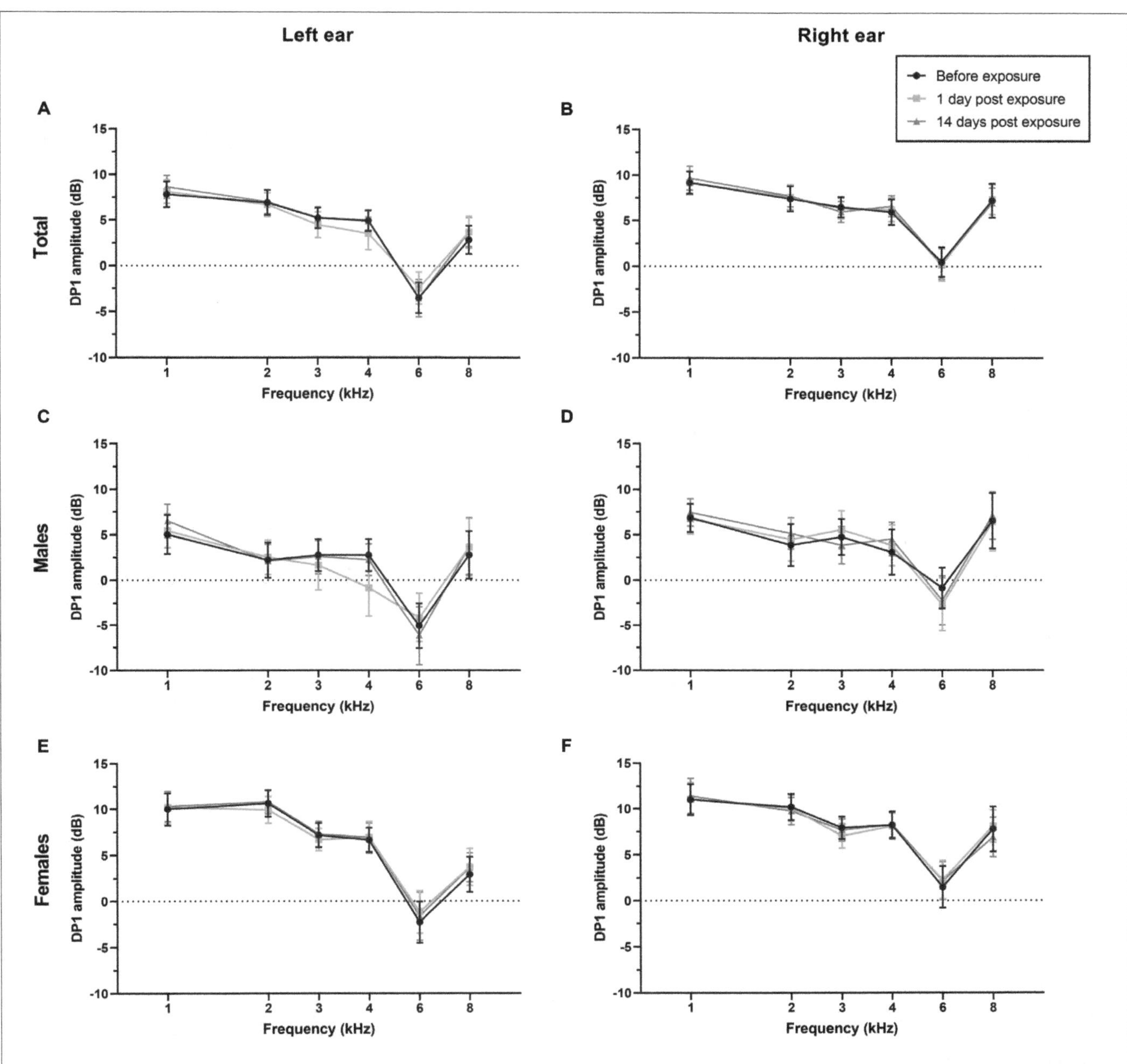

FIGURE 4 | Effects of noise exposure on DPOAE. There were no statistically significant differences in the DPOAE amplitudes of either ear at frequencies of 1–8 kHz in the overall sample **(A,B)**, in males specifically **(C,D)**, or in females specifically **(E,F)** among baseline (black), 1 day after outdoor music festival noise exposure (orange) and 14 days (blue) after exposure. Analyses were performed by the two-way repeated measures ANOVA.

Le Prell et al., 2012), in this study, we did not detect any audiometric TTS, DPOAE amplitude decrement (a reflection of hair cell function), or alteration in MOC efferent nerve function or speech recognition ability amid noise for either males or females after outdoor festival noise exposure (see **Figures 3–5** and **Table 2**). The only significant changes were the reversible decrement of ABR wave I amplitude at 1 day after exposure (see **Figure 6**).

The inconsistent effects on auditory function among studies with quantified exposure doses are probably due to the following reasons: (1) the different timepoints after noise exposure to follow-up auditory examinations, as Le Prell et al. (2012) showed that most TTSs recovered within 4 h after exposure; (2) the different doses of acute noise exposure between studies, since TTSs were detected in studies with higher noise exposure doses [approximately 100 dB(A) TWA] (Ramakers et al., 2016) but not with approximately 90 dB(A) TWA exposure (Grinn et al., 2017); (3) these data also provided important insight into the high variability across individuals in vulnerability to TTSs after music exposure. Thus, it is necessary to conduct more prospective

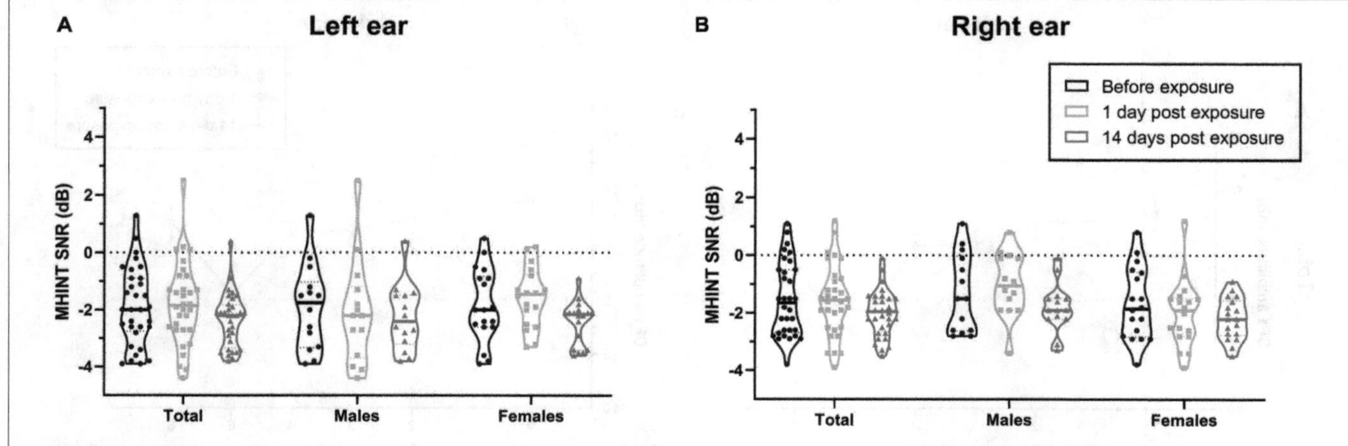

FIGURE 5 | Effects of noise exposure on MHINT. There were no statistically significant differences in the SNRs of MHINT in the overall sample, in males specifically, or in females specifically among baseline (black), 1 day after outdoor music festival noise exposure (orange) and 14 days (blue) after exposure for the left ear **(A)** or the right ear **(B)**. Analyses were performed by the two-way repeated measures ANOVA.

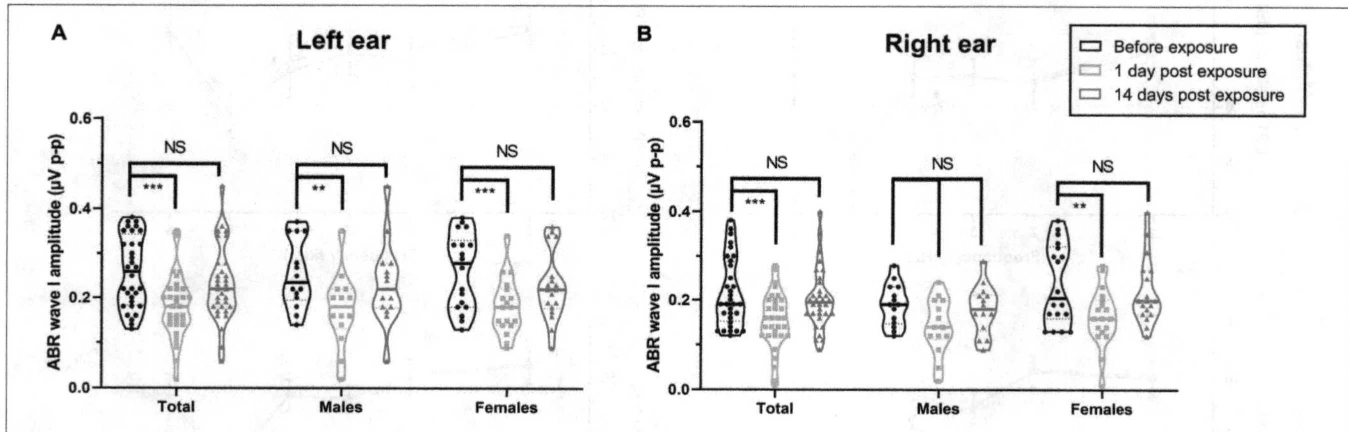

FIGURE 6 | Effects of noise exposure on ABR wave I amplitudes. The peak amplitude of wave I significantly decreased at 1 day after outdoor music festival noise exposure (orange) and recovered to the baseline level (black) at 14 days after exposure (blue) in the left **(A)** and right **(B)** ears of total participants and of females specifically, as well as in the left ear of males, but not in the right ear of males. Analyses were performed by the two-way repeated measures ANOVA. NS, no significance. $^{**}P < 0.01$, $^{***}P < 0.001$.

studies with measurable exposure doses to determine which level of recreational noise exposure doses would induce the temporary or permanent auditory impairment.

Optimal Metrics for the Assessment of Cochlear Synaptopathy and "Hidden Hearing Loss" in Humans

Numerous recent animal studies in mice (Kujawa and Liberman, 2009), rats (Lobarinas et al., 2017), guinea pigs (Shi et al., 2016), and rhesus monkeys (Valero et al., 2017) have demonstrated that moderate noise exposure that does not induce a PTS or hair cell death could result in cochlear synaptopathy, manifested as loss of a subset of synaptic connections between inner hair cells and afferent nerves and decreased ABR wave I amplitude in response to suprathreshold stimulus (Lobarinas et al., 2017), which is widely accepted as the primary cause of HHL. In humans, direct evidence of cochlear synaptopathy is based on extraction of the temporal bones (Viana et al., 2015; Wu et al., 2019); however, noise exposure history and auditory examination data are not always available for these tissues. To date, it is still unclear whether noise-induced cochlear synaptopathy occurs in humans and whether there are optimal audiological measurements to assess cochlear synaptopathy and HHL. According to previous studies, candidate metrics include ABR, the middle-ear muscle reflex (MEMR), envelope-following responses (EFR), and extended high-frequency (EHF) audiograms (Bramhall et al., 2019).

Most human studies used the amplitudes of ABR wave I or electrocochleogram peak I to indicate cochlear synaptopathy. Some previous studies on normal-hearing young veterans (Bramhall et al., 2017) and college music students (Liberman et al., 2016) have suggested that individuals with high doses of reported noise exposure may have a reduction in ABR

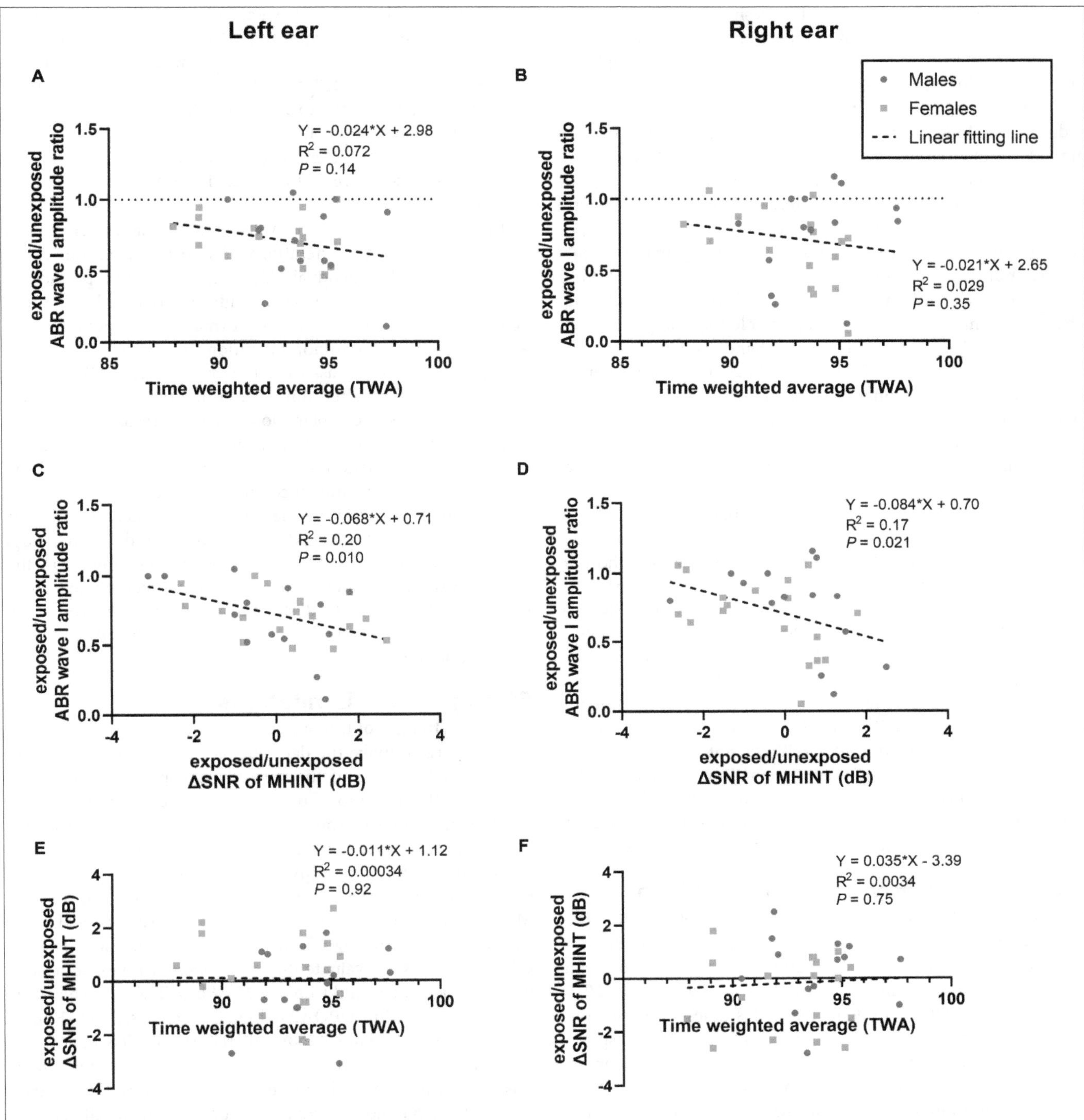

FIGURE 7 | Correlations of noise exposure, ABR wave I, and MHINT. Neither the exposed/unexposed ABR wave I amplitude ratio **(A,B)** nor the SNR changes (ΔSNR) of the MHINT **(E,F)** significantly correlated with time-weighted average (TWA) noise exposure, whereas the exposed/unexposed ABR wave I amplitude ratio significantly correlated with the ΔSNR of MHINT **(C,D)** for the left ear and right ear. Males are in blue, females are in pink, and lines of fit for the overall sample are in black.

wave I amplitude or ratio of the summating potential to the action potential; however, other recent studies did not find significant correlations between noise exposure history and electrophysiological metrics related to cochlear synaptopathy (Grinn et al., 2017; Prendergast et al., 2017a; Guest et al., 2018). Many factors may underlie the discordant conclusion of those studies, including the difficulty in quantification of self-reported lifetime noise exposure and the large individual variability of ABR wave I amplitudes in humans (Bharadwaj et al., 2019; Bramhall et al., 2019).

Benefiting from the perspective design of our study, we were able to perform a self-comparison by normalizing the post exposure ABR wave I amplitude to the baseline amplitude within each individual, as most animal studies did (Kujawa and Liberman, 2009). We were surprised to find a transient reduction in ABR wave I amplitude at 1 day after exposure with almost complete recovery at 14 days after exposure (see **Figure 6** except for the right ear of male participants), which appears to be the temporary functional alteration of cochlear synapses and AN fibers, rather than the permanent loss of synaptic connections in previous animal studies. An explanation might be that humans are more resistant to noise-induced cochlear damage than experimental animals. Cochlear synaptopathy was observed in mice, rats, and guinea pigs at levels of approximately 100, 106, and 109 dB SPL octave band exposure for 2 h (Kujawa and Liberman, 2009; Shi et al., 2016; Lobarinas et al., 2017), while rhesus monkeys were more resistant to cochlear synaptopathy than rodents (Valero et al., 2017), resulting in predictions that the human ear is quite "robust" and resistant to damage from daily noise exposure. In contrast, another perspective study did not detect electrophysiological deficits at 1 day after acute recreational noise exposure (Grinn et al., 2017). The inconsistence might be due to the lower exposure doses [92.7 ± 7.7 dB(A) for 3.3 ± 0.9 h] in their study than those in our study (TWA range 93.2 ± 2.4 dB(A) for 7.34 ± 0.63 h).

In general, our results indicated that suprathreshold ABR wave I amplitude might be a proper auditory electrophysiology metric to detect the cochlear synaptic dysfunction. However, we failed to find a significant correlation between the sound exposure doses and any temporary or sustainable auditory function changes, although the ABR wave I amplitude alteration showed a trend of correlation with TWA without statistical significance (see **Figures 7A,B**). A potential explanation was the variable susceptibility of cochlear synaptopathy among individuals, since a previous study in mice suggested that decreasing sound levels by 3 dB can eliminate synaptic injury (Fernandez et al., 2015).

The Risk of Recreational Noise-Induced Cochlear Synaptopathy and Auditory Perceptual Disorder

Noise-induced cochlear synaptopathy was expected to induce not only neural deficits but also suprathreshold speech-processing abilities, especially in noisy environments (Skoe et al., 2019; Washnik et al., 2020). Previous animal studies indicated that AN fibers with lower spontaneous rates and higher response thresholds seemed to be more vulnerable to noise damage (Furman et al., 2013; Liberman and Kujawa, 2017). Thus, speech recognition in noise tests has been used to research cochlear synaptopathy in many human studies. Liberman et al. (2016) assessed the word recognition performance of 34 normal-hearing participants aged 18–41 years and found that participants with high risk of noise damage performed more poorly in the presence of ipsilateral noise. In contrast, a number of recent studies failed to reveal the significant association between noise exposure and auditory behavioral function in humans. A study including 138 normal-hearing participants aged 18–36 years reported little relation between lifetime noise exposure and a series of perceptual behavioral measures (Prendergast et al., 2017b). Several other studies reported no relation between noise exposure, ABR wave I amplitude, and speech recognition in noise in humans with clinically normal hearing (Grinn et al., 2017; Yeend et al., 2017; Guest et al., 2018). However, it is necessary to note that the different procedures of speech-in-noise tests used in various studies might have different degrees of listening task difficulty, which makes it complicated to compare performances in speech perception from one study to another.

In our study, we used the MHINT SNR changes after noise exposure to assess the alterations of speech recognition ability in noise for each individual. Although our results provide no evidence that acute noise exposure induces any speech perceptual deficit in noisy environments for normal-hearing young adults, we found that even minor alterations in speech recognition ability in noise were associated with transient ABR wave I amplitude changes after noise exposure (see **Figures 7C,D**). There might be some explanations for these results: (1) speech-in-noise performances could not directly represent the cochlear synaptic or AN function as the ABR wave I, (2) the speech-in-noise ability might be influenced by confounding central factors such as attention, working memory, and language in addition to peripheral effects (Yeend et al., 2017), and (3) the large individual variability of SNRs changes among subjects in this study. Thus, our findings indicated that the recreational noise-induced cochlear synaptic dysfunction could probably contribute to at least a bit of change in auditory perception ability in noisy background in humans.

Strengths and Limitations

The main strength of this study was that prospective design and self-comparison make the data reliable. To our knowledge, this current study is one of the very few prospective studies that focused on the recreational noise-induced cochlear synaptopathy or HHL in humans. Another strength was the well-measured noise exposure level for each participant using the individual sound dosimeter in this study, which provides the accurate noise exposure doses. Moreover, we attempted to detect the effect on MOC efferent functional changes of acute recreational noise exposure, though no significance was found. Here we chose the CS on TEOAEs to evaluate the MOC efferent reflex because of its reliability (Stuart and Cobb, 2015). Since TEOAE is biased to low frequencies while DPOAE to high frequencies, DPOAE could be a choice in future noise-induced HHL studies. There are some other limitations. We did not perform the EHF audiograms in this study, which might be more sensitive to NIHL (Mehrparvar et al., 2011). We did not exclude participants with self-reported tinnitus in this study, while attenuated wave I amplitudes have been observed in normal human listeners with tinnitus compared with non-tinnitus controls (Schaette and McAlpine, 2011; Gu et al., 2012). The extent to which tinnitus is a symptomatic manifestation of noise-induced synaptopathy remains unclear.

In general, larger sample sizes and additional candidate cochlear synaptopathy-related metrics such as the compound action potential wave AP, ABR wave V amplitudes, EHF audiograms, EFRs, MEMR, and more auditory processing tests are needed to investigate the correlations in the future.

CONCLUSION

Benefiting from the prospective design of this study, we were able to catch the transient ABR wave I amplitude decrement at 1 day post acute recreational noise exposure in normal hearing young adults. Our results indicated that the ABR wave I amplitude might be a sensitive metric to detect the noise-induced cochlear synaptopathy in humans, which also contributes to speech recognition ability in noise. Nevertheless, it should be noted that, although wave I of the ABR is the most direct non-invasive measure of cochlear synaptic and AN fidelity in humans, one of the obstacles for the use of the ABR to identify synaptopathy in humans is that wave I amplitude is highly variable across individuals. Overall, our study provides an insight into the potential recreational noise-induced cochlear synaptopathy and auditory speech perceptual difficulty in noisy backgrounds. With the increased prevalence of HHL, more attention should be paid to the prevention of recreational noise exposure-induced hearing impairment in humans.

AUTHOR CONTRIBUTIONS

QW, ZH, and HW contributed to the conception and design of the study. LY, YH, and XW organized the database. QW and MQ performed the statistical analysis. QW and LY wrote the first draft of the manuscript. MQ and XW wrote sections of the manuscript. All authors contributed to manuscript revision, read, and approved the submitted version.

ACKNOWLEDGMENTS

We thank all the participants in this study for their time and cooperation. We also thank the undergraduate student Jiejing Zhang from the Zhejiang Chinese Medical University for assistance in the noise exposure measurement.

REFERENCES

Bharadwaj, H. M., Mai, A. R., Simpson, J. M., Choi, I., Heinz, M. G., and Shinn-Cunningham, B. G. (2019). Non-invasive assays of cochlear synaptopathy - candidates and considerations. *Neuroscience* 407, 53–66. doi: 10.1016/j.neuroscience.2019.02.031

Bramhall, N., Beach, E. F., Epp, B., Le Prell, C. G., Lopez-Poveda, E. A., Plack, C. J., et al. (2019). The search for noise-induced cochlear synaptopathy in humans: mission impossible? *Hear. Res.* 377, 88–103. doi: 10.1016/j.heares.2019.02.016

Bramhall, N. F., Konrad-Martin, D., Mcmillan, G. P., and Griest, S. E. (2017). Auditory brainstem response altered in humans with noise exposure despite normal outer hair cell function. *Ear. Hear.* 38, e1–e12.

Delhez, A., Lefebvre, P., Péqueux, C., Malgrange, B., and Delacroix, L. (2020). Auditory function and dysfunction: estrogen makes a difference. *Cell Mol. Life Sci.* 77, 619–635. doi: 10.1007/s00018-019-03295-y

Eichwald, J., Scinicariello, F., Telfer, J. L., and Carroll, Y. I. (2018). Use of personal hearing protection devices at loud athletic or entertainment events among adults - United States, 2018. *MMWR Morb. Mortal. Wkly Rep.* 67, 1151–1155. doi: 10.15585/mmwr.mm6741a4

Fernandez, K. A., Jeffers, P. W. C., Lall, K., Liberman, M. C., and Kujawa, S. G. (2015). Aging after noise exposure: acceleration of cochlear synaptopathy in "Recovered". *Ears. J. Neurosci.* 35, 7509–7520. doi: 10.1523/jneurosci.5138-14.2015

Furman, A. C., Kujawa, S. G., and Liberman, M. C. (2013). Noise-induced cochlear neuropathy is selective for fibers with low spontaneous rates. *J. Neurophysiol.* 110, 577–586. doi: 10.1152/jn.00164.2013

Grinn, S. K., Wiseman, K. B., Baker, J. A., and Le Prell, C. G. (2017). Hidden hearing loss? No effect of common recreational noise exposure on cochlear nerve response amplitude in humans. *Front. Neurosci.* 11:465. doi: 10.3389/fnins.2017.00465

Gu, J. W., Herrmann, B. S., Levine, R. A., and Melcher, J. R. (2012). Brainstem auditory evoked potentials suggest a role for the ventral cochlear nucleus in tinnitus. *J. Assoc. Res. Otolaryngol.* 13, 819–833. doi: 10.1007/s10162-012-0344-1

Guest, H., Munro, K. J., Prendergast, G., Millman, R. E., and Plack, C. J. (2018). Impaired speech perception in noise with a normal audiogram: no evidence for cochlear synaptopathy and no relation to lifetime noise exposure. *Hear. Res.* 364, 142–151. doi: 10.1016/j.heares.2018.03.008

Hoffman, H. J., Dobie, R. A., Losonczy, K. G., Themann, C. L., and Flamme, G. A. (2017). Declining prevalence of hearing loss in US adults aged 20 to 69 years. *JAMA Otolaryngol. Head Neck Surg.* 143, 274–285. doi: 10.1001/jamaoto.2016.3527

Kohrman, D., Wan, G., Cassinotti, L., and Corfas, G. (2020). Hidden hearing loss: a disorder with multiple etiologies and mechanisms. *Cold Spring Harb. Perspect. Med.* 10:a035493. doi: 10.1101/cshperspect.a035493

Kraaijenga, V. J. C., Van Munster, J., and Van Zanten, G. A. (2018). Association of behavior with noise-induced hearing loss among attendees of an outdoor music festival: a secondary analysis of a randomized clinical trial. *JAMA Otolaryngol. Head Neck Surg.* 144, 490–497. doi: 10.1001/jamaoto.2018.0272

Kujawa, S. G., and Liberman, M. C. (2009). Adding insult to injury: cochlear nerve degeneration after "temporary" noise-induced hearing loss. *J. Neurosci.* 29, 14077–14085. doi: 10.1523/jneurosci.2845-09.2009

le Clercq, C. M. P., Goedegebure, A., Jaddoe, V. W. V., Raat, H., Baatenburg De Jong, R. J., and Van Der Schroeff, M. P. (2018). Association between portable music player use and hearing loss among children of school age in the netherlands. *JAMA Otolaryngol. Head Neck Surg.* 144, 668–675. doi: 10.1001/jamaoto.2018.0646

Le Prell, C. G., Dell, S., Hensley, B., Hall, J. W. III, Campbell, K. C., Antonelli, P. J., et al. (2012). Digital music exposure reliably induces temporary threshold shift in normal-hearing human subjects. *Ear. Hear.* 33, e44–e58.

Liberman, L. D., Suzuki, J., and Liberman, M. C. (2015). Dynamics of cochlear synaptopathy after acoustic overexposure. *J. Assoc. Res. Otolaryngol.* 16, 205–219. doi: 10.1007/s10162-015-0510-3

Liberman, M. C., Epstein, M. J., Cleveland, S. S., Wang, H., and Maison, S. F. (2016). Toward a differential diagnosis of hidden hearing loss in humans. *PLoS One* 11:e0162726. doi: 10.1371/journal.pone.0162726

Liberman, M. C., and Kujawa, S. G. (2017). Cochlear synaptopathy in acquired sensorineural hearing loss: manifestations and mechanisms. *Hear. Res.* 349, 138–147. doi: 10.1016/j.heares.2017.01.003

Lobarinas, E., Spankovich, C., and Le Prell, C. G. (2017). Evidence of "hidden hearing loss" following noise exposures that produce robust TTS and ABR wave-I amplitude reductions. *Hear. Res.* 349, 155–163. doi: 10.1016/j.heares.2016.12.009

Mehraei, G., Hickox, A. E., Bharadwaj, H. M., Goldberg, H., Verhulst, S., Liberman, M. C., et al. (2016). Auditory brainstem response latency in noise as a marker of cochlear synaptopathy. *J. Neurosci.* 36, 3755–3764. doi: 10.1523/jneurosci.4460-15.2016

Mehrparvar, A. H., Mirmohammadi, S. J., Ghoreyshi, A., Mollasadeghi, A., and Loukzadeh, Z. (2011). High-frequency audiometry: a means for early diagnosis of noise-induced hearing loss. *Noise Health* 13, 402–406. doi: 10.4103/1463-1741.90295

Meng, Z., Zheng, Y., Liu, S., Wang, K., Kong, X., Tao, Y., et al. (2012). Reliability and validity of the chinese (mandarin) tinnitus handicap inventory. *Clin. Exp. Otorhinolaryngol.* 5, 10–16. doi: 10.3342/ceo.2012.5.1.10

Murphy, W. J., Eichwald, J., Meinke, D. K., Chadha, S., and Iskander, J. (2018). CDC grand rounds: promoting hearing health across the lifespan. *MMWR Morb. Mortal Wkly Rep.* 67, 243–246. doi: 10.15585/mmwr.mm6708a2

Neitzel, R. L., and Fligor, B. J. (2019). Risk of noise-induced hearing loss due to recreational sound: review and recommendations. *J. Acoust. Soc. Am.* 146:3911. doi: 10.1121/1.5132287

Peng, J. H., Tao, Z. Z., and Huang, Z. W. (2007). Risk of damage to hearing from personal listening devices in young adults. *J. Otolaryngol.* 36, 181–185.

Pouryaghoub, G., Mehrdad, R., and Pourhosein, S. (2017). Noise-induced hearing loss among professional musicians. *J. Occup. Health* 59, 33–37. doi: 10.1539/joh.16-0217-oa

Prendergast, G., Guest, H., Munro, K. J., Kluk, K., Léger, A., Hall, D. A., et al. (2017a). Effects of noise exposure on young adults with normal audiograms I: electrophysiology. *Hear. Res.* 344, 68–81. doi: 10.1016/j.heares.2016.10.028

Prendergast, G., Millman, R. E., Guest, H., Munro, K. J., Kluk, K., Dewey, R. S., et al. (2017b). Effects of noise exposure on young adults with normal audiograms II: behavioral measures. *Hear. Res.* 356, 74–86. doi: 10.1016/j.heares.2017.10.007

Ramakers, G. G., Kraaijenga, V. J., Cattani, G., Van Zanten, G. A., and Grolman, W. (2016). Effectiveness of earplugs in preventing recreational noise-induced hearing loss: a randomized clinical trial. *JAMA Otolaryngol. Head Neck Surg.* 142, 551–558. doi: 10.1001/jamaoto.2016.0225

Schaette, R., and McAlpine, D. (2011). Tinnitus with a normal audiogram: physiological evidence for hidden hearing loss and computational model. *J. Neurosci.* 31, 13452–13457. doi: 10.1523/jneurosci.2156-11.2011

Schink, T., Kreutz, G., Busch, V., Pigeot, I., and Ahrens, W. (2014). Incidence and relative risk of hearing disorders in professional musicians. *Occup. Environ. Med.* 71, 472–476. doi: 10.1136/oemed-2014-102172

Sergeyenko, Y., Lall, K., Liberman, M. C., and Kujawa, S. G. (2013). Age-related cochlear synaptopathy: an early-onset contributor to auditory functional decline. *J. Neurosci.* 33, 13686–13694. doi: 10.1523/jneurosci.1783-13.2013

Shi, L., Chang, Y., Li, X., Aiken, S. J., Liu, L., and Wang, J. (2016). Coding deficits in noise-induced hidden hearing loss may stem from incomplete repair of ribbon synapses in the cochlea. *Front. Neurosci.* 10:231. doi: 10.3389/fnins.2016.00231

Skoe, E., Camera, S., and Tufts, J. (2019). Noise exposure may diminish the musician advantage for perceiving speech in noise. *Ear. Hear.* 40, 782–793. doi: 10.1097/aud.0000000000000665

Stamper, G. C., and Johnson, T. A. (2015). Auditory function in normal-hearing. Noise-exposed human ears. *Ear. Hear.* 36, 172–184. doi: 10.1097/aud.0000000000000107

Stuart, A., and Cobb, K. M. (2015). Reliability of measures of transient evoked otoacoustic emissions with contralateral suppression. *J. Commun. Disord.* 58, 35–42. doi: 10.1016/j.jcomdis.2015.09.003

Tronstad, T. V., and Gelderblom, F. B. (2016). Sound exposure during outdoor music festivals. *Noise Health* 18, 220–228. doi: 10.4103/1463-1741.189245

Valero, M. D., Burton, J. A., Hauser, S. N., Hackett, T. A., Ramachandran, R., and Liberman, M. C. (2017). Noise-induced cochlear synaptopathy in rhesus monkeys (*Macaca mulatta*). *Hear. Res.* 353, 213–223. doi: 10.1016/j.heares.2017.07.003

Viana, L. M., O'malley, J. T., Burgess, B. J., Jones, D. D., Oliveira, C. A., Santos, F., et al. (2015). Cochlear neuropathy in human presbycusis: confocal analysis of hidden hearing loss in post-mortem tissue. *Hear. Res.* 327, 78–88. doi: 10.1016/j.heares.2015.04.014

Wang, Q., Wang, X., Yang, L., Han, K., Huang, Z., and Wu, H. (2021). Sex differences in noise-induced hearing loss: a cross-sectional study in China. *Biol. Sex Differ.* 12:24. doi: 10.1186/s13293-021-00369-0

Washnik, N. J., Bhatt, I. S., Phillips, S. L., Tucker, D., and Richter, S. (2020). Evaluation of cochlear activity in normal-hearing musicians. *Hear. Res.* 395:108027. doi: 10.1016/j.heares.2020.108027

Wong, L. L., Soli, S. D., Liu, S., Han, N., and Huang, M. W. (2007). Development of the mandarin hearing in noise test (MHINT). *Ear. Hear.* 28, 70s–74s.

Wu, P. Z., Liberman, L. D., Bennett, K., De Gruttola, V., O'malley, J. T., and Liberman, M. C. (2019). Primary neural degeneration in the human cochlea: evidence for hidden hearing loss in the aging ear. *Neuroscience* 407, 8–20. doi: 10.1016/j.neuroscience.2018.07.053

Yao, C., Ma, A. K., Cushing, S. L., and Lin, V. Y. W. (2017). Noise exposure while commuting in Toronto - a study of personal and public transportation in Toronto. *J. Otolaryngol. Head Neck Surg.* 46:62.

Yeend, I., Beach, E. F., Sharma, M., and Dillon, H. (2017). The effects of noise exposure and musical training on suprathreshold auditory processing and speech perception in noise. *Hear. Res.* 353, 224–236. doi: 10.1016/j.heares.2017.07.006

Zhang, N., Liu, S., Xu, J., Liu, B., Qi, B., Yang, Y., et al. (2010). Development and applications of alternative methods of segmentation for mandarin hearing in noise test in normal-hearing listeners and cochlear implant users. *Acta Otolaryngol.* 130, 831–837. doi: 10.3109/00016480903493758

5

The Relationship Between Hearing Loss and Cognitive Impairment in a Chinese Elderly Population

Xinxing Fu[1,2,3], Bo Liu[1]*, Shuo Wang[1]*, Robert H. Eikelboom[2,3,4] and Dona M. P. Jayakody[2,3,5]*

[1] Beijing Institute of Otolaryngology, Otolaryngology-Head and Neck Surgery, Beijing Tongren Hospital, Capital Medical University, Beijing, China, [2] Medical School, The University of Western Australia, Crawley, WA, Australia, [3] Ear Science Institute Australia, Subiaco, WA, Australia, [4] Department of Speech Language Pathology and Audiology, University of Pretoria, Pretoria, South Africa, [5] WA Centre for Health and Ageing, The University of Western Australia, Crawley, WA, Australia

***Correspondence:**
Xinxing Fu
xinxing.fu@research.uwa.edu.au
Bo Liu
trliubo@139.com
Shuo Wang
shannonwsh@aliyun.com

Objectives: The objective of the study was to investigate the association between untreated age-related hearing loss and cognitive impairment in Mandarin-speaking older adults living in China.

Methods: Older adults (293; 111 males, $M = 70.33 \pm 4.90$ years; 182 females, $M = 69.02 \pm 4.08$ years) were recruited. All participants completed a pure tone audiometric hearing assessment, Hearing Impairment-Montreal Cognitive Assessment Test (HI-MoCA), and a computerized neuropsychology test battery (CANTAB). The Mandarin version of the De Jong Gierveld Loneliness Scale was used to measure the loneliness, and the Mandarin version of the 21-item Depression Anxiety Stress Scale (DASS-21) was used to measure the current severity of a range of symptoms common to depression, stress, and anxiety of the participants.

Results: A multiple stepwise regression analysis showed that the average of four mid-frequency thresholds in the better ear was related to CANTAB Paired Associates Learning ($\beta = 0.20$, $p = 0.002$), and the global cognitive function score (HI-MoCA) ($\beta = -0.25$, $p < 0.001$). The average of three high frequencies in the better ear was significantly associated with CANTAB Delayed Matching to Sample ($\beta = -0.16$, $p = 0.008$), and Spatial Working Memory ($\beta = 0.17$, $p = 0.003$).

Conclusion: The results revealed a significant relationship between age-related hearing loss and cognitive impairment in Mandarin-speaking older adults. These research outcomes have clinical implications specifically for hearing health care professionals in China and other populations that speak a tonal language, especially when providing hearing rehabilitation.

Keywords: age-related hearing loss (ARHL), cognitive impairment, depression, loneliness, tonal language

INTRODUCTION

An estimated 1.57 billion people worldwide had hearing loss in 2019, accounting for 20.3% of the global population (Haile et al., 2021). Approximately one-third of people over 65 years of age are affected by disabling hearing loss. Hearing loss hampers effective communication, which can have a significant impact on the activities of daily life causing feelings of loneliness, isolation, and frustration (Ciorba et al., 2012). Depression, anxiety, and stress are also associated with untreated hearing loss (Jayakody et al., 2018a).

Studies conducted with non-tonal language speakers have established a relationship between untreated age-related hearing loss and cognitive impairment and dementia (Deal et al., 2015; Jayakody et al., 2018b). Those with mild, moderate, and severe hearing loss are two to five times more likely to develop dementia compared with those with normal hearing sensitivity (Lin et al., 2011).

Approximately 50% of the population of the world speaks a tonal language, e.g., Mandarin, Cantonese. In tonal languages, changes in pitch (tone) at the monosyllabic level convey lexical meaning of a word. As pitch is the important factor here, tonal language perception can be equated with music perception. This view is supported by evidence that speaking tonal language leads to enhanced pitch perception in music. The benefits of music training and tonal language experience are bidirectional, and a background in either domain improves processing in the other domain (Ngo et al., 2016). Furthermore, playing a musical instrument may have the benefits on slowing age-related cognitive decline (Balbag et al., 2014). This may be explained by the fact that playing a musical instrument trains executive function involving different cognitive functions of the brain, including memory, visual, and executive functions (Mansky et al., 2020).

There is also psychophysiological evidence that suggests that a tonal language background maybe associated with enhanced general cognitive abilities. A study conducted by using the Corsi blocks tapping test has shown that the Cantonese speakers had a superior working memory related to pitch perception relative to English speakers (Bidelman et al., 2013).

Therefore, it is possible to hypothesize that tonal language speakers are likely to have better working memory in their later life compared with non-tonal language older adults. As hearing sensitivity is strongly associated with age, this raises the question whether speaking a tonal language is a protective factor for cognitive decline in older adults.

There are a handful of studies that have investigated the associations between cognitive function and untreated hearing loss in tonal language speakers. However, these studies have reported conflicting findings. Luo et al. (2018) reported that the prevalence of dementia was 0.61 (95% CI = 0.53–0.71%) with hearing impairment, whereas Gyanwali et al. (2020) failed to find an independent association between hearing loss and dementia ($p > 0.05$).

An analysis of the cognitive assessments utilized in studies that investigated the association between hearing loss and cognitive impairment/dementia in tonal language speakers have not thoroughly assessed cognition, or often used verbally loaded test materials that rely on audition, i.e., some of the materials are presented orally–aurally. For example, a population-based study of age-related hearing loss and dementia in Taiwan was only able to assess the cognitive status of the participants as impaired or normal by psychiatric diagnosis, not enabling a full quantitative analysis (Su et al., 2017). A cohort study investigated the association between hearing loss with cognitive function in a Han Chinese cohort using a standardized neurocognitive battery (Ren et al., 2019). However, as both of these studies used verbal language instructions, it is possible that the hearing loss of the participants had an impact on their cognitive performance, causing an overestimate on the degree of cognition impairment (Dupuis et al., 2015).

The underlying mechanism between hearing loss and cognitive impairment is yet to be established. However, the posited underlying factors of this mechanism may include low education, hypertension, obesity, smoking, depression, physical inactivity, and low social contact (Livingston et al., 2017).

Therefore, this study explored the potential association between hearing loss and cognitive impairment in Mandarin-speaking older adults in China using a non-verbal cognitive assessment test battery, controlling for a number of potential confounders.

MATERIALS AND METHODS

Participants were recruited through social media advertisements, flyers, and community centers in Beijing. Ethics approval for this study was obtained from The University of Western Australia—Human Research Ethics Committee (RA/4/20/5538) and Beijing Tongren Hospital, Capital Medical University (TRECKY2019-090). All procedures were carried out in accordance with these approvals, and the participants all provided written informed consent.

Inclusion criteria: Native Mandarin speakers, aged 60 years and above with hearing impairment were invited to participate in the study. Exclusion criteria: Those not in general state of good health or unable to perform tasks required in the cognition evaluation session due to an underlying physical or mental condition, or those who had previously worn or currently wearing hearing aids or a hearing implant were excluded from the study. Those who could not complete the Motor Screening Task (MOT) module of the Cambridge Neuropsychological Test Battery (CANTAB) (Cambridge Cognition Ltd., 2014) due to inability to follow instructions, or dexterity problems were also excluded from the study.

Measure and Procedure

The assessment methods comprised measurements of hearing ability, cognition function, loneliness, and mental health status.

After enrollment, all participants completed a baseline questionnaire capturing demographic information, and data on alcohol consumption (never, less than 14, 15–28, 29–42, or 43 or more standard drinks per week), smoking (never, past, current, or exposed to second-hand smoking), self-reported chronic disease history (heart disease, stroke, high cholesterol, atherosclerosis, hypertension, diabetes, frequent childhood ear infections, trauma to ear or head, and depression), leisure activities, as well as marital status and living arrangements. Leisure activities were classified into recreational, intellectual, physical, and social categories (Leung et al., 2010). Living arrangements were recorded as living with spouse, living with children, or living alone, and marital status as single, married, widowed, or divorced.

Hearing Assessment

Pure-tone audiometry (PTA) was assessed with an audiometer (Conera Audiometer, GN Otometrics Ltd., Denmark) and supra-aural earphone (TDH-39). For all participants, bilateral air-conduction thresholds were measured at 0.25, 0.5, 1, 2, 4, 6, and 8 kHz; and bone-conduction thresholds were measured at 0.5, 1, 2, and 4 kHz, through standard audiometric assessment conducted by a qualified audiologist in a soundproof booth at the audiology center of the Beijing Institute of Otolaryngology.

Evaluation of hearing loss was deployed by two different methods: the traditional four frequency average of hearing thresholds at 0.5, 1, 2, and 4 kHz, and the three high frequency average of hearing thresholds at 4, 6, and 8 kHz in the better ear, noted, respectively, as 4FA and 3HFA. These were analyzed as continuous variables. For the purpose of summarizing the hearing loss of the study cohort, the 4FA hearing loss was classified using the World Health Organization (WHO) grades of hearing impairment (Humes, 2019), respectively, normal hearing—less than 20 dB HL; mild hearing loss—20 to < 35 dB HL; moderate hearing loss—35 to < 50 dB HL; moderately severe hearing loss—50 to < 65 dB HL; severe hearing loss—65 to < 80 dB HL; profound hearing loss—80 to < 95 dB HL; complete hearing loss—95 dB HL or greater in the better ear.

Cognitive Assessment

The global cognitive functions of the subjects were tested using the Montreal Cognitive Assessment Test (MoCA) for the hearing impaired. A Mandarin version of the MoCA (version 7.2) was adapted (Nasreddine et al., 2005), which was converted into a timed PowerPoint (Microsoft Corp., Redmond, Washington, United States) presentation, here named HI-MoCA (Hearing impaired-MoCA), with all the verbal instructions replaced with visual instructions (Lin et al., 2017).

For the visuospatial and executive tasks, an answer sheet was given to the subject to be completed as instructed. For all other tasks, the subjects were asked to verbally answer or respond. For example, for the memory recall section, a series of words were presented at a rate of 2 s per word (truck, banana, violin, desk, and green), comparable to the standard verbal administration of the original MoCA. In the attention tasks, for both the forward and backward order digits repetition, all the numbers were presented at a rate of 1.5 s (compared with one digit per second in the original MoCA). For the digits series task, requiring the participant to identify the digit 1 among a string of digits from 0 to 9 by tapping the table, the HI-MoCA visually presented a series of numbers at a rate of 1.5 s between numbers for the subject to observe and respond to by tapping the table. In the language task, both sentences are presented for 9 s.

All the HI-MoCA tests were administered by an audiologist, who received formal training from a senior neurology physician with advanced clinical experience and completed the certificated training course via the MoCA website.

Non-verbal cognition was assessed using the Cambridge Neuropsychological Test Automated Battery (CANTAB) (Campos-Magdaleno et al., 2020). The CANTAB software was installed on a laptop with an integrated touch screen (IBM, Yoga S, with Windows 10.1 platform).

Evaluation of cognitive function for this study was focused on working and episode memory, processing speed, and spatial information processing. Therefore, the relevant test items were chosen from the CANTAB test battery, including delayed matching to sample (DMS), paired associates learning (PAL), and spatial working memory (SWM), respectively. Assessment commenced with a test of motor function, to qualify the participant for further assessment.

Motor Screening Task

The motor screening task provides a general assessment of whether vision, sensorimotor deficits, or lack of comprehension, which, if present, would limit the collection of valid data from the participant (Cambridge Cognition Ltd., 2014). It involved the selection of colored crosses in different positions on the screen as quickly and accurately as possible by the participant. MST outcome measures assess the speed of response and the accuracy of pointing of the participant.

Delayed Matching to Sample

The DMS test assesses both simultaneous visual matching ability and short-term visual recognition memory, for non-verbalizable patterns (Cambridge Cognition Ltd., 2014). DMS is primarily sensitive to damage in the medial temporal lobe area, with some input from the frontal lobes (Olsen et al., 2009). The participant is shown a complex visual pattern (the sample) and four response patterns. The task of the participant is to identify the response pattern that is identical to the sample pattern. Response patterns will be shown simultaneously with the sample pattern, whereas in others, a delay (of 0, 4, or 12 s) is introduced. DMS outcome measures include latency (the speed of response of the participant), the percentage of correct patterns selected, and a statistical measure giving the probability of an error after a correct or incorrect response. The DMS parallel mode was administered for all the subjects, including three practice trials and 20 assessment trials. The average administration time is around 8 min. Percentage of correct patterns selected by the participant was analyzed in this study (Cambridge Cognition Ltd., 2014).

Paired Associates Learning

The PAL test assesses episodic visuospatial memory, learning, and association ability (Cambridge Cognition Ltd., 2014). This test is primarily sensitive to changes in medial temporal lobe functioning (Cambridge Cognition Ltd., 2014). In this task, six to eight white boxes are displayed on a computer screen. These briefly reveal a pattern which varies in shape and color. The task of the participant is to remember the pattern revealed and match it to the pattern that appears in the middle of the screen by touching the box that contains the correct pattern. The task is made progressively difficult by presenting 1, 2, 3, 6, and 8 patterns to the participant. Outcome measures include the errors made by the participant, the number of trials required to locate the pattern(s) correctly, memory scores, and stages completed. The PAL clinical mode was administered for all the subjects with up to eight stages depending on the performance of the subjects; each stage may have up to 10 trials (attempts) in total. The average administration time is around 10 min but is greatly affected by the degree of impairment of the subject and the number of repeat presentations that are required. PAL errors (total shapes) and PAL errors (six shapes) were analyzed in this study (Cambridge Cognition Ltd., 2014).

Spatial Working Memory

The SWM test requires retention and manipulation of visuospatial information. This self-ordered test has obvious executive function demands and provides a measure of non-verbal working memory, visuospatial working memory, and strategy use (Cambridge Cognition Ltd., 2014). SWM is a sensitive measure of frontal lobe and "executive" dysfunction. The task of the participant was to locate tokens hidden in increasing number of boxes (3, 4, 6, and 8). Each box contained only one token per sequence. Searching a box more than once during a sequence results in a "within search error" and revisiting a box in which a token has been found before incurs a "between search error." A "strategy" score, calculated for the more difficult six- and eight-box levels, represented the use of an efficient strategy based on predetermined sequence. Poor use of strategy is reflected in higher strategy scores and vice versa. Three main outcome measures, spatial working memory within errors, between errors, and strategy scores, were calculated for the purpose of this study. The SWM clinical mode was administered for all the subjects with 16 stages, including four practices and 12 assessment trials. The average administration time is around 9 min but is also affected by the degree of impairment of the subjects.

Loneliness Measurement

The Mandarin version of the six-item De Jong Gierveld Loneliness Scale was used to measure the loneliness of the subjects (Leung et al., 2008; Yang et al., 2018; Fung et al., 2019). In this six-item scale, three statements are made about emotional loneliness and three about social loneliness. There are negatively (items 1, 2, and 3) and positively (items 4, 5, and 6) worded items, scored 1 point for "Yes" and "More or less" answers, and 0 points for "No" answers to questions 1–3; scored 1 point for "More or less" and "No" answers, and 0 points for "Yes" answers to questions 4–6.

Assessment of Depression, Anxiety, and Stress

The Depression Anxiety Stress Scales (DASS-21) is a questionnaire to assess the symptoms of depression, anxiety, and stress (Chan et al., 2012; Wang K. et al., 2016). The 21 items on the questionnaire comprise a set of three self-reported scales designed to assess depression, anxiety, and stress status of subjects. The seven elements on each scale are graded on a Likert scale from 0 to 3 (0: "Did not apply to me at all," 1: "Applied to me to some degree or some of the time," 2: "Applied to me to a considerable degree or a good part of the time," and 3: "Applied to me very much or most of the time"). Depression, anxiety, and stress scores are determined by summarizing the scores of the related items (Lovibond and Lovibond, 1995). As the DASS-21 is a shorter version of the 42-item original DASS, the score for each subscale is multiplied by two to calculate the final score.

Statistics Analysis

All statistical analyses were performed using SPSS version 25 (SPSS Inc., Chicago, IL, United States). A multiple forward stepwise regression analysis was used to examine the relationship between cognitive functions and other variables, including age, gender, smoking and alcohol consumption, chronic medical history, education years, loneliness and mental health, and PTA thresholds of better ear average across 500 Hz–8 kHz. The different CANTAB modules and HI-MoCA scores were entered as dependent variables, respectively. The collinearity tests were examined during each stepwise regression analysis.

At each step of the regression analysis, variables were added based on *p*-values, and the Akaike Information Criterion (AIC) was used to set a limit on the total number of variables included in the final model. The criteria of entry of each variable was a probability of $F \leq 0.05$ and removal of each variable a probability of $F \geq 0.10$.

RESULTS

Descriptive Data

The demographic information, cognitive function scores, and other descriptive data of this study population are presented in **Table 1**, including the age, gender, education years, hearing threshold, smoking status, alcohol intake, history of chronic disease, depression, anxiety, and stress status of the participants. A total of 293 Mandarin speakers aged between 60 and 87 years were included in the study. The study cohort consisted of 111 males (mean age = 70.33 ± 4.90 years) and 182 females (mean age = 69.02 ± 4.08 years).

For descriptive purposes, the better ear 4FA was used to group the participants; 65 had normal hearing, 106 had mild hearing loss, 54 had moderate hearing loss, 34 had moderately severe hearing loss, 31 had severe hearing loss, and three had profound hearing loss, as shown in **Table 1**.

Regression Analysis

The multiple stepwise regression analyses revealed that the better ear 4FA significantly predicted HI-MoCA scores ($p < 0.001$), PAL error for 6 shapes ($p < 0.05$), and that the better ear 3HFA significantly predicted SWM within error ($p < 0.05$) and DMS correct percent ($p < 0.05$). The detailed results are shown in **Table 2**. Only the last model of the stepwise regression is shown. Each model of forward stepwise regression for HI-MoCA, SWM between error, SWM within error, SWM strategy, PAL error (all shapes), PAL error (six shapes), DMS correct percent are, respectively, shown in **Supplementary Tables 1–7**.

DISCUSSION

This study investigated the association between hearing loss and global cognitive abilities (HI-MoCA) and multiple domains of non-verbal cognitive abilities in Mandarin-speaking older adults. To the best of our knowledge, this is the first study to elucidate the association between hearing loss and cognitive function by using the hearing impairment version MoCA and a non-verbal neurocognitive assessment tool with tonal language participants.

Our results are consistent with previous cross-sectional studies of pure-tone audiometric hearing loss and cognitive decline and impairment in non-tonal language speakers (Gussekloo et al., 2005; Deal et al., 2015; Jayakody et al., 2018b). Our results revealed that both mid-frequency hearing sensitivity and self-reported hearing loss were significantly associated with HI-MoCA score.

As shown in **Table 2**, self-reported hearing loss was significantly associated with both HI-MoCA ($\beta = 0.18, p = 0.004$) and PAL error (six shapes) ($\beta = -0.16$, $p = 0.009$). This finding suggests that self-reported hearing loss may be a useful indicator when evaluating the relationship between hearing loss and cognitive impairment. This finding accords with another study, which showed that self-reported hearing loss was significantly associated with both baseline and follow-up cognitive impairment (Amieva et al., 2015).

Our results also showed that the age-related hearing loss significantly associated with poor performance on some of the cognitive domains, specifically DMS (short-term visual memory) and PAL (episodic visuospatial memory). Prior studies have noted that episodic memory impairments are one of the earliest signs of amnestic mild cognitive impairment, Alzheimer's disease, and other dementias (Wang P. et al., 2016).

Short-term visual memory function in this study was assessed using DMS module of the CANTAB test battery. Linear regression showed that while high-frequency hearing in the better ear was significantly associated with the DMS score, mid-frequency hearing was not associated with the DMS score. This finding is consistent with previous research (Jayakody et al., 2018b) on non-tonal language speakers. A possible explanation for this is that presbycusis usually begins with reduced hearing sensitivity in the higher frequencies while remaining relatively better in the low and mid-frequency range. Consequently, the association between DMS and mid-frequency hearing impairment was not observed in the regression analysis.

Visual memory and learning ability were measured by PAL task of CANTAB test battery. There was a significant positive correlation between mid-frequency hearing in (4FA) in the better ear, and PAL error (six shapes). Previous studies have also demonstrated that performance on the PAL task is highly associated with cognition impairment, and can differentiate subjects with Alzheimer's disease from normal controls with high sensitivity and specificity (Hicks et al., 2020). However, no significant association was found between PAL scores (all shapes) and hearing loss.

Two types of leisure activities (intelligent and social) were observed in the regression model to be associated with PAL error (all shapes), but not PAL error (6 shapes). Prior studies that have noted the importance of participation in leisure activities, which

TABLE 1 | Descriptive data of the participants.

Characteristics	All subjects
	$N = 293$
Male sex, no. (%)	111 (37.9%)
Smoking, no. (%)	107 (36.5%)
Alcohol consumption[a], no. (%)	279 (95.2%)
Vascular disease[b], no. (%)	231 (78.8%)
Diabetes, no. (%)	66 (22.5%)
Frequent childhood ear infections, no. (%)	13 (4.4%)
Depression clinically diagnosed, no. (%)	10 (3.4)
Self-report HL, no. (%)	212 (72.4%)
Noise exposure, no. (%)	52 (17.7%)
Living alone, no. (%)	17 (5.8%)
Single or divorced, no. (%)	33 (11.3%)
Age (years)	69.52 ± 4.45
Education (years)	12.98 ± 2.84
Hearing loss classification, no. (%)	
Normal hearing	65 (22.2%)
Mild hearing loss	106 (36.2%)
Moderate hearing loss	54 (18.4%)
Moderately severe hearing loss	34 (11.6%)
Severe hearing loss	31 (10.6%)
Profound hearing loss	3 (1.0%)
4FA (dB HL)	36.94 ± 18.78
3HFA (dB HL)	52.31 ± 20.17
Emotional loneliness	0.92 ± 0.84
Social loneliness	1.11 ± 1.18
Loneliness	2.03 ± 1.59
Depression	3.65 ± 5.22
Anxiety	5.98 ± 5.58
Stress	6.45 ± 6.70
Recreational activities score	14.5 ± 10.68
Intellectual activities score	20.87 ± 12.72
Physical activities score	21.15 ± 11.06
Social activities score	2.11 ± 2.79
HI-MoCA score	25.00 ± 2.63
SWM between error	35.99 ± 16.25
SWM within error	6.83 ± 5.49
SWM strategy	34.64 ± 5.21
PAL error (all shapes)	32.54 ± 26.66
PAL error (six shapes)	7.60 ± 7.66
DMS correct percent	79.43 ± 11.75

The data are presented as means ± standard deviations, unless otherwise indicated.

4FA: four frequencies (500 Hz, 1, 2, and 4 kHz) average of pure tone hearing thresholds of the better ear; 3HFA: three high frequencies (4, 6, and 8 kHz) average of pure tone hearing thresholds of the better ear; HI-MoCA, hearing impaired-Montreal cognitive assessment test; PAL, paired associates learning; DMS, delayed matching to sample; SWM, spatial working memory.

[a]Alcohol consumption reference is never or less than 14 standard drinks per week.

[b]Vascular disease indicates any one of heart disease, stroke, high cholesterol, atherosclerosis, or hypertension.

has been associated with the reduced risk of cognitive impairment after controlling for age, gender, and education (Verghese et al., 2003). In this study, information regarding four categories of leisure activities was collected by a questionnaire. It is difficult to explain this result that why PAL error (all shapes) and PAL error (six shapes) showed different regression outcomes, but it may be related to the high level of difficultly of the PAL eight shapes task. Participants sometimes took a very long time on the task and lost their patience, and the results are likely to be inaccurate and unreliable.

Spatial working memory requires retention and manipulation of visuospatial information. The SWM task has notable demands on executive function and provides a measure of strategy as well as working memory. This study showed that high frequency hearing is significantly associated with SWM within error, but not with mid-frequency hearing. This result may be explained, as noted earlier, by the fact that high frequencies show a decrease in sensitivity at least a decade earlier than for the mid-frequency speech frequencies (Salvi et al., 2018). However, neither 4HA nor 3HFA were associated with SWM between error and SWM strategy. This finding is contrary to a previous study which has suggested that both the SWM errors and strategy score are associated with mid-frequency hearing (Jayakody et al., 2018b).

Education was significantly associated with almost all the cognitive-dependent variables, including HI-MoCA and CANTAB DMS, PAL, and SWM. These results corroborate the findings of a great deal of the previous work in this field. Lower rates of late-life dementia are associated with higher education levels during earlier life (Livingston et al., 2017). Early education may promote the development during a sensitive period of childhood that protect against late-life cognitive decline (Zahodne et al., 2015).

Another important finding was that social loneliness and overall loneliness (social and emotional) were significantly associated with both SWM between error and SWM strategy. Several reports have shown that both loneliness and social isolation are associated with cognitive decline (Donovan et al., 2017; Lara et al., 2019). The literature does not testify the causal relationship between loneliness and cognitive function. Loneliness may lead to cognitive decline, perhaps from limited social interactions, but it is also possible that cognitive impairment may lead to limited social interactions and further loneliness (Boss et al., 2015).

TABLE 2 | Multiple stepwise regression between CANTAB/HI-MoCA scores and other variables.

Dependent variable	Independent variables	R^2	Adjusted R^2	B	β	*t*	Sig.	95% Confidence interval for B	
								Lower bound	Upper bound
HI-MoCA score	4FA	0.09	0.08	−0.04	−0.25	−4.03	0.000	−0.05	−0.02
	Self-report HL			1.04	0.18	2.88	0.004	0.33	1.75
	Education years			0.14	0.15	2.63	0.009	0.04	0.24
SWM between error	Age	0.09	0.08	0.76	0.21	3.69	0.000	0.36	1.17
	Social loneliness			−5.24	−0.38	−3.46	0.001	−8.22	−2.26
	Loneliness			2.69	0.26	2.41	0.017	0.49	4.89
SWM within error	3HFA	0.04	0.04	0.05	0.17	2.99	0.003	0.02	0.08
	Education years			0.26	0.14	2.34	0.020	0.04	0.48
SWM strategy	Social loneliness	0.06	0.05	−2.02	−0.46	−3.99	0.000	−3.01	−1.02
	Loneliness			1.19	0.36	3.11	0.002	0.44	1.94
	Anxiety			−0.13	−0.14	−2.29	0.023	−0.24	−0.02
PAL error (All shapes)	Education years	0.11	0.09	−1.58	−0.17	−2.95	0.003	−2.63	−0.53
	Intelligent activities			−0.35	−0.16	−2.89	0.004	−0.58	−0.11
	Gender			8.93	0.16	2.82	0.005	2.70	15.15
	Social activities			1.37	0.14	2.52	0.012	0.30	2.45
	Living arrangements			14.96	0.13	2.32	0.021	2.25	27.67
PAL error (6 shapes)	4FA	0.08	0.07	0.08	0.20	3.16	0.002	0.03	0.13
	Self-report HL			−2.78	−0.16	−2.64	0.009	−4.86	−0.71
	Depression			0.19	0.13	2.31	0.021	0.03	0.36
	Education years			−0.32	−0.12	−2.09	0.038	−0.63	−0.02
DMS correct percent	3HFA	0.12	0.10	−0.09	−0.16	−2.66	0.008	−0.16	−0.02
	Education years			0.57	0.14	2.43	0.016	0.11	1.03
	Age			−0.31	−0.12	−2.02	0.045	−0.62	−0.01
	Anxiety			−0.26	−0.12	−2.22	0.027	−0.49	−0.03
	Gender			−2.88	−0.12	−2.06	0.040	−5.64	−0.13

4FA, four frequencies (500 Hz, 1, 2, and 4 kHz) average of pure-tone hearing thresholds of the better ear; HI-MoCA, hearing impaired-Montreal cognitive assessment; PAL, paired associates learning; DMS, delayed matching to sample; SWM, spatial working memory. 3HFA, three high frequencies (4, 6, and 8 kHz) average of pure-tone hearing thresholds of the better ear.

Between 20 and 40% of the elderly in Western countries are reported to be lonely (Savikko et al., 2005), and the prevalence of loneliness has increased from 16 to 30% from 1992 to 2000 (Yang and Victor, 2008), possibly due to the impact of the "empty-nester" phenomenon that had impact on that (Fung et al., 2019). However, among the participants in this study, only 5.8% lived alone, the majority living with their children and even grandchildren. In China, elderly people tend to live with their children, playing an important role in caring for their grandchildren. This living arrangement is likely to have an impact on mental wellbeing and cognitive functioning (Mazzuco et al., 2017), as well as possible decreasing of loneliness and social isolation. This contrasts with the prevailing culture in Western countries, where parents tend to live alone after children move out of home, and they tend to live in residential aged-care facilities later in life; however, less than 2% of the subjects of this study population lived in aged-care centers.

Clinical Implications

This study contributes evidence to the growing global body of evidence that hearing loss and cognitive decline are significantly associated, also in Mandarin-speaking older adults. While the risk of hearing loss to cognition has not been determined, the association is something that hearing health professionals need to bear in mind when managing and counseling their patients.

Limitations

One of the limitations in this study is that the age of participants recruited generally reflected their level of hearing loss and that there were relatively fewer participants with increasing severity of hearing loss. However, this is consistent with the prevalence of hearing loss in the population in relation to age. This study was designed as a longitudinal study, so as to examine the association between ARHL and cognitive decline over time. Another potential limitation is that participant fatigue may have affected some of the more strenuous tests.

Future Directions

These findings warrant longitudinal studies to better understand the association between hearing loss and cognitive impairment over time and also to investigate how confounding factors contribute to the cognitive functions overall. Recent studies have studied the impact of hearing aids and cochlear implantation on cognitive functions of older adults with hearing loss (Jayakody et al., 2017, 2020; Kramer et al., 2018; Maharani et al., 2018). The results indicate that hearing rehabilitation has some degree of impact on improving cognitive functions. Based on the findings, we recommend a randomized control trial investigating the impact of hearing rehabilitation on the cognitive functions of Mandarin-speaking older adults.

CONCLUSION

This study provides more evidence for the association between hearing loss and cognitive impairment in Mandarin-speaking older adults. This study revealed that the hearing loss has a significant relationship with cognitive impairment in a Chinese-speaking population.

AUTHOR CONTRIBUTIONS

DJ and XF designed the experiments. XF carried out the experiments and wrote the manuscript. XF, BL, SW, RE, and DJ analyzed the experimental results. RE, DJ, BL, and SW reviewed the manuscript. All authors contributed to the article and approved the submitted version.

REFERENCES

Amieva, H., Ouvrard, C., Giulioli, C., Meillon, C., Rullier, L., and Dartigues, J. F. (2015). Self-reported hearing loss, hearing aids, and cognitive decline in elderly adults: a 25-year study. *J. Am. Geriatr. Soc.* 63, 2099–2104. doi: 10.1111/jgs.13649

Balbag, M. A., Pedersen, N. L., and Gatz, M. (2014). Playing a musical instrument as a protective factor against dementia and cognitive impairment: a population-based twin study. *Int. J. Alzheimers Dis.* 2014:836748. doi: 10.1155/2014/836748

Bidelman, G. M., Hutka, S., and Moreno, S. (2013). Tone language speakers and musicians share enhanced perceptual and cognitive abilities for musical pitch: evidence for bidirectionality between the domains of language and music. *PLoS One* 8:e60676. doi: 10.1371/journal.pone.0060676

Boss, L., Kang, D. H., and Branson, S. (2015). Loneliness and cognitive function in the older adult: a systematic review. *Int. Psychoger.* 27, 541–553. doi: 10.1017/s1041610214002749

Cambridge Cognition Ltd (2014). *CANTABeclipse Test Administration Guide.* Cambridge: Cambridge Cognition Limited.

Campos-Magdaleno, M., Leiva, D., Pereiro, A. X., Lojo-Seoane, C., Mallo, S. C., Facal, D., et al. (2020). Changes in visual memory in mild cognitive impairment: a longitudinal study with CANTAB. *Psychol. Med.* 51, 2465–2475. doi: 10.1017/s0033291720001142

Chan, R. C., Xu, T., Huang, J., Wang, Y., Zhao, Q., Shum, D. H., et al. (2012). Extending the utility of the depression anxiety stress scale by examining its psychometric properties in Chinese settings. *Psychiatry Res.* 200, 879–883. doi: 10.1016/j.psychres.2012.06.041

Ciorba, A., Bianchini, C., Pelucchi, S., and Pastore, A. (2012). The impact of hearing loss on the quality of life of elderly adults. *Clin. Interv. Aging* 7, 159–163. doi: 10.2147/cia.S26059

Deal, J. A., Sharrett, A. R., Albert, M. S., Coresh, J., Mosley, T. H., Knopman, D., et al. (2015). Hearing impairment and cognitive decline: a pilot study conducted within the atherosclerosis risk in communities neurocognitive study. *Am. J. Epidemiol.* 181, 680–690. doi: 10.1093/aje/kwu333

Donovan, N. J., Wu, Q., Rentz, D. M., Sperling, R. A., Marshall, G. A., and Glymour, M. M. (2017). Loneliness, depression and cognitive function in older U.S. adults. *Int. J. Geriatr. Psychiatry* 32, 564–573. doi: 10.1002/gps.4495

Dupuis, K., Pichora-Fuller, M. K., Chasteen, A. L., Marchuk, V., Singh, G., and Smith, S. L. (2015). Effects of hearing and vision impairments on the montreal cognitive assessment. *Neuropsychol. Dev. Cogn. Section B Aging, Neuropsychol. Cogn.* 22, 413–437. doi: 10.1080/13825585.2014.968084

Fung, A. W. T., Lee, A. T. C., Cheng, S. T., and Lam, L. C. W. (2019). Loneliness interacts with family relationship in relation to cognitive function in Chinese older adults. *Int. Psychogeriatr.* 31, 467–475. doi: 10.1017/S1041610218001333

Gussekloo, J., de Craen, A. J., Oduber, C., van Boxtel, M. P., and Westendorp, R. G. (2005). Sensory impairment and cognitive functioning in oldest-old subjects: the leiden 85+ study. *Am. J. Geriatr. Psychiatry* 13, 781–786. doi: 10.1176/appi.ajgp.13.9.781

Gyanwali, B., Hilal, S., Venketasubramanian, N., Chen, C., and Loo, J. H. Y. (2020). Hearing handicap in Asian patients with dementia. *Am. J. Otolaryngol.* 41:102377. doi: 10.1016/j.amjoto.2019.102377

Haile, L. M., Kamenov, K., Briant, P. S., Orji, A. U., Steinmetz, J. D., Abdoli, A., et al. (2021). Hearing loss prevalence and years lived with disability, 1990–2019: findings from the global burden of disease study 2019. *Lancet* 397, 996–1009. doi: 10.1016/S0140-6736(21)00516-X

Hicks, E. B., Ahsan, N., Bhandari, A., Ghazala, Z., Wang, W., Pollock, B. G., et al. (2020). Associations of visual paired associative learning task with global cognition and its potential usefulness as a screening tool for Alzheimer's dementia. *Int. Psychogeriatr.* doi: 10.1017/s1041610220003841 [Epub ahead of print].

Humes, L. E. (2019). The world health organization's hearing-impairment grading system: an evaluation for unaided communication in age-related hearing loss. *Int. J. Audiol.* 58, 12–20. doi: 10.1080/14992027.2018.1518598

Jayakody, D. M. P., Almeida, O. P., Ford, A. H., Atlas, M. D., Lautenschlager, N. T., Friedland, P. L., et al. (2020). Hearing aids to support cognitive functions of older adults at risk of dementia: the HearCog trial- clinical protocols. *BMC Geriatr.* 20:508. doi: 10.1186/s12877-020-01912-1

Jayakody, D. M. P., Almeida, O. P., Speelman, C. P., Bennett, R. J., Moyle, T. C., Yiannos, J. M., et al. (2018a). Association between speech and high-frequency hearing loss and depression, anxiety and stress in older adults. *Maturitas* 110, 86–91. doi: 10.1016/j.maturitas.2018.02.002

Jayakody, D. M. P., Friedland, P. L., Eikelboom, R. H., Martins, R. N., and Sohrabi, H. R. (2018b). A novel study on association between untreated hearing loss and cognitive functions of older adults: baseline non-verbal cognitive assessment results. *Clin. Otolaryngol.* 43, 182–191. doi: 10.1111/coa.12937

Jayakody, D. M. P., Friedland, P. L., Nel, E., Martins, R. N., Atlas, M. D., and Sohrabi, H. R. (2017). Impact of cochlear implantation on cognitive functions of older adults: pilot test results. *Otol. Neurotol.* 38, e289–e295. doi: 10.1097/mao.0000000000001502

Kramer, S., Vasil, K. J., Adunka, O. F., Pisoni, D. B., and Moberly, A. C. (2018). Cognitive functions in adult cochlear implant users, cochlear implant candidates, and normal-hearing listeners. *Laryngoscope Investig Otolaryngol.* 3, 304–310. doi: 10.1002/lio2.172

Lara, E., Caballero, F. F., Rico-Uribe, L. A., Olaya, B., Haro, J. M., Ayuso-Mateos, J. L., et al. (2019). Are loneliness and social isolation associated with cognitive decline? *Int. J. Geriatr. Psychiatry* 34, 1613–1622. doi: 10.1002/gps.5174

Leung, G. T., de Jong Gierveld, J., and Lam, L. C. (2008). Validation of the Chinese translation of the 6-item de jong gierveld loneliness scale in elderly Chinese. *Int. Psychogeriatr.* 20, 1262–1272. doi: 10.1017/s1041610208007552

Leung, G. T., Fung, A. W., Tam, C. W., Lui, V. W., Chiu, H. F., Chan, W. M., et al. (2010). Examining the association between participation in late-life leisure activities and cognitive function in community-dwelling elderly Chinese in hong kong. *Int. Psychogeriatr.* 22, 2–13. doi: 10.1017/S1041610209991025

Lin, F. R., Metter, E. J., O'Brien, R. J., Resnick, S. M., Zonderman, A. B., and Ferrucci, L. (2011). Hearing loss and incident dementia. *Arch. Neurol.* 68, 214–220. doi: 10.1001/archneurol.2010.362

Lin, V. Y. W., Chung, J., Callahan, B. L., Smith, L., Gritters, N., Chen, J. M., et al. (2017). Development of cognitive screening test for the severely hearing impaired: hearing-impaired MoCA. *Laryngoscope* 127, S4–S11. doi: 10.1002/lary.26590

Livingston, G., Sommerlad, A., Orgeta, V., Costafreda, S. G., Huntley, J., Ames, D., et al. (2017). Dementia prevention, intervention, and care. *Lancet* 390, 2673–2734. doi: 10.1016/s0140-6736(17)31363-6

Lovibond, P. F., and Lovibond, S. H. (1995). The structure of negative emotional states: comparison of the depression anxiety stress scales (DASS) with the beck depression and anxiety inventories. *Behav. Res. Ther.* 33, 335–343. doi: 10.1016/0005-7967(94)00075-u

Luo, Y., He, P., Guo, C., Chen, G., Li, N., and Zheng, X. (2018). Association between sensory impairment and dementia in older adults: evidence from China. *J. Am. Geriatr. Soc.* 66, 480–486. doi: 10.1111/jgs.15202

Maharani, A., Dawes, P., Nazroo, J., Tampubolon, G., and Pendleton, N. (2018). Longitudinal relationship between hearing aid use and cognitive function in older americans. *J. Am. Geriatr. Soc.* 66, 1130–1136. doi: 10.1111/jgs.15363

Mansky, R., Marzel, A., Orav, E. J., Chocano-Bedoya, P. O., Grünheid, P., Mattle, M., et al. (2020). Playing a musical instrument is associated with slower cognitive decline in community-dwelling older adults. *Aging Clin. Exp. Res.* 32, 1577–1584. doi: 10.1007/s40520-020-01472-9

Mazzuco, S., Meggiolaro, S., Ongaro, F., and Toffolutti, V. (2017). Living arrangement and cognitive decline among older people in Europe. *Ageing Soc.* 37, 1111–1133. doi: 10.1017/S0144686X16000374

Nasreddine, Z. S., Phillips, N. A., Bédirian, V., Charbonneau, S., Whitehead, V., Collin, I., et al. (2005). The montreal cognitive assessment, MoCA: a brief screening tool for mild cognitive impairment. *J. Am. Geriatr. Soc.* 53, 695–699. doi: 10.1111/j.1532-5415.2005.53221.x

Ngo, M. K., Vu, K. P., and Strybel, T. Z. (2016). Effects of music and tonal language experience on relative pitch performance. *Am. J. Psychol.* 129, 125–134. doi: 10.5406/amerjpsyc.129.2.0125

Olsen, R. K., Nichols, E. A., Chen, J., Hunt, J. F., Glover, G. H., Gabrieli, J. D., et al. (2009). Performance-related sustained and anticipatory activity in human medial temporal lobe during delayed match-to-sample. *J. Neurosci.* 29, 11880–11890. doi: 10.1523/jneurosci.2245-09.2009

Ren, F., Luo, J., Ma, W., Xin, Q., Xu, L., Fan, Z., et al. (2019). Hearing loss and cognition among older adults in a Han Chinese cohort. *Front. Neurosci.* 13:632. doi: 10.3389/fnins.2019.00632

Salvi, R., Ding, D., Jiang, H., Chen, G. D., Greco, A., Manohar, S., et al. (2018). Hidden age-related hearing loss and hearing disorders: current knowledge and future directions. *Hearing Balance Commun.* 16, 74–82. doi: 10.1080/21695717.2018.1442282

Savikko, N., Routasalo, P., Tilvis, R. S., Strandberg, T. E., and Pitkälä, K. H. (2005). Predictors and subjective causes of loneliness in an aged population. *Arch. Gerontol. Geriatr.* 41, 223–233. doi: 10.1016/j.archger.2005.03.002

Su, P., Hsu, C. C., Lin, H. C., Huang, W. S., Yang, T. L., Hsu, W. T., et al. (2017). Age-related hearing loss and dementia: a 10-year national population-based study. *Eur. Arch. Otorhinol.* 274, 2327–2334. doi: 10.1007/s00405-017-4471-5

Verghese, J., Lipton, R. B., Katz, M. J., Hall, C. B., Derby, C. A., Kuslansky, G., et al. (2003). Leisure activities and the risk of dementia in the elderly. *N. Engl. J. Med.* 348, 2508–2516. doi: 10.1056/NEJMoa022252

Wang, K., Shi, H. S., Geng, F. L., Zou, L. Q., Tan, S. P., Wang, Y., et al. (2016). Cross-cultural validation of the depression anxiety stress scale-21 in China. *Psychol Assess* 28, e88–e100. doi: 10.1037/pas0000207

Wang, P., Li, J., Li, H. J., Huo, L., and Li, R. (2016). Mild cognitive impairment is not "Mild" at all in altered activation of episodic memory brain networks: evidence from ale meta-analysis. *Front Aging Neurosci* 8:260. doi: 10.3389/fnagi.2016.00260

Yang, F., Zhang, J., and Wang, J. (2018). Correlates of loneliness in older adults in shanghai, China: does age matter? *BMC Geriatr.* 18:300. doi: 10.1186/s12877-018-0994-x

Yang, K., and Victor, C. (2008). The prevalence of and risk factors for loneliness among older people in China. *Ageing Soc.* 28, 305–327. doi: 10.1017/S0144686X07006848

Zahodne, L. B., Stern, Y., and Manly, J. J. (2015). Differing effects of education on cognitive decline in diverse elders with low versus high educational attainment. *Neuropsychology* 29, 649–657. doi: 10.1037/neu0000141

6

Middle Ear Surgeries for Chronic Otitis Media Improve Cognitive Functions and Quality of Life of Age-Related Hearing Loss Patients

Juanjuan Gao†*, Junyan Chen*†*, Jia Xu, Sichao Liang and Haijin Yi**

Department of Otolaryngology, Head and Neck Surgery, Beijing Tsinghua Changgung Hospital, School of Clinical Medicine, Tsinghua University, Beijing, China

Correspondence:
Haijin Yi
dl7599@163.com

†*These authors share first authorship*

Age-related hearing loss (ARHL) may limit communication, which is closely associated with cognitive decline of the elderly and negatively affects their quality of life. In ARHL patients who suffer chronic otitis media (COM), hearing impairment may worsen and negatively affect the cognition and quality of life. It is currently unknown whether restoration of the conductive hearing in the mixed hearing loss through middle ear surgeries can improve both the cognitive function and quality of life of the ARHL patients. Therefore, in the present study, the ARHL patients were followed up for 6 months after middle ear surgeries for COM, and both the cognitive functions and quality of life of the patients were assessed using Montreal Cognitive Assessment and Glasgow Benefit Inventory. It was found that both the cognitive functions and quality of life were improved 6 months after middle ear surgeries. In conclusion, hearing recovery after middle ear surgeries could improve cognitive functions and quality of life of ARHL patients with COM, and surgical intervention is, hence, recommended for COM.

Keywords: middle ear surgeries, chronic otitis media, age-related hearing loss, cognition functions, quality of life

INTRODUCTION

With global aging, the number of age-related diseases is increasing. According to the WHO, hearing loss is the second cause of disability throughout the world, over 42% of which is age-related hearing loss (ARHL) (WHO, Deafness and hearing loss, 2021). ARHL, which is also called presbycusis and characterized by progressive bilateral, symmetrical, sensorineural hearing loss, may limit communication and has a close relationship with cognitive decline and even dementia (Fortunato et al., 2016; Griffiths et al., 2020), negatively affecting the quality of life. However, the exact mechanisms related to the relationship between hearing loss and cognitive impairment are still unclear. One of the mechanisms is that the impoverished environment caused by auditory deprivation can negatively change brain structure and function, leading to cognitive impairment (Peelle et al., 2011; Mamo et al., 2019; Griffiths et al., 2020; Häggström et al., 2020).

To date, the treatment of hearing impairment in senile population is hearing aids and cochlear implantation. Cochlear implantation is indicated for patients with severe to profound sensorineural hearing loss who cannot benefit from hearing aids (Clark et al., 2012). Moreover, among the elderly with hearing impairment who are indicated for hearing aid intervention, two thirds did not wear hearing aids (Fischer et al., 2011). According to the Global Burden of Disease in 2019, over 65% of the elderly aged above 60 years experienced hearing impairment. Furthermore, it has been shown that the prevalence of chronic otitis media (COM) is 10.5% in China in those aged more than 60 years (Ren and Chen, 2016). In the meantime, many old people with presbycusis may also suffer from COM that can ultimately result in mixed hearing loss (i.e., combination of conductive hearing loss and presbycusis), which makes hearing of the elderly much worse. In ARHL patients who also suffer COM, they mainly present with symptoms of hearing loss, recurrent otorrhea, and tinnitus, and it may be more inconvenient to wear hearing aids, especially when otorrhea occurs. Under both ARHL and COM, the hearing impairment may worsen, and thus, negatively affect the cognition and quality of life.

However, it is currently unknown whether correction of the conductive hearing in the mixed hearing loss through middle ear surgeries can improve both the cognitive function and quality of life of the ARHL patients.

Therefore, the aim of the present study was to investigate whether middle ear surgeries could improve the cognitive functions and quality of life in elderly patients who suffered both ARHL and COM, and to further investigate the mechanisms related to the relationship between hearing loss and cognitive impairment.

SUBJECTS AND METHODS

Subjects

Patients aged over 60 years who were diagnosed with both ARHL and COM and underwent tympanoplasty under general anesthesia by experienced otologists in our department from January 2015 to December 2020 were included in this study. The purpose of the study was explained to the patients, and informed consents were obtained from all the participants. The protocol was approved by the Ethics Committee of Beijing Tsinghua Changgung Hospital.

Exclusion criteria: (1) patients who were not benefited from middle ear surgeries [i.e., improvement of the hearing thresholds less than 15 dB or improvement of the maximum speech discrimination score (SDSmax) less than 10%]; (2) patients who had moderate, severe, or profound ARHL and are not benefited from middle ear surgeries; (3) patients who suffered active COM or were complicated by cholesteatoma; (4) patients who had history of middle ear surgeries or were combined with middle ear tumors; (5) patients who had received hearing aids before; (6) patients who had visual impairment that limited the cognitive test; and (7) patients who suffered from diseases that may interfere the cognition or quality of life during the 6-month follow-up after operation, such as cerebrovascular disease, craniocerebral trauma, schizophrenia, sudden hearing loss, severe tinnitus, etc.

Patients included in our study were examined by the same audiologist. Pure tone audiometry (PTA), SDSmax tests, and temporal bone high-resolution CT (HRCT) were carried out before operation and 6 months after operation, respectively. The average hearing threshold was calculated based on all PTA frequencies at the surgical side. Hearing loss was categorized based on the classification proposed by the WHO (World report on hearing, 2021): normal hearing, less than 20 dB HL; mild hearing loss, 20–35 dB HL; moderate hearing loss, 35–50 dB HL; moderately severe hearing loss, 50–65 dB; severe hearing loss, 65–80 dB HL; profound hearing loss, 80–95 dB HL; and complete or total hearing loss, 95 dB or greater.

Intervention

The continuity of the ossicular chain was checked by temporal bone HRCT before operation. During operation, we attempted to preserve the ossicular chain if the mobility was good (type I tympanoplasty). Ossicular chain reconstruction during tympanoplasty was performed when the incus was eroded (partial ossicular replacement prosthesis, PORP) or the stapes was eroded (total ossicular replacement prosthesis, TORP). Perforation of the tympanic membrane was repaired using a fascia graft and/or tragus cartilage.

Outcomes

Cognitive performance was assessed using Montreal Cognitive Assessment (MoCA), by a separate observer. The MoCA consists of seven subsections, including Visuospatial/Executive, Naming, Memory, and Delayed Recall, Attention, Language, Abstraction, and Orientation. According to the answers, the total score ranges from 0 to 30.

Quality of life was assessed using Glasgow Benefit Inventory 9. Glasgow Benefit Inventory is a kind of questionnaire covering 18 questions, which addresses changes in quality of life after operation. The scores for each question range from 1 to 5: 1, the worst change; 5, the best change; and 3, no change. The numerical data from the questionnaire were then converted to a GBI index score ranging from -100 (the worst outcome) to $+100$ (the best outcome). GBI consists of three subscales: general subscale scores, social support scores, and physical health scores. The Glasgow Benefit Inventory is a systematic review of the use and value of an otorhinolaryngological generic patient-recorded outcome measure.

The MoCA assessment was performed before middle ear surgeries and 6 months after operation, respectively, and the scores were compared. The GBI assessment was performed 6 months after operation.

Statistics

Quantitative data were expressed as mean $\pm$ standard deviation (SD). The parametric data were compared using the paired t-test, and $p < 0.05$ was considered statistically significant. Concerning multivariate analysis for improvement of the total MoCA scores and the seven subsection scores, $p < 0.025$ was considered statistically significant (one-tailed test). Pearson's correlation analysis was performed to determine the correlation between hearing improvement and MoCA/GBI. SPSS 22.0 program (SPSS Inc., Chicago, IL, United States) and GraphPad Prism 6.05 software (GraphPad Software, Inc., La Jolla, United States) were used for statistical analysis.

RESULTS

Demographic and Treatment of the Patients

A total number of 29 patients, including 23 females and six males, were enrolled in the study. The age of the subjects ranged from 60 to 74 years, with a mean age of 65.6 ± 4.7 years. All patients were diagnosed with ARHL and COM, and underwent tympanoplasty. The demographic features and treatments of the subjects are shown in **Table 1**.

Surgery Outcomes of the Patients

To intuitively evaluate the surgery outcomes, all patients underwent temporal bone HRCT before and after operation. Tympanoplasty in the present study could reconstruct the middle ear into a normal anatomical structure to the maximum extent (**Figures 1, 2**).

The preoperative and postoperative hearing function is shown in **Table 2**. The decrease in air–bone-gap (ABG) (dB) at 6 months after operation was found to be statistically significant (**Table 2**).

TABLE 1 | Demographics properties and treatment for all patients included.

Demographics properties and treatment for patients	
Parameters	***n***
Age in years (mean ± SD)	65.6 ± 4.7
Sex	
Female	23
Male	6
ARHL with COM	
Right ear	18
Left ear	11
Treatment	
Type I tympanoplasty	20
Tympanoplasty with PORP	8
Tympanoplasty with TORP	1

The preoperative and postoperative SDSmax is shown in **Table 3**. The improvement in SDSmax at 6 months after operation was found to be statistically significant (**Table 3**).

The Preoperative and Postoperative MoCA Total Scores Were Significantly Different

The MoCA assessment was performed before operation and 6 months after operation, respectively. The preoperative and postoperative MoCA total scores and subsection scores were compared (**Table 4**). Concerning the total MoCA scores, before operation, the mean score was 21.9 ± 4.7, and it increased to 23.9 ± 4.1 at 6 months after operation, with significant difference ($p < 0.0001$). As shown in **Table 3**, of the subsections, the language capacity was significantly improved ($p < 0.0001$). Furthermore, the Visuospatial/Executive, Memory and Delayed Recall, and Attention were also improved, with $p < 0.05$.

The multivariate analysis showed that improvement of the seven subsections at 6 months after operation was included as an independent variable, and improvement of MoCA scores was the dependent variable (**Table 5**). Our results suggested that all the improvement of Visuospatial/Executive, Naming, Language, and Abstraction had moderate correlation with MoCA improvement. Furthermore, improvement of Visuospatial/Executive, Naming, Language, and Abstraction was associated with MoCA improvement.

According to the results of paired *t*-test, it was found that the subsections of Language and Visuospatial/Executive were associated with the total MoCA improvement.

The Preoperative and Postoperative Glasgow Benefit Inventory Scores Were Significantly Different

The GBI assessment was performed 6 months after operation. The average benefit at 6 months after operation was found to be +22.8 ± 16, suggesting that the overall quality of life of the patients was significantly improved after operation. The three subscales of GBI were analyzed separately, with general benefit of

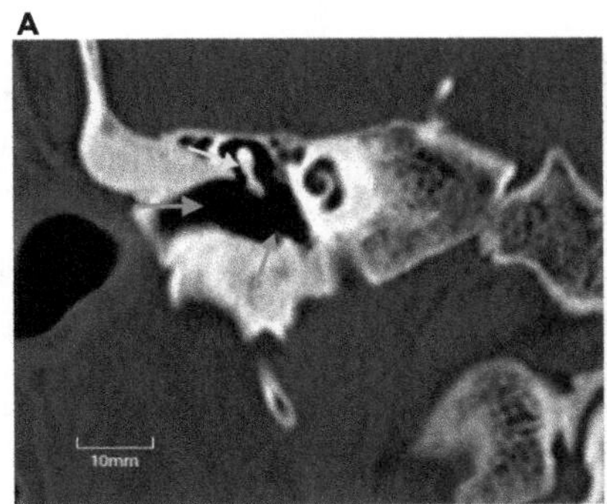

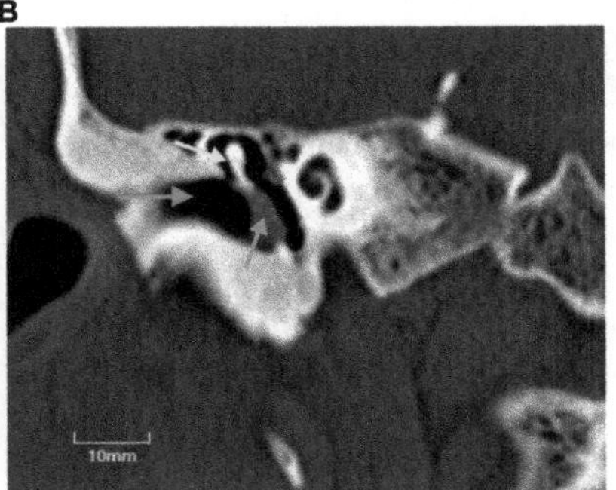

FIGURE 1 | Temporal bone high-resolution CT (HRCT) before and after operation. **(A)** HRCT before operation. **(B)** HRCT after operation. Perforation of the tympani membrane (green arrow in **A**) was repaired using a tragus cartilage (green arrow in **B**), and the middle ear was reconstructed to a normal anatomical structure to the maximum extent. Red arrow, external auditory canal; yellow arrow, malleus.

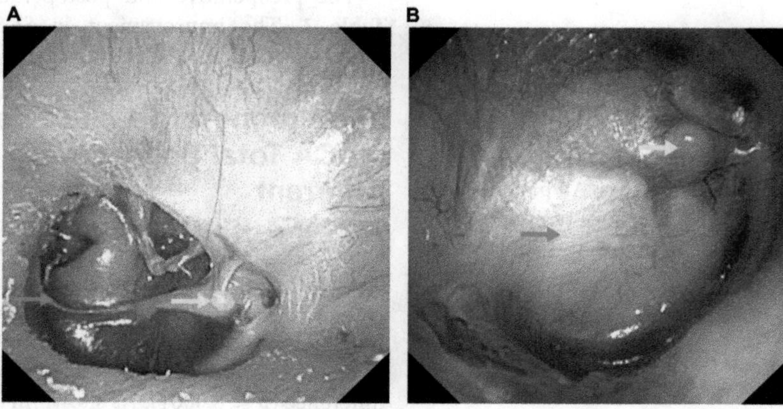

FIGURE 2 | Endoscopic pictures before and after operation. **(A)** Endoscopic picture before operation. **(B)** Endoscopic picture after operation. Perforation of the tympani membrane (red arrow in **A**) was repaired using a tragus cartilage (red arrow in **B**) and healed well. Yellow arrow, lateral process of the malleus.

TABLE 2 | Comparison of PTA preoperation and 6 months postoperation.

	Preop (dB)	Postop (dB)	*P*
BC threshold	35.1 ± 6.7	34.9 ± 6.3	0.2144
AC threshold	71.3 ± 13.6	41.5 ± 8.3	<0.0001
ABG	36.2 ± 10.9	6.6 ± 4.4	<0.0001
Hearing gain		29.6 ± 8.1	

Paired t test. Means ± SD. SD, Standard deviation; BC, bone conduction; AC, air conduction; ABG, air-bone-gap; Hearing gain, postoperative ABG − preoperative ABG.

TABLE 3 | Comparison of SDSmax preoperation and 6 months postoperation.

	Preop (%)	Postop (%)	*P* value
SDSmax	73.9 ± 21.0	94.0 ± 4.8	<0.0001
SDSmax gain		20.1 ± 17.1	

Paired t test. Means ± SD. SDSmax gain, postoperative SDSmax − preoperative SDSmax; Preop, preoperation; Postop, postoperation.

+21.4 ± 21.1, social benefit of 40.8 ± 28.4, and physical benefit of 10.3 ± 13.7.

Hearing Improvement Was Correlated With Cognitive Improvement and Improvement of Quality of Life

To explore whether cognitive improvement or improvement of quality of life is correlated with hearing improvement, Pearson's correlation analysis was performed. As shown in **Table 4**, a significant correlation between hearing improvement and the increase in MoCA scores was revealed (**Table 6**). A correlation between hearing improvement and GBI scores was also indicated (**Table 6**).

DISCUSSION

In the present study, it was found that cognitive functions were improved after tympanoplasty for ARHL and COM. ARHL is a highly prevalent disability in later life, affecting the cognitive capacity of the elderly and even leading to dementia, which has posed a serious threat to quality of life (Griffiths et al., 2020). Furthermore, when ARHL is combined with COM, hearing of the patients will be worse, and it is quite inconvenient to wear hearing aids.

Although tympanoplasty and hearing aids can both improve hearing, they are quite different from each other. Fischer et al. (2011) found that nearly two-thirds of the hearing loss patients did not wear hearing aids because of discomfort, cost, inconvenience, etc (van den Brink et al., 1996; Meyer and Hickson, 2012). Tympanoplasty conducted in the present study not only reconstructed the middle ear to a normal anatomical structure to the maximum extent but also relieved the discomfort, such as otorrhea and tinnitus. Whether hearing aids can positively influence cognitive functions of the elderly with hearing impairment is a mooting question. Mulrow et al. (1990) evaluated the cognitive performance of 188 hearing loss patients who received hearing aids or not. During a 4-month follow-up, it was concluded that cognitive functions were significantly improved in patients receiving hearing aids compared with those assigned to the waiting list (Mulrow et al., 1990). However, in a multicenter double-blind randomized placebo-controlled trial conducted by Nguyen et al. (2017), 51 hearing loss patients with Alzheimer's disease (AD) were followed up for 6 months to determine the cognitive benefit of hearing aids. The change from baseline of the Alzheimer's Disease Assessment Scale—Cognitive subscale was assessed, and it was found that cognitive functions were not improved by hearing aids (Nguyen et al., 2017). Although many studies have proven that hearing loss is associated with cognitive decline, it is difficult to obtain a consistent relationship between the use of hearing aids and cognitive improvement in ARHL patients. Nevertheless, the results of our study may explain this paradox.

In the current study, after a 6-month follow-up, it was found that the cognitive functions, especially the language capacity, were significantly improved in the ARHL patients with COM after tympanoplasty. The main difference between hearing aids

TABLE 4 | Comparison between preop and postop MoCA scores.

	Preop	Postop	*P* value	*P* value summary
Total	21.9 ± 4.7	23.9 ± 4.1	<0.0001	****
Visuospatial/Executive	2.9 ± 1.3	3.1 ± 1.2	0.0116	*
Naming	2.4 ± 0.6	2.5 ± 0.6	0.0831	ns
Memory and delayed recall	2.8 ± 1.3	3.1 ± 1.4	0.0173	*
Attention	5.2 ± 1.2	5.3 ± 1.0	0.0433	*
Language	1.9 ± 0.6	2.7 ± 0.5	<0.0001	****
Abstraction	1.1 ± 0.6	1.2 ± 0.7	0.1609	ns
Orientation	5.8 ± 0.5	5.9 ± 0.3	0.1609	ns

*Means ± SD, *P < 0.05, ****P < 0.0001, paired t test.*

TABLE 5 | Multivariate analysis for improvement of the total MoCA scores and the seven subsection scores.

	Multivariate analysis	
	Pearson correlation (r)	*P* value (one-tailed)
Visuospatial/ Executive gain	0.4838	0.0039
Naming gain	0.4475	0.0075
Memory and delayed recall gain	0.2052	0.1428
Attention gain	0.2604	0.0862
Language gain	0.4080	0.0140
Abstraction gain	0.5399	0.0013
Orientation gain	0.2376	0.1073

The improvement of the seven subsections 6 months after operation were included as independent variables, and improvement of MoCA scores was the dependent variable. Subsections gain (Visuospatial/Executive gain, Naming gain, Memory and Delayed recall gain, Attention gain, Language gain, Abstraction gain, Orientation gain): postoperative subsection score – preoperative subsection score. $p < 0.025$ was considered statistically significant (one tail test).

TABLE 6 | Correlation coefficients between hearing improvement and cognitive improvement/quality of life improvement in the present study.

	Correlation coefficient (r)	
	MoCA gain	GBI scores
Hearing gain	0.546	0.603
SDSmax gain	0.760	0.840

Pearson's correlation analysis. Hearing gain, postoperative ABG-preoperative ABG; SDSmax gain, postoperative SDSmax – preoperative SDSmax; MoCA gain, postoperative total MoCA score-preoperative total MoCA score.

and surgeries is that hearing improvement is lasting for the patients receiving surgeries, while it is discontinuous for hearing aid users (Fischer et al., 2011). Until now, the underlying mechanisms related to hearing loss and cognitive decline are unclear, and there are various hypotheses (Lin and Albert, 2014; Fulton et al., 2015; Wayne and Johnsrude, 2015; Stahl, 2017), such as cognitive load hypothesis, common cause hypothesis, and cascade hypothesis. Our study supports the cascade hypothesis (Uchida et al., 2019). The cascade hypothesis pointed out that the impoverished auditory signals can cause brain neuropathological alterations (Xie, 2016; Park et al., 2018); thus, constant hearing input is necessary for hearing loss patients to maintain or restore cognitive functions. In our study, by surgeries, the hearing stimulations are lasting for the patients, and thus, the cognition functions are significantly improved. However, the cognitive benefit is uncertain for hearing aid users because of the discontinuous hearing improvement. The same explanation may also apply to cochlear implantation, in which the hearing signals are discontinued while resting or swimming.

Furthermore, we also assessed the quality of life of the patients at 6 months after operation by Glasgow Benefit Inventory, a well-established validated questionnaire used to measure the results of surgical interventions. GBI is widely used to assess the QoL of the patients after ENT surgeries with good reliability. Furthermore, GBI, Chinese version, has also been evaluated by Yang et al. (2020), with good validity and reliability. Previous studies have shown that poor social relationships are a risk factor for incident dementia in later life (Kuiper et al., 2015; Livingston et al., 2017). In our study, patients showed a significantly positive benefit after tympanoplasty, with scores of more than +22.8, especially in social support scores (+40.8 ± 28.4). The results proved that hearing improvement improved social interactions, which may prevent cognitive decline (Hsiao et al., 2018; Qiu and Fratiglioni, 2018).

Therefore, for ARHL patients with COM, active surgical intervention for COM is recommended because hearing improvement may result in cognitive improvement and improvement of quality of life. Because tympanoplasty is performed under general anesthesia, surgical complications seem to be the greatest concern. Vartiainen and Karjalainen (1985) illustrated that no severe complications occurred in the perioperative period of patients aged 60 years. In our study, there were also no severe complications found perioperatively.

Although it was found that tympanoplasty could improve both cognitive functions and quality of life, some limitations must be considered in the present study. First, the sample size in the study was relatively small. However, as there are few similar studies, it adds important knowledge to the current field. Second, the current research focused on the relationship between hearing improvement after middle ear surgeries and cognitive functions/quality of life. The correlation between relief of other discomforts and cognitive functions, such as otorrhea and tinnitus, was not studied. In the future studies, we will conduct COM-specific questionnaires

(Wang et al., 2003; Yang et al., 2020) on the patients and further explore the relationships between them.

AUTHOR CONTRIBUTIONS

HY conceptualized and designed the study and approved the final version of the manuscript. JG prepared the draft of the manuscript and made revisions. JC followed up of patients and handled the acquisition of the data. JX and SL performed the analysis and interpretation of the data. All authors contributed to the article and approved the submitted version.

REFERENCES

Clark, J. H., Yeagle, J., Arbaje, A. I., Lin, F. R., Niparko, J. K., and Francis, H. W. (2012). Cochlear implant rehabilitation in older adults: literature review and proposal of a conceptual framework [J]. *J. Am. Geriat. Soc.* 60, 1936–1945. doi: 10.1111/j.1532-5415.2012.04150.x

Fischer, M. E., Cruickshanks, K. J., Wiley, T. L., Klein, B. E., Klein, R., and Tweed, T. S. (2011). Determinants of hearing aid acquisition in older adults [J]. *Am. J. Public Health* 101, 1449–1455. doi: 10.2105/ajph.2010.300078

Fortunato, S., Forli, F., Guglielmi, V., De Corso, E., Paludetti, G., Berrettini, S., et al. (2016). review of new insights on the association between hearing loss and cognitive decline in ageing [J]. *Acta Otorhinolaryngol. Ital.* 36, 155–166.

Fulton, S. E., Lister, J. J., Bush, A. L., Edwards, J. D., and Andel, R. (2015). Mechanisms of the hearing-cognition relationship [J]. *Sem. Hear.* 36, 140–149. doi: 10.1055/s-0035-1555117

Griffiths, T. D., Lad, M., Kumar, S., Holmes, E., McMurray, B., Maguire, E. A., et al. (2020). How can hearing loss cause dementia? [J]. *Neuron* 108, 401–412.

Häggström, J., Hederstierna, C., Rosenhall, U., Östberg, P., and Idrizbegovic, E. (2020). Prognostic value of a test of central auditory function in conversion from mild cognitive impairment to dementia [J]. *Audiol. Neurootol.* 25, 276–282. doi: 10.1159/000506621

Hsiao, Y. H., Chang, C. H., and Gean, P. W. (2018). Impact of social relationships on Alzheimer's memory impairment: mechanistic studies [J]. *J. Biomed. Sci.* 25:3. doi: 10.1186/s12929-018-0404-x

Kuiper, J. S., Zuidersma, M., Oude Voshaar, R. C., Zuidema, S. U., van den Heuvel, E. R., Stolk, R. P., et al. (2015). Social relationships and risk of dementia: a systematic review and meta-analysis of longitudinal cohort studies [J]. *Ageing Res. Rev.* 22, 39–57. doi: 10.1016/j.arr.2015.04.006

Lin, F. R., and Albert, M. (2014). Hearing loss and dementia - who is listening? [J]. *Aging Ment. Health* 18, 671–673.

Livingston, G., Sommerlad, A., Orgeta, V., Costafreda, S. G., Huntley, J., Ames, D., et al. (2017). Dementia prevention, intervention, and care [J]. *Lancet* 390, 2673–2734.

Mamo, S. K., Reed, N. S., Sharrett, A. R., Albert, M. S., Coresh, J., Mosley, T. H., et al. (2019). Relationship between domain-specific cognitive function and speech-in-noise performance in older adults: the atherosclerosis risk in communities hearing pilot study [J]. *Am. J. Audiol.* 28, 1006–1014. doi: 10.1044/2019_AJA-19-00043

Meyer, C., and Hickson, L. (2012). What factors influence help-seeking for hearing impairment and hearing aid adoption in older adults? [J]. *Int. J. Audiol.* 51, 66–74.

Mulrow, C. D., Aguilar, C., Endicott, J. E., Tuley, M. R., Velez, R., Charlip, W. S., et al. (1990). Quality-of-life changes and hearing impairment. A randomized trial [J]. *Ann. Intern. Med.* 113, 188–194. doi: 10.7326/0003-4819-113-3-188

Nguyen, M. F., Bonnefoy, M., Adrait, A., Gueugnon, M., Petitot, C., Collet, L., et al. (2017). Efficacy of hearing aids on the cognitive status of patients with alzheimer's disease and hearing loss: a multicenter controlled randomized trial [J]. *J. Alzheimers Dis.* 58, 123–137. doi: 10.3233/JAD-160793

Park, S. Y., Kim, M. J., Kim, H. L., Kim, D. K., Yeo, S. W., and Park, S. N. (2018). Cognitive decline and increased hippocampal p-tau expression in mice with hearing loss [J]. *Behav. Brain Res.* 342, 19–26. doi: 10.1016/j.bbr.2018.01.003

Peelle, J. E., Troiani, V., Grossman, M., and Wingfield, A. (2011). Hearing loss in older adults affects neural systems supporting speech comprehension [J]. *J. Neurosci.* 31, 12638–12643.

Qiu, C., and Fratiglioni, L. (2018). Aging without dementia is achievable: current evidence from epidemiological research [J]. *J. Alzheimers Dis.* 62, 933–942. doi: 10.3233/jad-171037

Ren, D. D., and Chen, Z. S. (2016). Etiological investigation and analysis on hearing loss of chinese people over 60 years old [J]. *Chin. J. Rehabil. Theory Pract.* 22:3.

Stahl, S. M. (2017). Does treating hearing loss prevent or slow the progress of dementia? Hearing is not all in the ears, but who's listening? [J]. *CNS Spectr.* 22, 247–250.

Uchida, Y., Sugiura, S., Nishita, Y., Saji, N., Sone, M., and Ueda, H. (2019). Age-related hearing loss and cognitive decline - The potential mechanisms linking the two [J]. *Auris Nasus Larynx* 46, 1–9. doi: 10.1016/j.anl.2018.08.010

van den Brink, R. H., Wit, H. P., Kempen, G. I., and van Heuvelen, M. J. (1996). Attitude and help-seeking for hearing impairment [J]. *Br. J. Audiol.* 30, 313–324.

Vartiainen, E., and Karjalainen, S. (1985). Surgery in elderly patients with chronic otitis media [J]. *Arch. Otolaryngol.* 111, 509–510. doi: 10.1001/archotol.1985.00800100057006

Wang, P. C., Chu, C. C., Liang, S. C., Tai, C. J., and Gliklich, R. E. (2003). Validation assessment of the Chinese-version Chronic Ear Survey: a comparison between data from English and Chinese versions [J]. *Ann. Otol. Rhinol. Laryngol.* 112, 85–90. doi: 10.1177/000348940311200116

Wayne, R. V., and Johnsrude, I. S. (2015). A review of causal mechanisms underlying the link between age-related hearing loss and cognitive decline [J]. *Ageing Res. Rev.* 23(Pt B), 154–166. doi: 10.1016/j.arr.2015.06.002

Xie, R. (2016). Transmission of auditory sensory information decreases in rate and temporal precision at the endbulb of Held synapse during age-related hearing loss [J]. *J. Neurophysiol.* 116, 2695–2705. doi: 10.1152/jn.00472.2016

Yang, R., Zhang, Y., Han, W., Li, Y., Li, S., Ke, J., et al. (2020). Measuring health-related quality of life in chronic otitis media in a Chinese population: cultural adaption and validation of the Zurich Chronic Middle Ear Inventory (ZCMEI-21-Chn) [J]. *Health Qual. Life Outcomes* 18:218.

7

The Correlation Between Hearing Loss, Especially High-Frequency Hearing Loss and Cognitive Decline Among the Elderly

Tongxiang Diao[1†], Xin Ma[1†], Junbo Zhang[2†], Maoli Duan[3,4] and Lisheng Yu[1*]*

[1] Department of Otolaryngology, Head and Neck Surgery, People's Hospital, Peking University, Beijing, China, [2] Department of Otolaryngology, Head and Neck Surgery, Peking University First Hospital, Beijing, China, [3] Department of Clinical Science, Intervention and Technology, Karolinska Institute, Stockholm, Sweden, [4] Department of Otolaryngology, Head and Neck Surgery & Audiology and Neurotology, Karolinska University Hospital, Karolinska Institute, Stockholm, Sweden

***Correspondence:**
Maoli Duan
maoli.duan@ki.se
Lisheng Yu
yulish68@163.com

† These authors have contributed equally to this work and share first authorship

Objective: The relation between cognition and hearing loss has been increasingly paid high attention, however, few studies have focused on the role of high-frequency hearing loss in cognitive decline. This study is oriented to role of hearing loss especially high-frequency hearing loss in cognitive impairment among elderly people (age $\geq$ 60 years).

Methods: The Montreal Cognitive Assessment Scale (MoCA) and pure tone audiometry were used to investigate the hearing loss and cognitive function of 201 elderly people older than 60 years. Factors possibly related to cognitive impairment including age, years of education, occupation, living conditions, history of otologic diseases, and high blood pressure were registered. This study consisted of two parts. First, univariate analysis and multiple linear regressions were performed to analyze the possible influencing factors of cognitive function among the 201 elderly people. Second, average hearing thresholds of low frequencies (250, 500 Hz), intermediate frequencies (1 k, 2 kHz), and high frequencies (4 k, 8 kHz) were calculated to screen out 40 cases with high-frequency hearing loss alone and 18 cases with normal hearing. Univariate analysis was used to compare the general condition, cognitive function, and each cognitive domain between the two groups, analyzing the relation between high-frequency hearing loss and cognitive function.

Result: We found that age, years of education, pure tone average (PTA), occupation, living condition, history of otologic diseases, years of self-reported hearing loss, and hypertension history were related to cognitive function. Furthermore, age, education experience, duration of self-reported hearing loss, and hypertension were independent factors ($p < 0.05$). PTA was negatively related with attention, orientation, and general cognition ($p < 0.05$). There were only 18 cases (9.0%) with normal hearing, and 40 cases (19.9%) with abnormal high-frequency hearing alone. The overall cognitive function showed no significant difference between them ($p > 0.05$); in contrast, the speech and abstract ability were significantly decreased in cases with high-frequency hearing loss ($p < 0.05$).

Conclusion: The increase of PTA among the elderly may affect the overall cognition by reducing attention and orientation. High-frequency hearing loss alone can affect the language and abstract ability to a certain extent, which is worthy of more attention.

Keywords: hearing loss, high-frequency hearing loss, cognition, language ability, abstract ability

INTRODUCTION

Hearing loss has become the third leading disability factor in the worldwide according to the latest researches, which is an important factor affecting human health, especially the health of the elderly (GBD 2016 Disease and Injury Incidence and Prevalence Collaborators, 2017). In recent years, the correlation between hearing loss and cognitive decline has attracted more and more attention. Numerous studies, including several systematic review articles and meta-analyses, have shown that hearing loss is remarkably related with cognitive dysfunction, impaired performance of various cognitive domains, and the occurrence of dementia (Thomson et al., 2017; Zheng et al., 2017; Ford et al., 2018; Loughrey et al., 2018). Cognitive impairment includes memory, learning, orientation, comprehension, judgment, calculation, language, visuospatial, analysis and problem-solving ability and is often accompanied by mental, behavioral, and personality abnormalities at a certain stage of the disease process (Arlington, 2013). A meta-analysis conducted by Loughrey et al. (2018) found that there was a significant association between age-related hearing loss (ARHL) and cognitive impairment [odds ratio, 1.22; 95% confidence interval (CI), 1.09–1.36] among the prospective cohort studies and a small but statistically significant association between ARHL and seven cognitive domains, such as episodic memory and processing speed, among the cohort studies (Loughrey et al., 2018). Meanwhile, a novel lifespan-based model of dementia risk was reported by the Lancet Commission on Dementia Prevention, Intervention, and Care and simultaneously published in *Lancet* at the 2017 Alzheimer's Association International Conference in London (Livingston et al., 2017). Hearing loss was positioned as the largest potentially modifiable risk factor for dementia among nine health and lifestyle factors. The Lancet Commission found that midlife hearing loss, if eliminated, might reduce the risk of dementia by 9%. The underlying causal mechanisms leading to the connection between the two are not well understood. Several possible relationships have been postulated. (1) cognitive load on perception hypothesis (cognitive decline may reduce the cognitive resources that are available for auditory perception, manifesting as hearing loss) (Lin et al., 2013); (2) sensory-deprivation hypothesis (hearing loss causes cognitive decline that is permanent) (Lindenberger and Baltes, 1994); (3) information-degradation hypothesis (hearing loss causes cognitive decline which is potentially remediable) (Pichora-Fuller, 2003); and (4) common cause hypothesis (a third factor causes both declines) (Baltes and Lindenberger, 1997).

However, most previous studies have focused on the correlation between speech-frequency hearing loss and cognitive function, while ignoring the importance of high-frequency hearing loss. Studies have shown that the incidence of high-frequency hearing loss is significantly higher than that of speech frequency (REF). Among people aged 20 to 29 years, the proportion of combined speech-frequency hearing loss is only 2.2%, whereas the proportion of high-frequency hearing loss can be as high as 7% (Hoffman et al., 2017). And this difference is more obvious in the elderly group. Among people aged 60 to 69 years, the incidence of speech-frequency hearing loss is 39.3%, and the proportion of high-frequency hearing loss can be as high as 68% (Hoffman et al., 2017). These data indicate that high-frequency hearing tends to decline earlier than speech-frequency hearing. Previously, it was believed that high-frequency hearing loss would not affect the daily life of the patients significantly. However, with the introduction of hidden hearing loss, the important role of high-frequency hearing in the speech recognition has attracted more and more attention (Monson et al., 2019). Some studies have already shown that high-frequency hearing is key for speech recognition, especially speech perception in noise (George et al., 2007; Motlagh Zadeh et al., 2019; Varnet et al., 2019). However, there is no study that has focused on the correlation between pure high-frequency hearing loss and cognitive function except for speech perception. This study chose the elderly as the subjects and studied the correlation between average of hearing loss, especially the degree of pure high-frequency hearing loss, and cognitive function to explore the relationship between hearing loss and cognitive decline and the underline mechanism, providing a theoretical basis for early detection and prevention of senile cognitive decline in clinical practice.

MATERIALS AND METHODS

Participants

A total of 201 elderly volunteers were enrolled in this study from the free clinic of 2019 Ear Day at Peking University People's Hospital. The detailed inclusion criteria were as follows: (1) age $\geq$ 60 years, (2) sensorineural hearing loss, and no significant difference in hearing threshold between two ears, (3) no history of otitis media, sudden deafness history, and acoustic neuroma, and (4) no mental illness history and could cooperate with the whole study process. All study subjects underwent pure tone audiometry test, otoscope examination, and cognitive function assessment. The basic information including sex, age, living condition, years of education, occupation, self-reported hearing loss, tinnitus, ear diseases history, and some chronic disease history (hypertension, diabetes, and hyperlipidemia) was collected by face-to-face survey with questionnaires. All included subjects and (or) their family members were asked to fill the questionnaire under the supervision of the same experienced physician.

Study Design

A questionnaire on cognitive function and influencing factors was designed according to previous study (Hugo and Ganguli, 2014). All the elderly participants were examined during the Ear Day free clinic. When the survey was completed, the questionnaires and related examination data were returned.

Cognitive Function Assessment

The cognitive function assessments of all participants were completed with a unified Montreal Cognitive Assessment Scale (MoCA) questionnaire survey, which was administered to assess the global cognitive level by the same neurologist. The MoCA scale consisted of eight several subtasks to assess different cognitive domains, of which the immediate memory subdomain is not scored. The other seven cognitive domains and corresponding scores were visuospatial and executive function for 5 points, language ability for 3 points, attention for 6 points, orientation for 6 points, delayed memory for 5 points, naming for 3 points, and abstract ability for 2 points (Nasreddine et al., 2005). Moreover, existing studies have shown that the scores of different cognitive domains of MoCA assessment result may represent the different cognitive function (Faria et al., 2020; Rossetto et al., 2020).

Auditory and Otoscope Tests

The pure tone audiometry and the otoscope examination were all completed in the ENT departments of Peking University People's Hospital. According to the World Health Organization criteria (1997), the average value of 500−, 1, 000−, 2, 000−, and 4,000-Hz air conduction pure tone average (PTA) hearing thresholds was used for defining the hearing loss degree, including normal hearing (≤25 dB), mild (26–40 dB), moderate (41–60 dB), severe (61–80 dB), and profound hearing loss (>80 dB). On the other hand, the average hearing thresholds of low frequencies (250, 500 Hz), intermediate frequencies (1 k, 2 kHz), and high frequencies (4 k, 8 kHz) were all calculated separately to select a group of subjects with hearing loss at only high frequencies (4 k, 8 kHz) (HHL group). Except for average hearing threshold of 4 and 8 k is greater than 25 dB, the hearing thresholds of other frequencies (250 Hz, 500 Hz, 1 k, 2 k) of patients in the HHL group are all not higher than 25 dB (HHL group).

Ethics Statement

The Peking University People's Hospital Ethical permission committee approved study (2019PHB084-01), and all subjects provided their informed consents.

TABLE 1 | Factors related to cognitive function among the elderly.

Univariable analysis			
Variable	**Number (percentage)**	**Cognitive function ($\bar{x} \pm \mu$)**	***p***
Sex (female)	101/201 (50.2%)	24.30 ± 3.80	0.139
Age (years)	201	−0.116 (−0.201, −0.030)	0.008*
Occupation			0.027*
Physical	137/201 (68.16%)	23.797 ± 4.0832	
Mental	64/201 (31.84%)	25.029 ± 3.4170	
Education experience (years)	201	0.417 (0.262, 0.572)	0.000*
Living situation			
Living with spouse	158/201 (78.61%)	25.006 ± 3.2644	0.028*
Others	43/201 (21.39%)	23.279 ± 4.7073	
Ear disease history	153/201 (76.1%)	24.3 ± 3.9	
No	37/201 (18.4%)	25.8 ± 2.8	0.044*
Otitis media	11/201 (5.5%)	25.7 ± 2.4	
Sudden deafness			
Hypertension	96/201 (47.8%)	24.000 ± 3.8906	0.022*
Diabetes	64/201 (31.84%)	24.094 ± 4.0147	0.153
Hyperlipidemia	99/201 (49.25%)	24.354 ± 3.5637	0.283
PTA			
≤25 dBHL	39/201 (19.40%)	39 25.051 ± 2.5950	
26–40 dBHL	65/201 (32.34%)	65 25.292 ± 3.7279	
41–60 dBHL	80/201 (39.80%)	80 24.375 ± 3.8397	0.016*
61–80 dBHL	17/201 (8.46%)	17 22.235 ± 4.0083	
Self-reported hearing loss	169/201 (84.08%)	24.497 ± 3.7783	0.270
Duration of self-reported hearing loss (years)			
≤5 y	153/201 (76.12%)	24.908 ± 3.4724	0.048*
>5 y	48/201 (23.88%)	23.708 ± 4.1767	
Multivariable analysis			
Variable	***B***	**95% CI**	***p***
Age	−0.191	(−0.271, −0.111)	0.000*
Education experience (years)	0.512	(0.361, 0.663)	0.000*
Duration of self-reported hearing loss (years)	−1.164	(−2.218, −0.111)	0.030*
Hypertension	−0.990	(−1.895, −0.086)	0.032*

* *Statistical significance.*

Statistical Analysis

Statistical analyses in this study were performed with SPSS 24.0 software package (IBM, Armonk, NY, United States). This study consisted of two parts. First, univariate analysis and multiple linear regressions were performed to analyze the possible influencing factors of cognitive function among the 201 elderly people. Second, average hearing thresholds of low frequencies (250, 500 Hz), intermediate frequencies (1 k, 2 kHz), and high frequencies (4 k, 8 kHz) were calculated to screen out 40 cases with high-frequency hearing loss alone (HHL) and 18 cases with absolutely normal hearing (NH). Univariate analysis was used to compare the general condition, cognitive function, and each cognitive domain between the two groups, analyzing the relation between high-frequency hearing loss and cognitive function. All the statistical significances were at the level $p < 0.05$.

RESULTS

Epidemiology and Clinical Characteristics of All the Participants

There were 201 participants (101 females, 50.2%; 100 males, 49.8%). The overall average age was 72.06 ± 5.90 years, with a range of 60 to 90 years. According to PTA values, the number of participants with normal hearing, mild, moderate, severe, and profound hearing loss were 39 (19.4%), 65 (32.3%), 80 (39.8%), 17 (8.5%), and 0 (0%), respectively. The overall average score of MoCA scale assessment was 24.64 ± 3.68, with a range of 11 to 30.

Factors Related to Cognitive Function in the Elderly

As shown in **Table 1**, the univariate analysis showed that age, education experience, occupation, living conditions, ear diseases history, hypertension, PTA, and years of self-reported hearing loss remarkably correlated with the results of cognitive assessment ($p < 0.05$). The above factors were all included in a multivariate analysis, which indicated that age, years of education, years of self-reported hearing loss, and hypertension were independent factors related to cognitive function ($p < 0.05$). The elderly with older age, shorter years of education, longer time of self-conscious hearing loss, and high blood pressure were more likely to be associated with cognitive dysfunction.

Correlation Between Pure Tone Average and Different Cognitive Domains Among the Elderly

Among the elderly people with different hearing levels, the comparisons of cognitive functions suggested that abstract and orientation abilities, and overall cognitive function all deteriorate with the increasing hearing loss degrees ($p < 0.05$). No other cognitive domains showed significant differences between these groups ($p > 0.05$) (**Table 2**).

Clinical Characteristics and Cognitive Function of Subjects in HHL Group

There were only 18 subjects (9.0%) with completely normal hearing levels (<25 dB) at all frequencies tested, including 0.25, 0.5, 1.0, 2.0, 3.0, 4.0, and 8.0 kHz (normal hearing group, NH group). On the other hand, the number of subjects with hearing loss (>25 dB) at only high frequencies (4.0 k and 8.0 kHz) was 40 (19.9%) (high-frequency hearing loss group, HHL group). As shown in **Table 3**, the overall PTA and the PTA at high frequencies (PTA-HF) were both significantly higher in the HHL group than in the NH group ($p = 0.013$ vs. $p < 0.001$). Meanwhile, no other basic information we studied showed significant differences between these two groups ($p > 0.05$). As shown in **Table 4** and **Figures 1**, **2**, the comparisons of cognitive function between these two groups suggested that the language and abstract ability scores were both significantly lower in the HHL group than in the NH group ($p = 0.027$ vs. $p = 0.005$). Meanwhile, no significant differences were found in other cognitive domains and overall cognitive function ($p > 0.05$).

DISCUSSION

As the aging problem increasing worldwide, hearing loss as one of the most common problems among the elderly has drawn more and more attention. Studies have shown that hearing loss is a modifiable age-associated condition linked to dementia (Livingston et al., 2017); however, the underlying mechanism of the association between hearing loss and cognitive decline remains unclear. Of all the 201 elderly participants in this study, only 18 had completely normal hearing. Among the remaining 183 participants, 143 had speech-frequency hearing loss (78.14%), and 40 had only high-frequency hearing loss (21.86%). In this study, we found that the hearing loss is related but not independent influencing factor of cognitive decline, which mainly affects cognitive function by affecting abstract and orientation ability. The age, years of education, years of self-reported hearing loss, and hypertension are independent factors related to the cognitive function of the elderly. In addition, although pure high-frequency hearing loss had no remarkable relevance with general cognitive function, it affected abstract and speech ability.

Related Factors of Cognitive Function Among the Elderly

The results of this study indicated that among the elderly, occupation, living conditions, ear diseases history, and PTA were the influencing but not independent influencing factors of cognitive function, whereas age, educational experience, years of self-reported hearing loss, and whether accompanied by hypertension were independent related factors of cognitive function. Among them, age is unchangeable, hypertension can be regulated by tertiary prevention, the years of education requires the joint efforts of the whole society, whereas the years of self-reported hearing loss is the only factor that can be changed by early hearing interventions.

As early as 2001, a clinical study conducted by Gomez et al. (2001) proposed that the degree of self-conscious hearing loss could be used as a simple way to self-evaluation of hearing level. Amieva et al. (2015) also proposed that self-reported hearing loss was an independent factor of the cognitive decline among the elderly, and the use of hearing aids can slow down the process of cognitive decline. From the behavior perspective, a number of elderly people with hearing loss often choose to avoid social activities because of the impact of hearing loss on communication, which leads to social isolation and coexistence of the decrease in communication between family and friends eventually leading to depression or cognitive impairment (Brink and Stones, 2007; Mick et al., 2014; Pichora-Fuller et al., 2015). From the neurological perspective, on the one hand, chronic hearing loss will lead to a decrease in the activity of the central auditory system, trigger the compensation mechanism, and ultimately lead to the associated disorder of the auditory center-limbic system and the disuse atrophy of the frontal lobe. On the other hand, hearing loss will cause the reduction of the cognitive capacity, which mainly represents the ability to minimize pathological damage by

TABLE 2 | Correlation between PTA and different cognitive domains among the elderly.

	PTA				*p*
	≤25 dBHL *n* = 39	26 ~ 40 dBHL *n* = 65	41 ~ 60 dBHL *n* = 80	61 ~ 80 dBHL *n* = 17	
Visual spatial and executive function	4.256 ± 0.8801	4.246 ± 1.1596	4.100 ± 1.0626	3.765 ± 1.0326	0.344
Naming	2.795 ± 0.4091	2.800 ± 0.4402	2.863 ± 0.4132	2.882 ± 0.3321	0.711
Attention	5.436 ± 0.9678	5.477 ± 0.8680	5.375 ± 0.8624	5.235 ± 1.1472	0.771
Language	2.231 ± 0.7420	2.169 ± 0.7618	1.988 ± 0.9345	1.941 ± 1.2976	0.384
Abstract	1.667 ± 0.5298	1.554 ± 0.6381	1.525 ± 0.6931	0.882 ± 0.7812	0.001*
Delayed memory	2.667 ± 1.3443	3.138 ± 1.4018	2.663 ± 1.7059	2.294 ± 1.7594	0.125
Orientation	6.000 ± 0.0000	5.908 ± 0.3411	5.863 ± 0.4132	5.235 ± 1.2005	0.000*
Total	25.051 ± 2.5950	25.29 ± 3.7279	24.375 ± 3.8397	22.235 ± 4.0083	0.016*

** Statistical significance.*

cognitive pregeneration processes or activation of compensatory mechanisms (Stern, 2002; Tun et al., 2009) in the central system. As theorized by the cognitive load hypothesis, that hearing loss leads to degraded auditory signals, greater cognitive resources being required for auditory perceptual processing, and diversion from other cognitive tasks to effortful listening, eventually resulting in cognitive reserve depletion (Tun et al., 2009).

However, there are several researchers who believe that the association between hearing loss and cognitive impairment is caused by overestimation, namely, overdiagnosis hypothesis, in which degraded hearing, rather than cognitive function, impacts performance on certain neuropsychological tests. First, despite that hearing loss usually occurs earlier than dementia or cognitive impairment, suggesting hearing loss may lead to dementia or cognitive impairment, it may also be due to the fact that patients with hearing loss usually receive more neuropsychological tests. Therefore, it is easier to diagnose the accompanying cognitive impairment (Fulton et al., 2015). Or more broadly speaking, hearing loss itself can cause bias in neuropsychological evaluations, because most neuropsychological evaluations need to be achieved through speech. Furthermore, as verbal instructions or tasks that rely considerably on hearing are used during cognitive assessments, individuals with hearing difficulty are sometimes at a disadvantage. The selection of tests for cognitive measures that are heavily loaded for verbal skills is not appropriate for individuals with hearing difficulty; however, even when the response mode of a measure is non-verbal, instructions for tasks can be complex or difficult to perceive for the hearing-impaired. Any degree of hearing loss can affect functioning and test performance for neuropsychological assessments (Hill-Briggs et al., 2007; Dupuis et al., 2015; Jorgensen et al., 2016).

TABLE 3 | The epidemiology and clinical characteristics of the HHL group and NH groups.

	Total (*n* = 58)	NH (*n* = 18)	HHL (*n* = 40)	*p*
Sex (female)	35	13/35 (37.14%)	22/35 (62.86%)	0.215
Age (years)	69.78 ± 2.96	69.17 ± 3.45	70.05 ± 2.72	0.297
PTA	21.96 ± 6.71	18.75 ± 7.30	23.41 ± 5.96	0.013*
PTA-HF	36.51 ± 13.92	21.81 ± 8.04	43.13 ± 10.50	<0.001*
Living situation				0.215
Living with spouse	8	1/8 (12.5%)	7/8 (87.5%)	
Others	50	17/50 (34.00%)	33/50 (66.00%)	
Education experience (years)	13.34 ± 2.91	13.06 ± 3.72	13.48 ± 2.52	0.667
Occupation				0.282
Physical	17	7/17 (41.18%)	10/17 (58.82%)	
Mental	40	10/40 (25.00%)	30/40 (75.00%)	
Self-reported hearing loss	22	8/22 (36.36%)	14/22 (63.64%)	0.493
Duration of self-reported hearing loss (years)				1.000
≤5y	52	16/52 (30.77%)	36/52 (69.23%)	
>5y	6	2/6 (33.33%)	4/6 (66.67%)	
Tinnitus	23	8/23 (34.78%)	15/23 (65.22%)	0.617
Hypertension	29	12/29 (41.38%)	17/29 (58.62%)	0.089
Diabetes	19	5/19 (26.32%)	14/19 (73.68%)	0.588
Hyperlipidemia	31	9/31 (29.03%)	22/31 (70.97%)	0.724

** Statistical significance.*

TABLE 4 | Cognitive function and different cognitive domains of the HHL and NH groups.

	Total (*n* = 58)	NH (*n* = 18)	HHL (*n* = 40)	*p*
Visual spatial and executive function	4.40 ± 0.82	4.44 ± 0.62	4.38 ± 0.90	0.767
Naming	2.79 ± 0.45	2.89 ± 0.32	2.75 ± 0.49	0.209
Attention	5.52 ± 0.86	5.56 ± 0.71	5.50 ± 0.93	0.823
Language	2.38 ± 0.67	2.67 ± 0.49	2.25 ± 0.71	0.027*
Abstract	1.72 ± 0.52	1.94 ± 0.24	1.63 ± 0.59	0.005*
Delayed memory	2.95 ± 1.29	2.78 ± 1.31	3.03 ± 1.29	0.504
Orientation	5.97 ± 0.18	6.00 ± 0.00	5.95 ± 0.22	0.160
Total	25.69 ± 2.64	26.17 ± 2.31	25.48 ± 2.78	0.361

** Statistical significance.*

Correlation Between Hearing Loss and Cognitive Function Among the Elderly

In this study, we found that hearing loss has significantly related to the cognitive decline, which is consistent with the previous study conducted by Lin et al. (2011), They found the annual hearing threshold of participants with dementia was higher than that of those without dementia, and the patients with severe

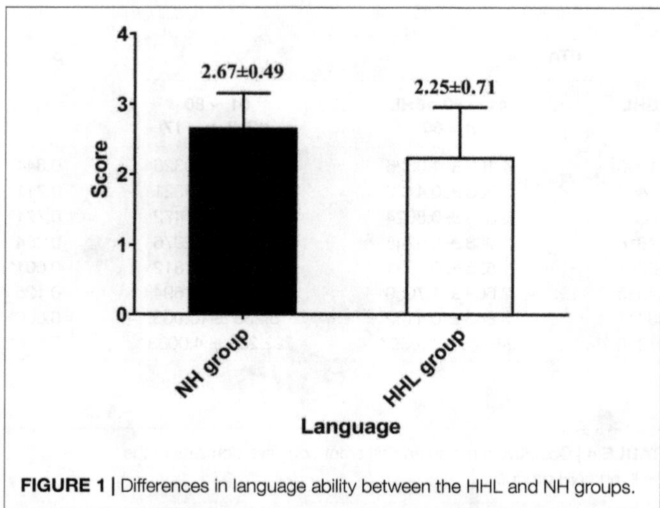

FIGURE 1 | Differences in language ability between the HHL and NH groups.

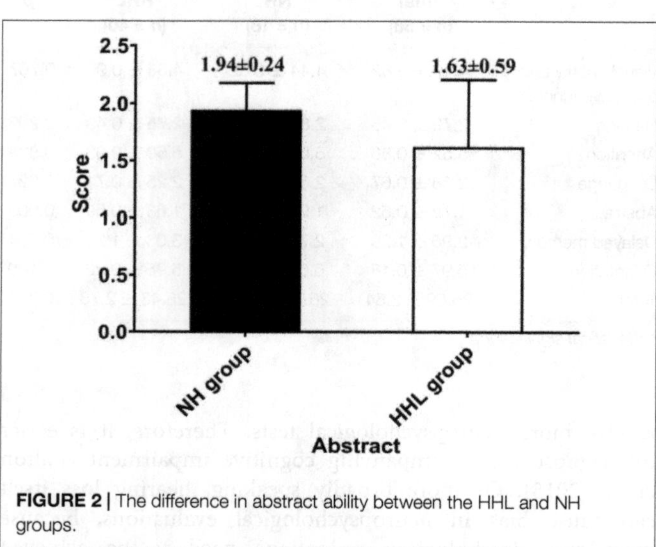

FIGURE 2 | The difference in abstract ability between the HHL and NH groups.

hearing loss suffering from dementia was 4.9 times of those with normal hearing.

In addition, our results suggested that the PTA has a significant correlation with orientation and abstract ability, indicating that hearing loss might affect the cognitive function by affecting orientation and abstract ability. Orientation is the ability of the individual to perceive signal and recognize the surrounding environment (time, place/space, and person) and one's own state (name, age, occupation, etc.). Hearing loss causes the decline of hearing sensitivity and the speech perception in noise (Yamasoba et al., 2013), consequently affects the individual's recognition of the surrounding environment and their own state, and ultimately leads to disorientation. It has shown that chronic hearing loss can lead to a decline of central auditory function (Peelle et al., 2011), activating the central compensation mechanism (Wild et al., 2012), and ultimately leading to the associated disorder of the auditory central-limbic system and the disuse atrophy of the frontal lobe (Wager et al., 2008; Lin et al., 2014). As we know, the frontal lobe is related to physical activities and mental activities such as judgment, predictability, emotion, and mood, which will reduce cognitive activity, increase the risk of depression, and lead to executive and emotional disorders. Liu et al. (2014) also found that the impairment of frontal lobe is more likely to be accompanied by the orientation and abstract disorders, which may be caused by the combined effects of nerve degeneration and vascular injury, which is consistent with the results of this study.

The Correlation Between High-Frequency Hearing Impairment and Cognitive Function

Presbycusis, the hearing of the old man, has been recognized since the late 19th century (Kearns, 1977), and the high frequency is first affected. Studies have shown that degenerative changes in the inner ear of aged humans and other mammals occur among the sensory hair cells, the primary sensory neurons or spiral ganglion cells, and the cells of the stria vascularis and spiral ligament including the vasculature (Keithley, 2020). Neural degeneration is a very common pathology of the aged inner ear, both in humans and other animals, and occurs in both the apical and basal cochlear turns (Makary et al., 2011; Viana et al., 2015). In fact, the magnitude of neuronal loss exceeds that of inner hair cell loss in both humans and other mammals (Chen et al., 2006; Wu et al., 2019). So we deemed that the pure high-frequency hearing loss of the elderly was more likely to be caused by neural degeneration. In 2020, a study conducted by Liu et al. on APP/PS1 Alzheimer's disease mice also found that the hearing loss appeared at high frequency as early as 2 months old, prior to the reported occurrence of spatial learning deficit at 6 to 7 months of age in this AD mouse model. The hearing loss was progressive and extended from high frequency to low frequency. We speculated that high-frequency hearing is more closely related to cognitive function (Liu et al., 2020).

The results of this study showed that pure high-frequency hearing loss has no obvious correlation with the general cognitive function, but was significantly related with the abstract and speech function; that is, early high-frequency hearing loss will affect the speech and abstract ability among the elderly. Some studies have already shown that the high-frequency sensitivity has a significant correlation with speech recognition ability, especially speech perception in noise (Monson et al., 2019),which is consistent with the results of this study. However, it is widely believed that the high-frequency hearing plays little or no role in speech perception, being beyond the information-bearing traditional "speech bandwidth." Therefore, although the incidence of high-frequency hearing loss is significantly higher than that of speech frequency, there are still few studies on the correlation between pure high-frequency hearing loss and cognitive decline except for the speech perception. Jung and Haier (2007) hypothesized that the neural basis of human intelligence is attributable to activities in the frontal–parietal functional network. In their hypothesis, collected visual and auditory information is processed in the occipital and temporal cortices and then fed forward to the parietal cortex where structural symbolism, abstraction, and elaboration emerge (Apostolova et al., 2006). Therefore, once the auditory function is damaged, it will affect the subsequent abstraction and elaboration emerge process, which is consistent with our results.

LIMITATIONS

Of course, this study also has some limitations. First, the 201 elderly volunteers were enrolled from the free clinic of 2019 Ear Day at Peking University People's Hospital, which would cause selection bias, resulting in the higher proportion of hearing loss in this study. Second, the sample size of this study is relatively small, only 40 cases of pure high-frequency hearing loss, and 18 cases of normal hearing. Finally, in this study, we chose only a general cognitive assessment scale, the MoCA scale, for ease of operation and separate scales for each cognitive domain, and cognitive behavioral tests will be added in subsequent studies.

CONCLUSION

Age, hypertension, years of self-reported hearing loss, and years of education are independent related factors for cognitive decline among the elderly. PTA was not an independent influencing factor of cognitive function, which may affect cognitive function by influencing orientation and abstract ability. Pure high-frequency hearing loss may affect the speech and abstract ability of elderly patients, but not significantly affect their global cognitive function. The early high-frequency hearing loss is not easy to be detected by the elderly, as it is relatively mild and does not significantly affect the cognitive ability. But as the result of this study, it may have a certain impact on the speech and abstract ability, which is necessary to be detected and prevented early.

AUTHOR CONTRIBUTIONS

TD, XM, JZ, MD, and LY contributed to the study conception and design. TD, XM, and JZ supervised this research and wrote the first draft of the manuscript. All authors contributed to the material preparation, data collection, and read and approved the final manuscript.

REFERENCES

Amieva, H., Ouvrard, C., Giulioli, C., Meillon, C., Rullier, L., and Dartigues, J. F. (2015). Self-reported hearing loss, hearing aids, and cognitive decline in elderly adults: a 25-year study. *J. Am. Geriatr. Soc.* 63, 2099–2104. doi: 10.1111/jgs.13649

Apostolova, L. G., Lu, P. H., Rogers, S., Dutton, R. A., Hayashi, K. M., Toga, A. W., et al. (2006). 3D mapping of mini-mental state examination performance in clinical and preclinical Alzheimer disease. *Alzheimer Dis. Assoc. Disord.* 20, 224–231. doi: 10.1097/01.wad.0000213857.89613.10

Arlington, V. A. (2013). *American Psychiatric Association: Diagnostic and Statistical Manual of Mental Disorders*, 5th Edn. Washington, DC: American Psychiatric Association.

Baltes, P. B., and Lindenberger, U. (1997). Emergence of a powerful connection between sensory and cognitive functions across the adult life span: a new window to the study of cognitive aging? *Psychol. Aging* 12, 12–21. doi: 10.1037//0882-7974.12.1.12

Brink, P., and Stones, M. (2007). Examination of the relationship among hearing impairment, linguistic communication, mood, and social engagement of residents in complex continuing-care facilities. *Gerontologist* 47, 633–641. doi: 10.1093/geront/47.5.633

Chen, M. A., Webster, P., Yang, E., and Linthicum, F. H. Jr. (2006). Presbycusic neuritic degeneration within the osseous spiral lamina. *Otol. Neurotol.* 27, 316–322. doi: 10.1097/00129492-200604000-00005

Dupuis, K., Pichora-Fuller, M. K., Chasteen, A. L., Marchuk, V., Singh, G., and Smith, S. L. (2015). Effects of hearing and vision impairments on the Montreal Cognitive Assessment. *Neuropsychol. Dev. Cogn. B Aging Neuropsychol. Cogn.* 22, 413–437. doi: 10.1080/13825585.2014.968084

Faria, A. L., Pinho, M. S., and Bermúdez, I. B. S. (2020). A comparison of two personalization and adaptive cognitive rehabilitation approaches: a randomized controlled trial with chronic stroke patients. *J. Neuroeng. Rehabil.* 17:78. doi: 10.1186/s12984-020-00691-5

Ford, A. H., Hankey, G. J., Yeap, B. B., Golledge, J., Flicker, L., and Almeida, O. P. (2018). Hearing loss and the risk of dementia in later life. *Maturitas* 112, 1–11. doi: 10.1016/j.maturitas.2018.03.004

Fulton, S. E., Lister, J. J., Bush, A. L., Edwards, J. D., and Andel, R. (2015). Mechanisms of the hearing-cognition relationship. *Semin. Hear.* 36, 140–149. doi: 10.1055/s-0035-1555117

GBD 2016 Disease and Injury Incidence and Prevalence Collaborators (2017). Global, regional, and national incidence, prevalence, and years lived with disability for 328 diseases and injuries for 195 countries, 1990-2016: a systematic analysis for the Global Burden of Disease Study 2016. *Lancet* 390, 1211–1259. doi: 10.1016/s0140-6736(17)32154-2

George, E. L., Zekveld, A. A., Kramer, S. E., Goverts, S. T., Festen, J. M., and Houtgast, T. (2007). Auditory and nonauditory factors affecting speech reception in noise by older listeners. *J. Acoust. Soc. Am.* 121, 2362–2375. doi: 10.1121/1.2642072

Gomez, M. I., Hwang, S. A., Sobotova, L., Stark, A. D., and May, J. J. (2001). A comparison of self-reported hearing loss and audiometry in a cohort of New York farmers. *J. Speech Lang. Hear. Res.* 44, 1201–1208. doi: 10.1044/1092-4388(2001/093)

Hill-Briggs, F., Dial, J. G., Morere, D. A., and Joyce, A. (2007). Neuropsychological assessment of persons with physical disability, visual impairment or blindness, and hearing impairment or deafness. *Arch. Clin. Neuropsychol.* 22, 389–404. doi: 10.1016/j.acn.2007.01.013

Hoffman, H. J., Dobie, R. A., Losonczy, K. G., Themann, C. L., and Flamme, G. A. (2017). Declining prevalence of hearing loss in US adults aged 20 to 69 years. *JAMA Otolaryngol. Head Neck Surg.* 143, 274–285. doi: 10.1001/jamaoto.2016.3527

Hugo, J., and Ganguli, M. (2014). Dementia and cognitive impairment: epidemiology, diagnosis, and treatment. *Clin. Geriatr. Med.* 30, 421–442. doi: 10.1016/j.cger.2014.04.001

Jorgensen, L. E., Palmer, C. V., Pratt, S., Erickson, K. I., and Moncrieff, D. (2016). The effect of decreased audibility on MMSE performance: a measure commonly used for diagnosing dementia. *J. Am. Acad. Audiol.* 27, 311–323. doi: 10.3766/jaaa.15006

Jung, R. E., and Haier, R. J. (2007). The parieto-frontal integration theory (P-FIT) of intelligence: converging neuroimaging evidence. *Behav. Brain Sci.* 30, 135–154; discussion 154–187. doi: 10.1017/s0140525x07001185

Kearns, J. R. (1977). Presbycusis. *Can. Fam. Physician* 23, 96–100.

Keithley, E. M. (2020). Pathology and mechanisms of cochlear aging. *J. Neurosci. Res.* 98, 1674–1684. doi: 10.1002/jnr.24439

Lin, F. R., Ferrucci, L., An, Y., Goh, J. O., Doshi, J., Metter, E. J., et al. (2014). Association of hearing impairment with brain volume changes in older adults. *Neuroimage* 90, 84–92. doi: 10.1016/j.neuroimage.2013.12.059

Lin, F. R., Metter, E. J., O'Brien, R. J., Resnick, S. M., Zonderman, A. B., and Ferrucci, L. (2011). Hearing loss and incident dementia. *Arch. Neurol.* 68, 214–220. doi: 10.1001/archneurol.2010.362

Lin, F. R., Yaffe, K., Xia, J., Xue, Q. L., Harris, T. B., Purchase-Helzner, E., et al. (2013). Hearing loss and cognitive decline in older adults. *JAMA Intern. Med.* 173, 293–299. doi: 10.1001/jamainternmed.2013.1868

Lindenberger, U., and Baltes, P. B. (1994). Sensory functioning and intelligence in old age: a strong connection. *Psychol. Aging* 9, 339–355. doi: 10.1037//0882-7974.9.3.339

Liu, J., Lei, S., Zhang, X. N., and Rehabilitation, D. O. (2014). Characteristics and related factors of montreal cognitive assessment for cognitive impairment after stroke. *Chin. J. Rehabil. Theory Pract.* 20, 554–557.

Liu, Y., Fang, S., Liu, L. M., Zhu, Y., Li, C. R., Chen, K., et al. (2020). Hearing loss is an early biomarker in APP/PS1 Alzheimer's disease mice. *Neurosci. Lett.* 717:134705. doi: 10.1016/j.neulet.2019.134705

Livingston, G., Sommerlad, A., Orgeta, V., Costafreda, S. G., Huntley, J., Ames, D., et al. (2017). Dementia prevention, intervention, and care. *Lancet* 390, 2673–2734. doi: 10.1016/s0140-6736(17)31363-6

Loughrey, D. G., Kelly, M. E., Kelley, G. A., Brennan, S., and Lawlor, B. A. (2018). Association of age-related hearing loss with cognitive function, cognitive impairment, and dementia: a systematic review and meta-analysis. *JAMA Otolaryngol. Head Neck Surg.* 144, 115–126. doi: 10.1001/jamaoto.2017.2513

Makary, C. A., Shin, J., Kujawa, S. G., Liberman, M. C., and Merchant, S. N. (2011). Age-related primary cochlear neuronal degeneration in human temporal bones. *J. Assoc. Res. Otolaryngol.* 12, 711–717. doi: 10.1007/s10162-011-0283-2

Mick, P., Kawachi, I., and Lin, F. R. (2014). The association between hearing loss and social isolation in older adults. *Otolaryngol. Head Neck Surg.* 150, 378–384. doi: 10.1177/0194599813518021

Monson, B. B., Rock, J., Schulz, A., Hoffman, E., and Buss, E. (2019). Ecological cocktail party listening reveals the utility of extended high-frequency hearing. *Hear. Res.* 381:107773. doi: 10.1016/j.heares.2019.107773

Motlagh Zadeh, L., Silbert, N. H., Sternasty, K., Swanepoel, W., Hunter, L. L., and Moore, D. R. (2019). Extended high-frequency hearing enhances speech perception in noise. *Proc. Natl. Acad. Sci. U.S.A.* 116, 23753–23759. doi: 10.1073/pnas.1903315116

Nasreddine, Z. S., Phillips, N. A., Bédirian, V., Charbonneau, S., Whitehead, V., Collin, I., et al. (2005). The montreal cognitive assessment, MoCA: a brief screening tool for mild cognitive impairment. *J. Am. Geriatr. Soc.* 53, 695–699. doi: 10.1111/j.1532-5415.2005.53221.x

Peelle, J. E., Troiani, V., Grossman, M., and Wingfield, A. (2011). Hearing loss in older adults affects neural systems supporting speech comprehension. *J. Neurosci.* 31, 12638–12643. doi: 10.1523/jneurosci.2559-11.2011

Pichora-Fuller, M. K. (2003). Cognitive aging and auditory information processing. *Int. J. Audiol.* 42(Suppl. 2), 2S26–2S32.

Pichora-Fuller, M. K., Mick, P., and Reed, M. (2015). Hearing, cognition, and healthy aging: social and public health implications of the links between age-related declines in hearing and cognition. *Semin. Hear.* 36, 122–139. doi: 10.1055/s-0035-1555116

Rossetto, F., Baglio, F., Massaro, D., Alberoni, M., Nemni, R., Marchetti, A., et al. (2020). Social cognition in rehabilitation context: different evolution of affective and cognitive theory of mind in mild cognitive impairment. *Behav. Neurol.* 2020:5204927. doi: 10.1155/2020/5204927

Stern, Y. (2002). What is cognitive reserve? Theory and research application of the reserve concept. *J. Int. Neuropsychol. Soc.* 8, 448–460.

Thomson, R. S., Auduong, P., Miller, A. T., and Gurgel, R. K. (2017). Hearing loss as a risk factor for dementia: a systematic review. *Laryngoscope Investig. Otolaryngol.* 2, 69–79. doi: 10.1002/lio2.65

Tun, P. A., McCoy, S., and Wingfield, A. (2009). Aging, hearing acuity, and the attentional costs of effortful listening. *Psychol. Aging* 24, 761–766. doi: 10.1037/a0014802

Varnet, L., Langlet, C., Lorenzi, C., Lazard, D. S., and Micheyl, C. (2019). High-frequency sensorineural hearing loss alters cue-weighting strategies for discriminating stop consonants in noise. *Trends Hear.* 23:2331216519886707. doi: 10.1177/2331216519886707

Viana, L. M., O'Malley, J. T., Burgess, B. J., Jones, D. D., Oliveira, C. A., Santos, F., et al. (2015). Cochlear neuropathy in human presbycusis: confocal analysis of hidden hearing loss in post-mortem tissue. *Hear. Res.* 327, 78–88. doi: 10.1016/j.heares.2015.04.014

Wager, T. D., Davidson, M. L., Hughes, B. L., Lindquist, M. A., and Ochsner, K. N. (2008). Prefrontal-subcortical pathways mediating successful emotion regulation. *Neuron* 59, 1037–1050. doi: 10.1016/j.neuron.2008.09.006

Wild, C. J., Yusuf, A., Wilson, D. E., Peelle, J. E., Davis, M. H., and Johnsrude, I. S. (2012). Effortful listening: the processing of degraded speech depends critically on attention. *J. Neurosci.* 32, 14010–14021. doi: 10.1523/jneurosci.1528-12.2012

Wu, P. Z., Liberman, L. D., Bennett, K., de Gruttola, V., O'Malley, J. T., and Liberman, M. C. (2019). Primary neural degeneration in the human cochlea: evidence for hidden hearing loss in the aging ear. *Neuroscience* 407, 8–20. doi: 10.1016/j.neuroscience.2018.07.053

Yamasoba, T., Lin, F. R., Someya, S., Kashio, A., Sakamoto, T., and Kondo, K. (2013). Current concepts in age-related hearing loss: epidemiology and mechanistic pathways. *Hear. Res.* 303, 30–38. doi: 10.1016/j.heares.2013.01.021

Zheng, Y., Fan, S., Liao, W., Fang, W., Xiao, S., and Liu, J. (2017). Hearing impairment and risk of Alzheimer's disease: a meta-analysis of prospective cohort studies. *Neurol. Sci.* 38, 233–239. doi: 10.1007/s10072-016-2779-3

8

A Review of Speech Perception of Mandarin-Speaking Children with Cochlear Implantation

*Qi Gao[1,2], Lena L. N. Wong[2] and Fei Chen[1]**

[1] *Department of Electrical and Electronic Engineering, Southern University of Science and Technology, Shenzhen, China,*
[2] *Faculty of Education, The University of Hong Kong, Pokfulam, Hong Kong SAR, China*

Correspondence:
Fei Chen
fchen@sustech.edu.cn

Objective: This paper reviewed the literature on the development of and factors affecting speech perception of Mandarin-speaking children with cochlear implantation (CI). We also summarized speech outcome measures in standard Mandarin for evaluating auditory and speech perception of children with CI.

Method: A comprehensive search of Google Scholar and PubMed was conducted from March to June 2021. Search terms used were speech perception/lexical tone recognition/auditory perception AND cochlear implant AND Mandarin/Chinese.

Conclusion: Unilateral CI recipients demonstrated continuous improvements in auditory and speech perception for several years post-activation. Younger age at implantation and longer duration of CI use contribute to better speech perception. Having undergone a hearing aid trial before implantation and having caregivers whose educational level is higher may lead to better performance. While the findings that support the use of CI to improve speech perception continue to grow, much research is needed to validate the use of unilateral and bilateral implantation. Evidence to date, however, revealed bimodal benefits over CI-only conditions in lexical tone recognition and sentence perception in noise. Due to scarcity of research, conclusions on the benefits of bilateral CIs compared to unilateral CI or bimodal CI use cannot be drawn. Therefore, future research on bimodal and bilateral CIs is needed to guide evidence-based clinical practice.

Keywords: cochlear implant, Mandarin, children, speech perception, outcome measures

INTRODUCTION

In Western societies, the advantages of bilateral cochlear implantation (CI) over unilateral CI for speech perception in quiet and in noise, preverbal communication development and sound localization in the pediatric population have been well demonstrated (Sparreboom et al., 2010). The effects of adding a contralateral hearing aid (HA) among children implanted in the other ear (i.e., bimodal stimulation) have been demonstrated through extensive comparative studies as well (e.g., Beijen et al., 2008). However, unilateral CI is still the norm in mainland China, with the other two modes of amplification gaining popularity in the past decade only. With emerging research on this topic and the gradual reduction in the age of implantation, it is necessary to synthesize new evidence regarding speech perception of Mandarin-speaking children with unilateral CI, bimodal stimulation and bilateral CIs in order to guide clinical application and identify knowledge gaps. This review attempts to cover areas not addressed in the review by Chen and Wong (2017).

The first multi-channel CI operation was conducted in mainland China in 1995 (Liang and Mason, 2013). Since then, CI has become a well-accepted intervention for patients with severe-to-profound hearing loss (HL), funded by local and the central government, due to its cost-effectiveness compared to no intervention or HA (Qiu et al., 2017). Han and Wang (2013) reported over 30,000 persons in mainland China have received CIs, and among them 85% were children. In several provinces, unilateral CI for pediatric population is included in the basic medical insurance scheme (Li J. N. et al., 2017). Despite the fact that CI penetration in the pediatric population is less than 5% (Liang and Mason, 2013), the rate of implantation is expected to grow with the number of qualified specialists and hearing service providers (Li J. N. et al., 2017).

Unlike English, Mandarin is a tonal language with four lexical tones that carry lexical meaning at the monosyllabic level. Lexical tone recognition plays an important role in Mandarin sentence perception (Fu et al., 1998). Superior sentence recognition was noted in normal-hearing (NH) individuals listening to vocoded speech and pediatric CI users when sentences were presented with natural tone contours compared to flattened or randomized tones in quiet, and greater benefit was observed in noise, suggesting the importance of lexical tone contour (Chen F. et al., 2014; Huang et al., 2020). In addition, CI users needed a greater fundamental frequency (F0) range to detect lexical tones at a comparable level as NH listeners (He et al., 2016). Mandarin vowels also convey more intelligibility information than consonants in sentence perception in a ratio of 3:1 compared to 2:1 in English (Chen F. et al., 2013). Furthermore, Mandarin listeners relied more heavily on temporal fine structure when recognizing sentences in competing speech compared with English native listeners who rely more on temporal envelope (Wang et al., 2014). As CIs provide limited access to temporal fine structure and pitch information because of the coarse frequency resolution, it is reasonable to speculate that some findings regarding speech perception among English-speaking CI users may not apply directly to the Mandarin-speaking CI population. Thus, there is a need to synthesize evidence from studies that targeted this population.

Prior to the review, standard Mandarin speech outcome measures are summarized, highlighting their use and limitations. We then reviewed the current evidence related to speech perception with CI and factors influencing speech perception among pediatric users who speak Mandarin as their first language. Evidence on unilateral, bimodal, and bilateral CI use will be presented in separate sections.

METHOD

Between March and June 2021, Google Scholar and PubMed were searched for relevant studies. The search terms were speech perception/lexical tone recognition/auditory perception AND cochlear implant AND Mandarin/Chinese. Due to the advancement of CI algorithms in the past two decades, we limited the search on publication year from 2000 onward. We focused on speech perception of participants with congenital HL, who spoke Mandarin as their first language and received CI. Only studies that were conducted in mainland China and published in English were included.

The search generated a total of 3954 records relevant to the topic. After removing duplicates, 3815 records remained. After screening the titles and/or abstracts, 3719 records were discarded because they were not published in peer-reviewed journals, written in English and/or involved irrelevant content. Among the 96 articles that were retrieved for full-text screening, 58 articles were further excluded because results from children and adults were not reported separately ($n = 25$), the studies were conducted outside of mainland China ($n = 19$), the studies did not focus on speech perception ($n = 10$), findings from non-CI participants were not reported separately ($n = 4$), and only an abstract was available ($n = 1$). Finally, 37 articles remained for review. A flowchart of the screening process can be found in **Figure 1**. Among the 37 articles, 30 studies targeted Mandarin-speaking children with unilateral CI, and 5 studies focused on Mandarin-speaking children with bimodal stimulation. One study considered both populations. One study was identified to be relevant to bilateral CI pediatric recipients.

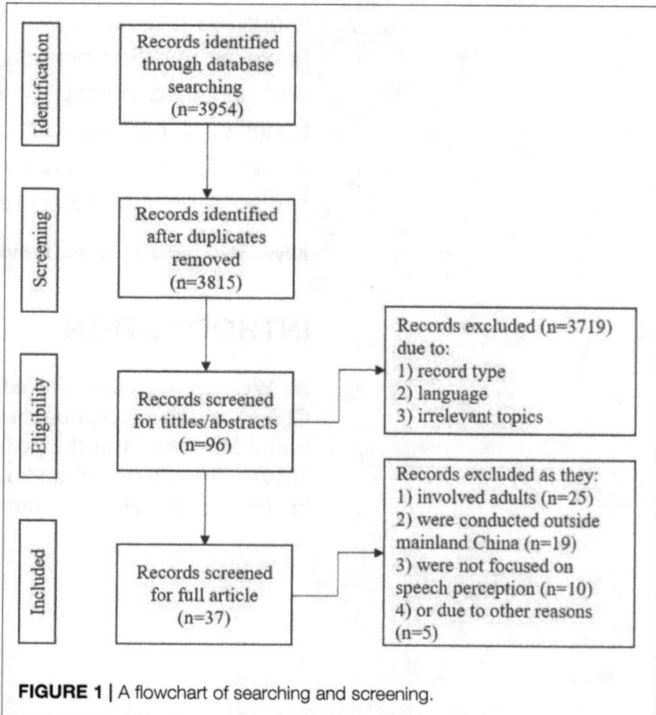

FIGURE 1 | A flowchart of searching and screening.

REVIEW

Auditory and Speech Perception Measures

When selecting outcome measures for children, it is important to take into account a variety of factors, including chronological age, developmental status, vocabulary and language competency. Age-appropriate auditory and speech perception outcomes may include self-report questionnaires and behavioral measures (see **Tables 1, 2** for a summary). Four parental questionnaires were identified, including the Meaningful Auditory Integration Scale (MAIS)/Infant-Toddler Meaningful Auditory Integration Scale (ITMAIS; Zheng et al., 2009c), the LittleEARS® Auditory Questionnaire (LEAQ; Wang et al., 2013), the Categories of Auditory Performance Questionnaire (CAPQ; Wang et al., 2020), and the Parent's Evaluation of Aural/Oral of Children (PEACH) rating scale (Zhang et al., 2021). These parental questionnaires could be utilized to evaluate preverbal, early auditory, and speech perception in children up to 6 years of age, when children have limited language skills and speech perception measures are difficult to administer. The IT-MAIS/MAIS, LEAQ and CAPQ have been used extensively in research institutes and clinics in China. Since the PEACH rating scale is newly developed, few studies have employed this measure.

Multiple measures were developed to evaluate the perception of phonemes, lexical tones, mono- and multi-syllables, and sentences in quiet and/or in noise. Considering the developmental capabilities of young children, the majority of tests are administered in a closed-set paradigm, in which children point to objects or select answers from a picture panel (**Figure 2**). Open-set tests are used for older children by requesting them to verbally repeat words they heard. Although materials developed by Sun et al. (1993) and Chen X. et al. (2007) are popular, they were mainly developed for use in rehabilitation. Thus, they are not presented in the summary table. Phoneme perception could be evaluated using the vowel (category 4) and consonant (category 5) sub-tests of the Mandarin Early Speech Perception (MESP) test (Zheng et al., 2009a). Lexical tone perception is evaluated using category 6 of the MESP test, the Mandarin Tone Identification Test (MTIT; Zhu et al., 2014), and tone test of the computerized Mandarin Pediatric Lexical Tone and Disyllabic-word Picture Identification Test in Noise (MAPPID-N; Yuen et al., 2009b). Syllable perception could be measured using the spondee perception (category 2) sub-test of the MESP test, disyllables test of the MAPPID-N, and Standard-Chinese version of the Lexical Neighborhood Test (LNT; Liu C. et al., 2011). Sentence recognition is evaluated using the Mandarin Pediatric Speech Intelligibility (MPSI) test (Zheng et al., 2009b), the Mandarin Bench–Kowal–Bamford sentences in noise test (MBKB-SIN; Xi et al., 2009), and the Mandarin version of the Hearing in Noise Test for Children (MHINT-C; Chen and Wong, 2020).

Accuracy of tests depends on the reliability and validity of speech outcome measures. Reliability of a speech test refers to how consistent it measures listeners' speech perception ability. The consistency across time, raters, and measurement itself are recognized as test–retest reliability, inter-rater reliability, and internal consistency, respectively. Validity refers to how accurate a speech test truly measures the listener's speech perception ability. These types of validity were commonly evaluated. Construct validity refers to the adherence of speech audiometry to existing theory or knowledge of speech perception. Content validity refers to the extent to which speech audiometry measures all aspects of speech perception. Criterion validity reflects how comparable the measure is to other valid speech audiometry.

All four self-report questionnaires considered one or two reliability assessments in the development process, in the form of internal consistency (Zheng et al., 2009c; Wang et al., 2013), test–retest reliability (Wang et al., 2020; Zhang et al., 2021), and inter-rater reliability (Wang et al., 2020). Criterion validity was assessed for the CAPQ and the PEACH rating scale.

Among the behavioral measures, item or list equivalence was mostly established by measuring psychometric functions and adjusting the intensity of corresponding mean recognition scores and/or mean slope at 50%. While inter-list or test-retest reliability was assessed for some measures (i.e., the MBKB-SIN and the MHINT-C), and certain criteria were applied in constructing the items (e.g., vocabulary, familiarity, phonetically balancing for phoneme distribution and lexical tones), other types of validity was seldom reported. In fact, normative data were mostly collected on NH listeners and researchers rarely validated these measures on listeners with HL or CI, whose performance varies greatly within the group and the error patterns in performance may differ from NH listeners (Li et al., 2016).

Outcomes With Unilateral Cochlear Implantation

The majority of CI users in mainland China are using unilateral implants. There are 31 studies examining outcomes from unilateral CI; among them, 16 are cross-sectional and 15 are longitudinal. Demographic factors were evaluated in both types of studies in order to explain performance variability. As all but one study on lexical tone perception have been reviewed by Chen and Wong (2017), they are not reviewed here. For this review, we focused on longitudinal studies on unilateral CI to synthesize evidence. A summary of results from cross-sectional studies can be found in **Supplementary Material**.

Longitudinal Studies on the Development of Auditory and Speech Perception

The 15 longitudinal studies focused on the developmental trajectory of children with congenital HL and used unilateral CI for not more than 7 years (see **Table 3** for a summary). The age of implantation ranged from an average of 1.58–8.86 years across studies. Auditory behavior, perception of phonemes, syllables and sentences in quiet and in noise were evaluated, demonstrating continuous improvement in early auditory behavior and early speech perception after the device activation, up to 5 years post implantation.

Data showed no or very low level of auditory skills pre-implant. After 6 months of CI use, these children could achieve a score of about 50~60% on the IT-MAIS/MAIS (Chen Y. et al., 2016; Lu and Qin, 2018; Li G. et al., 2020) and reach

TABLE 1 | Parental questionnaires.

Studies	Test name	Test materials	Content	Reliability and validity reported	Target age (years)
Zheng et al., 2009c	The IT-MAIS The MAIS	10 items in 3 categories on a 5-point scale	Self-report about device/vocal behavior and device use; spontaneous detection of and response to sounds; spontaneous and meaningful recognition and discrimination of sounds	Internal consistency (Cronbach's $\alpha = 0.96$; Guttmann's split-half coefficient = 0.96), item reliability (Pearson's r with other items and overall scores = 0.70–0.89)	IT-MAIS: 2–3 MAIS: ≥ 3
Wang et al., 2013	The LEAQ	35 yes-or-no questions	Observed receptive, semantic and early expressive language skills, such as response to a familiar voice or whether simple questions can be understood	Predictability (Guttman's lambda = 0.882), internal consistency (Cronbach's $\alpha = 0.945$; Spearman–Brown split-half coefficient = 0.914), validity (Pearson's r between age and total scores = 0.841)	<2
Wang et al., 2020	The CAPQ	10 categories from Level 0 to Level 9	Hierarchical categories on children's auditory abilities, ranging from Level 0 indicating no awareness of environmental sounds to Level 9 indicating the ability to use the phone with unknown speakers in unpredictable context.	Test-retest reliability (Spearman's r coefficient = 0.981), inter-rater reliability (Pearson's $r = 0.983$) and criterion validity (Pearson's r with the LEAQ: $r = 0.721$)	0–6 (tested[1])
Zhang et al., 2021	The PEACH rating scale	12 items on a 5-point scale	Aural/oral behaviors in real-world quiet and noisy listening conditions, such as being able to follow simple instructions in a quiet or noisy situation	Test–retest reliability (Cronbach's $\alpha = 0.98$; correlation coefficient[2]: $r = 0.96$) and validity (correlation coefficient[2] with the PCDI: $r = 0.42$)	<4

The CAPQ, The Categories of Auditory Performance questionnaire; The IT-MAIS, Infant-Toddler Meaningful Auditory Integration Scale; The LEAQ, The LittleEARS® Auditory Questionnaire; The MAIS, The Meaningful Auditory Integration Scale; The PCDI, Putonghua Communicative Development Inventory; The PEACH rating scale, The Parent's Evaluation of Aural/Oral of Children Rating Scale.

[1] *The study did not indicate the target age and thus the age range of participants in the study is reported.*

[2] *The study did not indicate the type of correlation analysis.*

TABLE 2 | Speech perception tests.

Studies	Test name	Type of test materials	Paradigm	Test in quiet and/or noise	Homogeneity	Target age (years)	Reliability and validity reported
Zheng et al., 2009a	The MESP test	A hierarchically structured test with six categories in speech sound and pattern, spondee, vowel, consonant and tone.	Closed-set recognition 12-AFC or other depending on the category	Quiet	Not reported	≥2	Not reported
Zheng et al., 2009b	The MPSI test	Sentences with 6–7 characters	Closed-set recognition 6-AFC	Quiet and/or in competing sentence at fixed SNRs from +10 to −10 dB	Not reported	3–6 (tested[1])	Not reported
Yuen et al., 2009b	The MAPPID-N	Disyllables and lexical tones	Closed-set recognition 8-AFC for Disyllable test 4-AFC for Lexical tone test	Speech spectrum shaped noise	Across items	4–9 (tested[1])	Not reported
Xi et al., 2009	MBKB-SIN	Sentences with 6–8 characters	Open-set recognition	Quiet and/or in four-talker babble noise	Across lists	4.5–6 (tested[1])	Test–retest reliability (critical difference: 24.6%)
Liu C. et al., 2011	The LNT	Easy and hard Monosyllables and disyllables	Open-set recognition	Quiet	Across lists	4–7 (tested[1])	Inter-rater reliability (consistency between two raters: 92.5–95%)
Zhu et al., 2014	The MTIT	Lexical tones	Closed-set recognition 4-AFC with 1 target word, 1 tone contrast and 2 unrelated distracters	Quiet and/or in speech spectrum shaped noise at fixed SNRs	Not reported	≥7	Internal consistency (Cronbach's α = 0.66-0.76), Test–retest reliability (intra-class correlation = 0.65–0.71), criterion validity [correlated with MPSI in quiet (Kendall's tau = 0.33) and in noise (Spearman's r = 0.71) (Zhu et al., 2016)]
Chen and Wong, 2020	The MHINT-C	Sentences with 10 characters	Open-set SRT	Quiet and/or in Steady-state-speech-spectrum-shaped noise at adaptive SNRs	Across lists	6–17 (tested[1])	Inter-list reliability (confidence intervals: ± 2.8 dB), response variability (1.90-2.0 dB)

AFC, alternative forced choice; MBKB-SIN, Mandarin Bench-Kowal-Bamford sentence in Noise Test; The LNT, the Standard-Chinese version of the Lexical Neighborhood Test; The MAPPID-N, The computerized Mandarin Pediatric Lexical Tone and Disyllabic-word Picture Identification Test in Noise; The MESP test, the Mandarin Early Speech Perception test; The MHINT-C, The Mandarin version of the Hearing in Noise Test for Children; The MPSI, The Mandarin Pediatric Speech Intelligibility test; The MTIT, The new Mandarin Tone Identification Test; SNR, Signal-to-noise ratio; SRT, Speech Recognition Threshold.

[1] *The study did not indicate the target age and thus the age range of participants in the study is reported.*

TABLE 3 | Longitudinal studies on speech perception with unilateral CI.

Studies	Participant characteristics	Outcome measures[1]	Overall results[1]
Chen X. et al., 2010 (*N* = 259)	AAI (years): *M* = 1.8, *R* = 0.7–3.0 Tested at baseline, 1-, 2-, 3-, 6-, 12-months post CI	The IT-MAIS	Early auditory skills improved significantly over time.
Zheng et al., 2011 (*N* = 39)	AAI (years): 1–2 (*n* = 4), 2–3 (*n* = 12), 3–4 (*n* = 12), 4–6 (*n* = 11) Tested at baseline, 3-, 6-, and 12-months post CI	The IT-MAIS The MESP test The MPSI test	Early pre-lingual auditory development and early speech perception were comparable to English-speaking children.
Li Y. et al., 2015 (*N* = 22)	AAI (years): *M* = 2.9, *R* = 1.1-5.7 Tested at baseline, 1-, 3-, 6-, 9-, 12-, 24-, and 36-months post CI	The MESP test	Speech performance through the first 3 years of implant use, with the median categories of MESP increased from a score of 0.23 indicating barely any speech detection at baseline to 5.57 suggesting phoneme, tone and word recognition 3 years later.
Liu et al., 2015a (*N* = 33)	AAI (years): *M* = 2.02, *SD* = 0.89, *R* = 0.5–3.83 Tested at baseline, 1-, 3-, 6-, 9-, 12-, 18-, and 24-months post CI	The LEAQ	Auditory preverbal skills improved significantly post CI in the first 2 years of use.
Liu et al., 2015b (*N* = 105)	AAI (years): *M* = 3.1, *SD* = 2.3, *R* = 0.9-15.5 Tested at 6-, 12-, 24-, 36-, 48-, 60-, 72-, and 84-months post CI	The LNT	Spoken word recognition improved significantly over time. The fastest improvement occurred in the first 36 months, after which it slowed down and peaked at 72 months post CI (81.7%).
Chen Y. et al., 2016 (N = 80)	AAI (years): M = 2.61, SD = 1.04, R = 0.93-5.00 Tested at baseline, 3-, 6-, and 12-months post CI	The IT-MAIS/ MAIS The MESP test The MPSI test	Significant progress in prelingual auditory, word and sentence recognition were observed during the first year of CI use. Mandarin-speaking children with CIs attained early speech perception results comparable to those of their English-speaking counterparts.
Guo et al., 2016 (*N* = 23)	AAI (years): *M* = 3.0, *R* = 1.08-5.67 Tested at 1-, 2-, 3-, and 4-years post CI	The MESP test	The proportion of participants having reached higher categories increased significantly during the 4 years post CI. The percentage of participants passing category 6 (tone perception) of the MESP increased from 9% at 1st year to 91% at 4th year post CI.
Liu et al., 2016 (*N* = 213)	AAI (years): The mean ranged from 2.49 to 3.15 in groups of different etiology. Tested at baseline and 1-year post CI	Mono-, di-syllable and sentence recognition	Significant improvement in recognition of monosyllabic, disyllabic words and sentences at 1 year post CI.
Li G. et al., 2017 (*N* = 143)	AAI (years): 1–2 (*n* = 34), 2–3 (*n* = 72), 3–4 (*n* = 37) Test at before, 2-, 6-, 12-, 24-, 36-, 48-months post CI	Tone perception subset in the MESP test	Mean identification score increased from approximately 68% to 79% by 4 years post CI.
Lu and Qin, 2018 (*N* = 132)	AAI (years): *M* = 3.4 *SD* = 1.35 Tested at baseline, 3-, 6-, 9-, 12-, 18-, and 24-months post CI	The IT-MAIS The MESP test	Significant improvements in early auditory and speech development that follow the normative developmental trajectories. However, there was still a gap (10–15%) compared with normative values.
Liu S. et al., 2019 (*N* = 98)	AAI (years): *M* = 8.86, *SD* = 3.66, *R* = 1.0–16.0 Tested at baseline, 3-, 6-, and 12-months post CI	Speech perception[2] The MAIS The CAPQ	The scores of all measures significantly improved at 1 year post CI.
Lyu et al., 2019 (*N* = 278)	AAI (years): *M* = 1.58, *R* = 0.5–3.0 Tested at baseline, 1-, 3-, 6-, 12-, 18-, 24-, 36-, 48-, 60-months post CI	The CAPQ	Scores improved during the 5 years post CI, although speech development lagged behind that of hearing.
Fan et al., 2020 (*N* = 52)	AAI (years): Median = 1.25, *R* = 0.83–5.66 Tested at baseline, 3-, 6-, 9-, 12-, 15-, 18-, 21- and 24-months post CI	Closed monosyllables and disyllables recognition The CAPQ	Auditory and speech perception improved significantly over the 24 months post CI period.
Jiang et al., 2020 (*N* = 100)	AAI (years): Median = 4.0, *R* = 3.0–7.0 Tested at 1 months, 1-, 2-, and 3-years post CI	The CAPQ	Significant improvements in the CAPQ scores at 3 years post CI. 60% of children reached Level 7 indicating children were able to use the telephone with a familiar talker at 3 years post CI.
Li G. et al., 2020 (*N* = 24)	Age at Switch-on: *M* = 2.1, *SD* = 0.47, *R* = 1.2–2.8 Tested at baseline, 3-, 6-, and 12-months post CI	The IT-MAIS	Children below 3 years of age had similar trajectories in early auditory developments to NH children.

AAI, Age at Implant; CI, Cochlear Implantation; M, Mean; N, The Number of Participants; R, Range; SD, Standard Deviation.
[1]Only outcome measures and results related to speech perception were reported.
[2]Speech perception here referred to Chinese auditory perception and open-set speech perception.

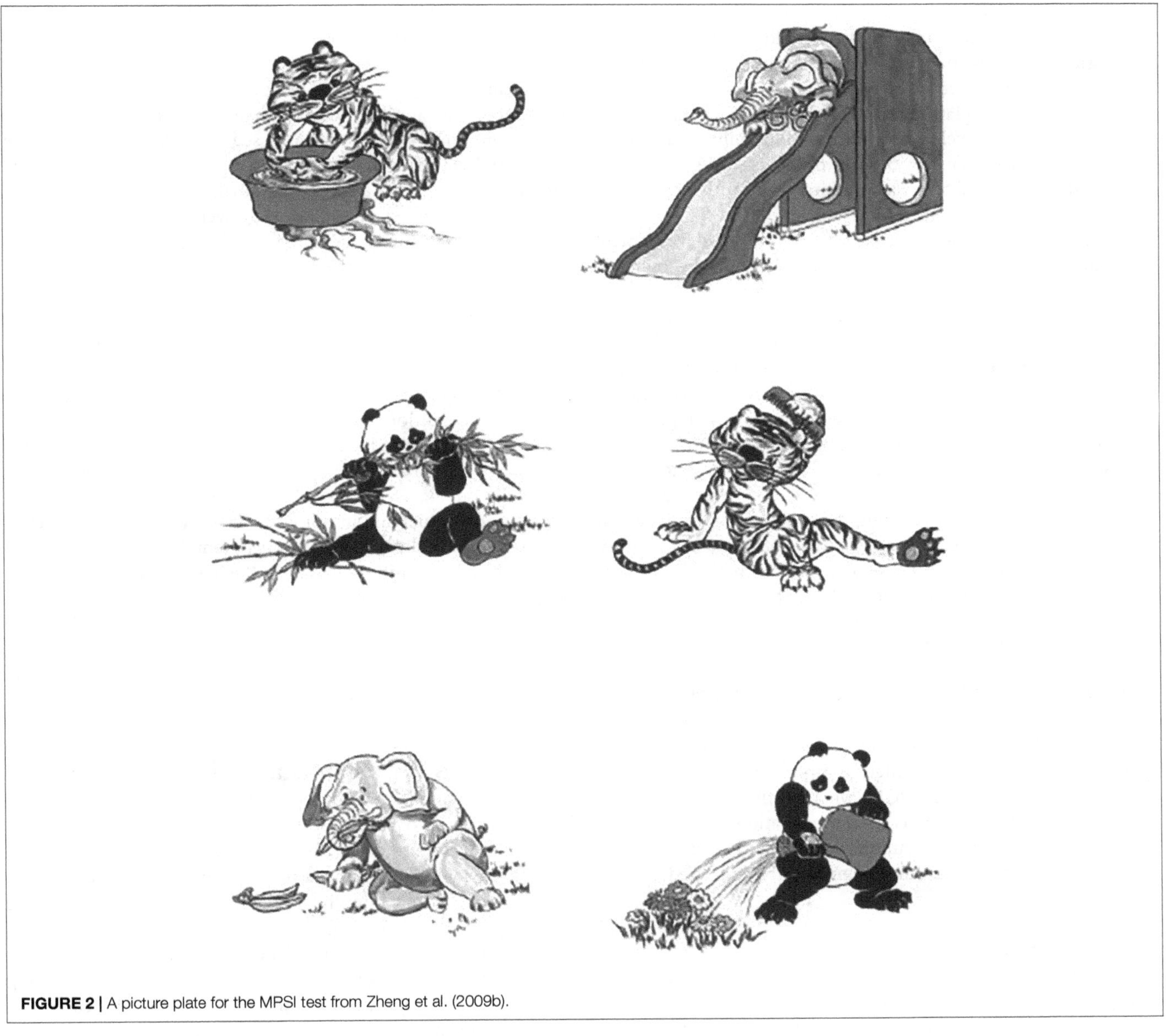

FIGURE 2 | A picture plate for the MPSI test from Zheng et al. (2009b).

category 3 (i.e., recognizes environmental sounds) on the CAPQ (Lyu et al., 2019; Chen Y. et al., 2020; Jiang et al., 2020). About 40∼88% of children reached category 2 (i.e., speech pattern perception) or higher on the MESP test (Zheng et al., 2011; Chen Y. et al., 2016; Guo et al., 2016; Lu and Qin, 2018). Approximately 7.9∼20.6% of children could obtain a score of 25∼42% for close-set sentence perception on the MPSI in quiet (Zheng et al., 2011; Chen Y. et al., 2016) and participants in Liu et al. (2015b) achieved an average score of 30.9% for mono- and disyllable recognition on the LNT. These results suggest that at 6 months post CI, children begin to develop closed-set word recognition and sentence recognition in quiet, as well as open-set word recognition in quiet. At 12 months post CI, children could obtain scores of about 70∼80% on the IT-MAIS/MAIS (Chen Y. et al., 2016, 2020; Lu and Qin, 2018; Li G. et al., 2020) and reach category 4 (i.e., discriminates at least two speech sounds) on the CAPQ (Lyu et al., 2019; Chen Y. et al., 2020; Jiang et al., 2020). More than half of the children could achieve category 4 (i.e., vowel perception) and category 5 (i.e., consonant perception) on the MESP test (Zheng et al., 2011; Chen Y. et al., 2016; Guo et al., 2016; Lu and Qin, 2018). About 33.9–56.7% of the children could achieve a mean score of 60–70% for closed-set sentence recognition on the MPSI test in quiet and a similar proportion of children could obtain a mean score of 46–59% on the MPSI test in noise (Zheng et al., 2011; Chen Y. et al., 2016). The mean recognition scores in monosyllables, disyllables and sentences increased significantly to 78.60, 88.57, and 89.79% respectively at 1-year post-operatively from a baseline of 13∼42% pre-implant (Liu et al., 2016). These results suggest that at one-year post-operation, children with unilateral CI could demonstrate a good ability to identify closed-set words and sentences in quiet; and some children could develop the ability to identify sentences in noise. Greatest improvement in open-set word recognition occurs between 1 and 3 years after surgery and then reaches a plateau at 48 months (Liu et al., 2015b). All children could develop tone recognition ability (category 6 of the MESP test) after 4 to 5 years of CI use, and 60–80% of children showed lexical tone recognition significantly higher than the chance level (Li G. et al., 2017).

From these findings, a clear trajectory of development on auditory behaviors and closed-set phoneme recognition is observed. However, there are few reports on sentence and open-set words recognition. Many studies (6 out of 15) reported findings from 1-year post-implantation, thus allowing insufficient time to develop mastery of complex grammatical skills and lexicons to be assessed in open-set word recognition tasks or sentence tests, which is more demanding than phoneme and closed-set word recognition. Longer follow-up period is necessary in order to observe the performance trajectory over time. In addition, considering various tests were used on participants with different demographic factors such as age at implantation (AAI) [e.g., mean AAI was 1.58 years in Lyu et al. (2019) and 8.86 years in Liu S. et al. (2019)], whether HAs were trialed pre-implant, and whether speech therapy was provided post-implant, performance varied across participants and studies, decreasing the ability of this review in generalizing findings.

Important Factors That Affect Speech Perception

A summary of frequently examined factors among studies can be found in **Table 4**. Details about less-frequently examined factors (≤3 studies) are presented in **Supplementary Materials**. AAI, duration of CI use (DCI), whether there was a pre-CI hearing aid trial (HAT), and caregiver education level (CEL) are discussed below and more than half of analyses that investigated these variables show that they significantly impacted speech perception outcomes.

Early AAI, similar to studies on an English-speaking population (see a review from, for example, Bruijnzeel et al., 2016; Sharma et al., 2020), is associated with enhanced speech perception in children. Seven longitudinal studies reported that early implantation contributed positively to prelingual auditory skills and early speech perception evaluated on the IT-MAIS/MAIS, the LEAQ, the MESP test, the MPSI test, and the LNT (Liu et al., 2015a; Chen Y. et al., 2016; Lu and Qin, 2018; Liu S. et al., 2019; Lyu et al., 2019; Fan et al., 2020; Jiang et al., 2020).

Longer DCI significantly contributes to better auditory skills and speech perception in all longitudinal studies. Open-set word recognition and sentence recognition were significantly correlated with longer DCI in cross-sectional studies, as reported in the previous review (Liu H. et al., 2013; Chen Y. et al., 2014). Lexical tone recognition, however, was not correlated with DCI in 4 out of 6 cross-sectional studies that conducted such analyses (Han et al., 2009; Li A. et al., 2014; Tao et al., 2015; Mao and Xu, 2017). Participants in studies that demonstrated a lack of effects of DCI used their devices longer (M = 2.36–6.50 years) than those in the two studies (Mean DCI = 1.27–1.64) that found significant correlations (Zhou et al., 2013; Chen Y. et al., 2014). The only study assessing the effect of DCI on Mandarin consonant contrast perception also showed no significant correlation (Liu Q. et al., 2013).

Having undergone a HAT before CI is a factor that positively influences the auditory development and speech perception. All longitudinal studies that assessed the relationship between receiving HAT prior to implantation and auditory scores showed significant effects (Chen X. et al., 2010; Lu and Qin, 2018; Fan et al., 2020; Jiang et al., 2020). However, mixed findings were reported among studies on early speech perception, with Zheng et al. (2011) and Fan et al. (2020) reporting significant effects of HAT on closed monosyllable and disyllable recognition and the MESP scores, but Chen Y. et al. (2016) and Lu and Qin (2018) did not observe such correlations with early speech perception. In a cross-sectional study, having undergone HAT was associated with better sentence recognition in noise, but not with sentence and tone recognition in quiet (Chen Y. et al., 2016).

Better caregiver's education contributed positively to preverbal auditory skills (Liu et al., 2015a), overall early speech perception (Chen Y. et al., 2015, 2016; Fan et al., 2020) and sentence perception in quiet and in noise (Chen Y. et al., 2014). However, Chen Y. et al. (2014) did not find parental education relate to lexical tone recognition in quiet. Such variables are specified as parents' education levels in Liu et al. (2015a) and maternal education level in Chen Y. et al. (2020, 2014, 2015) and therefore cannot be directly compared. Interestingly, Fan et al. (2020) found that children who were cared for by their mothers exhibited better closed monosyllable recognition rates, than those who were cared for by their grandparents.

Outcomes With Bimodal Stimulation

With improving socioeconomics and greater recognition of the importance of binaural hearing, bimodal stimulation is gradually becoming a key focus of researchers, clinicians and parents in mainland China. Bimodal stimulation refers to the combination of a CI in the implanted ear and a HA in the non-implanted ear. Adding a contralateral HA allows unilateral CI users to exploit the residual hearing in the non-implanted ear, reducing auditory deprivation and enabling binaural hearing (Hurley, 1999; Polonenko et al., 2018). Bimodal benefits in sound localization, music perception, and speech perception for non-tonal language speakers such as English have been established by a huge body of evidence (Ching et al., 2007). For example, speech perception in noise could be enhanced through binaural summation, head shadow effect, and squelch effect (Lotfi et al., 2019).

The contribution of the F0 in the low-frequency range is important for Mandarin perception. Thus, a contralateral HA that delivers amplification in this frequency range may produce unique bimodal benefits for the Mandarin-speaking population. One longitudinal and five cross-sectional studies were identified through the literature search, comparing speech perception with bimodal stimulation and CI only condition (see **Table 5** for a summary).

Chen Y. et al. (2020) was the only study that retrospectively compared the auditory skills of children with unilateral CI and bimodal stimulation during the 24 months post CI. The AAI in

TABLE 4 | Frequently examined factors that affect speech perception of children with unilateral CI.

Studies	Participant characteristics	Outcome measures[1]	Analysis method	AAT	AAI	CEL	DCI	HAT	PHL
Han et al., 2009 (*N* = 20)	AAI: *M* = 5.2, *SD* = 3.8, *R* = 1.3–13.5 years	Lexical tone recognition in quiet	Least-squared linear fit	√*	√*	–	√	–	–
Chen X. et al., 2010 (*N* = 259)	AAI: M = 1.8, *R* = 0.7–3.0 years Tested at baseline, 1-, 2-, 3-, 6-, 12-months post CI	The IT-MAIS	ANOVA and *t* test	–	√	–	√*	√*	–
Zhu et al., 2011 (*N* = 37)	AAI: *M* = 4.2, *R* = 1.2–17.5 years (Group 1: Congenitally deafened children)	Open-set disyllables recognition	Multiple linear regression	√	√*	–	–	–	–
		Sentences recognition		√*	√*	–	–	–	–
Zheng et al., 2010 (*N* = 25)	AAI: *M* = 3.39, *R* = 1.5–9.1 years	The MESP test	DNR	–	√	–	√	–	–
Zheng et al., 2011 (*N* = 39)	AAI: 1–2 years (*n* = 4), 2–3 years (*n* = 12), 3–4 years (*n* = 12), 4–6 years (*n* = 11) Tested at baseline, 3-, 6-, and 12-months post CI	The IT-MAIS	Pearson's correlation and χ^2 test of independence	–	√*	–	–	√*	–
		The MESP and MPSI test		–	–	–	–	√*	–
Liu H. et al., 2013 (*N* = 230)	AAI: *M* = 3.9, *SD* = 3.0, *R* = 0.9-16.0 years	Open-set word recognition	Stepwise multiple regression	–	√*	–	√*	–	–
Liu Q. et al., 2013 (*N* = 41)	AAI: *M* = 2.0, *SD* = 0.74, *R* = 0.83–4.17 years	Mandarin consonant contrast perception	Linear regression	√	√*	–	√	–	√
Zhou et al., 2013 (*N* = 110)	AAI: *M* = 3.96, *SD* = 2.70, *R* = 1.11–12.95 years	Lexical tone recognition in quiet	Step-wise linear regression	√	√	-	√*	-	-
Li A. et al., 2014 (*N* = 20)	AAI: *M* = 4.1, *R* = 2.0–6.7 years	Lexical tone recognition in quiet	Linear regression	√*	√*	–	√	–	√
Chen Y. et al., 2014 (*N* = 96)	AAI: *M* = 2.72, *SD* = 1.03, *R* = 0.69–5.00 years	Lexical tone perception in quiet	Step-wise multiple linear regression	–	√	√	√*	√	√
		Sentence perception in quiet		–	√	√*	√*	√	√
		Sentence perception in noise		–	√	√*	√*	√*	√*
Chen Y. et al., 2015[2] (*N* = 115)	AAI: *M* = 2.67, *SD* = 1.08, *R* = 0.69–5.00 years	Overall speech perception[3]	Structural equation modeling	–	√*	√*	–	√*	√
Li Y. et al., 2015 (*N* = 22)	AAI: *M* = 2.9, *R* = 1.1–5.7 years Tested at baseline and 1-, 3-, 6-, 9-, 12-, 24-, and 36-months post CI	The MESP test	Repeated-measure ANOVA	–	√*	–	√*	–	–
Liu et al., 2015a[4] (*N* = 33)	AAI: *M* = 2.02, *SD* = 0.89, *R* = 0.5–3.83 years Tested at baseline, 1-, 3-, 6-, 9-, 12-, 18-, and 24-months post CI	The LEAQ	ANOVA	–	√*	√*	√*	–	–
Liu et al., 2015b (*N* = 105)	AAI: *M* = 3.1, *SD* = 2.3, *R* = 0.9–15.5 years Tested at 6-, 12-, 24-, 36-, 48-, 60-, 72-, 84-months post CI	Open-set word recognition	ANOVA	–	√*	–	√*	–	–

(Continued)

TABLE 4 | (Continued)

Studies	Subject characteristics	Outcome measures[1]	Analysis method	AAT	AAI	CEL	DCI	HAT	PHL
Tao et al., 2015 ($N = 21$)	AAI: $M = 4.3$, $R = 2–12$ years (Prelingual group)	Lexical tone perception in quiet	Linear regression	–	–	–	√	–	–
Chen Y. et al., 2016 ($N = 80$)	AAI: $M = 2.61$ $SD = 1.04$, $R = 0.93–5.00$ years Tested at baseline, 3-, 6-, and 12-months post CI	Overall speech perception[3]	Hierarchical linear modeling	–	√*	√*	√*	√	√*
Mao and Xu, 2017[5] ($N = 66$)	AAI: $M = 2.97$, $SD = 3.05$, $R = 0.6–16.50$ years	Lexical tone recognition in quiet and in noise	Linear correlation	√	√*	–	√	–	–
Li G. et al., 2017 ($N = 143$)	AAI: 1–2 years: $n = 34$; 2-3 years: $n = 72$; 3–4 years: $n = 37$ Test at baseline, 2-, 6-, 12-, 24-, 36-, and 48-months post CI	Tone perception subset in the MESP test	Two-sample t test	–	√	–	√*	–	–
Lu and Qin, 2018[6] ($N = 132$)	AAI: $M = 3.4$ $SD = 1.35$ years Tested at baseline, 3-, 6-, 9-, 12-, 18-, and 24-months post CI	The IT-MAIS	Multiple linear and logistic regression	–	√*	–	√*	√*	√*
		The MESP test		–	√*	–	√*	√	√*
Liu S. et al., 2019 ($N = 98$)	AAI: $M = 8.86$, $SD = 3.66$, $R = 1.0–16.0$ years Tested at baseline, 3-, 6-, and 12-months post CI	The MAIS, the CAPQ and speech perception[7]	ANOVA	–	√*	–	√*	–	–
Lyu et al., 2019 ($N = 278$)	AAI: $M = 1.58$, $R = 0.5–3.0$ years Tested at baseline, 1-, 3-, 6-, 12-, 18-, 24-, 36-, 48-, and 60-months post CI	The CAPQ	t test and linear regression	–	√	–	√*	–	–
Fan et al., 2020[8] ($N = 52$)	AAI: Median = 1.25, $R = 0.83–5.66$ years Tested at baseline, 3-, 6-, 9-, 12-, 15-, 18-, 21- and 24-months post CI	Closed-set monosyllables Closed-set disyllables The CAPQ	Generalized estimating equation	–	√*	√*	√*	√*	√
Jiang et al., 2020 ($N = 100$)	AAI: Median = 4.0, $R = 3.0–7.0$ years Tested at 1 months, 1-, 2-, and 3-years post CI	The CAPQ	Mann-Whitney test	–	√*	–	√*	√*	–
Li G. et al., 2020 ($N = 24$)	Age at Switch-on: $M = 2.1$, $SD = 0.47$, $R = 1.2–2.8$ years Tested at baseline, 3-, 6-, and 12-months post CI	The IT-MAIS	Mann-Whitney test	–	√	–	√*	–	–

AAI, Age at Implant; AAT, Age at Testing; ANOVA, Analysis of Variance; CEL, Caregiver's Educational Level; CI, Cochlear Implantation; DCI, Duration of CI use; DNR, Did not report the statistical test used; HAT, Hearing Aid Trial; M, Mean; N, The Number of Participants; PHL, Pre-implant Hearing Level; R, Range; SD, Standard Deviation.

'√' shows that this study examined the corresponding factor and found a significant correlation. '√' shows that this study examined the corresponding factor but no significant relationship was found. '–' shows that this study did not examine the corresponding factor.*

1 Only outcome measures and results related to speech perception were reported.

2 In Chen Y. et al. (2015), 5 children used a HA in the non-implanted ear and were tested with both CI and HA on.

3 Overall speech perception referred to a single composite score was generated by combining results from MAIS, the MESP test and the MPSI test using the principal component analysis.

4 In Liu et al. (2015a), 1 child received bilateral CIs.

5 In Mao and Xu (2017), the significance for AAI became non-significant after correction for multiple comparisons.

6 In Lu and Qin (2018), only results at 1 year post CI were presented due to space limitation.

7 Speech perception here referred to Chinese auditory perception and open-set speech perception.

8 6. In Fan et al. (2020), 9 (18.4%) children used bilateral CIs and 11 (22.4%) children used CI + HA.

TABLE 5 | Speech perception of children with bimodal stimulation.

Studies	Participant characteristics	Device settings	Outcome measures[1]	Overall results
Yuen et al., 2009a ($N = 15$)	Age (years): $M = 10.2$, $R = 5.1–14.3$ DCI (years): $M = 2.3$, $R = 0.3$-6.7	HA fitting was optimization based on the NAL-RP prescription formula	Lexical tones and disyllabic words in quiet and in noise (The MAPPID-N) Test settings: CI-only, CI + HA	Significant bimodal benefits[2] in lexical tone recognition in quiet and in noise, and disyllabic words in noise when speech and noise both presented from the front.
Cheng et al., 2018 ($N = 35$)	AAI (years): $M = 2.9$, $R = 0.9–7.0$ DCI (years): $M = 3.5$, $R = 0.6–8.1$ DHA (years): $M = 2.7$, $R = 0.5–9.0$	Participants used their clinical settings for CI and HA	Mandarin tone recognition in quiet Vowel recognition in quiet Consonant recognition in quiet Sentence recognition in quiet Test settings: CI-only, CI + HA	Significant bimodal benefits for tone recognition in quiet (Tone 2), but not for vowel, consonant or sentence recognition in quiet.
Liu Y. W. et al., 2019 ($N = 11$)	Age (years): $M = 8.2$, $R = 6.0–12.5$ DCI (years): $M = 4.5$, $R = 2.0–8.0$ DHA (years): $M = 4.0$, $R = 0.5–8.0$	Participants used their clinical settings for CI and HA	Sentence recognition in steady-state noise and in a competing talker Test settings: CI-only, CI + HA	With 2-keywords scoring, no bimodal benefit in steady-state noise and female competing talker. Bimodal stimulation resulted in better scores than the CI-only condition. With 5-keywords scoring, significant bimodal benefits were observed.
Chen Y. et al., 2020 ($N = 28$)	AAI (years): $M = 1.47$, $SD = 0.57$ Tested at first mapping, 0.5-, 1-, 3-, 6-, 12-, 18-, and 24-months after	CI mapping and HA fitting were carried out by experienced clinicians	The IT-MAIS The CAPQ Test settings: CI + HA for the bimodal group	The bimodal group demonstrated significantly higher scores at baseline, 3-, and 6-months on the IT-MAIS and from 3- to 24 months on the CAPQ compared to the unilateral CI group.
Zhang et al., 2020a ($N = 14$)	AAI (years): $M = 1.96$, $R = 0.9$-3.3 DCI (years): $M = 3.59$, $R = 2.3$-5.2 Bimodal duration (years): $M = 3.23$, $R = 1.7–5.0$	Participants used their daily settings for CI and HA	Lexical tone recognition in quiet and in speech spectrum-shaped noise at + 5 dB Test settings: CI-only, CI + HA	Significant improvement was seen in the CI + HA condition over the CI-only condition for lexical tone recognition in noise.
Zhang et al., 2020b ($N = 16$)	AAI (years): $M = 1.91$, $R = 0.9–3.3$ DCI (years): $M = 3.45$, $R = 2.1–5.1$ DHA (years): $M = 3.45$, $R = 1.7–5.3$	Not mentioned	An identification task with a set of synthetic tone-pair continuum (T1-T2) A discrimination task with same stimuli Test settings: CI-only, CI + HA	Significant bimodal benefits in lexical tone categorization were found over the CI-only condition.

AAI, Age at implant; CI, Cochlear Implantation; DCI, Duration of CI use; DHA, Duration of hearing aid use; HA, Hearing Aid; M, Mean; N, The number of participants; R, Range; SD, Standard deviation; T, Tone.

[1] *Only outcome measures and results related to speech perception are reported.*

[2] *Bimodal benefits are measured as a comparison between CI + HA condition over CI-only condition for all studies except Chen Y. et al. (2020) where the comparison was made with a group of participants using unilateral CI.*

TABLE 6 | Factors that affect speech perception of children with bimodal stimulation.

Studies	Participant characteristics	Outcome measures	Test setting	Analysis method	AAT	AAI	DCI	DHA	DOB	DOD	PTA
Yuen et al., 2009a[1] (N = 15)	Age (years): M = 10.2, R = 5.1–14.3 DCI (years): M = 2.3, R = 0.3–6.7	Lexical tone recognition in quiet and in noise	Bimodal benefits	Pearson's correlation	–	–	–	–	–	–	√
		Disyllable recognition in noise			–	–	–	–	–	–	√*
Cheng et al., 2018[2] (N = 35)	AAI (years): M = 2.9, R = 0.9–7.0 DCI (years): M = 3.5, R = 0.6–8.1 DHA (years): M = 2.7, R = 0.5–9.0	Tone recognition in quiet	CI + HA	Pearson's correlation	√	√*	√*	√	–	√	√
		Vowel recognition in quiet			√	√	√	√	–	√	√
		Consonant recognition in quiet			√	√*	√	√	–	√*	√
		Sentence recognition in quiet			√	√	√	√	–	√	√*
Liu Y. W. et al., 2019[3] (N = 11)	Age (years): M = 8.2, R = 6.0–12.5 DCI (years): M = 4.5, R = 2.0–8.0 DHA (years): M = 4.0, R = 0.5–8.0	Sentence recognition in noise	CI + HA	Pearson's correlation	√	–	√	√	–	√	√*
Zhang et al., 2020a[4] (N = 14)	AAI (years): M = 1.96, R = 0.9–3.3 DCI (years): M = 3.59, R = 2.3–5.2 Bimodal duration (years): M = 3.23, R = 1.7–5.0	Lexical tone recognition in quiet	CI + HA	Multivariate regression	√	√	√*	–	√	–	√
			Bimodal benefits		√	√	√	–	√*	–	√*
		Lexical tone recognition in noise	CI + HA		√	√	√	–	√	–	√
			Bimodal benefits		√	√	√	–	√*	–	√

AAI, Age at Implant; AAT, Age at Testing; CI, Cochlear Implantation; DCI, Duration of CI use; DHA, Duration of Hearing Aid use; DOB, Duration of Bimodal use; DOD, Duration of Deafness; HA, Hearing aid; M, Mean; N, The number of participants; PTA, Pure Tone Average; R, Range; SD, Standard Deviation.

'√' Shows that this study examined the corresponding factor and found a significant correlation. '√' Shows that this study examined the corresponding factor but no significant relationship was found. '–' Shows that this study did not examine the corresponding factor.*

[1] *In Yuen et al. (2009a), PTA referred to aided threshold at 250 and 500 Hz of the non-implanted ear.*

[2] *In Cheng et al. (2018), PTA referred to unaided PTA at 500, 1000, and 2000 Hz.*

[3] *In Liu Y. W. et al. (2019), PTA referred to unaided thresholds in the non-implanted ear at 500 Hz and averaged across all frequencies. The significance was found with bimodal SRTs when the target and masker gender was both male.*

[4] *In Zhang et al. (2020a), PTA referred to three factors including unaided PTA at 125, 250, and 500 Hz, five-frequencies unaided PTA and five-frequencies aided PTA (250–4000 Hz). The significance was only found for the first factor.*

the bimodal group and unilateral CI group was on average of 1.47 and 1.58 years respectively. The bimodal group had better averaged scores compared with the unilateral CI group on the IT-MAIS and CAPQ obtained during follow-up period. The bimodal group obtained nearly full scores on the IT-MAIS faster than the unilateral CI group (18 months vs. 24 months post-implantation). Also, they outperformed the unilateral CI group from 3-months post CI on the CAPQ.

Four out of seven studies evaluated lexical tone perception in quiet and/or in noise. Three of these studies focused on bimodal benefits on lexical tone identification (Yuen et al., 2009a; Cheng et al., 2018; Zhang et al., 2020a), specified as the performance differences of bimodal stimulation (i.e., CI + HA) condition over CI-only condition. All studies found significant bimodal benefits in lexical tone recognition in quiet and/or in noise. Although significant improvement in the recognition of Tone 2 in quiet with bimodal stimulation was noted in Cheng et al. (2018), a ceiling effect was evident where listeners performed nearly perfectly regardless of conditions (CI + HA or CI-only). Zhang et al. (2020a) showed bimodal benefits in lexical tone recognition in speech spectrum-shaped noise at +5 dB but not in quiet, whereas Yuen et al. (2009a) also found significant bimodal benefits in lexical tone recognition when speech was presented from the front and noise from the CI side. Zhang et al. (2020b) investigated categorial perception using synthetic tone-pair continuums, showing enhanced categorical perception in Tone 1–2 continuums with bimodal stimulation compared to CI-only condition.

Vowel, consonant, disyllable and sentence recognition was assessed in three studies (Yuen et al., 2009a; Cheng et al., 2018; Liu Y. W. et al., 2019). Yuen et al. (2009a) reported significant benefits in disyllable recognition when speech was presented from the front and noise was presented on the CI side. Vowel, consonant and sentence recognition were measured in quiet and no significant bimodal benefits were found (Cheng et al., 2018). Liu Y. W. et al. (2019) compared speech reception thresholds (SRTs) in different maskers with and without HAs using 2-keywords scoring. While performance in steady-state noise (SSN) and the female competing talker did not differ, SRTs with bimodal listening was worse when competing and target voices were the same, indicating bimodal interference. In the second experiment of this study, using 5-keywords scoring, a significant bimodal benefit in SRTs in the presence of SSN was evident, indicating bimodal benefits in more challenging tasks.

Four out of six studies examined the correlation between demographic factors and speech perception (Yuen et al., 2009a; Cheng et al., 2018; Liu Y. W. et al., 2019; Zhang et al., 2020a). A summary of these studies can be found in **Table 6**. Effects of hearing thresholds in the non-implanted ear were examined in all four studies. Significant correlations were found between low-frequency hearing thresholds in the non-implanted ear and disyllables recognition in noise (Yuen et al., 2009a), lexical tone recognition in noise (Zhang et al., 2020a); and sentence recognition in quiet (Cheng et al., 2018) and in noise (Liu Y. W. et al., 2019) (please see **Table 6**). Similar to studies in unilateral CI use, age at testing, AAI and DCI were examined. Cheng et al. (2018) found that AAI significantly correlated with lexical tone and consonant recognition in quiet with bimodal stimulation. Cheng et al. (2018) and Zhang et al. (2020a) both found that DCI significantly correlated with lexical tone recognition in quiet with bimodal stimulation. Duration of deafness was examined in two studies, but only Cheng et al. (2018) found bimodal stimulation significantly correlated with consonant recognition in quiet. Duration of bimodal use was examined in Zhang et al. (2020a) only and the study revealed that bimodal CI was significantly related to lexical tone recognition both in quiet and in noise.

Overall, Mandarin-speaking children with bimodal stimulation seem to outperform unilateral CI users in the development of auditory skills post-implantation, demonstrated as higher scores on the IT-MAIS and CAP during the 24 months post CI (Chen Y. et al., 2020). Better lexical tone recognition in quiet and/or noise is noted with bimodal stimulation, compared to the CI-only condition. Bimodal benefits in speech perception may be related to the task difficulty and more benefits are noted in more challenging situations such as in noise. Apart from lexical tone identification and sentence perception in noise, there is only one study each concerning vowel, consonant and disyllable recognition in quiet, long-term speech perception and the effect of duration of bimodal use. In addition, HA optimization before testing was performed only in Yuen et al. (2009a), which makes comparison with other studies difficult. Therefore, more studies are needed to understand the benefits of bimodal CI compared with unilateral CI.

Outcomes With Bilateral Cochlear Implantations

Although bilateral CIs have been found to improve speech recognition in noisy conditions over unilateral CI among English-speaking populations (e.g., Asp et al., 2015), reports on bilateral CIs in mainland China did not emerge until 2018. Long et al. (2018) was the only study we identified that investigated the development of early auditory skills in 19 children with simultaneous bilateral CIs. The averaged age at implant was 1.89 years. Participants exhibited continuous improvement in overall LEAQ scores and categorial scores in receptive, semantic auditory behavior and expressive language skills during the 2-year post CI. Children with bilateral CIs obtained significantly higher scores at 1-, 3-, and 6-months post CI than those using unilateral CI (data from Liu et al., 2015a) and the difference nearly disappeared at 24 months post CI. This is possibly due to both groups performing at ceiling. They also found that children whose caregivers have better education and those implanted early tended to exhibit higher LEAQ scores.

CONCLUSION

This paper reviewed the literature on speech perception of Mandarin-speaking children with congenital HL and who used CI. Important factors that contribute to individual variations in speech perception outcomes were discussed.

Unilateral CI recipients demonstrated continuous improvements in auditory and speech perception for several years post-activation. Younger AAI and longer DCI contribute to better speech perception. Having undergone a HAT before implantation and having caregivers whose educational level is higher may lead to better performance. While the findings that support the use of CI to improve speech perception continue to grow, much research is needed to validate the use of bimodal and bilateral implantation. Evidence to date, however, revealed bimodal benefits over CI-only conditions in lexical tone recognition and sentence perception in noise. Due to scarcity of research, conclusions on the benefits of bilateral CIs compared to unilateral CI or bimodal CI use cannot be drawn. Therefore, future research on bimodal and bilateral CIs is needed to guide evidence-based clinical practice.

AUTHOR CONTRIBUTIONS

QG contributed to the literature review and manuscript drafting. LW contributed to providing review comments. FC contributed to manuscript drafting. All the authors contributed to the article and approved the submitted version.

REFERENCES

Asp, F., Mäki-Torkko, E., Karltorp, E., Harder, H., Hergils, L., Eskilsson, G., et al. (2015). A longitudinal study of the bilateral benefit in children with bilateral cochlear implants. *Int. J. Audiol.* 54, 77–88. doi: 10.3109/14992027.2014.973536

Beijen, J.-W., Mylanus, E. A. M., Leeuw, A. R., and Snik, A. F. M. (2008). Should a hearing aid in the contralateral ear be recommended for children with a unilateral cochlear implant? *Ann. Otol. Rhinol. Laryngol.* 117, 397–403. doi: 10.1177/000348940811700601

Bruijnzeel, H., Ziylan, F., Stegeman, I., Topsakal, V., and Grolman, W. (2016). A systematic review to define the speech and language benefit of early (<12 Months) pediatric cochlear implantation. *Audiol. Neurootol.* 21, 113–126. doi: 10.1159/000443363

Chen, F., Wong, L. L., and Wong, E. Y. (2013). Assessing the perceptual contributions of vowels and consonants to Mandarin sentence intelligibility. *J. Acoust. Soc. Am.* 134, EL178–EL184. doi: 10.1121/1.4831541

Chen, F., Wong, L. L. N., and Hu, Y. (2014). Effects of lexical tone contour on mandarin sentence intelligibility. *J. Speech Lang. Hear. Res.* 57, 338–345. doi: 10.1044/1092-4388(2013/12-0324)

Chen, X., Liu, H., and Chen, A. (2007). The formation of auditory and visual material in Chinese utilized in aural rehabilitation for hearing impaired children. *J. Audiol. Speech Pathol.* 24, 316–318.

Chen, X., Liu, S., Liu, B., Mo, L., Kong, Y., Liu, H., et al. (2010). The effects of age at cochlear implantation and hearing aid trial on auditory performance of Chinese infants. *Acta Laryngol.* 130, 263–270. doi: 10.3109/00016480903150528

Chen, Y., Huang, M., Li, B., Wang, Z., Zhang, Z., Jia, H., et al. (2020). Bimodal stimulation in children with bilateral profound sensorineural hearing loss: a suitable intervention model for children at the early developmental stage. *Otol. Neurotol.* 41, 1357–1362. doi: 10.1097/MAO.0000000000002812

Chen, Y., Wong, L. L., Chen, F., and Xi, X. (2014). Tone and sentence perception in young Mandarin-speaking children with cochlear implants. *Int. J. Pediatr. Otorhinolaryngol.* 78, 1923–1930. doi: 10.1016/j.ijporl.2014.08.025

Chen, Y., Wong, L. L., Zhu, S., and Xi, X. (2015). A structural equation modeling approach to examining factors influencing outcomes with cochlear implant in mandarin-speaking children. *PLoS One* 10:e0136576. doi: 10.1371/journal.pone.0136576

Chen, Y., Wong, L. L., Zhu, S., and Xi, X. (2016). Early speech perception in Mandarin-speaking children at one-year post cochlear implantation. *Res. Dev. Disabil.* 49-50, 1–12. doi: 10.1016/j.ridd.2015.11.021

Chen, Y., and Wong, L. L. N. (2017). Speech perception in Mandarin-speaking children with cochlear implants: a systematic review. *Int. J. Audiol.* 56, S7–S16. doi: 10.1080/14992027.2017.1300694

Chen, Y., and Wong, L. L. N. (2020). Development of the mandarin hearing in noise test for children. *Int. J. Audiol.* 59, 707–712. doi: 10.1080/14992027.2020.1750717

Cheng, X., Liu, Y., Wang, B., Yuan, Y., Galvin, J. J. III, Fu, Q.-J., et al. (2018). The benefits of residual hair cell function for speech and music perception in pediatric bimodal cochlear implant listeners. *Neural Plast.* 2018:4610592. doi: 10.1155/2018/4610592

Ching, T. Y., van Wanrooy, E., and Dillon, H. (2007). Binaural-bimodal fitting or bilateral implantation for managing severe to profound deafness: a review. *Trends Amplif.* 11, 161–192. doi: 10.1177/1084713807304357

Fan, X., Sui, R., Qi, X., Yang, X., Wang, N., Qin, Z., et al. (2020). Analysis of the developmental trajectory and influencing factors of auditory and speech functions after cochlear implantation in Mandarin Chinese speaking children. *Acta Laryngol.* 140, 501–508. doi: 10.1080/00016489.2020.1736622

Fu, Q. J., Zeng, F. G., Shannon, R. V., and Soli, S. D. (1998). Importance of tonal envelope cues in Chinese speech recognition. *J. Acoust. Soc. Am.* 104, 505–510. doi: 10.1121/1.423251

Guo, Q., Li, Y., Fu, X., Liu, H., Chen, J., Meng, C., et al. (2016). The relationship between cortical auditory evoked potentials (CAEPs) and speech perception in children with Nurotron(§) cochlear implants during four years of follow-up. *Int. J. Pediatr. Otorhinolaryngol.* 85, 170–177. doi: 10.1016/j.ijporl.2016.03.035

Han, D., Liu, B., Zhou, N., Chen, X., Kong, Y., Liu, H., et al. (2009). Lexical tone perception with HiResolution and HiResolution 120 sound-processing strategies in pediatric Mandarin-speaking cochlear implant users. *Ear Hear.* 30, 169–177. doi: 10.1097/AUD.0b013e31819342cf

Han, D. Y., and Wang, C. C. (2013). The current status and focus of cochlear implantation. *Chin. Sci. J. Hear. Speech Rehabil.* 5, 330–334.

He, A., Deroche, M. L., Doong, J., Jiradejvong, P., and Limb, C. J. (2016). Mandarin tone identification in cochlear implant users using exaggerated pitch contours. *Otol. Neurotol.* 37, 324–331. doi: 10.1097/MAO.0000000000000980

Huang, W., Wong, L. L. N., Chen, F., Liu, H., and Liang, W. (2020). Effects of fundamental frequency contours on sentence recognition in mandarin-speaking children with cochlear implants. *J. Speech Lang. Hear. Res.* 63, 3855–3864. doi: 10.1044/2020_JSLHR-20-00033

Hurley, R. (1999). Onset of auditory deprivation. *J. Am. Acad. Audiol.* 10, 529–534.

Jiang, F., Alimu, D., Qin, W. Z., and Kupper, H. (2020). Long-term functional outcomes of hearing and speech rehabilitation efficacy among paediatric cochlear implant recipients in Shandong, China. *Disabil. Rehabil.* 43, 2860–2865. doi: 10.1080/09638288.2020.1720317

Li, A., Wang, N., Li, J., Zhang, J., and Liu, Z. (2014). Mandarin lexical tones identification among children with cochlear implants or hearing aids. *Int. J. Pediatr. Otorhinolaryngol.* 78, 1945–1952. doi: 10.1016/j.ijporl.2014.08.033

Li, G., Soli, S. D., and Zheng, Y. (2017). Tone perception in Mandarin-speaking children with cochlear implants. *Int. J. Audiol.* 56, S49–S59. doi: 10.1080/14992027.2017.1324643

Li, G., Zhao, F., Tao, Y., Zhang, L., Yao, X., and Zheng, Y. (2020). Trajectory of auditory and language development in the early stages of pre-lingual children post cochlear implantation: a longitudinal follow up study. *Int. J. Pediatr. Otorhinolaryngol.* 128:109720. doi: 10.1016/j.ijporl.2019.109720

Li, J. N., Chen, S., Zhai, L., Han, D. Y., Eshraghi, A. A., Feng, Y., et al. (2017). The advances in hearing rehabilitation and cochlear implants in China. *Ear Hear.* 38, 647–652. doi: 10.1097/AUD.0000000000000441

Li, Y., Dong, R., Zheng, Y., Xu, T., Zhong, Y., Fong, S. Y., et al. (2015). Speech performance in pediatric users of nurotron (R) Venus cochlear implants. *Int. J. Pediatr. Otorhinolaryngol.* 79, 1017–1023. doi: 10.1016/j.ijporl.2015.04.016

Li, Y., Wang, S., Su, Q., Galvin, J. J., and Fu, Q. J. (2016). Validation of list equivalency for Mandarin speech materials to use with cochlear implant listeners. *Int. J. Audiol.* 56, S31–S40. doi: 10.1080/14992027.2016.1204564

Liang, Q., and Mason, B. (2013). Enter the dragon–China's journey to the hearing world. *Cochlear Implants Int.* 14 Suppl. 1, S26–S31. doi: 10.1179/1467010013Z.00000000080

Liu, C., Liu, S., Zhang, N., Yang, Y., Kong, Y., and Zhang, L. (2011). Standard-chinese lexical neighborhood test in normal-hearing young children. *Int. J. Pediatr. Otorhinolaryngol.* 75, 774–781. doi: 10.1016/j.ijporl.2011.03.002

Liu, H., Jin, X., Li, J., Liu, L., Zhou, Y., Zhang, J., et al. (2015a). Early auditory preverbal skills development in Mandarin speaking children with cochlear implants. *Int. J. Pediatr. Otorhinolaryngol.* 79, 71–75. doi: 10.1016/j.ijporl.2014.11.010

Liu, H., Liu, H. X., Kang, H. Y., Gu, Z., and Hong, S. L. (2016). Evaluation on health-related quality of life in deaf children with cochlear implant in China. *Int. J. Pediatr. Otorhinolaryngol.* 88, 136–141. doi: 10.1016/j.ijporl.2016.06.027

Liu, H., Liu, S., Kirk, K. I, Zhang, J., Ge, W., Zheng, J., et al. (2015b). Longitudinal performance of spoken word perception in Mandarin pediatric cochlear implant users. *Int. J. Pediatr. Otorhinolaryngol.* 79, 1677–1682. doi: 10.1016/j.ijporl.2015.07.023

Liu, H., Liu, S., Wang, S., Liu, C., Kong, Y., Zhang, N., et al. (2013). Effects of lexical characteristics and demographic factors on Mandarin Chinese open-set word recognition in children with cochlear implants. *Ear Hear.* 34, 221–228. doi: 10.1097/AUD.0b013e31826d0bc6

Liu, Q., Zhou, N., Berger, R., Huang, D., and Xu, L. (2013). Mandarin consonant contrast recognition among children with cochlear implants or hearing aids and normal-hearing children. *Otol. Neurotol.* 34, 471–476. doi: 10.1097/MAO.0b013e318286836b

Liu, S., Wang, F., Chen, P., Zuo, N., Wu, C., Ma, J., et al. (2019). Assessment of outcomes of hearing and speech rehabilitation in children with cochlear implantation. *J. Otol.* 14, 57–62. doi: 10.1016/j.joto.2019.01.006

Liu, Y. W., Tao, D. D., Chen, B., Cheng, X., Shu, Y., Galvin, J. J. III, et al. (2019). Factors affecting bimodal benefit in pediatric mandarin-speaking Chinese cochlear implant users. *Ear Hear.* 40, 1316–1327. doi: 10.1097/AUD.0000000000000712

Long, Y., Liu, H., Li, Y., Jin, X., Zhou, Y., Li, J., et al. (2018). Early auditory skills development in Mandarin speaking children after bilateral cochlear implantation. *Int. J. Pediatr. Otorhinolaryngol.* 114, 153–158. doi: 10.1016/j.ijporl.2018.08.039

Lotfi, Y., Hasanalifard, M., Moossavi, A., Bakhshi, E., and Ajaloueyan, M. (2019). Binaural hearing advantages for children with bimodal fitting. *Int. J. Pediatr. Otorhinolaryngol.* 121, 58–63. doi: 10.1016/j.ijporl.2019.02.043

Lu, X., and Qin, Z. (2018). Auditory and language development in Mandarin-speaking children after cochlear implantation. *Int. J. Pediatr. Otorhinolaryngol.* 107, 183–189. doi: 10.1016/j.ijporl.2018.02.006

Lyu, J., Kong, Y., Xu, T. Q., Dong, R. J., Qi, B. E., Wang, S., et al. (2019). Long-term follow-up of auditory performance and speech perception and effects of age on cochlear implantation in children with pre-lingual deafness. *Chin. Med. J.* 132, 1925–1934. doi: 10.1097/CM9.0000000000000370

Mao, Y., and Xu, L. (2017). Lexical tone recognition in noise in normal-hearing children and prelingually deafened children with cochlear implants. *Int. J. Audiol.* 56(suppl. 2), S23–S30. doi: 10.1080/14992027.2016.1219073

Polonenko, M. J., Papsin, B. C., and Gordon, K. A. (2018). Limiting asymmetric hearing improves benefits of bilateral hearing in children using cochlear implants. *Sci. Rep.* 8:13201. doi: 10.1038/s41598-018-31546-8

Qiu, J., Yu, C., Ariyaratne, T. V., Foteff, C., Ke, Z., Sun, Y., et al. (2017). Cost-effectiveness of pediatric cochlear implantation in rural China. *Otol. Neurotol.* 38, e75–e84. doi: 10.1097/MAO.0000000000001389

Sharma, S. D., Cushing, S. L., Papsin, B. C., and Gordon, K. A. (2020). Hearing and speech benefits of cochlear implantation in children: a review of the literature. *Int. J. Pediatr. Otorhinolaryngol.* 133:109984. doi: 10.1016/j.ijporl.2020.109984

Sparreboom, M., van Schoonhoven, J., van Zanten, B. G., Scholten, R. J., Mylanus, E. A., Grolman, W., et al. (2010). The effectiveness of bilateral cochlear implants for severe-to-profound deafness in children: a systematic review. *Otol. Neurotol.* 31, 1062–1071. doi: 10.1097/MAO.0b013e3181e3d62c

Sun, X., Gao, C., and Yuan, H. (1993). *Assessment of Hearing and Speech Rehabilitation for Children with Hearing Impairment.* Changchun: Jilin Educational Audio-Visual Publishing Co.

Tao, D. D., Deng, R., Jiang, Y., Galvin, J. J., Fu, Q. J., and Chen, B. (2015). Melodic pitch perception and lexical tone perception in Mandarin-speaking cochlear implant users. *Ear Hear.* 36, 102–110. doi: 10.1097/AUD.0000000000000086

Wang, D., Kates, J., and Hansen, J. (2014). "Investigation of the relative perceptual importance of temporal envelope and temporal fine structure between tonal and non-tonal languages," in *Proceedings of the INTERSPEECH-2014*, Singapore. doi: 10.21437/Interspeech.2014-123

Wang, L., Shen, M., Liang, W., Dao, W., Zhou, L., Zhu, M., et al. (2020). Validation of the Mandarin versions of CAP and SIR. *Int. J. Pediatr. Otorhinolaryngol.* 139:110413. doi: 10.1016/j.ijporl.2020.110413

Wang, L., Sun, X., Liang, W., Chen, J., and Zheng, W. (2013). Validation of the Mandarin version of the LittlEARS(R) auditory questionnaire. *Int. J. Pediatr. Otorhinolaryngol.* 77, 1350–1354. doi: 10.1016/j.ijporl.2013.05.033

Xi, X., Chen, A. T., Li, J., Ji, F., Hong, M. D., Hanekom, J., et al. (2009). Standardized Mandarin sentence perception in babble noise test materials for children. *J. Audiol. Speech Pathol.* 17, 318–322.

Yuen, K. C., Cao, K. L., Wei, C. G., Luan, L., Li, H., Zhang, Z.-Y., et al. (2009a). Lexical tone and word recognition in noise of Mandarin-speaking children who use cochlear implants and hearing aids in opposite ears. *Cochlear Implants Int.* 10 Suppl. 1, 120–129. doi: 10.1179/cim.2009.10.Supplement-1.120

Yuen, K. C., Luan, L., Li, H., Wei, C. G., Cao, K. L., Yuan, M., et al. (2009b). Development of the computerized Mandarin pediatric lexical tone and disyllabic-word picture identification test in noise (MAPPID-N). *Cochlear Implants Int.* 10 Suppl. 1, 138–147. doi: 10.1179/cim.2009.10.Supplement-1.138

Zhang, H., Zhang, J., Ding, H., and Zhang, Y. (2020a). Bimodal benefits for lexical tone recognition: an investigation on Mandarin-speaking preschoolers with a cochlear implant and a contralateral hearing aid. *Brain Sci.* 10:238. doi: 10.3390/brainsci10040238

Zhang, H., Zhang, J., Peng, G., Ding, H., and Zhang, Y. (2020b). Bimodal benefits revealed by categorical perception of lexical tones in Mandarin-speaking kindergarteners with a cochlear implant and a contralateral hearing aid. *J. Speech, Lang.* 63, 4238–4251. doi: 10.1044/2020_JSLHR-20-00224

Zhang, V., Xu, T., Ching, T., and Chen, X. (2021). The Chinese version of the parents' evaluation of aural/oral performance of children (PEACH) rating scale for infants and children with normal hearing. *Int. J. Audiol.* 16, 1–7. doi: 10.1080/14992027.2021.1922768

Zheng, Y., Soli, S. D., Meng, Z., Tao, Y., Wang, K., Xu, K., et al. (2010). Assessment of Mandarin-speaking pediatric cochlear implant recipients with the Mandarin Early Speech Perception (MESP) test. *Int. J. Pediatr. Otorhinolaryngol.* 74, 920–925. doi: 10.1016/j.ijporl.2010.05.014

Zheng, Y., Meng, Z. L., Wang, K., Tao, Y., Xu, K., and Soli, S. D. (2009a). Development of the Mandarin early speech perception test: children with normal hearing and the effects of dialect exposure. *Ear Hear.* 30, 600–612. doi: 10.1097/AUD.0b013e3181b4aba8

Zheng, Y., Soli, S. D., Tao, Y., Xu, K., Meng, Z., Li, G., et al. (2011). Early prelingual auditory development and speech perception at 1-year follow-up in Mandarin-speaking children after cochlear implantation. *Int. J. Pediatr. Otorhinolaryngol.* 75, 1418–1426. doi: 10.1016/j.ijporl.2011.08.005

Zheng, Y., Soli, S. D., Wang, K., Meng, J., Meng, Z., Xu, K., et al. (2009b). Development of the Mandarin pediatric speech intelligibility (MPSI) test. *Int. J. Audiol.* 48, 718–728. doi: 10.1080/14992020902902658

Zheng, Y., Soli, S. D., Wang, K., Meng, J., Meng, Z., Xu, K., et al. (2009c). A normative study of early prelingual auditory development. *Audiol. Neurootol.* 14, 214–222. doi: 10.1159/000189264

Zhou, N., Huang, J., Chen, X., and Xu, L. (2013). Relationship between tone perception and production in prelingually deafened children with cochlear implants. *Otol. Neurotol.* 34, 499–506. doi: 10.1097/MAO.0b013e318287ca86

Zhu, M., Fu, Q. J., Galvin, J. J. III, Jiang, Y., Xu, J., Xu, C., et al. (2011). Mandarin Chinese speech recognition by pediatric cochlear implant users. *Int. J. Pediatr. Otorhinolaryngol.* 75, 793–800. doi: 10.1016/j.ijporl.2011.03.009

Zhu, S., Wong, L., Chen, F., Chen, Y., and Wang, B. (2016). Known-groups and concurrent validity of the mandarin tone identification test (MTIT). *PLoS One* 11:e0155595. doi: 10.1371/journal.pone.0155595

Zhu, S. F., Wong, L. N., and Chen, F. (2014). Development and validation of a new Mandarin tone identification test. *Int. J. Pediatr. Otorhinolaryngol.* 78, 2174–2182. doi: 10.1016/j.ijporl.2014.10.004

9

The Neural Processing of Vocal Emotion after Hearing Reconstruction in Prelingual Deaf Children: A Functional Near-Infrared Spectroscopy Brain Imaging Study

Yuyang Wang[1], Lili Liu[2], Ying Zhang[3], Chaogang Wei[1], Tianyu Xin[1], Qiang He[3], Xinlin Hou[2] and Yuhe Liu[1]**

[1] Department of Otolaryngology, Head and Neck Surgery, Peking University First Hospital, Beijing, China, [2] Department of Pediatrics, Peking University First Hospital, Beijing, China, [3] Department of Otolaryngology, Head and Neck Surgery, The Second Hospital of Hebei Medical University, Shijiazhuang, China

***Correspondence:**
Xinlin Hou
houxinlin66@163.com
Yuhe Liu
liuyuhefeng@163.com

As elucidated by prior research, children with hearing loss have impaired vocal emotion recognition compared with their normal-hearing peers. Cochlear implants (CIs) have achieved significant success in facilitating hearing and speech abilities for people with severe-to-profound sensorineural hearing loss. However, due to the current limitations in neuroimaging tools, existing research has been unable to detail the neural processing for perception and the recognition of vocal emotions during early stage CI use in infant and toddler CI users (ITCI). In the present study, functional near-infrared spectroscopy (fNIRS) imaging was employed during preoperative and postoperative tests to describe the early neural processing of perception in prelingual deaf ITCIs and their recognition of four vocal emotions (fear, anger, happiness, and neutral). The results revealed that the cortical response elicited by vocal emotional stimulation on the left pre-motor and supplementary motor area (pre-SMA), right middle temporal gyrus (MTG), and right superior temporal gyrus (STG) were significantly different between preoperative and postoperative tests. These findings indicate differences between the preoperative and postoperative neural processing associated with vocal emotional stimulation. Further results revealed that the recognition of vocal emotional stimuli appeared in the right supramarginal gyrus (SMG) after CI implantation, and the response elicited by fear was significantly greater than the response elicited by anger, indicating a negative bias. These findings indicate that the development of emotional bias and the development of emotional perception and recognition capabilities in ITCIs occur on a different timeline and involve different neural processing from those in normal-hearing peers. To assess the speech perception and production abilities, the Infant-Toddler Meaningful Auditory Integration Scale (IT-MAIS) and Speech Intelligibility Rating (SIR) were used. The results revealed no significant differences between preoperative and postoperative tests. Finally, the correlates of the neurobehavioral results were investigated, and the results demonstrated that the preoperative response of the right SMG to anger stimuli was significantly and positively correlated with the evaluation of postoperative behavioral outcomes. And the postoperative response of the right SMG to anger stimuli was significantly and negatively correlated with the evaluation of postoperative behavioral outcomes.

Keywords: vocal emotion, cochlear implant, prelingual deaf, infant and toddler, functional near-infrared spectroscopy

INTRODUCTION

Emotional communication is a universal form of expression that enables people to overcome language and cultural barriers (Thompson and Balkwill, 2006; Bryant and Barrett, 2008; Pell et al., 2009). Deficits in vocal emotion perception (facial expressions are not always visible in many environments) not only affect the quality of life and social interactions among adults but also potentially affect the cognitive and social development of infants and toddlers (Denham et al., 1990). Responding to emotional stimuli is one of the first developmental milestones, and has higher credibility in infants and toddlers, who have immaturely perception and cognition. Meanwhile, in other research, newborns have been shown to have a preference for the infant-directed speech of female voices, which can be attributed to infant-directed speech generally conveying more emotion and information, compared with the suppressed emotion expression in most adult communication (Glenn and Cunningham, 1983; Cooper and Aslin, 1989; Pegg et al., 1992). These findings revealed that the perception and recognition of vocal emotions are significant factors during cognition and communication in early life. Numerous studies have shown that establishing a strong emotional connection with adults is crucial for the physical and intellectual development of infants and toddlers (Ainsworth and Bell, 1970; Drotar and Sturm, 1988). The perception of vocal emotion is likely to be a more significant factor during early infant development because the auditory system develops earlier than the visual system (Gottlieb, 1971; Kasatkin, 1972). However, infants and toddlers with hearing loss face difficulties in emotional communications (Ludlow et al., 2010; Most and Michaelis, 2012).

Many studies have examined the neural processing for vocal emotions in infants with normal hearing, which may provide a reference for the neural processing associated with hearing loss. Information regarding the neural processing mechanism of vocal emotion was also reported in neonates (Zhang et al., 2017, 2019; Zhao et al., 2019). The results showed that vocal emotions enhance the activation of the right superior temporal gyrus (STG), the left superior frontal gyrus (SFG), and the left angular gyrus, which may indicate the regions associated with the neural processing of vocal emotional perception during neonatal development. Moreover, happiness elicited increased neural responses in the right STG and the right inferior frontal gyrus (IFG) as compared to fear and anger, and these results also indicate that neonates' response to positive vocal emotions takes precedence over negative vocal emotions, which is contrary to the negative biases observed in adult studies. Up to now, very little is known about the neural processes of vocal emotion in infants and toddlers with normal hearing. Studies have shown that infants younger than 6 months show a preferential response to positive emotions received through vocal emotional stimuli (Farroni et al., 2007; Vaish et al., 2008; Rigato et al., 2010). This result is supported by Trainor et al. (2000), who demonstrated that infants are more inclined to listen to infant-directed speech associated with positive emotions than to infant-direct speech associated with negative emotions. Conversely, negative bias refers to the priority processing of negative information in the brain, which typically appears in infants between 6 and 12 months of age (Peltola et al., 2009; Grossmann et al., 2010; Hoehl and Striano, 2010). The findings of these previous studies seem to indicate that emotional preferences are different at different stages of human development.

Emotions are expressed through a combination of numerous acoustic cues (Linnankoski et al., 2005; Sauter et al., 2010). Hearing loss will affect the perception and recognition of emotions in speech, including cochlear implant (CI) users (Most et al., 1993; Ludlow et al., 2010; Wiefferink et al., 2013; Chatterjee et al., 2015), because the reduction of acquired acoustic cues makes it difficult to distinguish acoustic emotions. Speech processing and adaptive behaviors in the social environment depend on the effective decoding of vocal emotions (Fruhholz and Grandjean, 2013), especially for deaf infants and toddlers who cannot recognize words and sentences (Eisenberg et al., 2010). Therefore, hearing loss in infants and toddlers can have long-term impacts on language learning, social functioning and psychological development (Wauters and Knoors, 2008; Schorr et al., 2009; Eisenberg et al., 2010; Geers et al., 2013). Previous studies have concluded that the auditory emotion recognition of children with severe-to-profound hearing loss is significantly worse than that of chronological- and mental-age-matched normal hearing children (Ludlow et al., 2010). However, no significant difference in auditory emotion recognition has been observed between children with mild-to-moderate hearing loss relative to their normal-hearing peers (Cannon and Chatterjee, 2019). Infants and toddlers with congenital severe-to-profound hearing loss represent good models for studying emotional recognition processes after hearing reconstruction. Observing differences in the perception and recognition of vocal emotion between children with congenital severe-to-profound hearing loss and normal-hearing children will help us to better understand the development of vocal emotion recognition during the early stages of life. However, little is known about the effects of severe-to-profound hearing loss and hearing reconstruction on the neural processing of vocal emotion in infants and toddlers.

To investigate these phenomena, neural data from early life stages should be included. To date, no brain imaging studies have focused on the vocal emotion processing that occurs in infants and toddlers with severe-to-profound hearing loss who received few vocal emotional cues from the social environment. The auditory perception of infants and toddlers with hearing loss can be reconstructed through the use of cochlear implants (CIs) (Zeng et al., 2008). The use of CIs is a world-recognized method for hearing reconstruction in individuals with severe-to-profound sensorineural hearing loss. The use of CI has significantly benefited children with severe to profound hearing loss in acoustic emotion recognition (Chatterjee et al., 2015). However there are still some imperfections in the sound collection, information processing and transmission of existing cochlear implant systems, such as the transmission of spectro-temporal fine structure information are degraded (Xu et al., 2009; Kang et al., 2010; Kong et al., 2011). The acoustic information received by CI users is decreased. Therefore, perceiving prosodic information is difficult for CI users compared to people with normal hearing (such as vocal emotion, music appreciation) (Jiam and Limb, 2020). And prosodic limitation will bring adverse consequences to the decoding and communication of vocal emotions for CI users (Planalp, 1996). But the neural mechanism of how CI users processing this severely reduced acoustic information after auditory cortex deprivation and remodeling remains unclear. For example, if the incomplete acoustic information can enable a specific emotional state to reproduce the experience in the sensory-motor system, this may involve embodied cognition theory (Damasio, 1989; Wilson, 2002; Niedenthal, 2007). In addition, the correlation between cortical activation elicited by these vocal emotional stimuli and postoperative behavioral outcomes remains to be studied. Part of the problem is the lack of neuroimaging tools suitable for early, repeatable measurements. Prelingual deaf infant and toddler CI users (ITCIs) represent a unique group of people who have experienced hearing loss and reconstruction, with limited hearing experience. Research on this group will bring new perspectives and supplement existing knowledge in this field.

In this study, we used functional near-infrared spectroscopy (fNIRS) to observe changes between the preoperative and early postoperative neural response to four vocal emotions in prelingual deaf ITCIs. The primary advantages of fNIRS include low invasiveness and the characteristics of optical principles, which are compatible with ITCI and allow for the safe and repeated use of fNIRS. In addition, the ability to use fNIRS without generating additional noise makes this a compatible evaluation modality for auditory tasks. fNIRS also offers higher spatial resolution than event-related potentials and can be easily adapted to accommodate the test subject's head and body movements (Piper et al., 2014; Saliba et al., 2016). The ability to collect data from low-attention and active infants and toddlers was further enhanced by the use of fNIRS. We tested the participants within 1 week prior to the CI operation (preoperative test) and within 1 week after turning the CI on (postoperative test). We presented four vocal emotional stimuli for the subjects, including fear (negative), anger (negative), happiness (positive), and neutral. The Infant-Toddler Meaningful Auditory Integration Scale (IT-MAIS)/MAIS (Zimmerman-Phillips et al., 1997) and Speech Intelligibility Rating (SIR) scales (Allen et al., 1998) were used to evaluate the participants' speech perception and expression abilities. This design allowed for three critical questions to be addressed. (1). How the neural processing (regions and intensity of cortical activation) for vocal emotional stimuli in prelingual deaf ITCI differ between preoperative and postoperative tests. (2). Whether vocal emotion recognition and bias exist in the processing of prelingual deaf ITCIs during preoperative and postoperative tests and whether these change following CI use (see Zhang et al., 2017, 2019). (3). Whether any correlations exist between the neural responses to vocal emotional stimuli and speech perception in prelingual deaf children and their expression abilities and how these differ between the preoperative and postoperative tests.

Although we make hypotheses based on the results of studies performed in people with normal hearing, our research is exploratory due to the lack of existing brain imaging studies evaluating the effects of severe-to-profound hearing loss on vocal emotional processing patterns. We hypothesized that the neural responses to the four vocal emotions in the preoperative test results of prelingual deaf ITCIs would not differ significantly due to the impacts of hearing loss, whereas the neural processing will differ from that observed for normal-hearing infants (Zhang et al., 2019). That is, the region and intensity of cortical activation should be different. The correlation between neural and behavioral results will be difficult to observe at this time due to the lack of sufficiently mature auditory cortex development. The hypothesis for postoperative test results was that differences would be observed in vocal emotion recognition ability and neural processing relative to those in the preoperative test. After the hearing is reconstructed, the auditory cortex receives better auditory stimulation. Because emotion recognition and positive bias could be observed in neonates as early as 0–4 days after birth in previous studies (Zhang et al., 2019), we expected that ITCIs would respond to the four vocal emotional stimuli in 0–7 days after the CI is activated, and a stronger neural response will be observed in the right temporal area, with a positive bias. That is, happiness will cause stronger activation of the cortex than other vocal emotions. However, fewer emotions will be recognized due to the limitation of CI itself, and the cortical activation region elicited by vocal emotional stimulation will be different from that of neonates with normal hearing, and the activating intensity will be weaker. We don't expect to find significant differences in preoperative and postoperative behavioral tests, but that overall performance on these assessments was being examined to determine if these common clinical assessments would be correlated with cortical activation. And we expected to observe a correlation between the neural response elicited by vocal emotional stimuli in the right temporal region and behavioral results at this time because the correlation between cortical activation elicited by auditory and visual stimulation and behavioral results has been observed in previous deaf adult studies (Anderson et al., 2019).

We hope that these results can establish a baseline for future research in this field.

MATERIALS AND METHODS

Participants

Twenty-two prelingual deaf infants and toddlers with bilateral severe-to-profound sensorineural hearing loss (10 girls; age: 13–38 months, mean: 22.5 ± 6.43 months) participated in this study (see **Table 1** for detailed information). All participants failed the first hearing screening of the otoacoustic emissions test combined with automatic auditory brainstem response 3–5 days after birth and failed the second hearing screening performed within 42 days of birth. All participants met the Chinese national guidelines for cochlear implantation (Editorial Board of Chinese Journal of Otorhinolaryngology Head and Neck Surgery et al., 2014). Before implantation, all participants were evaluated for auditory ability: The click auditory brainstem response thresholds for both ears were above 90 dB nHL; and the auditory steady-state response was above 90 dB nHL in response to frequency thresholds of 2 kHz and above. Cooperating with a pure tone audiometry test or auditory word recognition test is difficult for the participants in this study because our participants lack sufficient auditory and speech skills and attention to understand and perform the test procedure. Therefore, they were assessed by unaided pediatric behavioral auditory testing (PBA), using thresholds above 80 dB HL, and aided pediatric behavioral auditory testing, using thresholds above 60 dB HL, for both ears. Participants also met the following criteria: (A) except for hearing, other physiological development was normal (including vision); (B) imaging examinations showed no deformities of the inner ear; (C) the postoperative X-ray examination did not reveal any abnormalities, and implanted electrodes were correctly located in the cochlea; (D) all impedances for all electrodes after surgery are within the normal range; (E) the clinical team evaluated the comfort and threshold levels of each electrode position according to standard clinical protocols; and (F) the participants were clinically asymptomatic (No abnormality or discomfort) at the two times of fNIRS recording.

Behavioral Measurements

At every visit, participants' auditory perception was assessed by the IT-MAIS/MAIS (Zimmerman-Phillips et al., 1997), and speech production was assessed by the SIR (Allen et al., 1998). These two tests reported by caregiver were widely used tools for screening and monitoring the hearing and speech development of infants and toddlers (Cavicchiolo et al., 2018; Lu and Qin, 2018; Yang et al., 2020). The IT-MAIS/MAIS assessment of auditory perception in infants and young children includes three dimensions: Adaptability to CI, auditory perception ability, and auditory recognition ability. The use of the IT-MAIS/MAIS enabled us to perform a more comprehensive assessment and monitoring of auditory development in infants and toddlers at earlier stages. To better measure the participant's hearing and speech abilities, we converted the scores of all assessments to a 0–100 scale. The total score of ITMAIS/MAIS is 40 points. We multiply the score by 2.5. There are 5 levels of SIR, and each level counts as 20 points.

fNIRS Experimental Stimuli and Procedure

The auditory stimuli program presented to ITCI users was generated by E-Prime (version 2.0, Psychology Software Tools, United States). Vocal emotional stimulation included four types: Fear, anger, happiness, and neutral. The vocal stimulation materials used in this study were obtained from the Chinese vocal emotional stimulation material database (Liu and Pell, 2012). We used infant-directed vocal emotional stimulation as the stimulus material because this stimulus does not require substantial auditory experience, and vocal emotional perception develops earlier than speech perception capabilities and has been shown to be effective even in neonates (Zhang et al., 2017, 2019). These vocal emotional stimuli are composed of pseudo-sentences, which are non-semantic but contain grammatical information and deliver vocal emotional information at the same time. Stimulation materials were read in infant-directed speech prosody by a native Chinese female. The recognition rate and emotional intensity of vocal emotional stimuli have been confirmed in our previous research (Zhang et al., 2019). Vocal emotional stimulation is presented in a block design, with 15-s sound presentation blocks interleaved with silent blocks of varying durations between 14 and 15 s. The four types of emotional prosodies were presented in random order. Each type of emotional prosody was repeated 10 times, and the entire stimulation program lasts approximately 20 min (**Figure 1A**).

Preoperative brain imaging using fNIRS was performed after the participant agreed to receive CI but before the operation when the participant was asleep. During the preoperative test, participants wore hearing aids on both sides during the test. Participants visited the hospital approximately 4 weeks after surgery to activate the CI, and fNIRS brain imaging was performed within 0–7 days after CI activation (mean: 5.727 ± 2.700 days). fNIRS were conducted in the hearing room of the Department of Otolaryngology Head and Neck Surgery, Peking University First Hospital. During the postoperative test, participants wore both CI and hearing aids. The sound was passively presented through a pair of speakers (Edifier R26T, Edifier, China). The speakers were placed 10 cm from the left and right ears of the participants (**Figure 1B**). To reflect the typical level of conversational speech, the sound pressure level was maintained at 60–65 dB SPL. To ensure the collection of fNIRS data, extra optical and acoustic signals were excluded to the greatest extent possible during the experiment, and the average background noise intensity was measured near 30 dB SPL. These data were measured in the listening position using a sound level meter (HS5633T, Hengsheng, China) during the experiment and in a quiet state, with participants absent. The fNIRS recording was performed with the participants in a quiet sleeping state, or in a quiet state of alert (see Cheng et al., 2012; Gomez et al., 2014; Zhang et al., 2019; **Figure 1B**). We recruited 30 ITCIs. ITCIs who started crying or were too active during fNIRS recording

TABLE 1 | Demographic and clinical information of participants.

Subject	Gender	Implanted-age (months)	Implantation side	Cochlear implant	Preoperative aided thresholds (Implanted side)	Preoperative aided thresholds (contralateral side)
1	Girl	23	Right	Nucleus CI-512	80	90
2	Girl	17	Right	Nucleus CI-512	70	60
3	Boy	21	Right	Nucleus CI-512	66	94
4	Girl	30	Right	Nucleus CI-512	100	100
5	Boy	34	Right	Nucleus CI-512	70	70
6	Boy	17	Right	Nucleus CI-512	65	65
7	Boy	16	Right	Nucleus CI-512	90	100
8	Boy	27	Right	Nucleus CI-512	70	80
9	Girl	16	Right	Nucleus CI-512	95	95
10	Boy	22	Right	Nucleus CI-512	98	98
11	Girl	23	Right	Nucleus CI-512	96	99
12	Girl	28	Right	Nucleus CI-512	94	96
13	Boy	15	Right	Nucleus CI-512	79	65
14	Boy	13	Right	Nucleus CI-512	71	86
15	Girl	16	Right	Nucleus CI-512	95	95
16	Girl	16	Right	Nucleus CI-512	100	100
17	Boy	38	Left	Nucleus CI-512	70	65
18	Girl	27	Left	Nucleus CI-512	70	75
19	Boy	25	Right	Nucleus CI-512	80	80
20	Boy	25	Right	Nucleus CI-512	90	90
21	Boy	26	Right	Nucleus CI-512	100	100
22	Girl	20	Right	Nucleus CI-512	60	60
Mean (SD)		22.5(6.43)			82.23(13.66)	84.68(14.70)

were not included in the analysis. Therefore, the final analysis was performed on a data set that included 22 participants.

fNIRS Data Recording

fNIRS was performed using a multichannel continuous-wave near-infrared optical imaging system (Nirsmart, Huichuang, China) to record fNIRS data in continuous-wave mode, as described in previous studies (Bu et al., 2018; Li et al., 2020). fNIRS recordings were generated using NIRScan software (Version 2.3.5.1a, Huichuang, China). Based on the results reported by previous studies on vocal emotions in infants (Benavides-Varela et al., 2011; Minagawa-Kawai et al., 2011; Sato et al., 2012) and adults (Bruck et al., 2011; Fruhholz et al., 2016) with normal hearing, as well as the remodeling known to occur in the cortex after cochlear implantation, we placed the optodes over the temporal, frontal, and central regions of the brain, using an elastic cap with a 46–50 cm diameter (Huichuang, China), using the international 10–20 system (Okamoto et al., 2004; **Figures 2A,B**). We used 20 optical emitters (intensity greater than 50 mW/wavelength) and 16 two-wavelength (760 and 850 nm) detectors to form 52 available channels (26 per hemisphere), with the optical source and detector at a distance of approximately 2.50 cm (see **Table 2** and **Figures 2C,D**).

fNIRS Data Preprocessing

Data preprocessing uses the Nirspark software package (version 6.12, Huichuang, China), run in MATLAB (R2017b, The MathWorks, United States). The following steps were used to preprocess the signal. (1) The task-unrelated time intervals were removed. (2) The task-unrelated artifacts were removed. (3) The light intensity was converted into optical density. (4) The data were band-pass filtered between 0.01 and 0.2 Hz to remove the task-unrelated effects of low-frequency drift and high-frequency neurophysiological noise. (5) Based on the Beer–Lambert law, the optical density was converted into oxyhemoglobin and deoxyhemoglobin concentrations. The hemodynamic response function initial time was set to -2 s, and the end time was set to 20 s (with "-2–0 s" as the reserved baseline state and "0–20 s" as the time for a single block paradigm). (6) With the "fear, angry, happy, neutral" duration set to 15 s, the oxyhemoglobin concentrations for each block paradigm were superimposed and averaged to generate a block average result. Because oxyhemoglobin is more sensitive to changes between conditions than deoxyhemoglobin and is typically associated with a better signal-to-noise ratio (Strangman et al., 2002), the subsequent statistical analysis only used oxyhemoglobin.

Statistical Analyses

The preprocessed fNIRS data and behavioral data were counted using SPSS software (version 21.0, SPSS company, United States). We conducted vocal emotional stimulation (fearful, angry, happy, and neutral) by time (preoperative and postoperative) repeated-measures analysis of variance for each channel. To investigate the specific period during which the vocal emotion recognition ability was generated, a one-way analysis of variance was performed on those channels with significant main effects.

A

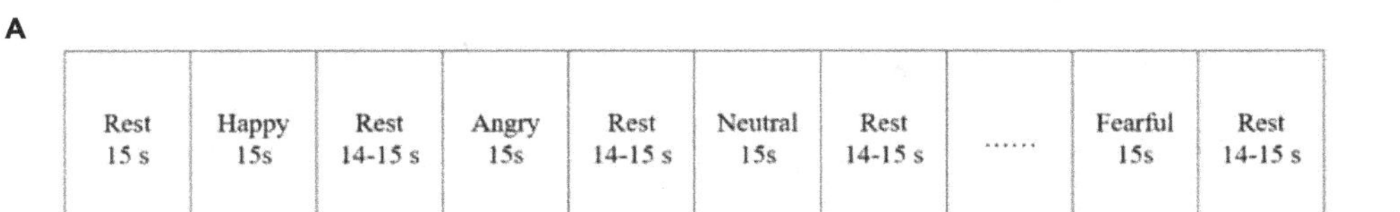

B

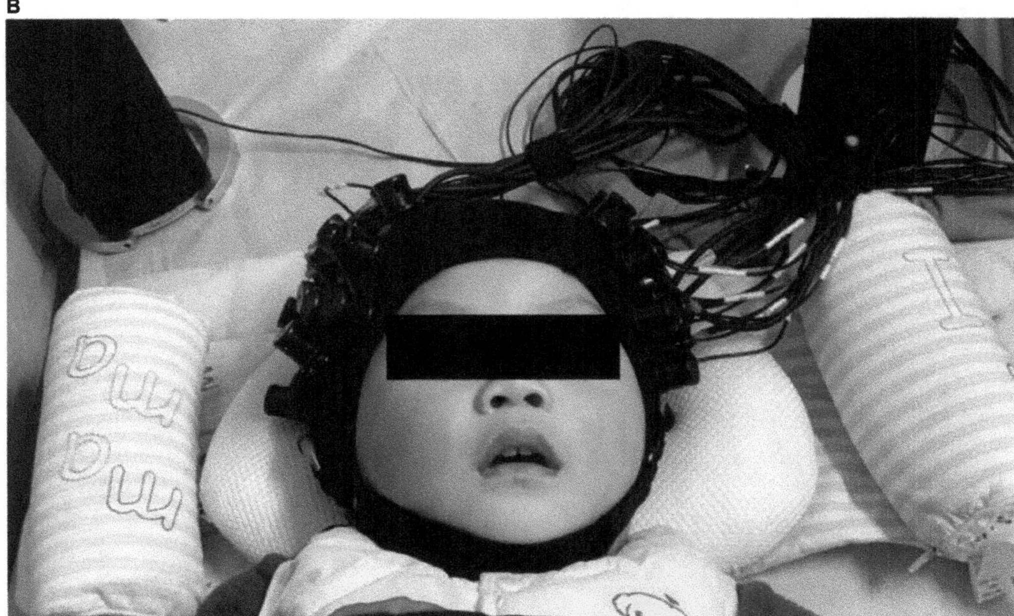

FIGURE 1 | fNIRS test procedures and environment. **(A)** A schematic representation of the block design used for the vocal emotional stimulation experimental procedure. **(B)** An example of the positioning of the participants during the fNIRS test. The test was conducted in a dark environment, and the lights in the room were switched off.

Levene's test was performed to detect the homogeneity of variance. When $p > 0.05$, variance was considered homogeneous. Follow-up analyses involved pairwise comparisons between the four emotional conditions, and the Bonferroni corrected method was used to correct for multiple comparisons between pairs. Pearson's correlational analysis was used to measure the correlation between cortical responses to vocal emotional stimuli and behavioral results. For all analyses, $p < 0.05$ was considered significant.

RESULTS

Behavioral Outcomes

We performed a one-way analysis of variance on the two behavioral outcomes, the IT-MAIS/MAIS and SIR tests, comparing the preoperative and postoperative performance. In the preoperative test, the participants' average score for the IT-MAIS/MAIS was 23.00, with a standard deviation of 17.41, and the average score for the SIR was 20, with a standard deviation of 0. In the postoperative test, the average score for the IT-MAIS/MAIS was 29.09, with a standard deviation of 24.00, and the average score for the SIR was 20.01, with a standard deviation of 4.26. No significant difference was identified between the behavioral results for either test ($p > 0.05$; **Figure 3**).

fNIRS

We analyzed changes in the oxyhemoglobin response for each channel in response to four types of vocal emotional stimuli during two periods using a repeated-measures analysis of variance. The results showed that the main effect of the period factor (preoperative and postoperative) was significant for channels 21 ($F = 5.970$, $p = 0.017$, $\eta^2 = 0.066$), 22 ($F = 5.217$, $p = 0.025$, $\eta^2 = 0.058$), 40 ($F = 4.829$, $p = 0.031$, $\eta^2 = 0.054$), 42 ($F = 4.885$, $p = 0.030$, $\eta^2 = 0.055$), and 47 ($F = 4.361$, $p = 0.040$, $\eta^2 = 0.049$; **Figures 4A–E**), whereas the main effect of vocal emotional stimulation (fearful, angry, happy, and neutral) was not significant ($F < 0.792$, $p > 0.502$, $\eta^2 < 0.028$), and the interaction between vocal emotional stimulation and period was not significant ($F < 1.418$, $p > 0.243$, $\eta^2 < 0.048$). However, in channel 30, the main effect of vocal emotional stimulation was significant ($F = 3.122$, $p = 0.030$, $\eta^2 = 0.100$), whereas the main effect of the period was not significant ($F = 0.220$, $p = 0.640$, $\eta^2 = 0.003$), and the interaction between vocal

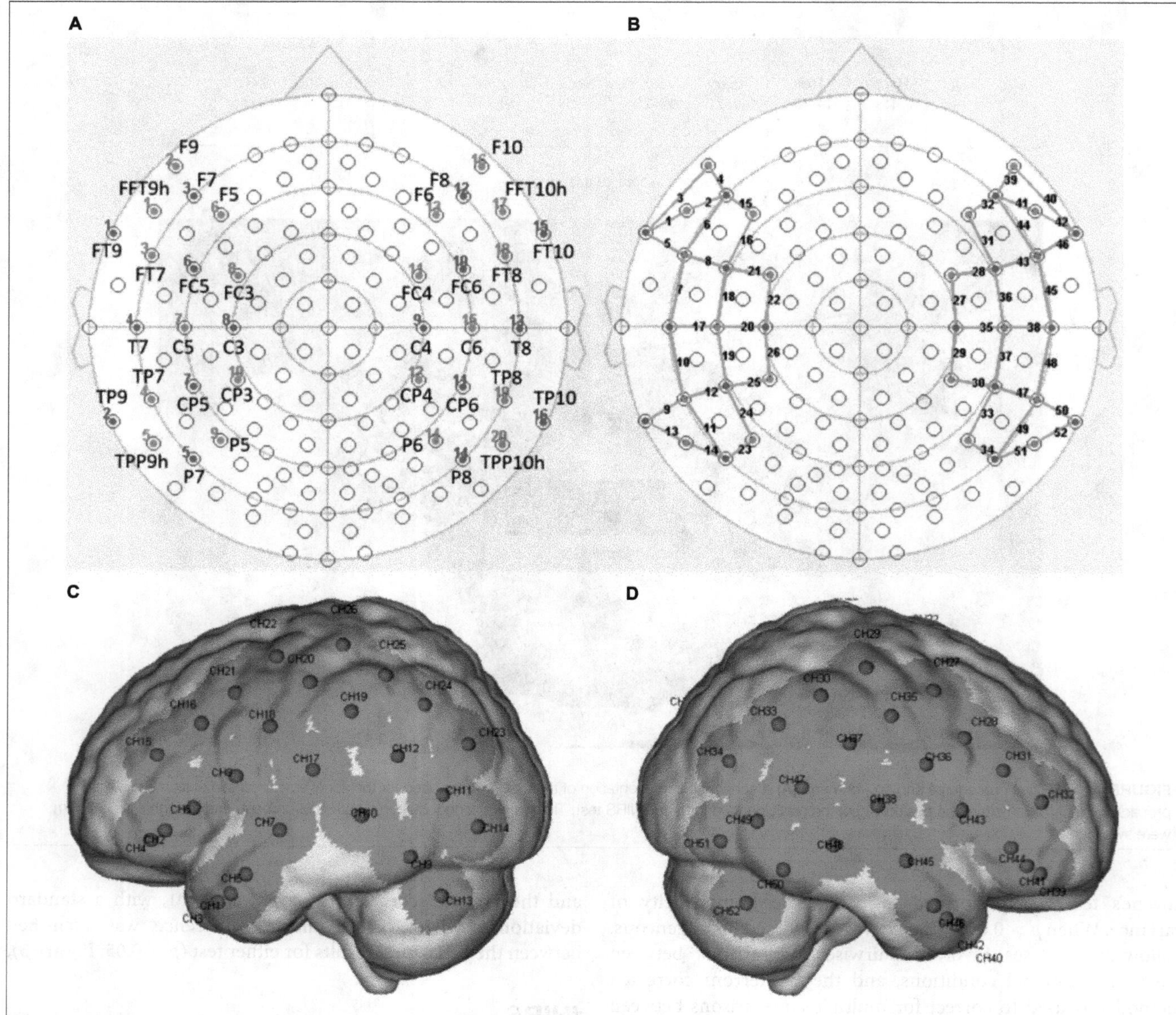

FIGURE 2 | The arrangement of the light sources and detectors and the positions of the detection channels. **(A)** The position of the light sources and detectors, arranged according to the 10–20 system, with red indicating a light source and blue indicating a detector. **(B)** A schematic representation of the positions of the detection channels (indicated by the green line) formed by the light sources and the detectors. **(C,D)** Schematic representations of the channel positions in the left **(C)** and right **(D)** hemispheres during fNIRS. Each gray dot represents the center of the detection channel.

emotional stimulation and period was not significant ($F = 2.072$, $p = 0.110$, $\eta^2 = 0.069$). Further pairwise comparison results showed that a significant difference between fear and anger ($p = 0.038$, Bonferroni corrected), and the cortical response when hearing a fear stimulus was greater than that hearing and anger stimulus (**Figure 4F**). The results of the one-way analysis of variance showed no significant difference in the response of channel 30 to the four vocal emotional stimuli in the preoperative test ($F = 1.689$, $p = 0.176$, $\eta^2 = 0.057$), whereas a significant difference was identified in the postoperative test ($F = 3.051$, $p = 0.033$, $\eta^2 = 0.098$). The cortical response to a fear stimulus was greater than that in response to an anger stimulus ($p = 0.022$, Bonferroni corrected). All statistical results were reported in **Table 3**.

Neuro-Behavioral Correction

Significant differences in the cortical response to different vocal emotional stimuli were identified in channel 30; therefore, the cortical data from channel 30 in response to the four vocal emotional stimuli were used to perform correlation analysis with the behavioral outcomes. The results showed that changes in the neural response to anger observed in channel 30 were significantly correlated with the IT-MAIS/MAIS results. A positive correlation was identified between the preoperative

TABLE 2 | Channels and corresponding brain regions.

Channel	Brodmann area	P	Channel	Brodmann area	P
1	Middle temporal gyrus	0.825	27	Pre-motor and supplementary motor cortex	0.858
2	Inferior prefrontal gyrus	0.987	28	Dorsolateral prefrontal cortex	0.579
3	Middle temporal gyrus	0.791	29	Supramarginal gyrus part of Wernicke's area	0.291
4	Inferior prefrontal gyrus	1	30	Supramarginal gyrus part of Wernicke's area	1
5	Middle temporal gyrus	0.796	31	Dorsolateral prefrontal cortex	0.451
6	Pars triangularis Broca's area	0.441	32	Dorsolateral prefrontal cortex	0.843
7	Middle temporal gyrus	0.822	33	Supramarginal gyrus part of Wernicke's area	0.645
8	Pre-motor and supplementary motor cortex	0.473	34	Angular gyrus, part of Wernicke's area	0.608
9	Fusiform gyrus	0.665	35	Pre-motor and supplementary motor cortex	0.315
10	Middle temporal gyrus	0.619	36	Pre-motor and supplementary motor cortex	0.739
11	Visual association cortex 3	0.487	37	Supramarginal gyrus part of Wernicke's area	0.927
12	Supramarginal gyrus part of Wernicke's area	0.399	38	Primary and auditory association cortex	0.616
13	Visual association cortex 3	0.579	39	Inferior prefrontal gyrus	0.886
14	Visual association cortex 3	0.732	40	Middle temporal gyrus	0.592
15	Dorsolateral prefrontal cortex	0.946	41	Inferior prefrontal gyrus	1
16	Dorsolateral prefrontal cortex	0.824	42	Middle temporal gyrus	0.806
17	Primary and auditory association cortex	0.396	43	Pars opercularis, part of Broca's area	0.505
18	Pre-motor and supplementary motor cortex	0.706	44	Inferior prefrontal gyrus	0.8
19	Supramarginal gyrus part of Wernicke's area	0.951	45	Middle temporal gyrus	1
20	Primary somatosensory cortex	0.318	46	Middle temporal gyrus	0.822
21	Pre-motor and supplementary motor cortex	0.656	47	Superior temporal Gyrus	0.816
22	Pre-motor and supplementary motor cortex	0.713	48	Middle temporal gyrus	0.876
23	Angular gyrus, part of Wernicke's area	0.718	49	Fusiform gyrus	0.611
24	Angular gyrus, part of Wernicke's area	0.508	50	Fusiform gyrus	0.526
25	Supramarginal gyrus part of Wernicke's area	1	51	Visual association cortex 3	0.746
26	Primary somatosensory cortex	0.303	52	Fusiform gyrus	0.814

cortical activation elicited by anger and the postoperative IT-MAIS/MAIS results ($r = 0.455$, $p = 0.033$, $n = 22$; **Figure 5A**). The results also showed a negative correlation between the postoperative cortical activation elicited by anger and the postoperative IT-MAIS/MAIS results ($r = -0.576$, $p = 0.005$, $n = 22$; **Figure 5B**). However, in response to other vocal emotional stimuli, no significant correlations with behavioral results were found ($p > 0.05$).

DISCUSSION

Although the perception and recognition of vocal emotions in neonates have been reported previously (Zhang et al., 2019), the present study is the first to focus on the perception and recognition of vocal emotions during the early period following CI operations in prelingual deaf infants and toddlers. We expected to describe the neural processing used in prelingual deaf infants and toddlers with vocal emotional stimuli and compared these before and early after surgery.

Regional Differences in Cortical Activation Elicited by Vocal Emotions Before and After Hearing Reconstruction

The neural responses to vocal emotional stimuli in the preoperative and postoperative fNIRS tests were significantly different for the left channels 21 and 22 [located in (pre-)SMA] and the right channels 40, 42, and 47 (located in STG and MTG) in the present study (**Figures 4A–E**). The neural response of the left (pre-)SMA to vocal emotional stimulation changed from preoperative activation to postoperative inhibition. By contrast, the neural responses of the right MTG and STG to

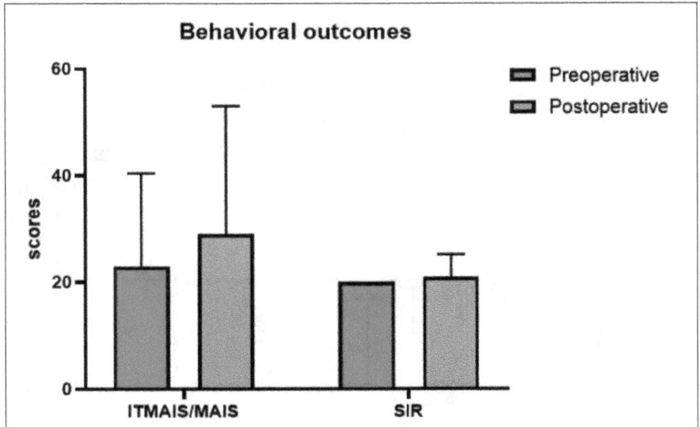

FIGURE 3 | Behavioral outcomes. The vertical axis is the score, and the horizontal axis is the test type. Red represents the preoperative test score, and blue represents the postoperative test score. The scores of the two tests did not differ significantly between the two periods.

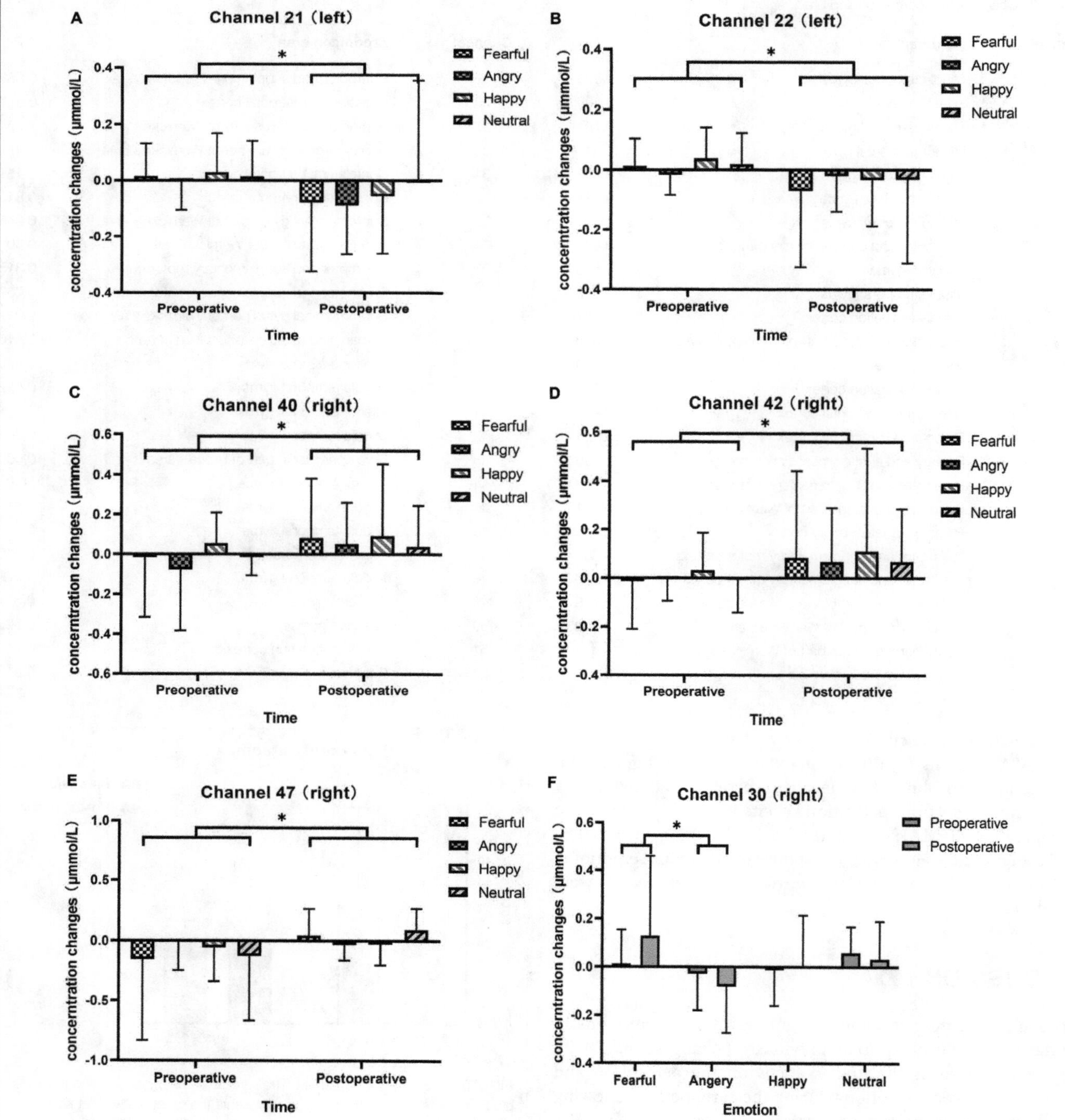

FIGURE 4 | Changes in the responses of cortical oxyhemoglobin to four vocal emotional stimuli (the white grid pattern represents fearful emotion, the gray grid pattern represents angry emotion, the white diagonal pattern represents happy emotion, and the gray diagonal pattern represents neutral emotion) in the two-period test (red represents the preoperative test, blue represents the postoperative test). The six subplots show channels 21, 22 (located in the left pre-motor and supplementary motor cortex), 30 (located in the right supramarginal gyrus of Wernicke's area), 40, 42 (located in the middle temporal gyrus), and 47 (located in the superior temporal gyrus). **(A,B)** In channels 21 and 22 (located in the left pre-motor and supplementary motor cortex), there is a significant difference in cortical activation elicited by vocal emotional stimulation in the preoperative and postoperative tests. **(C,D)** In channels 40 and 42 (located in the right middle temporal gyrus), there is a significant difference in cortical activation elicited by vocal emotional stimulation in the preoperative and postoperative tests. **(E)** In channel 47 (located in the right superior temporal gyrus), there is a significant difference in cortical activation elicited by vocal emotional stimulation in the preoperative and postoperative tests. **(F)** In channel 30 (located in the right supramarginal gyrus of Wernicke' s area), cortical activation elicited by fear is significantly different than that elicited by anger. *$p < 0.05$.

TABLE 3 | Statistical results of fNIRS test.

Channel	Emotion			Pre- and post-operation			Interaction		
	F	*p*	η^2	*F*	*p*	η^2	*F*	*p*	η^2
1	0.096	0.962	0.003	3.461	0.066	0.040	0.680	0.567	0.024
2	0.814	0.490	0.028	0.287	0.594	0.003	0.378	0.769	0.013
3	1.016	0.390	0.035	0.003	0.955	<0.001	0.526	0.666	0.018
4	0.648	0.586	0.023	1.232	0.270	0.014	0.868	0.461	0.030
5	0.066	0.978	0.002	1.251	0.267	0.015	0.268	0.848	0.009
6	1.142	0.337	0.039	1.600	0.209	0.019	0.483	0.695	0.017
7	1.407	0.246	0.048	0.685	0.410	0.008	1.047	0.376	0.036
8	1.536	0.211	0.052	1.008	0.318	0.012	1.875	0.140	0.063
9	0.599	0.617	0.021	0.203	0.653	0.002	0.353	0.787	0.012
10	0.986	0.404	0.034	0.265	0.608	0.003	0.936	0.427	0.032
11	0.559	0.644	0.020	0.422	0.518	0.005	0.316	0.814	0.011
12	2.278	0.085	0.075	1.282	0.261	0.015	0.912	0.439	0.032
13	2.149	0.100	0.071	0.087	0.769	0.001	0.231	0.874	0.008
14	0.613	0.608	0.021	0.033	0.857	<0.001	0.516	0.673	0.018
15	1.979	0.123	0.066	0.267	0.607	0.003	0.566	0.639	0.020
16	1.593	0.197	0.054	2.023	0.159	0.024	1.301	0.280	0.044
17	1.137	0.339	0.039	0.144	0.705	0.002	0.815	0.489	0.028
18	0.545	0.653	0.019	0.093	0.762	0.001	0.542	0.655	0.019
19	0.686	0.563	0.024	1.199	0.277	0.014	2.236	0.090	0.074
20	0.653	0.583	0.023	0.262	0.610	0.003	0.476	0.700	0.017
21	0.545	0.653	0.019	5.970	0.017	0.066	0.454	0.715	0.016
22	0.264	0.851	0.009	5.217	0.025	0.058	0.575	0.633	0.020
23	0.218	0.884	0.008	0.471	0.494	0.006	0.375	0.772	0.013
24	1.862	0.142	0.062	0.071	0.791	0.001	0.343	0.795	0.012
25	0.810	0.492	0.028	0.082	0.775	0.001	0.167	0.918	0.006
26	0.398	0.755	0.014	2.188	0.143	0.025	0.593	0.621	0.021
27	0.863	0.464	0.030	0.651	0.422	0.008	0.516	0.673	0.018
28	0.340	0.796	0.012	0.031	0.862	<0.001	0.584	0.627	0.020
29	1.176	0.324	0.040	0.154	0.696	0.002	0.839	0.476	0.029
30	3.122	0.030	0.100	0.220	0.640	0.003	2.072	0.110	0.069
31	1.454	0.233	0.049	2.582	0.112	0.030	1.197	0.316	0.041
32	0.033	0.992	0.001	2.580	0.112	0.030	0.571	0.636	0.020
33	2.083	0.109	0.069	<0.001	0.988	<0.001	1.495	0.222	0.051
34	2.528	0.063	0.083	0.012	0.915	<0.001	0.615	0.607	0.021
35	2.175	0.097	0.072	1.220	0.273	0.014	0.643	0.589	0.022
36	1.954	0.127	0.065	0.383	0.538	0.005	0.465	0.708	0.016
37	2.351	0.078	0.077	0.319	0.574	0.004	0.291	0.832	0.010
38	0.140	0.936	0.005	0.326	0.569	0.004	0.195	0.899	0.007
39	1.319	0.274	0.045	0.753	0.388	0.009	0.526	0.666	0.018
40	0.792	0.502	0.028	4.829	0.031	0.054	0.338	0.798	0.012
41	0.690	0.561	0.024	0.032	0.858	<0.001	0.477	0.699	0.017
42	0.270	0.847	0.010	4.885	0.030	0.055	0.028	0.994	0.001
43	0.130	0.942	0.005	0.385	0.537	0.005	0.685	0.564	0.024
44	1.431	0.240	0.049	1.013	0.317	0.012	0.906	0.442	0.031
45	1.109	0.350	0.038	0.330	0.567	0.004	1.048	0.376	0.036
46	1.343	0.266	0.046	1.950	0.166	0.023	0.498	0.685	0.017
47	0.107	0.956	0.004	4.361	0.040	0.049	1.418	0.243	0.048
48	0.258	0.856	0.009	0.153	0.697	0.002	0.878	0.456	0.030
49	1.859	0.143	0.062	0.066	0.797	0.001	2.405	0.073	0.079
50	1.898	0.136	0.063	0.062	0.804	0.001	2.020	0.117	0.067
51	0.120	0.948	0.004	2.624	0.109	0.030	0.624	0.601	0.022
52	0.436	0.728	0.015	0.031	0.860	<0.001	0.965	0.413	0.033

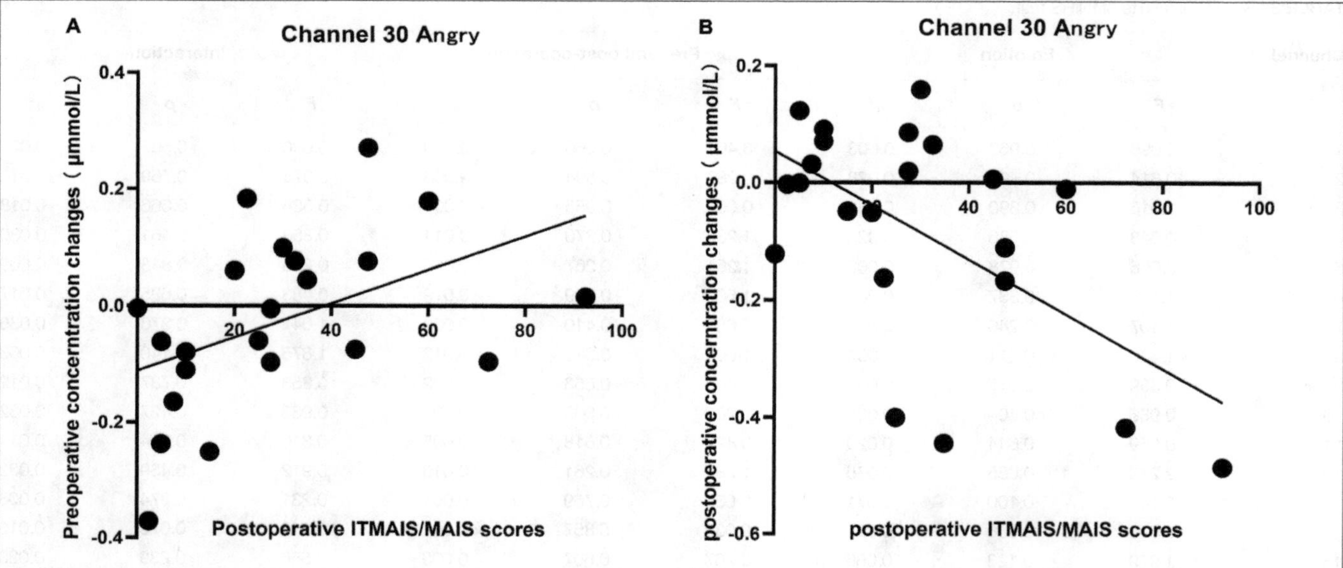

FIGURE 5 | Correlation between the changes in the cortical oxyhemoglobin response to angry vocal emotions in channel 30 (located in the right supramarginal gyrus of Wernicke's area) and the changes in the IT-MAIS/MAIS score. **(A)** A positive correlation was observed between preoperative neural responses to postoperative behavioral outcomes (Pearson's correlation coefficient, $r = 0.455$, $p = 0.033$, $n = 22$). **(B)** A negative correlation was observed between the postoperative neural responses to postoperative behavioral outcomes (Pearson's correlation coefficient, $r = -0.576$, $p = 0.005$, $n = 22$).

vocal emotional stimuli changed from preoperative inhibition to postoperative activation. To our best knowledge, this is the first observation to describe the neural processing of vocal emotional stimulation in prelingual deaf infants and toddlers, which revealed changes from the abnormal neural processing under hearing loss conditions to temporal auditory cortex processing after hearing reconstruction, which more closely resembled the normal processing locations. Previous studies have shown that the activity of the (pre-)SMA participates in emotional regulation initiated by the frontal lobe region and can affect the subcortical structures related to emotional regulation. The function of the (pre-)SMA is to reconceptualize and express information, which depends on language processing, memory tasks and embodied cognition (Kohn et al., 2014). The theory of embodied cognition and embodied emotion processing can help understand this result. The perceptual, motor, and emotional nervous systems are highly interconnected. The neuronal response of a system can reconnect neurons that were active during the initial experience through a cascade effect, reproducing the experience in multiple modes (Damasio, 1989; Wilson, 2002; Niedenthal, 2007). This theory suggests that the preoperative auditory emotional cognitive task processing is achieved by recruiting the SMA to reconceptualize the limited auditory perception information and activate the original neural state (obtained through a variety of channels, such as facial expressions, movements, and limited vocal emotional information) of the emotional information in memory. When postoperative hearing is reconstructed, the right MTG and STG will be recruited for the processing of vocal emotional cognitive tasks, which is in line with the lateralization theory of the brain, in which the right temporal area is the dominant area of emotion and prosody (Arimitsu et al., 2011; Güntürkün et al., 2020. Previous studies in people with normal hearing also observed a strong response for the right MTG and STG under vocal emotional stimulation (Zhang et al., 2017, 2019). These results show that the neural processing for vocal emotional stimulation in ITCIs gradually developed into a model similar to that observed in people with normal hearing. However, CI users have been described as having difficulty with the perception and recognition of vocal emotions compared with normal-hearing peers, which would impact the quality of life (Schorr et al., 2009).

Differences in Vocal Emotion Recognition and Bias Before and After Hearing Reconstruction

In the preoperative fNIRS test, no significant difference in the neural response was identified for any area in response to the four vocal emotional stimuli. In the postoperative test, a significant difference was identified between the neural responses to fear and anger stimuli in channel 30 (located in the right SMG), and the response of fear was stronger than that of anger (**Figure 4F**). The activities of the SMG are related to the enhancement of the auditory perception of vocal emotion (Kochel et al., 2015). The results of previous studies on neonates with normal hearing also indicated that the right SMG responds strongly to fear (Zhang et al., 2017, 2019). Our results are not completely consistent with previous studies on neonates with normal hearing. Specifically, in our study, prelingual deaf ITCIs recognized fewer types of emotions than normal-hearing neonates, and differences in emotional neural responses only appeared in the right SMG, not in the right MTG or STG. Previous results have shown that at this very early stage, the participants are still in the process of remodeling from the abnormal neural processing to normal neural processing, similar to that observed in people with normal hearing. This also may be due to the limitations of CI itself, or the difference in vocal cues of anger and fear (Jiam et al., 2017). Under these conditions, ITCI's still developing auditory system and brain may encounter greater difficulties in completing vocal emotional neural processing. Interestingly, although prelingual deaf ITCIs appear to be less well-developed than normal-hearing neonates in terms of vocal emotion recognition, they showed a negative bias toward vocal emotional stimuli. Previous studies performed in people with normal hearing suggested that the development of negative bias occurred at 6 months after birth (Farroni et al., 2007; Vaish et al., 2008; Peltola et al., 2009; Grossmann et al., 2010; Hoehl and Striano, 2010; Rigato et al., 2010). The result of this study may indicate that the development of emotional bias occurs independent of any specific sensory systems. The development of emotional bias in this study may benefit from facial or physical emotional stimulation, and multiple perception modalities might promote the development of emotional bias. This result supports the view of human infants' differential treatment of environmental threats, which is considered to be a mechanism conducive to evolution (Vaish et al., 2008).

Differences in Correlation Between Cortical Activation Elicited by Vocal Emotions Before and After Hearing Reconstruction and Behavioral Outcomes

Finally, we tested the correlation between the preoperative and postoperative neural response levels to the four emotions in channel 30 (located in the right SMG) and the preoperative and postoperative IT-MAIS/MAIS and SIR scores (**Figure 5**). We found that among the four emotions, only the neural response elicited by anger was significantly correlated with hearing ability (measured by IT-MAIS/MAIS which is reported by caregiver). The preoperative neural response was positively correlated with the postoperative hearing ability, whereas the postoperative neural response was negatively correlated with the postoperative hearing ability. We found that postoperative emotion recognition was elicited by an increased neural response to fear emotions and the inhibition of the neural response to anger emotions. This finding indicates that in the preoperative abnormal vocal emotional neural processing when the cortex is less strongly inhibited by anger stimuli, the abnormal processing is less well-developed, which improves the postoperative auditory ability. In the relatively normal vocal emotion neural processing after surgery, the enhanced inhibition of cortical response elicited by anger correlated with the better development of vocal emotion recognition abilities and better auditory function.

In this study, fNIRS was used to compare the differences between preoperative and postoperative vocal emotion discrimination ability and related neural mechanisms in prelingual deaf infants and toddlers. In addition, huge individual differences in the effects of CI were observed. Although the current preoperative examination can provide a basis for identifying CI candidates, no objective examination method exists to provide a reliable basis for how much these candidates can benefit from CI (Zhao et al., 2020). We also explored the possibility of using fNIRS as an objective, preoperative neuroimaging tool to monitor the early postoperative effects of CI prelingual deaf infants and toddlers.

LIMITATIONS

This study has some limitations. First, the sample size included in this study was small, which makes studying the influences of differences in patient fixed factors that may exist within the group difficult to perform. In future studies, larger sample sizes are necessary to confirm our conclusions. Second, the detection range of fNIRS only includes the cortical areas and cannot show changes in activity among deeper structures. In future research, combinations of other neuroimaging methods that are suitable for repeated measurement will be necessary to study the origins of changes throughout the entire vocal emotional cognitive network both before and after CI implantation in prelingual deaf ITCIs. To observe the initial changes after cochlear implantation, this study selected vocal emotional stimulation, which requires less auditory experience and develops earlier than other auditory processing systems. Although studies have confirmed that the cognitive abilities of vocal emotional stimulation are related to future speech abilities, whether this correlation is stable remains unclear, and more long-term follow-up studies remain necessary to confirm this.

CONCLUSION

In this study, we used fNIRS to monitor changes in neural processing for vocal emotional stimulation in prelingual deaf ITCIs before and after surgery. In addition, we explored the correlation between neural responses to vocal emotional stimulation and postoperative effects. The behavioral assessment showed no difference between the postoperative scores and the preoperative scores. However, significant differences between the preoperative and postoperative neural processing of the vocal emotional cognitive task were found during the neural assessment. A changing trend from the recruitment of the left (pre-)SMA during preoperative hearing loss to the recruitment of the right MTG and STG after hearing reconstruction was observed. We also found no significant difference in the response of each area to each emotional stimulus before the operation, whereas a negative bias was found in the right SMG after the operation. And there is a significantly stronger cortical response elicited by fear relative to anger that was identified after the operation. Finally, we found that the cortical response to anger in the right SMG was significantly correlated with the early

CI behavioral results. Our research supplements the early stage data regarding the vocal emotion perception and recognition differences in CI users and broadens our horizons for future research in this field. This study provides more meaningful consultation suggestions for CI candidates and provides a basis for early and personalized rehabilitation strategies for CI users.

AUTHOR CONTRIBUTIONS

YW: experimental design, data collection, data processing, and manuscript writing. LL: data processing. YZ, CW, TX, and QH: data collection. XH and YL: experimental design, test task writing, and project implementation management. All authors contributed to the article and approved the submitted version.

REFERENCES

Ainsworth, M. D., and Bell, S. M. (1970). Attachment, exploration, and separation: illustrated by the behavior of one-year-olds in a strange situation. *Child Dev.* 41, 49–67.

Allen, M. C., Nikolopoulos, T. P., and O'Donoghue, G. M. (1998). Speech intelligibility in children after cochlear implanation. *Otol. Neurotol.* 19, 742–746.

Anderson, C. A., Wiggins, I. M., Kitterick, P. T., and Hartley, D. E. (2019). Pre-operative brain imaging using functional near-infrared spectroscopy helps predict cochlear implant outcome in deaf adults. *J. Assoc. Res. Otolaryngol.* 20, 511–528.

Arimitsu, T., Uchida-Ota, M., Yagihashi, T., Kojima, S., Watanabe, S., Hokuto, I., et al. (2011). Functional hemispheric specialization in processing phonemic and prosodic auditory changes in neonates. *Front. Psychol.* 2:202. doi: 10.3389/fpsyg.2011.00202

Benavides-Varela, S., Gomez, D. M., and Mehler, J. (2011). Studying neonates' language and memory capacities with functional near-infrared spectroscopy. *Front. Psychol.* 2:64. doi: 10.3389/fpsyg.2011.00064

Bruck, C., Kreifelts, B., and Wildgruber, D. (2011). Emotional voices in context: a neurobiological model of multimodal affective information processing. *Phys. Life Rev.* 8, 383–403. doi: 10.1016/j.plrev.2011.10.002

Bryant, G., and Barrett, H. C. (2008). Vocal emotion recognition across disparate cultures. *J. Cogn. Cult.* 8, 135–148. doi: 10.1163/156770908x289242

Bu, L., Wang, D., Huo, C., Xu, G., Li, Z., and Li, J. (2018). Effects of poor sleep quality on brain functional connectivity revealed by wavelet-based coherence analysis using NIRS methods in elderly subjects. *Neurosci. Lett.* 668, 108–114. doi: 10.1016/j.neulet.2018.01.026

Cannon, S. A., and Chatterjee, M. (2019). Voice emotion recognition by children with mild-to-moderate hearing loss. *Ear Hear.* 40, 477–492. doi: 10.1097/AUD.0000000000000637

Cavicchiolo, S., Mozzanica, F., Guerzoni, L., Murri, A., Dall'Ora, I., Ambrogi, F., et al. (2018). Early prelingual auditory development in Italian infants and toddlers analysed through the Italian version of the infant-toddler meaningful auditory integration scale (IT-MAIS). *Eur. Arch. Otorhinolaryngol.* 275, 615–622. doi: 10.1007/s00405-017-4847-6

Chatterjee, M., Zion, D. J., Deroche, M. L., Burianek, B. A., Limb, C. J., Goren, A. P., et al. (2015). Voice emotion recognition by cochlear-implanted children and their normally-hearing peers. *Hear. Res.* 322, 151–162. doi: 10.1016/j.heares.2014.10.003

Cheng, Y., Lee, S. Y., Chen, H. Y., Wang, P. Y., and Decety, J. (2012). Voice and emotion processing in the human neonatal brain. *J. Cogn. Neurosci.* 24, 1411–1419. doi: 10.1162/jocn_a_00214

Cooper, R. P., and Aslin, R. N. (1989). The language environment of the young infant: implications for early perceptual development. *Can. J. Psychol.* 43, 247–265. doi: 10.1037/h0084216

Damasio, A. R. (1989). Time-locked multiregional retroactivation: a systems-level proposal for the neural substrates of recall and recognition. *Cognition* 33, 25–62. doi: 10.1016/0010-0277(89)90005-x

Denham, S. A., McKinley, M., Couchoud, E. A., and Holt, R. (1990). Emotional and behavioral predictors of preschool peer ratings. *Child Dev.* 61, 1145–1152.

Drotar, D., and Sturm, L. (1988). Prediction of intellectual development in young children with early histories of nonorganic failure-to-thrive. *J. Pediatr. Psychol.* 13, 281–296. doi: 10.1093/jpepsy/13.2.281

Editorial Board of Chinese Journal of Otorhinolaryngology Head and Neck Surgery, Chinese Medical Association Otorhinolaryngology Head and Neck Surgery Branch, and Professional Committee of Hearing and Speech Rehabilitation of China Disabled Rehabilitation Association (2014). Guidelines for cochlear implant work (2013). *Chin. J. Otorhinolaryngol. Head Neck Surg.* 49, 89–95. doi: 10.3760/cma.j.issn.1673-0860.2014.02.001

Eisenberg, N., Spinrad, T. L., and Eggum, N. D. (2010). Emotion-related self-regulation and its relation to children's maladjustment. *Annu. Rev. Clin. Psychol.* 6, 495–525. doi: 10.1146/annurev.clinpsy.121208.131208

Farroni, T., Menon, E., Rigato, S., and Johnson, M. H. (2007). The perception of facial expressions in newborns. *Eur. J. Dev. Psychol.* 4, 2–13. doi: 10.1080/17405620601046832

Fruhholz, S., and Grandjean, D. (2013). Multiple subregions in superior temporal cortex are differentially sensitive to vocal expressions: a quantitative meta-analysis. *Neurosci. Biobehav. Rev.* 37, 24–35. doi: 10.1016/j.neubiorev.2012.11.002

Fruhholz, S., Trost, W., and Kotz, S. A. (2016). The sound of emotions-towards a unifying neural network perspective of affective sound processing. *Neurosci. Biobehav. Rev.* 68, 96–110. doi: 10.1016/j.neubiorev.2016.05.002

Geers, A. E., Davidson, L. S., Uchanski, R. M., and Nicholas, J. G. (2013). Interdependence of linguistic and indexical speech perception skills in school-age children with early cochlear implantation. *Ear Hear.* 34, 562–574. doi: 10.1097/AUD.0b013e31828d2bd6

Glenn, S. M., and Cunningham, C. C. (1983). What do babies listen to most? A developmental study of auditory preferences in nonhandicapped infants and infants with Down's syndrome. *Dev. Psychol.* 19, 332–337. doi: 10.1037/0012-1649.19.3.332

Gomez, D. M., Berent, I., Benavides-Varela, S., Bion, R. A., Cattarossi, L., Nespor, M., et al. (2014). Language universals at birth. *Proc. Natl. Acad. Sci. U.S.A.* 111, 5837–5841. doi: 10.1073/pnas.1318261111

Gottlieb, G. (1971). *Ontogenesis of Sensory Function in Birds and Mammals.* New York, NY: Academic Press.

Grossmann, T., Oberecker, R., Koch, S. P., and Friederici, A. D. (2010). The developmental origins of voice processing in the human brain. *Neuron* 65, 852–858. doi: 10.1016/j.neuron.2010.03.001

Güntürkün, O., Ströckens, F., and Ocklenburg, S. (2020). Brain lateralization: a comparative perspective. *Physiol. Rev.* 100, 1019–1063. doi: 10.1152/physrev.00006.2019

Hoehl, S., and Striano, T. (2010). The development of emotional face and eye gaze processing. *Dev. Sci.* 13, 813–825. doi: 10.1111/j.1467-7687.2009.00944.x

Jiam, N. T., Caldwell, M., Deroche, M. L., Chatterjee, M., and Limb, C. J. (2017). Voice emotion perception and production in cochlear implant users. *Hear. Res.* 352, 30–39. doi: 10.1016/j.heares.2017.01.006

Jiam, N. T., and Limb, C. (2020). Music perception and training for pediatric cochlear implant users. *Expert Rev. Med. Devices* 17, 1193–1206. doi: 10.1080/17434440.2020.1841628

Kang, S. Y., Colesa, D. J., Swiderski, D. L., Su, G. L., Raphael, Y., and Pfingst, B. E. (2010). Effects of hearing preservation on psychophysical responses to cochlear implant stimulation. *J. Assoc. Res. Otolaryngol.* 11, 245–265.

Kasatkin, N. I. (1972). First conditioned reflexes and the beginning of the learning process in the human infant. *Adv. Psychobiol.* 1, 213–257.

Kochel, A., Schongassner, F., Feierl-Gsodam, S., and Schienle, A. (2015). Processing of affective prosody in boys suffering from attention deficit hyperactivity disorder: a near-infrared spectroscopy study. *Soc. Neurosci.* 10, 583–591. doi: 10.1080/17470919.2015.1017111

Kohn, N., Eickhoff, S. B., Scheller, M., Laird, A. R., Fox, P. T., and Habel, U. (2014). Neural network of cognitive emotion regulation–an ALE meta-analysis and MACM analysis. *Neuroimage* 87, 345–355. doi: 10.1016/j.neuroimage.2013.11.001

Kong, Y.-Y., Mullangi, A., Marozeau, J., and Epstein, M. (2011). Temporal and spectral cues for musical timbre perception in electric hearing. *J. Speech Lang. Hear. Res.* 54, 981–994.

Li, Q., Feng, J., Guo, J., Wang, Z., Li, P., Liu, H., et al. (2020). Effects of the multisensory rehabilitation product for home-based hand training after stroke on cortical activation by using NIRS methods. *Neurosci. Lett.* 717:134682. doi: 10.1016/j.neulet.2019.134682

Linnankoski, I., Leinonen, L., Vihla, M., Laakso, M.-L., and Carlson, S. (2005). Conveyance of emotional connotations by a single word in English. *Speech Commun.* 45, 27–39. doi: 10.1016/j.specom.2004.09.007

Liu, P., and Pell, M. D. (2012). Recognizing vocal emotions in Mandarin Chinese: a validated database of Chinese vocal emotional stimuli. *Behav. Res. Methods* 44, 1042–1051. doi: 10.3758/s13428-012-0203-3

Lu, X., and Qin, Z. (2018). Auditory and language development in Mandarin-speaking children after cochlear implantation. *Int. J. Pediatr. Otorhinolaryngol.* 107, 183–189. doi: 10.1016/j.ijporl.2018.02.006

Ludlow, A., Heaton, P., Rosset, D., Hills, P., and Deruelle, C. (2010). Emotion recognition in children with profound and severe deafness: do they have a deficit in perceptual processing? *J. Clin. Exp. Neuropsychol.* 32, 923–928. doi: 10.1080/13803391003596447

Minagawa-Kawai, Y., van der Lely, H., Ramus, F., Sato, Y., Mazuka, R., and Dupoux, E. (2011). Optical brain imaging reveals general auditory and language-specific processing in early infant development. *Cereb. Cortex* 21, 254–261. doi: 10.1093/cercor/bhq082

Most, T., and Michaelis, H. (2012). Auditory, visual, and auditory–visual perceptions of emotions by young children with hearing loss versus children with normal hearing. *J. Speech Lang. Hear. Res.* 55, 1148–1162. doi: 10.1044/1092-4388(2011/11-0060)

Most, T., Weisel, A., and Zaychik, A. (1993). Auditory, visual and auditory-visual identification of emotions by hearing and hearing-impaired adolescents. *Br. J. Audiol.* 27, 247–253. doi: 10.3109/03005369309076701

Niedenthal, P. M. (2007). Embodying emotion. *Science* 316, 1002–1005. doi: 10.1126/science.1136930

Okamoto, M., Dan, H., Sakamoto, K., Takeo, K., Shimizu, K., Kohno, S., et al. (2004). Three-dimensional probabilistic anatomical cranio-cerebral correlation via the international 10-20 system oriented for transcranial functional brain mapping. *Neuroimage* 21, 99–111. doi: 10.1016/j.neuroimage.2003.08.026

Pegg, J. E., Werker, J. F., and McLeod, P. J. (1992). Preference for infant-directed over adult-directed speech: evidence from 7-week-old infants. *Infant Behav. Dev.* 15, 325–345. doi: 10.1016/0163-6383(92)80003-d

Pell, M. D., Monetta, L., Paulmann, S., and Kotz, S. A. (2009). Recognizing emotions in a foreign language. *J. Nonverbal Behav.* 33, 107–120.

Peltola, M. J., Leppanen, J. M., Maki, S., and Hietanen, J. K. (2009). Emergence of enhanced attention to fearful faces between 5 and 7 months of age. *Soc. Cogn. Affect. Neurosci.* 4, 134–142. doi: 10.1093/scan/nsn046

Piper, S. K., Krueger, A., Koch, S. P., Mehnert, J., Habermehl, C., Steinbrink, J., et al. (2014). A wearable multi-channel fNIRS system for brain imaging in freely moving subjects. *Neuroimage* 85(Pt 1), 64–71. doi: 10.1016/j.neuroimage.2013.06.062

Planalp, S. (1996). Varieties of cues to emotion in naturally occurring situations. *Cogn. Emot.* 10, 137–154.

Rigato, S., Farroni, T., and Johnson, M. H. (2010). The shared signal hypothesis and neural responses to expressions and gaze in infants and adults. *Soc. Cogn. Affect. Neurosci.* 5, 88–97. doi: 10.1093/scan/nsp037

Saliba, J., Bortfeld, H., Levitin, D. J., and Oghalai, J. S. (2016). Functional near-infrared spectroscopy for neuroimaging in cochlear implant recipients. *Hear. Res.* 338, 64–75. doi: 10.1016/j.heares.2016.02.005

Sato, H., Hirabayashi, Y., Tsubokura, H., Kanai, M., Ashida, T., Konishi, I., et al. (2012). Cerebral hemodynamics in newborn infants exposed to speech sounds: a whole-head optical topography study. *Hum. Brain Mapp.* 33, 2092–2103. doi: 10.1002/hbm.21350

Sauter, D. A., Eisner, F., Calder, A. J., and Scott, S. K. (2010). Perceptual cues in nonverbal vocal expressions of emotion. *Q. J. Exp. Psychol. (Hove)* 63, 2251–2272. doi: 10.1080/17470211003721642

Schorr, E. A., Roth, F. P., and Fox, N. A. (2009). Quality of life for children with cochlear implants: perceived benefits and problems and the perception of single words and emotional sounds. *J. Speech Lang. Hear. Res.* 52, 141–152. doi: 10.1044/1092-4388(2008/07-0213)

Strangman, G., Culver, J. P., Thompson, J. H., and Boas, D. A. (2002). A quantitative comparison of simultaneous BOLD fMRI and NIRS recordings during functional brain activation. *Neuroimage* 17, 719–731. doi: 10.1006/nimg.2002.1227

Thompson, W. F., and Balkwill, L.-L. (2006). Decoding speech prosody in five languages. *Semiotica* 2006, 407–424.

Trainor, L. J., Austin, C. M., and Desjardins, R. N. (2000). Is infant-directed speech prosody a result of the vocal expression of emotion? *Psychol. Sci.* 11, 188–195. doi: 10.1111/1467-9280.00240

Vaish, A., Grossmann, T., and Woodward, A. (2008). Not all emotions are created equal: the negativity bias in social-emotional development. *Psychol. Bull.* 134, 383–403. doi: 10.1037/0033-2909.134.3.383

Wauters, L. N., and Knoors, H. (2008). Social integration of deaf children in inclusive settings. *J. Deaf Stud. Deaf Educ.* 13, 21–36. doi: 10.1093/deafed/enm028

Wiefferink, C. H., Rieffe, C., Ketelaar, L., De Raeve, L., and Frijns, J. H. (2013). Emotion understanding in deaf children with a cochlear implant. *J. Deaf Stud. Deaf Educ.* 18, 175–186. doi: 10.1093/deafed/ens042

Wilson, M. (2002). Six views of embodied cognition. *Psychon. Bull. Rev.* 9, 625–636. doi: 10.3758/bf03196322

Xu, L., Zhou, N., Chen, X., Li, Y., Schultz, H. M., Zhao, X., et al. (2009). Vocal singing by prelingually-deafened children with cochlear implants. *Hear. Res.* 255, 129–134.

Yang, F., Zhao, F., Zheng, Y., and Li, G. (2020). Modification and verification of the infant-toddler meaningful auditory integration scale: a psychometric analysis combining item response theory with classical test theory. *Health Qual. Life Outcomes* 18:367. doi: 10.1186/s12955-020-01620-9

Zeng, F. G., Rebscher, S., Harrison, W., Sun, X., and Feng, H. (2008). Cochlear implants: system design, integration, and evaluation. *IEEE Rev. Biomed. Eng.* 1, 115–142. doi: 10.1109/RBME.2008.2008250

Zhang, D., Chen, Y., Hou, X., and Wu, Y. J. (2019). Near-infrared spectroscopy reveals neural perception of vocal emotions in human neonates. *Hum. Brain Mapp.* 40, 2434–2448. doi: 10.1002/hbm.24534

Zhang, D., Zhou, Y., Hou, X., Cui, Y., and Zhou, C. (2017). Discrimination of emotional prosodies in human neonates: a pilot fNIRS study. *Neurosci. Lett.* 658, 62–66. doi: 10.1016/j.neulet.2017.08.047

Zhao, C., Chronaki, G., Schiessl, I., Wan, M. W., and Abel, K. M. (2019). Is infant neural sensitivity to vocal emotion associated with mother-infant relational experience? *PLoS One* 14:e0212205. doi: 10.1371/journal.pone.0212205

Zhao, E. E., Dornhoffer, J. R., Loftus, C., Nguyen, S. A., Meyer, T. A., Dubno, J. R., et al. (2020). Association of patient-related factors with adult cochlear implant speech recognition outcomes: a meta-analysis. *JAMA Otolaryngol. Head Neck Surg.* 146, 613–620.

Zimmerman-Phillips, S., Osberger, M., and Robbins, A. (1997). *Infant-Toddler: Meaningful Auditory Integration Scale (IT-MAIS).* Sylmar, LA: Advanced Bionics Corporation.

10

Auditory Sensory Gating in Children with Cochlear Implants: A P50-N100-P200 Study

Yan-Xin Chen[1], Xin-Ran Xu[1], Shuo Huang[1], Rui-Rui Guan[1], Xiao-Yan Hou[1], Jia-Qiang Sun[1], Jing-Wu Sun[1*] and Xiao-Tao Guo[1,2*]*

[1] *Department of Otolaryngology-Head and Neck Surgery, The First Affiliated Hospital of USTC, Division of Life Sciences and Medicine, University of Science and Technology of China, Hefei, China,* [2] *CAS Key Laboratory of Brain Function and Diseases, School of Life Sciences, University of Science and Technology of China, Hefei, China*

***Correspondence:**
Jia-Qiang Sun
sunjq0605@126.com
Jing-Wu Sun
entsun@ustc.edu.cn
Xiao-Tao Guo
gxt2012@mail.ustc.edu.cn

Background: While a cochlear implant (CI) can restore access to audibility in deaf children, implanted children may still have difficulty in concentrating. Previous studies have revealed a close relationship between sensory gating and attention. However, whether CI children have deficient auditory sensory gating remains unclear.

Methods: To address this issue, we measured the event-related potentials (ERPs), including P50, N100, and P200, evoked by paired tone bursts (S1 and S2) in CI children and normal-hearing (NH) controls. Suppressed amplitudes for S2 compared with S1 in these three ERPs reflected sensory gating during early and later phases, respectively. A Swanson, Nolan, and Pelham IV (SNAP-IV) scale was performed to assess the attentional performance.

Results: Significant amplitude differences between S1 and S2 in N100 and P200 were observed in both NH and CI children, indicating the presence of sensory gating in the two groups. However, the P50 suppression was only found in NH children and not in CI children. Furthermore, the duration of deafness was significantly positively correlated with the score of inattention in CI children.

Conclusion: Auditory sensory gating can develop but is deficient during the early phase in CI children. Long-term auditory deprivation has a negative effect on sensory gating and attentional performance.

Keywords: auditory sensory gating, cochlear implant, P50, N100, P200, attentional dysfunction

INTRODUCTION

There is a close link between cognitive decline and hearing loss (Dye and Hauser, 2014; Heinrichs-Graham et al., 2021). Patients with hearing loss face the risk of delays in multiple cognitive functions, such as working memory and executive function (Lieu et al., 2020). Specifically, attention-deficit disorders are more commonly reported in deaf children compared with normal-hearing (NH) peers (Hall et al., 2018). As one of the most successful neural prostheses developed to date, cochlear implants (CIs) help not only to restore hearing of deaf children, thereby supporting speech communication, but also to enhance their cognitive abilities (Kral et al., 2019). For example, CI children showed an improvement in non-verbal cognitive functions and working memory at

6 months after CI surgery (Shin et al., 2007). However, CIs still cannot ensure optimal cognitive outcomes (Kral et al., 2019). There is a great variation in the attentional performances of CI children (Surowiecki et al., 2002). Both preschoolers and school-aged children with CIs were found to face a greater risk of deficits in the attention domain compared with NH children (Kronenberger et al., 2014). Nearly 40% of CI children attending mainstream classes could not pass the test of attention (Mukari et al., 2007), which may result in poor educational performance. However, the related neural mechanism underlying poor attentional performance in CI children remains unclear.

Previous evidence has shown that sensory gating is involved in early information processing of auditory attention (Wan et al., 2008). Sensory gating refers to the brain's ability to filter repetitive irrelevant stimuli (Chien et al., 2019), which is mainly assessed by P50 suppression. As a "pre-attentive" process, P50 sensory gating manifests in the central nervous system modulating its sensitivity to incoming stimuli (Braff and Geyer, 1990), protecting the brain from information overload (Adler et al., 1982). The P50 is a positive component of auditory event-related potentials (ERPs) and usually occurs at about 50 ms after stimuli onset. It has been supposed to be generated from the thalamo-cortical projection to the auditory cortex (Sharma et al., 2009). In a paired-click paradigm, two successive P50 responses are usually evoked by an initial stimulus (S1) and a shortly following identical stimulus (S2). (Fruhstorfer et al., 1970). Normal P50 suppression is characterized by a reduction in P50 amplitude for S2 compared with S1. A higher ratio (S2/S1) or smaller difference in these two P50 amplitudes suggests weaker sensory gating associated with diminished cognitive functioning, such as attention (Lijffijt et al., 2009).

Given that sensory gating is regarded as a multistage process (Boutros et al., 1999), previous studies have also paid attention to the later phases of auditory processing reflected by the N100 and P200 (Rosburg, 2018). The N100 is a negative component appearing about 100 ms after the onset of the auditory stimulus, and the P200 is a positive component appearing about 200 ms. The N100 and P200 components are mainly generated in the primary auditory cortex (Hegerl and Juckel, 1993). These two components have been proposed to involve distinct neural activities (Boutros et al., 2004; Chien et al., 2019) and thus be related to different functions (Lijffijt et al., 2009). Unlike the P50 involving the early phase of information processing, the N100 and P200 are considered to reflect triggering and allocation of attention, respectively (Shen et al., 2020). Thus, different phases of auditory information filtering should be investigated by the P50-N100-P200 complex.

There is a maturational course of sensory gating in typically developing children (Davies et al., 2009). Compared with adults, children always show immature sensory gating ability as revealed by longer P50 latencies (Hunter et al., 2012). With increasing age, young children (1–8 years of age) demonstrate a rapid decrease in latency (Freedman et al., 1987). The latency may stabilize at the pre-adolescent stage (9–12 years of age) and remain stable into adulthood. Brinkman and Stauder (2007) also found a negative correlation between age and the P50 amplitude ratio, indicating age-related sensory gating abilities. However, further analysis revealed that a significant difference in gating ratios was only found between the youngest children group (5–7 years of age) and the other three groups (8–9, 10–12, and 18–30 years of age) and not among the latter three groups. These findings imply that sensory gating may mature around the age of 8 years.

Sensory gating has been reported to be deficient in many neurological diseases (Gjini et al., 2011; Micoulaud-Franchi et al., 2015). Patients with schizophrenia (Smucny et al., 2013) or autism spectrum disorders (Crasta et al., 2021) showed reduced gating abilities reflected by abnormal P50, N100, and/or P200 amplitude ratios. This ineffective inhibitory modulation of sensory information may imply an imbalance of neuronal excitation/inhibition in this population (Culotta and Penzes, 2020). The inhibitory system is thought to be the underlying mechanism in modulating sensory gating (Adler et al., 1982). Evidence has also demonstrated that peripheral auditory deafferentation or sensorineural hearing loss negatively affects inhibitory mechanisms, reflected by a reduction of inhibitory inputs and subsequent imbalance between excitatory and inhibitory systems (Campbell et al., 2020a). The properties of the inhibitory synapses in the central auditory system are changed by auditory deprivation (Takesian et al., 2012). The inhibitory activity decreases, followed by an increase in the excitability of both midbrain and cortical neurons. Synaptic changes induced by early hearing loss contribute to auditory processing deficits and may be persistent even after auditory intervention (Takesian et al., 2009). Therefore, for deaf children who experience early auditory deprivation, it is unclear whether auditory sensory gating is deficient (no or reduced inhibition of repetitive irrelevant stimuli) after cochlear implantation.

In this study, we assessed auditory sensory gating in CI children by measuring the amplitude (gating) ratios of P50, N100, and P200 responses to paired tone bursts (S1 and S2). The attentional performance was also evaluated using the Swanson, Nolan, and Pelham IV (SNAP-IV) scale. We hypothesized that the sensory gating ability could develop after cochlear implantation but still be deficient because of long-term auditory deprivation. Therefore, we predicted that P50, N100, and/or P200 suppression would be poorer in CI children than in NH peers.

MATERIALS AND METHODS

Participants

Twenty-four native Chinese children, including 12 prelingually deafened children with unilateral Med-El CI devices [6 females, age range: 4–8 years; mean age ± standard deviation (SD): 6.01 ± 1.33 years] and 12 NH children (4 females, age range: 3.5–8.5 years; mean age ± SD: 6.59 ± 1.54 years), participated in this study. Eleven CI children did not pass the neonatal evoked otoacoustic emission test and were diagnosed with congenital sensorineural hearing loss. The other child was found to have profound sensorineural hearing loss before the age of 15 months. Two CI children had worn hearing aids before cochlear implantation. The auditory and speech abilities of CI children were evaluated by Categories of Auditory Performance (CAP), Speech Intelligibility Rate (SIR), and

TABLE 1 | Demographic information of the cochlear implant users.

Subject	Gender	Age at test (years)	CI use (years)	ABR threshold (dB nHL)		CI processor	Implant type	Age at CI (years)		MAIS	SIR	CAP
				left	right			left	right			
1	M	5.33	4.08	95	>95	Opus 1	CONCERTO	/	1.25	33	3	8
2	M	7.92	2.42	>95	>95	Opus 1	SONATA	/	5.50	31	3	6
3	M	4.00	2.00	>95	>95	Opus 2xs	SONATA	/	2.00	21	2	6
4	F	6.42	2.84	>95	>95	Opus 2xs	SONATA	3.58	/	37	5	8
5	M	4.58	2.00	>95	>95	Opus 2xs	SONATA	2.58	/	34	4	6
6	F	6.67	4.34	>95	>95	Opus 2xs	SONATA	/	2.33	38	5	7
7	M	4.83	3.83	>95	>95	Opus 2xs	SONATA	/	1.00	35	4	7
8	F	5.17	3.42	>95	>95	Opus 2xs	SONATA	/	1.75	40	5	8
9	F	7.83	6.41	>95	>95	Opus 1	SONATA	/	1.42	37	5	8
10	M	7.42	0.50	95	>95	Opus 2xs	CONCERTO	6.92	/	36	4	8
11	F	5.25	2.17	>95	>95	Opus 1	SONATA	/	3.08	34	3	6
12	F	6.75	5.25	>95	>95	Opus 2xs	SONATA	/	1.50	38	3	8

ABR, auditory brainstem response; CAP, categories of auditory performance; CI, cochlear implant; F, female; M, male; MAIS, meaningful auditory integration scale; nHL, normal hearing level; and SIR, speech intelligibility rate.

Meaningful Auditory Integration Scale (MAIS; Peixoto et al., 2013). The scores of these three scales and more detailed information for CI children are listed in **Table 1**. The NH children did not have a history of hearing loss. The two groups were matched in terms of years of education, family incomes and levels of parental education. They had normal vision and no history of neurological or psychiatric illness. The protocols and experimental procedures in this study were reviewed and approved by Anhui Provincial Hospital Ethics Committee. Each participant's guardians had filled out an informed consent carefully before the experiment.

Sensory Gating Paradigm

In the electroencephalography (EEG) experiment, the tone burst (1,000 Hz, 30 ms duration, 4 ms linear rise/fall time) was used as the auditory stimulus to evoke the P50, N100, and P200 components. Tone bursts were presented in pairs: a conditioning stimulus (S1) and a testing stimulus (S2) with an interstimulus interval of 500 ms and an interpair interval of 8 s through two loudspeakers placed at ± 45° azimuth, at a distance of 100 cm in front of the participants. The stimuli were delivered at an intensity of 80 dB SPL. For each participant, the experiment consisted of two blocks with 200 pairs of tone bursts in total and lasted for 30 min. The sound stimuli were generated by Adobe Audition 3.0 software (Adobe Systems Incorporated, San Jose, CA, United States) and presented by E-Prime 3.0 software (Psychological Software Tools, Pittsburgh, PA, United States).

Attention Assessment

A Swanson, Nolan, and Pelham IV (SNAP-IV) scale was used to assess the attentional performances of NH and CI subjects. This rating scale was usually used to evaluate attentional deficits in patients with ADHD (Swanson et al., 2001). The SNAP-IV includes 26 items divided into three subscales: inattention (9 items), hyperactivity/impulsivity (9 items), and oppositional (8 items) (Swanson et al., 2001). Parents were asked to rate the items according to the daily performance of their children by selecting one of four grades (not at all, just a little, quite a bit, very much). A Higher score indicated more severe symptoms.

Electroencephalography Recording

The EEG was recorded from a cap with 64 Ag/AgCl electrodes (SynAmps RT, Curry, United States) that were placed at the scalp according to the international 10–20 system. Another two electrodes were located at the left and right mastoids. The reference and ground electrodes were placed on the tip of the nose and the forehead, respectively. Vertical and horizontal electrooculography (EOG) signals were obtained by bipolar electrodes above and below the left eye and lateral to the outer canthi of both eyes, respectively. The EEG data were sampled at 500 Hz and filtered online between 0.05 and 100 Hz. Electrode resistances were kept under 5 kΩ. Each child was asked to watch a silent cartoon sitting on a soft couch and ignore the auditory stimuli.

Data Analysis

Offline analysis of EEG data was conducted by EEGLAB 13.0.0b in Matlab R2013b (The Mathworks, Natick, MA, United States). Data were filtered with a bandpass setting of 10–100 Hz for the P50 component and with a bandpass setting of 4–30 Hz for the N100 and P200 components. The epochs were set at 400 ms, starting at 100 ms before the onset of the stimulus. Baseline correction was performed relative to a baseline of −100 to 0 ms. The independent component analysis was used to remove the eye movement, heartbeat, and CI artifacts from the EEG signals (Hongmei and Nan, 2017). Independent components reflecting these artifacts were identified and removed by visual inspection of the component's properties, including the waveform, 2-D voltage map, and spectrum (Gilley et al., 2006). After artifact removal, segments containing voltage deviations exceeding ± 100 μV on any channels except for EOG channels were rejected.

The ERPs evoked by S1 and S2 were calculated by averaging individual trials. The P50 component was defined as the most

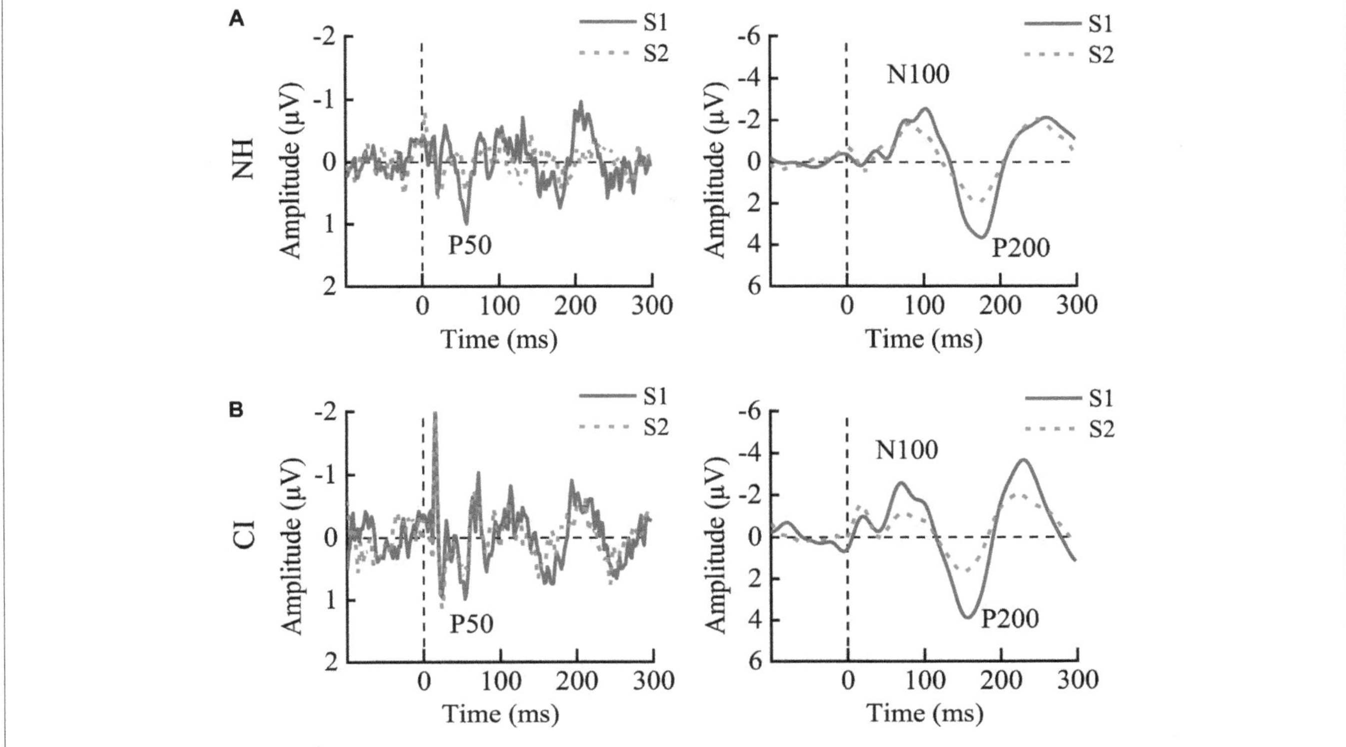

FIGURE 1 | Grand average event-related potentials in response to S1 (blue solid line) and S2 (red dashed line) at site Cz. Both **(A)** children with normal hearing (NH) and **(B)** those with cochlear implants (CIs) showed robust P50, N100, and P200 components.

positive peak between 40 and 100 ms after stimulus onset. The N100 and P200 components were determined as the most negative and positive peaks after P50 between 80 and 150 ms and between 120 and 250 ms, respectively (Crasta et al., 2021). The amplitude of P50, N100, or P200 was determined by the peak-to-peak amplitude between the peak of P50, N100, or P200 and its preceding peak with reversal polarity. The gating ratio between P50, N100, or P200 amplitude for S2 and that for S1 (S2/S1) was used to evaluate the sensory gating ability: A lower gating ratio indicated robust gating, and a higher ratio indicated attenuated gating. The electrode Cz was selected for illustration.

Statistical Methods

One NH child and one CI child who had no robust N100 and P200 components were removed from further N100-P200 analysis. To assess whether auditory sensory gating existed in both groups, we compared the amplitude differences of P50, N100, and P200 in response to S1 with those to S2 using repeated measures analysis of variance (ANOVA) with stimulus (S1 and S2) as the within-subject factor. The differences in gating ratios, amplitudes, peak latencies, and SNAP-IV scores between two groups were further evaluated by a one-way ANOVA with group (NH and CI) as the between-subject factor. The Pearson's correlation was performed to assess the relationship among the gating ratios, scores of inattention, and onset or duration of deafness or CI use.

RESULTS

Absence of P50 Suppression in Cochlear Implant Children

The grand average ERPs in response to S1 and S2 for two groups at the representative electrode Cz are shown in **Figure 1**. NH children showed significantly smaller amplitudes of P50 [$F_{(1,11)}$ = 39.251, $p < 0.001$], N100 [$F_{(1,10)}$ = 8.391, p = 0.016], and P200 [$F_{(1,10)}$ = 9.196, p = 0.013] in response to S2 than those to S1, indicating the presence of robust P50, N100, and P200 suppression. CI children showed similar amplitudes of P50 [$F_{(1,11)}$ = 0.348, p = 0.567] but significantly smaller amplitudes of N100 [$F_{(1,10)}$ = 8.126, p = 0.017] and P200 [$F_{(1,10)}$ = 8.019, p = 0.018] for S1 compared with S2 (**Figures 2A–C**, left).

Higher P50 Ratio but Similar N100 and P200 Ratios in Cochlear Implant Children Compared With Normal Hearing Children

We further assessed whether the gating ratios, amplitudes, and peak latencies of P50, N100, and P200 differed between NH and CI children. CI children showed a significantly higher P50 gating ratio than NH children did [$F_{(1,22)}$ = 13.450, p = 0.001] (**Figure 2A**, middle). However, no significant difference in N100 [$F_{(1,20)}$ = 0.855, p = 0.366] or P200 [$F_{(1,20)}$ = 0.047, p = 0.831] gating ratios was found between these two groups (**Figures 2B,C**, middle).

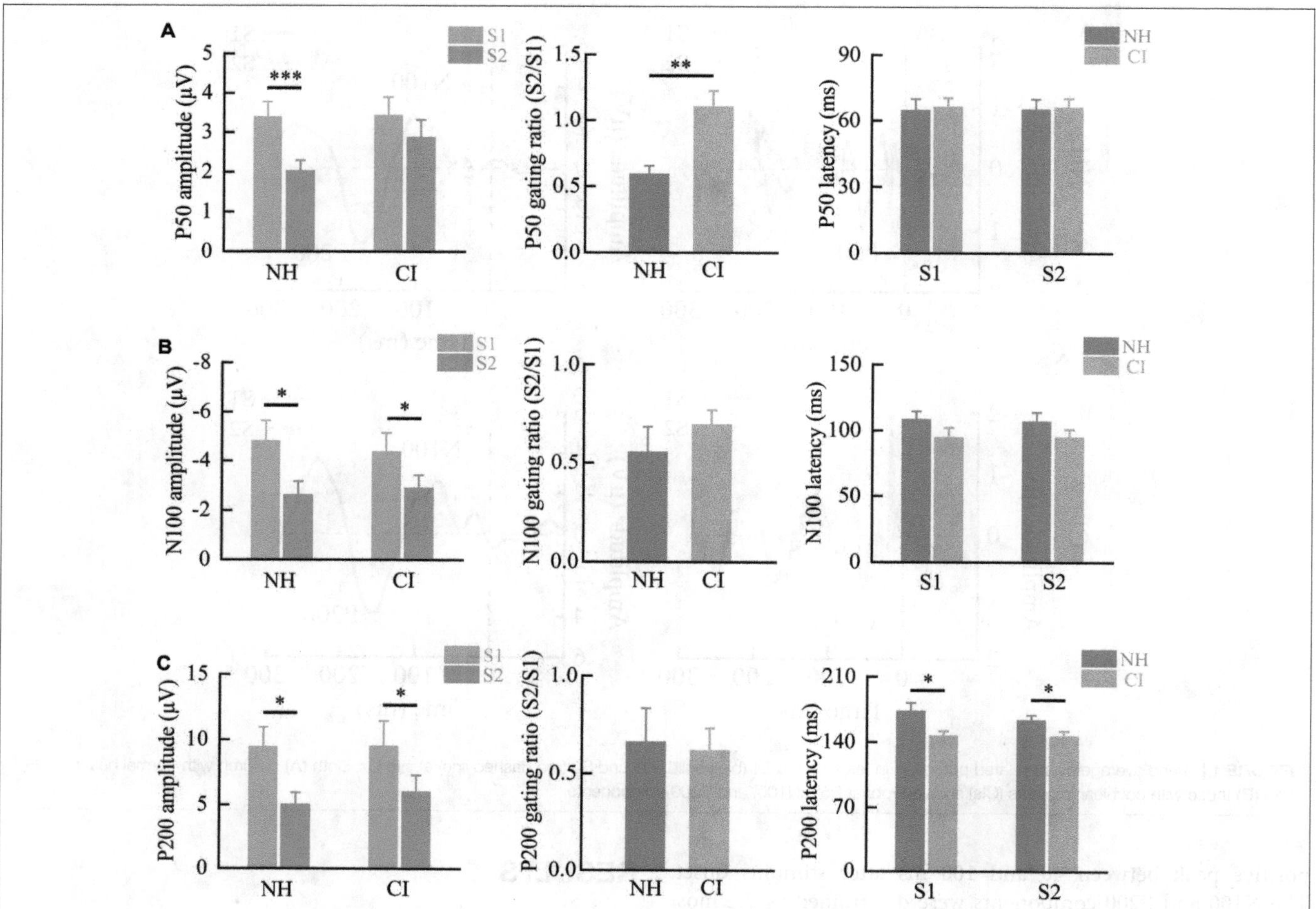

FIGURE 2 | Auditory sensory gating at the **(A)** P50, **(B)** N100, and **(C)** P200 for children with NH and those with CIs. (Left) The amplitudes of N100 and P200 in response to S2 were significantly smaller than those to S1, indicating the presence of the auditory sensory gating in both NH and CI children. However, P50 suppression only existed in NH and not in CI children. (Middle) CI children showed similar N100 and P200 suppression ratios (S2/S1) but a higher P50 ratio compared with NH children. (Right) The P200 latencies in CI children were significantly shorter than those in NH children. Vertical bars represent the standard error. ***p < 0.001, **p < 0.01, and *p < 0.05.

There was no significant difference in P50 [S1: $F_{(1,22)} = 0.026$, $p = 0.873$; S2: $F_{(1,22)} = 3.704$, $p = 0.067$], N100 [S1: $F_{(1,20)} = 0.138$, $p = 0.714$; S2: $F_{(1,20)} = 0.131$, $p = 0.721$], or P200 amplitudes [S1: $F_{(1,20)} < 0.001$, $p = 0.979$; S2: $F_{(1,20)} = 0.367$, $p = 0.551$] between NH and CI children. Peak latencies of P50 [S1: $F_{(1,22)} = 0.037$, $p = 0.848$; S2: $F_{(1,22)} = 0.016$, $p = 0.899$] and N100 [S1: $F_{(1,20)} = 1.917$, $p = 0.181$; S2: $F_{(1,20)} = 1.657$, $p = 0.213$] were similar between the two groups (**Figures 2A,B**, right). However, CI children showed shorter P200 peak latencies [S1: $F_{(1,20)} = 6.155$, $p = 0.022$; S2: $F_{(1,20)} = 4.448$, $p = 0.048$] than NH children did (**Figure 2C**, right).

Relationships Among Gating Ratios, Attentional Performance, and Onset or Duration of Deafness or Cochlear Implant Use

No significant difference in scores of inattention [$F_{(1,22)} = 0.004$, $p = 0.949$], hyperactivity/impulsivity [$F_{(1,22)} = 0.037$, $p = 0.849$], or opposition [$F_{(1,22)} = 0.692$, $p = 0.414$] was found between NH and CI groups (**Figure 3A**). In CI children, the score of inattention was significantly positively correlated with the duration of deafness [$R = 0.588$, $p = 0.044$] (**Figure 3B**). No other significant correlations were found (all $p > 0.05$).

DISCUSSION

In this study, we assessed auditory sensory gating in CI children. CI children showed robust N100 and P200 suppression but no P50 suppression. Furthermore, the duration of deafness was positively correlated with the score of inattention. Our results demonstrate that auditory sensory gating can develop in CI children but is deficient during the early phase. Long-term auditory deprivation negatively affects the restoration of auditory sensory gating and attentional performance.

Cochlear implant children showed auditory gating as revealed by the N100 and P200 suppression, indicating that the CI

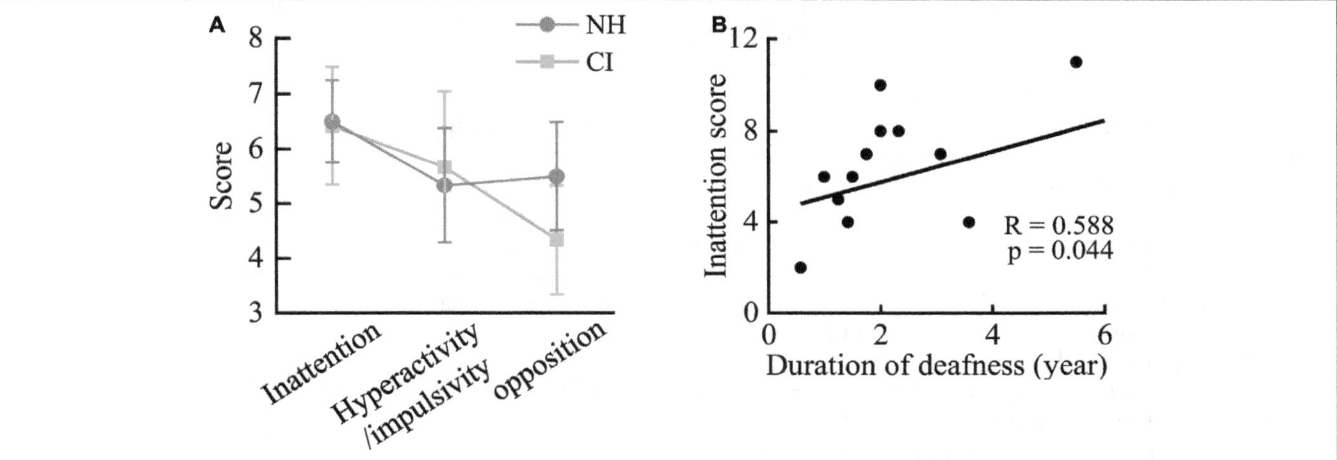

FIGURE 3 | The negative effect of long-term auditory deprivation on the attentional performance. **(A)** There was no significant difference in subscale scores of inattention, hyperactivity/impulsivity and oppositional between NH and CI children. **(B)** The score of inattention was significantly positively correlated with the duration of deafness in CI children. Vertical bars represent the standard error.

helps to rehabilitate the auditory sensory gating abilities of deaf children. The precise organization of neuronal circuits in the mature brain is established by developmental processes that involve reorganization and fine tuning of immature synaptic networks (Kandler, 2004). The maturation of the auditory system requires stimulation. Auditory deprivation may keep the synapses immature until the cochlear implantation helps to restore hearing and get rid of this frozen state (Sharma et al., 2002a). These activity-dependent processes may include improvement in synaptic efficacy and increased myelination (Gordon et al., 2003). The auditory system may rapidly develop within a critical period of 3–6 months after cochlear implantation and enter a maturation period after 12 months (Ni et al., 2021). Most CI children in our study received implantation before 3.5 years old and still had high plasticity of the auditory cortex (Manrique et al., 1999). Therefore, sensory gating can develop and be functional in CI children, though its developmental trajectory may be delayed. Considered as an automatic and involuntary first part in the attentional processes, sensory gating may prevent limited attentional resources from being disturbed by repetitive irrelevant stimuli and protect CI children from later attentional dysfunction (Hutchison et al., 2017).

Interestingly, compared with NH children, CI children showed similar gating ratios at the N100 and P200 but no robust P50 suppression, indicating deficient sensory gating during the early phase. There are two functionally distinct generators that are related to the P50 suppression, the temporal lobe and the frontal lobe (Weisser et al., 2001; Korzyukov et al., 2007; Campbell et al., 2020b). A considerable body of invasive and non-invasive research on sensory gating suggests that the auditory P50 response may be explained by contributions from the bilateral temporal lobes, including the left and right superior temporal gyri (STG; Lee et al., 1984; Liegeois-Chauvel et al., 1994; Knott et al., 2009; Mayer et al., 2009). In addition to the bilateral temporal lobes, the prefrontal source is usually attributed to the reduction of amplitudes to repeated stimuli (Grunwald et al., 2003; Korzyukov et al., 2007). In an MEG study on M50, the neuromagnetic counterpart of the P50 component, the prefrontal region was found to suppress the activity of the bilateral STG within the auditory M50 network (Josef Golubic et al., 2014). Similar to the P50 component, the N100 and P200 gating responses involve the activation of inhibitory frontal and temporo-prefrontal networks (Campbell et al., 2020b). However, functions of strong suppression regions may be differential. The P50 gating may work as a bottom-up process, while the N100 and P200 are mainly concerned with top-down processes (Boutros et al., 2013). Incoming sensory inputs first activate automatic central inhibitory mechanisms prior to top-down cognitive involvement (Javitt and Freedman, 2015). Evidence suggests that the N100 and P200 gating may be more susceptible to attention compared with early P50 gating (Rosburg et al., 2009). For the absence of P50 suppression and the presence of robust N100 and P200 suppression in CI children, we infer that the multi-stage inhibitory networks are damaged by auditory deprivation at the early stage but can be compensated for at the later stage by top-down modulation. We also found a positive correlation between the score of inattention and the duration of deafness. These findings suggest that long-term auditory deprivation has a negative effect on both early sensory gating and attentional functions. We did not find significant correlations between the gating ratio and the attention performance. The possible reason is that the Swanson, Nolan, and Pelham IV (SNAP-IV) scale for assessment of the attentional performance depending on parents' daily observation is relatively subjective. However, an objective and more accurate method for young children with hearing disability is indeed lacking.

Our previous study found that when dealing with complex speech sounds, CI children showed smaller and slower mismatch negativity (MMN) and even an absence of the late discriminative negativity (LDN) compared with NH children (Hu et al., 2021). Contrary to these late-latency ERPs, the robust P50-N100-P200 responses could be evoked by simple tone bursts, reflecting early processes of acoustic analysis. Compared with NH children, CI children showed similar P50 amplitudes but significantly different P50 amplitude ratios, suggesting that the brain can encode the acoustic features of novel sounds but has difficulty in inhibiting the neural response to repetitive irrelevant sounds (S2). The inhibitory system is thought to be the underlying mechanism in modulating sensory gating (Adler et al., 1982). Therefore, auditory deprivation may reduce the inhibitory activity, resulting in persistent higher excitability to repetitive irrelevant sounds during the early phase of information processing.

There are still some limitations to this study. First, while we tried to recruit CI children with consistent conditions (such as brand of CI devices), inhomogeneous aspects of CI children were still present. For example, two CI children had fitted hearing aids before cochlear implantation. We cannot separate the effect of early hearing aid fitting from that of CI use on the development of sensory gating. Therefore, a more detailed grouping method should be considered based on a larger sample size. Second, there was a lack of children implanted with the CI devices before the age of 12 months. Previous findings have shown the positive effect of early CI use on auditory rehabilitation (Sharma et al., 2002b; Dettman et al., 2007). Although we did not find correlations between the onset age of CI use and the P50-N100-P200 gating ratio, there is a possibility that earlier cochlear implantation (<12 months) may result in better rehabilitation of auditory sensory gating.

CONCLUSION

The CI helps to restore auditory sensory gating in prelingually deafened children. However, this gating ability is deficient in CI children during the early phase. Long-term auditory deprivation adversely affects auditory sensory gating and attentional performance.

AUTHOR CONTRIBUTIONS

Y-XC, J-QS, J-WS, and X-TG conceived and designed the experiments. Y-XC, X-RX, X-YH, R-RG, and J-WS recruited the participants. Y-XC and X-TG performed the data acquisition. Y-XC, SH, J-WS, and X-TG analyzed the data. All authors wrote the manuscript and approved the final article.

ACKNOWLEDGMENTS

The authors thank all participants for their participation in this research.

REFERENCES

Adler, L. E., Pachtman, E., Franks, R. D., Pecevich, M., Waldo, M. C., and Freedman, R. (1982). Neurophysiological evidence for a defect in neuronal mechanisms involved in sensory gating in schizophrenia. *Biol. Psychiatry* 17, 639–654.

Boutros, N. N., Belger, A., Campbell, D., D'Souza, C., and Krystal, J. (1999). Comparison of four components of sensory gating in schizophrenia and normal subjects: a preliminary report. *Psychiatry Res.* 88, 119–130. doi: 10.1016/s0165-1781(99)00074-8

Boutros, N. N., Gjini, K., Eickhoff, S. B., Urbach, H., and Pflieger, M. E. (2013). Mapping repetition suppression of the P50 evoked response to the human cerebral cortex. *Clin. Neurophysiol.* 124, 675–685. doi: 10.1016/j.clinph.2012.10.007

Boutros, N. N., Korzyukov, O., Jansen, B., Feingold, A., and Bell, M. (2004). Sensory gating deficits during the mid-latency phase of information processing in medicated schizophrenia patients. *Psychiatry Res.* 126, 203–215. doi: 10.1016/j.psychres.2004.01.007

Braff, D. L., and Geyer, M. A. (1990). Sensorimotor gating and schizophrenia. Human and animal model studies. *Arch. Gen. Psychiatry* 47, 181–188. doi: 10.1001/archpsyc.1990.01810140081011

Brinkman, M. J., and Stauder, J. E. (2007). Development and gender in the P50 paradigm. *Clin, Neurophysiol.* 118, 1517–1524. doi: 10.1016/j.clinph.2007.04.002

Campbell, J., Nielsen, M., Bean, C., and LaBrec, A. (2020a). Auditory gating in hearing loss. *J. Am. Acad. Audiol.* 31, 559–565. doi: 10.1055/s-0040-1709517

Campbell, J., Nielsen, M., LaBrec, A., and Bean, C. (2020b). Sensory inhibition is related to variable speech perception in noise in adults with normal hearing. *J. Speech Lang. Hear. Res.* 63, 1595–1607. doi: 10.1044/2020_JSLHR-19-00261

Chien, Y. L., Hsieh, M. H., and Gau, S. S. (2019). P50-N100-P200 sensory gating deficits in adolescents and young adults with autism spectrum disorders. *Prog. Neuropsychopharmacol. Biol. Psychiatry* 95:109683. doi: 10.1016/j.pnpbp.2019.109683

Crasta, J. E., Gavin, W. J., and Davies, P. L. (2021). Expanding our understanding of sensory gating in children with autism spectrum disorders. *Clin. Neurophysiol.* 132, 180–190. doi: 10.1016/j.clinph.2020.09.020

Culotta, L., and Penzes, P. (2020). Exploring the mechanisms underlying excitation/inhibition imbalance in human iPSC-derived models of ASD. *Mol. Autism.* 11:32. doi: 10.1186/s13229-020-00339-0

Davies, P. L., Chang, W. P., and Gavin, W. J. (2009). Maturation of sensory gating performance in children with and without sensory processing disorders. *Int. J. Psychophysiol.* 72, 187–197. doi: 10.1016/j.ijpsycho.2008.12.007

Dettman, S. J., Pinder, D., Briggs, R. J., Dowell, R. C., and Leigh, J. R. (2007). Communication development in children who receive the cochlear implant younger than 12 months: risks versus benefits. *Ear Hear* 28(2 Suppl), 11S–18S. doi: 10.1097/AUD.0b013e31803153f8

Dye, M. W., and Hauser, P. C. (2014). Sustained attention, selective attention and cognitive control in deaf and hearing children. *Hear Res.* 309, 94–102. doi: 10.1016/j.heares.2013.12.001

Freedman, R., Adler, L. E., and Waldo, M. (1987). Gating of the auditory evoked potential in children and adults. *Psychophysiology* 24, 223–227. doi: 10.1111/j.1469-8986.1987.tb00282.x

Fruhstorfer, H., Soveri, P., and Jarvilehto, T. (1970). Short-term habituation of the auditory evoked response in man. *Electroencephalogr. Clin. Neurophysiol.* 28, 153–161. doi: 10.1016/0013-4694(70)90183-5

Gilley, P. M., Sharma, A., Dorman, M., Finley, C. C., Panch, A. S., and Martin, K. (2006). Minimization of cochlear implant stimulus artifact in cortical auditory evoked potentials. *Clin. Neurophysiol.* 117, 1772–1782. doi: 10.1016/j.clinph.2006.04.018

Gjini, K., Burroughs, S., and Boutros, N. N. (2011). Relevance of attention in auditory sensory gating paradigms in schizophrenia a pilot study. *J. Psychophysiol.* 25, 60–66. doi: 10.1027/0269-8803/a000042

Gordon, K. A., Papsin, B. C., and Harrison, R. V. (2003). Activity-dependent developmental plasticity of the auditory brain stem in children who use cochlear implants. *Ear Hear* 24, 485–500. doi: 10.1097/01.AUD.0000100203.65990.D4

Grunwald, T., Boutros, N. N., Pezer, N., von Oertzen, J., Fernandez, G., Schaller, C., et al. (2003). Neuronal substrates of sensory gating within the human brain. *Biol. Psychiatry* 53, 511–519. doi: 10.1016/s0006-3223(02)01673-6

Hall, W. C., Li, D., and Dye, T. D. V. (2018). Influence of hearing loss on child behavioral and home experiences. *Am. J. Public Health* 108, 1079–1081. doi: 10.2105/AJPH.2018.304498

Hegerl, U., and Juckel, G. (1993). Intensity dependence of auditory evoked potentials as an indicator of central serotonergic neurotransmission: a new hypothesis. *Biol. Psychiatry* 33, 173–187. doi: 10.1016/0006-3223(93)90137-3

Heinrichs-Graham, E., Walker, E. A., Eastman, J. A., Frenzel, M. R., Joe, T. R., and McCreery, R. W. (2021). The impact of mild-to-severe hearing loss on the neural dynamics serving verbal working memory processing in children. *Neuroimage Clin.* 30:102647. doi: 10.1016/j.nicl.2021.102647

Hongmei, H., and Nan, L. (2017). Reduction of facial nerve stimulation artifacts in electrically evoked auditory bralnstem responses based on independent component analysis. *J. Electron. Sci. Tech.* 30, 57–60.

Hu, Z., Sun, J. Q., Guan, R. R., Chen, L., Sun, J. W., and Guo, X. T. (2021). Deficient sensory and cognitive processing in children with cochlear implants: an event-related potential study. *Hear Res.* 408:108295. doi: 10.1016/j.heares.2021.108295

Hunter, S. K., Mendoza, J. H., D'Anna, K., Zerbe, G. O., McCarthy, L., Hoffman, C., et al. (2012). Antidepressants may mitigate the effects of prenatal maternal anxiety on infant auditory sensory gating. *Am. J. Psychiatry* 169, 616–624. doi: 10.1176/appi.ajp.2012.11091365

Hutchison, A. K., Hunter, S. K., Wagner, B. D., Calvin, E. A., Zerbe, G. O., and Ross, R. G. (2017). Diminished infant p50 sensory gating predicts increased 40-month-old attention. Anxiety/Depression, and externalizing symptoms. *J. Atten. Disord.* 21, 209–218. doi: 10.1177/1087054713488824

Javitt, D. C., and Freedman, R. (2015). Sensory processing dysfunction in the personal experience and neuronal machinery of schizophrenia. *Am. J. Psychiatry* 172, 17–31. doi: 10.1176/appi.ajp.2014.13121691

Josef Golubic, S., Aine, C. J., Stephen, J. M., Adair, J. C., Knoefel, J. E., and Supek, S. (2014). Modulatory role of the prefrontal generator within the auditory M50 network. *Neuroimage* 92, 120–131. doi: 10.1016/j.neuroimage.2014.02.013

Kandler, K. (2004). Activity-dependent organization of inhibitory circuits: lessons from the auditory system. *Curr. Opin. Neurobiol.* 14, 96–104. doi: 10.1016/j.conb.2004.01.017

Knott, V., Millar, A., and Fisher, D. (2009). Sensory gating and source analysis of the auditory P50 in low and high suppressors. *Neuroimage* 44, 992–1000. doi: 10.1016/j.neuroimage.2008.10.002

Korzyukov, O., Pflieger, M. E., Wagner, M., Bowyer, S. M., Rosburg, T., Sundaresan, K., et al. (2007). Generators of the intracranial P50 response in auditory sensory gating. *Neuroimage* 35, 814–826. doi: 10.1016/j.neuroimage.2006.12.011

Kral, A., Dorman, M. F., and Wilson, B. S. (2019). Neuronal development of hearing and language: cochlear implants and critical periods. *Annu. Rev. Neurosci.* 42, 47–65. doi: 10.1146/annurev-neuro-080317-061513

Kronenberger, W. G., Beer, J., Castellanos, I., Pisoni, D. B., and Miyamoto, R. T. (2014). Neurocognitive risk in children with cochlear implants. *JAMA Otolaryngol. Head Neck Surg.* 140, 608–615. doi: 10.1001/jamaoto.2014.757

Lee, Y. S., Lueders, H., Dinner, D. S., Lesser, R. P., Hahn, J., and Klem, G. (1984). Recording of auditory evoked potentials in man using chronic subdural electrodes. *Brain* 107(Pt 1), 115–131. doi: 10.1093/brain/107.1.115

Liegeois-Chauvel, C., Musolino, A., Badier, J. M., Marquis, P., and Chauvel, P. (1994). Evoked potentials recorded from the auditory cortex in man: evaluation and topography of the middle latency components. *Electroencephalogr. Clin. Neurophysiol.* 92, 204–214. doi: 10.1016/0168-5597(94)90064-7

Lieu, J. E. C., Kenna, M., Anne, S., and Davidson, L. (2020). Hearing loss in children: a review. *JAMA* 324, 2195–2205. doi: 10.1001/jama.2020.17647

Lijffijt, M., Lane, S. D., Meier, S. L., Boutros, N. N., Burroughs, S., Steinberg, J. L., et al. (2009). P50, N100, and P200 sensory gating: relationships with behavioral inhibition, attention, and working memory. *Psychophysiology* 46, 1059–1068. doi: 10.1111/j.1469-8986.2009.00845.x

Manrique, M., Cervera-Paz, F. J., Huarte, A., Perez, N., Molina, M., and Garcia-Tapia, R. (1999). Cerebral auditory plasticity and cochlear implants. *Int. J. Pediatr. Otorhinolaryngol.* 49(Suppl. 1), S193–S197. doi: 10.1016/s0165-5876(99)00159-7

Mayer, A. R., Hanlon, F. M., Franco, A. R., Teshiba, T. M., Thoma, R. J., Clark, V. P., et al. (2009). The neural networks underlying auditory sensory gating. *Neuroimage* 44, 182–189. doi: 10.1016/j.neuroimage.2008.08.025

Micoulaud-Franchi, J. A., Vaillant, F., Lopez, R., Peri, P., Baillif, A., Brandejsky, L., et al. (2015). Sensory gating in adult with attention-deficit/hyperactivity disorder: event-evoked potential and perceptual experience reports comparisons with schizophrenia. *Biol. Psychol.* 107, 16–23. doi: 10.1016/j.biopsycho.2015.03.002

Mukari, S. Z., Ling, L. N., and Ghani, H. A. (2007). Educational performance of pediatric cochlear implant recipients in mainstream classes. *Int. J. Pediatr. Otorhinolaryngol.* 71, 231–240. doi: 10.1016/j.ijporl.2006.10.005

Ni, G., Zheng, Q., Liu, Y., Zhao, Y., Yue, T., Han, S., et al. (2021). Objective electroencephalography-based assessment for auditory rehabilitation of pediatric cochlear implant users. *Hear Res* 404, 108211. doi: 10.1016/j.heares.2021.108211

Peixoto, M. C., Spratley, J., Oliveira, G., Martins, J., Bastos, J., and Ribeiro, C. (2013). Effectiveness of cochlear implants in children: long term results. *Int. J. Pediatr. Otorhinolaryngol.* 77, 462–468. doi: 10.1016/j.ijporl.2012.12.005

Rosburg, T. (2018). Auditory N100 gating in patients with schizophrenia: a systematic meta-analysis. *Clin. Neurophysiol.* 129, 2099–2111. doi: 10.1016/j.clinph.2018.07.012

Rosburg, T., Trautner, P., Elger, C. E., and Kurthen, M. (2009). Attention effects on sensory gating–intracranial and scalp recordings. *Neuroimage* 48, 554–563. doi: 10.1016/j.neuroimage.2009.06.063

Sharma, A., Dorman, M. F., and Spahr, A. J. (2002b). A sensitive period for the development of the central auditory system in children with cochlear implants: implications for age of implantation. *Ear Hear* 23, 532–539. doi: 10.1097/00003446-200212000-00004

Sharma, A., Dorman, M., Spahr, A., and Todd, N. W. (2002a). Early cochlear implantation in children allows normal development of central auditory pathways. *Annu. Otol. Rhinol. Laryngol. Suppl.* 189, 38–41. doi: 10.1177/00034894021110s508

Sharma, A., Nash, A. A., and Dorman, M. (2009). Cortical development, plasticity and re-organization in children with cochlear implants. *J. Commun. Disord.* 42, 272–279. doi: 10.1016/j.jcomdis.2009.03.003

Shen, C. L., Chou, T. L., Lai, W. S., Hsieh, M. H., Liu, C. C., Liu, C. M., et al. (2020). P50, N100, and P200 auditory sensory gating deficits in schizophrenia patients. *Front. Psychiatry* 11, 868. doi: 10.3389/fpsyt.2020.00868

Shin, M. S., Kim, S. K., Kim, S. S., Park, M. H., Kim, C. S., and Oh, S. H. (2007). Comparison of cognitive function in deaf children between before and after cochlear implant. *Ear Hear* 28(2 Suppl), 22S–28S. doi: 10.1097/AUD.0b013e318031541b

Smucny, J., Olincy, A., Eichman, L., Lyons, E., and Tregellas, J. J. S. R. (2013). Early sensory processing deficits predict sensitivity to distraction in schizophrenia. *Schizophr Res/* 147, 196–200. doi: 10.1016/j.schres.2013.03.025

Surowiecki, V. N., Sarant, J., Maruff, P., Blamey, P. J., Busby, P. A., and Clark, G. M. (2002). Cognitive processing in children using cochlear implants: the relationship between visual memory, attention, and executive functions and developing language skills. *Ann. Otol. Rhinol. Laryngol. Suppl.* 189, 119–126. doi: 10.1177/00034894021110s524

Swanson, J. M., Kraemer, H. C., Hinshaw, S. P., Arnold, L. E., Conners, C. K., Abikoff, H. B., et al. (2001). Clinical relevance of the primary findings of the MTA: success rates based on severity of ADHD and ODD symptoms at the end of treatment. *J. Am. Acad. Child Adolesc. Psychiatry* 40, 168–179. doi: 10.1097/00004583-200102000-00011

Takesian, A. E., Kotak, V. C., and Sanes, D. H. (2009). Developmental hearing loss disrupts synaptic inhibition: implications for auditory processing. *Future Neurol.* 4, 331–349. doi: 10.2217/FNL.09.5

Takesian, A. E., Kotak, V. C., and Sanes, D. H. (2012). Age-dependent effect of hearing loss on cortical inhibitory synapse function. *J. Neurophysiol.* 107, 937–947. doi: 10.1152/jn.00515.2011

Wan, L., Friedman, B. H., Boutros, N. N., and Crawford, H. J. (2008). P50 sensory gating and attentional performance. *Int. J. Psychophysiol.* 67, 91–100. doi: 10.1016/j.ijpsycho.2007.10.008

Weisser, R., Weisbrod, M., Roehrig, M., Rupp, A., Schroeder, J., and Scherg, M. (2001). Is frontal lobe involved in the generation of auditory evoked P50? *Neuroreport* 12, 3303–3307. doi: 10.1097/00001756-200110290-00031

11

Alterations of Regional Homogeneity in Children with Congenital Sensorineural Hearing Loss: A Resting-State fMRI Study

Pingping Guo[1†], Siyuan Lang[2†], Muliang Jiang[2*], Yifeng Wang[3], Zisan Zeng[2], Zuguang Wen[4], Yikang Liu[5] and Bihong T. Chen[6]

[1] Department of Medical Ultrasound, Affiliated Tumor Hospital of Guangxi Medical University, Nanning, China, [2] Department of Radiology, First Affiliated Hospital of Guangxi Medical University, Nanning, China, [3] Institute of Brain and Psychological Sciences, Sichuan Normal University, Chengdu, China, [4] Department of Radiology, Seventh Affiliated Hospital of Sun Yat-sen University, Shenzhen, China, [5] Department of Otorhinolaryngology Head and Neck Surgery, First Affiliated Hospital of Guangxi Medical University, Nanning, China, [6] Department of Diagnostic Radiology, City of Hope National Medical Center, Duarte, CA, United States

****Correspondence:***
Muliang Jiang
jmlgxmu@gmail.com

[†] These authors have contributed equally to this work

Background: Brain functional alterations have been observed in children with congenital sensorineural hearing loss (CSNHL). The purpose of this study was to assess the alterations of regional homogeneity in children with CSNHL.

Methods: Forty-five children with CSNHL and 20 healthy controls were enrolled into this study. Brain resting-state functional MRI (rs-fMRI) for regional homogeneity including the Kendall coefficient consistency (KCC-ReHo) and the coherence-based parameter (Cohe-ReHo) was analyzed and compared between the two groups, i.e., the CSNHL group and the healthy control group.

Results: Compared to the healthy controls, children with CSNHL showed increased Cohe-ReHo values in left calcarine and decreased values in bilateral ventrolateral prefrontal cortex (VLPFC) and right dorsolateral prefrontal cortex (DLPFC). Children with CSNHL also had increased KCC-ReHo values in the left calcarine, cuneus, precentral gyrus, and right superior parietal lobule (SPL) and decreased values in the left VLPFC and right DLPFC. Correlations were detected between the ReHo values and age of the children with CSNHL. There were positive correlations between ReHo values in the pre-cuneus/pre-frontal cortex and age ($p < 0.05$). There were negative correlations between ReHo values in bilateral temporal lobes, fusiform gyrus, parahippocampal gyrus and precentral gyrus, and age ($p < 0.05$).

Conclusion: Children with CSNHL had RoHo alterations in the auditory, visual, motor, and other related brain cortices as compared to the healthy controls with normal hearing. There were significant correlations between ReHo values and age in brain regions involved in information integration and processing. Our study showed promising data using rs-fMRI ReHo parameters to assess brain functional alterations in children with CSNHL.

Keywords: congenital sensorineural hearing loss, kendall coefficient consistency, coherence-based regional homogeneity, functional magnetic resonance imaging, neuroimaging

INTRODUCTION

Congenital sensorineural hearing loss (CSNHL) is a disabling disease characterized by lack of sound stimulation and hearing loss at birth (Harlor and Bower, 2009; Tan et al., 2013). Hearing loss not only affects language but also causes changes to motor function and cognition (Lin et al., 2013). Cross-modal plasticity with enhanced sensory modes such as vision has been implicated in the effort to compensate for the hearing loss (Lee et al., 2001; Bavelier and Neville, 2002; Lomber et al., 2010). As a result, auditory cortex in both humans and animals with congenital deafness may remain relatively normal without degeneration or atrophy through non-sound stimulus from vision, movement, and perception (Stanton and Harrison, 2000). Nevertheless, it is unclear how brain function may be altered due to hearing loss and how brain neuroplasticity with other sensory modes may compensate for hearing deprivation in children with CSNHL.

Advanced neuroimaging has made possible for assessing *in vivo* brain structure and function (Mayer and Trezek, 2018). Resting-state functional brain MRI (rs-fMRI) is a functional imaging technique based on the blood-oxygen-level-dependent (BOLD) method to assess brain regional alterations when not performing a task (Mirzaei and Adeli, 2016). BOLD-fMRI indirectly reflects the intrinsic brain activity in the *infraslow frequency band (< 0.1 Hz)* (Biswal et al., 1995). Compared to the task-based fMRI, rs-fMRI can detect brain functional changes and core brain networks (Buckner, 2013). *Therefore, rs-fMRI has been used to study various conditions including attention deficit disorder, social anxiety disorder, epilepsy, and blindness* (Plichta et al., 2009; Fair et al., 2010; Bedny et al., 2011; Liu et al., 2015, 2017) *for functional connectivity between the whole brain and certain preset regions of interest* (Calamante et al., 2013). However, the connectivity analysis does not usually reflect brain regional changes that are specific to the conditions under scrutiny such as hearing loss (Greicius et al., 2007). These is an unmet need to assess specific brain regions involved in hearing, vision, motor, and cognition in order to understand the effect of hearing loss on brain structure and function in children with CSNHL.

Regional homogeneity (ReHo) can be calculated based on the Kendall coefficient consistency (KCC-ReHo) from rs-fMRI, which measures the similarity of the time series of a given voxel to those of its nearest neighbors (Zang et al., 2004; Zuo et al., 2013). A prior study by Wolak et al. (2019) found that hearing development and language processing were affected by hearing loss as indicated by changes in the KCC-ReHo values. However, KCC-ReHo is known to be susceptible to random noise caused by phase delay in the time span (Ou et al., 2018). A similar method, i.e., the coherent-based ReHo (Cohe-ReHo) method, has been used to detect the regional synchronization of rs-fMRI signals. *Compared to KCC-ReHo, Cohe-ReHo is not sensitive to noise* (Liu et al., 2010) *and has been successfully utilized to detect brain regional alterations for various disorders* (Guo et al., 2012; Liu et al., 2012, 2018; Zhou et al., 2019). Therefore, both KCC-ReHo and Cohe-ReHo are useful parameters and are complimentary for assessing brain functional alterations.

In this study, we analyzed rs-fMRI for both KCC-ReHo and Cohe-ReHo to assess the differences in brain regional activity between the children with CSNHL and the healthy controls with normal hearing. We used the rs-fMRI approach because it was feasible and practical for children with CSNHL who may not be able to perform any tasks in the MRI scanner while under sedation. We hypothesized that children with CSNHL would have alterations of ReHo values, especially in specific brain regions associated with hearing, vision, motor, and executive control, when compared to the healthy controls.

MATERIALS AND METHODS

Participants

Children with CSNHL who were right-handed and who had no treatment for hearing loss were recruited from our outpatient subspecialty clinic for hearing loss from January 2017 to October 2019. Children with normal hearing serving as healthy controls were recruited from the community. Part of this cohort was included in our previously published study of white matter microstructural analysis of diffusion tensor imaging (Jiang et al., 2019). However, we have not published any rs-fMRI data from this cohort.

Inclusion criteria included right-handed children with CSNHL diagnosed by both hearing screening tests at 3 and 42 days after birth and bilateral auditory brainstem response (ABR) > 91 db. Exclusion criteria included the following: severe neurological disorders such as epilepsy and congenital leukodystrophy, conditions with impaired cognition such as autism and severe hyperactivity syndrome, history of treatment for ear-related diseases such as infection, history of using hearing aids, and history of contraindications for MRI such as having a cardiac pacer and orbital metal. For rs-fMRI scans, all participants were sedated with 10% oral chloral hydrate in a dosage of 0.3–0.5 ml per kg of body weight with the maximal dosage of 80 ml. All children were under the care of a pediatrician or a pediatric nurse practitioner while under sedation for the brain MRI scan. No adverse effect was noted from the oral sedation in our cohort. The study was approved by the local ethics committee and institutional review board for research in our hospital. Informed consent was signed by all participants' legal guardians.

Resting-State Functional Brain MRI Acquisition

Rs-fMRI scans were obtained on the same Siemens Verio 3T scanner (Siemens Healthcare, Erlangen, Germany). Soft earplugs and foam pads were used to reduce the scanner noise and head motion. The rs-fMRI scans were obtained when the children were asleep after oral sedation. Gradient-echo planar imaging sequence for rs-fMRI was acquired for all participants with the following parameters: repetition time/echo time = 2,000/30 ms, 30 slices, 64×64 matrix, 90° flip angle, 24 cm field of view (FOV), 4 mm slice thickness, 0.4 mm gap, and 250 volumes (500 s).

Resting-State Functional Brain MRI Data Processing

Rs-fMRI data were preprocessed with DPARSF package based on the MATLAB platform (Chao-Gan and Yu-Feng, 2010).

Briefly, the first 10 volumes were discarded for signal stabilization and subject adaptation, which was followed by slice timing and spatial realignment. Subjects with excessive head motion (translational and rotational displacement exceeded 2.0 mm or 2.0°) were excluded.

All images were normalized to the standard space on the Montreal Neurological Institute (MNI) template and were resampled to $3 \times 3 \times 3$ mm^3. The MNI template has been known to be appropriate for normalizing brains from young children to adolescence (Chen et al., 2017, 2018). *Subsequently, linear trend, white matter signal, cerebrospinal fluid signal, and Friston 24 motion parameters were used as regressors to reduce effects of head movement and non-neuronal information* (Yan et al., 2013). Band-pass (0.01–0.08 Hz) filtering was then conducted.

The KCC-ReHo values of the pre-defined band time series of each voxel in the entire brain relative to the nearest 27 voxels were calculated with the REST plus software.[1] The resulting data were further spatially smoothed using a 6-mm isotropic full width at half maximum (FWHM) Gaussian kernel to generate the ReHo map.

In addition to the KCC-ReHo values, a second set of ReHo values, i.e., the Cohe-ReHo, were calculated with the following three steps in the REST plus software (Liu et al., 2010). First, the power spectrum of time series in each voxel was estimated with the Welch's modified periodogram averaging method. Second, the coherences between time series in each voxel and its nearest 27 voxels were estimated. Third, the 27 coherence values were averaged to represent the Cohe-ReHo of the center voxel. To eliminate the differences in the overall level of the whole brain ReHo value among the individuals, the ReHo value of each voxel was divided by the mean value of the whole brain signal amplitude. The resulting data were further spatially smoothed using a 6-mm isotropic FWHM Gaussian kernel to generate the ReHo maps for statistical analysis.

Statistical Analysis

The demographic data were analyzed with SPSS Version 16 (SPSS, Inc., Chicago, IL, United States). Two-sample *T*-test was performed to detect the differences in ReHo values between the CSNHL group and the healthy control group using REST plus. Age, gender, and mean framewise displacement (Mean FD) were considered as covariates for estimating their effects on group difference independently. Alphasim correction was used for multiple comparisons with voxel-level significance set at $p < 0.01$ and cluster-level significance set at $p < 0.05$ (Zhou et al., 2019). We chose more lenient *p*-values for multiple comparison because of our intent to identify preliminary results for hypothesis generating, to balance α and β errors in statistical analysis, and to verify the results with two ReHo indices. All significant clusters were reported on the MNI coordinates, and the *T*-values of the peak voxel were determined.

We conducted Pearson correlation analysis between ReHo values and age with REST plus software. Focusing on the positive and negative correlation peaks, the signals in the spheres with a radius of 6 mm were extracted, and age-related scatter plots were presented.

[1] http://restfmri.net/forum/restplus

RESULTS

A total of 45 children with CSNHL and 20 healthy controls were recruited into this study. The participants ranged from 0.5 to 16 years of age. There were no significant differences in gender ($p = 0.60$), age ($p = 0.33$), or head movement parameters ($p = 0.11$) between the CSNHL group and the healthy control group (**Table 1**).

Regional Homogeneity Results

There were significantly increased Cohe-ReHo values in left calcarine and decreased values in bilateral ventrolateral prefrontal cortex (VLPFC) and right dorsolateral prefrontal cortex (DLPFC) in the CSNHL group when compared to the healthy control group with corrected $p < 0.05$ for all clusters (**Table 2** and **Figure 1A**).

There were significantly increased KCC-ReHo values in the left calcarine, left cuneus, left precentral, and right superior parietal lobule (SPL) and decreased values in left VLPFC and right DLPFC in the CSNHL group when compared to the healthy control group with corrected $p < 0.05$ for all clusters (**Table 2** and **Figure 1B**).

Correlation Between Regional Homogeneity Values and Age

Significant correlations were detected between ReHo values in certain brain regions and the age of children with CSNHL with Alphasim- corrected $p < 0.01$ at the voxel level and $p < 0.05$ at the cluster level. There was no correlation between the ReHo values and age in the healthy control group after Alphasim correction ($p > 0.05$).

The correlation between the KCC-ReHo values and age and the correlation between the Cohe-ReHo and age were similar in the children with CSNHL. There were significant correlations between ReHo values and age in the following brain regions: prefrontal cortex (PFC), posterior cingulate cortex (PCC)/precuneus, bilateral fusiform/parahippocampal gyrus,

TABLE 1 | Participant information.

	CSNHL (*n* = 45)	HC (*n* = 20)	*p*
Age (years ± SD)	4.82 ± 2.64(range 1.5–13)	5.66 ± 3.36 (range 0.5–16)	0.33
Gender (Male/Female)	25/20	13/7	0.60
Handedness	45 right-handed	19 right-handed	
Mean FD	0.15 ± 0.07	0.19 ± 0.10	0.11
dB HL			
Left ear (dB)	105.01 ± 8.13 (97–120)		
Right ear (dB)	99.91 ± 8.74 (92–120)		

CSNHL, congenital sensorineural hearing loss; HL, hearing loss; dB, decibel; HC, healthy control; Mean FD, mean framewise displacement.

TABLE 2 | Differences in regional homogeneity (ReHo) values between the congenital sensorineural hearing loss (CSNHL) group and the healthy control (HC) group.

Index	Breakpoint cluster region (BCR)	Cluster size	Coordinate (mm)			*t*-value
			X	Y	Z	
Cohe-ReHo	**CSNHL > HC**					
	Left calcarine	190	−15	−57	9	4.96
	CSNHL < HC					
	Left VLPFC	737	−12	36	−6	−4.30
	Right VLPFC	352	30	48	6	−3.90
	Right DLPFC	222	12	51	30	−4.38
KCC-ReHo	**CSNHL > HC**					
	Left calcarine	146	−15	−57	9	4.88
	Left cuneus	164	−9	−78	30	3.62
	Left precentral	158	−48	−3	48	5.30
	Right SPL	196	48	−45	63	4.36
	CSNHL < HC					
	Left VLPFC	661	−36	36	9	−5.40
	Right DLPFC	702	12	54	24	−4.68

VLPFC, ventrolateral prefrontal cortex; DLPFC, dorsolateral prefrontal cortex; SPL, superior parietal lobule. All clusters were corrected with $p < 0.05$.

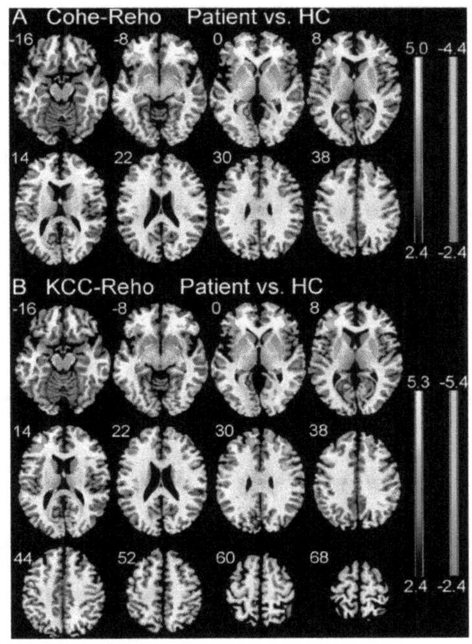

FIGURE 1 | Comparison of regional homogeneity (ReHo) values between the patient group with CSNHL and the healthy control (HC) group. **(A)** Comparison of coherence-based regional homogeneity (Cohe-ReHo) values between the CSNHL group and the HC group. **(B)** Comparison of Kendall coefficient consistency (KCC-ReHo) values between the CSNHL group and the HC group.

and precentral gyrus. Among them, PFC and PCC/precuneus were positively correlated with age, with the strongest point located at the right VLPFC. Bilateral temporal lobe fusiform gyrus/parahippocampal gyrus and precentral gyrus were negatively correlated with age, with the strongest point located in the right fusiform gyrus (**Table 3** and **Figure 2**). The mean ReHo values in each of the brain regions were extracted for both the CSNHL group and the healthy control group. Their relationships with age were presented in **Figure 3**.

DISCUSSION

To the best of our knowledge, our study was the first to assess brain regional Cohe-ReHo alterations in children with CSNHL. We found de-synchronization of brain regional activity showing different ReHo values in different brain regions of the deaf children. In addition, we also found significant correlations between the ReHo values and age in children with CSNHL.

Our findings of increased KCC-ReHo values in left calcarine and left cuneus in the CSNHL group as compared to the healthy control group were generally in line with literature. Calcarine and cuneus as parts of occipital lobe belong to the visual cortex and are involved in visual processing. Bavelier et al. (2006) reported that deaf patients had better visual performance than those with normal hearing, especially in tasks requiring higher attention. A higher KCC-ReHo value in the right occipital lobe has been found by Xia et al. (2017) in children with CSNHL. Shiell et al. (2015) suggested that early auditory deprivation may lead to functional reorganization of the auditory cortex and may enhance interactions between auditory and visual brain regions. Converging evidence from our data and other's observations supports the notion for cross-modal reorganization of auditory-related brain regions for the hearing impaired. Audio-visual

TABLE 3 | Correlation between regional homogeneity (ReHo) values and age in children with congenital sensorineural hearing loss (CSNHL).

Index	Breakpoint cluster region (BCR)	Cluster size	Coordinate (mm)			*t*-value
			X	Y	Z	
Cohe-ReHo						
	PFC	6,189	48	36	33	7.13
	PCC/precuneus	707	15	−75	60	4.81
	Right fusiform/parahippocampal	519	39	−33	−21	−4.76
	Left fusiform/parahippocampal	632	−18	−27	−18	−4.58
	Precentral gyrus	1,218	21	−27	69	−4.64
KCC-ReHo						
	PFC	5,230	−48	33	−12	7.11
	PCC/precuneus	449	15	−75	60	4.64
	Right fusiform/parahippocampal	401	39	−36	−18	−5.46
	Left fusiform/parahippocampal	358	−39	−21	−18	−4.58
	Precentral gyrus	1,480	18	−30	66	−5.43

PFC, prefrontal cortex; PCC, posterior cingulate cortex: KCC-ReHo, Kendall coefficient consistency; Cohe-ReHo, coherence-based regional homogeneity.

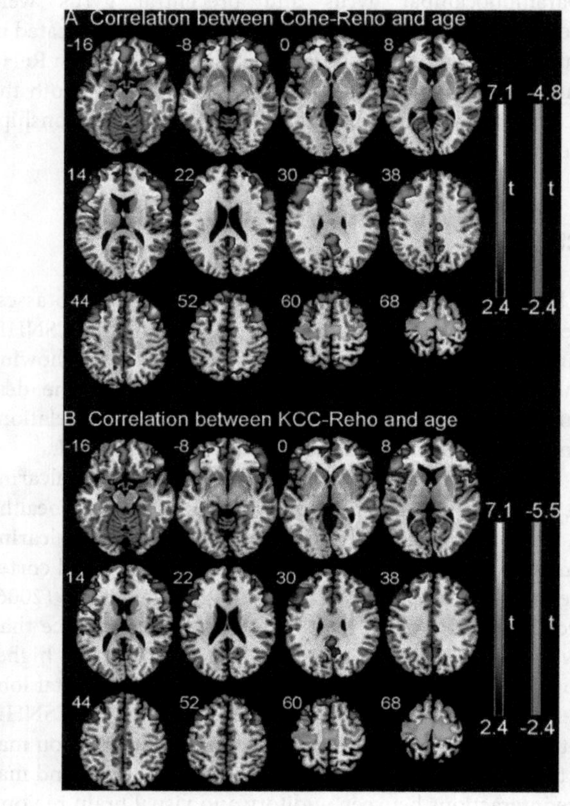

FIGURE 2 | Correlation between regional homogeneity (ReHo) values and age in children with congenital sensorineural hearing loss (CSNHL). Positive correlations were indicated in red color, and negative correlations were indicated in blue color. **(A)** Correlation between coherence-based regional homogeneity (Cohe-ReHo) values and age. **(B)** Correlation between Kendall coefficient consistency (KCC-ReHo) values and age.

modal reorganization is one type of the cross-modal patterns for which the deaf children may mobilize more visual resources to compensate for deprivation of sound stimuli (Bavelier et al., 2006; Xia et al., 2017).

Precentral gyrus is the primary motor cortex, and it is an important structure for autonomous movement (Rivara et al., 2003). Westermann and Reck Miranda (2004) and Shi et al. (2016) showed that infants learn language by learning the connections between sounds and actions needed for pronunciation, indicating that the synchronicity between the auditory and motor cortex may be critical in language development. For children with CSNHL, deprivation of sound and desynchronization of cortex may motivate and enhance additional sensory and motor stimuli. Therefore, it was not surprising to see our data showing increased brain activity in the motor-related cortex, i.e., precentral gyrus, which may be part of the efforts to compensate for the hearing loss.

SPL is a brain region important for cognitive and motion-related process operating as a transmitter of somatosensory, visual motor integration, and visual spatial attention (Corbetta et al., 1995; Parks and Madden, 2013). Iacoboni et al. (1999) reported that SPL could encode motion perception such as finger movements. Sign language has been used by school-age children with CSNHL for communication, and these children may activate their motor cortex through hand and finger movement (Hari et al., 1998). In line with the abovementioned studies, our results of showing increased ReHo values in the SPL may reflect the brain functional neuroplasticity to integrate the visual function and motor function through sign language.

Our study showed decreased ReHo in bilateral VLPFC and right DLPFC, which were components of the executive control network implicated in initiating and modulating cognitive function. These brain regions contain multi-sensory cells that can receive various types of afferent stimuli (Sugihara et al., 2006). Published literature has suggested that DLPFC is related to auditory spatial processing (Klaus and Schutter, 2018), while VLPFC is responsible for receiving the input of auditory cortex for non-spatial acoustic processing (Romanski et al., 1999). A prior study of amnestic mild cognitive impairment showed decreased ReHo in DLPFC and decreased local connectivity (Zhen et al., 2018). We speculated that the lack of sound stimulation may have weakened the functional integration of VLPFC and DLPFC as reflected by reduced ReHo values in these brain regions.

Our study showed both similarities and differences in the ReHo alterations between the Cohe-ReHo and the KCC-ReHo methods. For instances, both methods showed increased values in the left calcarine and decreased values in VLPFC and DLPFC. However, the KCC-ReHo method identified increased values in additional brain regions such as cuneus, precentral gyrus, and SPL, which are related to motor cortex and neuroplasticity. The mechanism underlying these results is not clear. We speculate that it might be due to the subtle variations in these two methods, such as calculation accuracy or threshold selection. Nevertheless, our pilot study identified these intriguing results, which should motivate more research to understand the implications of ReHo alterations from these two methods on functional adaptation and cross-modal plasticity for the children with hearing impairment.

We found a positive correlation between the ReHo value of PFC and PCC/precuneus with age in children with CSNHL. For our cohort, hearing deprivation became apparent at birth. Therefore, their age indicated the duration of their hearing loss and older children suffered from longer duration of hearing loss than the younger ones. We speculate that the positive correlation between ReHo and age may imply the occurrence of more brain alterations in older children due to the longer duration of their hearing loss.

Prior studies have shown that prefrontal cortex is essential in auditory cognition because it receives information from a wide range of auditory regions (Rowe et al., 2008). On the other hand, as a node in the default mode network, PCC/precuneus can simultaneously communicate with various brain networks involved in multiple brain functions such as cognition and motor (Rolls, 2019) while receiving sensory input from brain auditory regions (Rowe et al., 2008; Tanabe and Sadato, 2009). Conway et al. (2011) considered that the lack of auditory input may have reduced auditory-frontal connectivity, which may affect the development of cognitive function and motor skills for

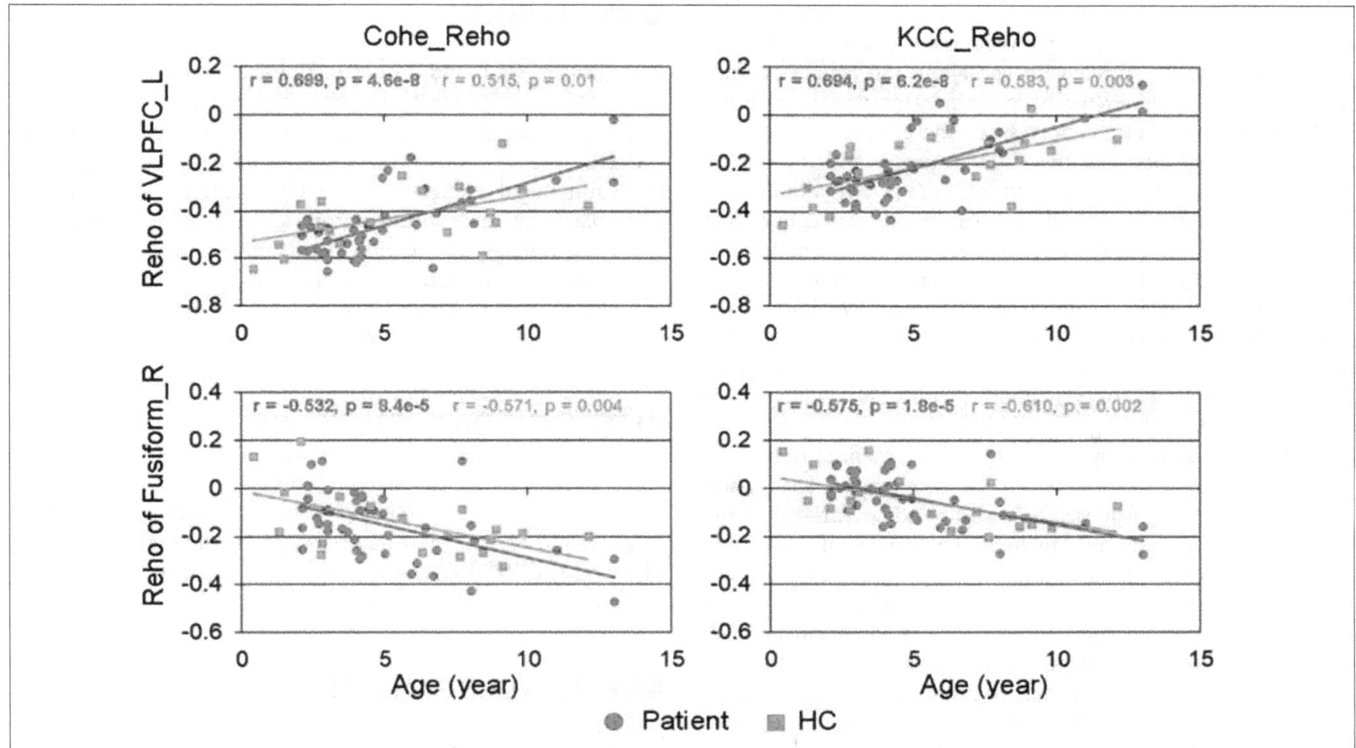

FIGURE 3 | Correlation between regional homogeneity (ReHo) values and age. The strongest positive correlation was located in the right ventrolateral prefrontal cortex (VLPFC), and the most negative correlation was located in the right fusiform gyrus.

the hearing impaired. In our study, with increasing age of the children with CSNHL along with longer duration of hearing loss, we should not be surprised to see increasing ReHo values as the children grow older, thus having a positive correlation between ReHo and age. We speculate that PFC and PCC/precuneus may need stronger information integration with more brain activity to cope with disruption of the normal physiological status in some brain regions due to prolonged hearing loss.

Our study showed that the ReHo values of bilateral temporal lobe fusiform gyrus/parahippocampal gyrus and precentral gyrus were negatively correlated with age. Temporal lobe fusiform gyrus and parahippocampal gyrus participate in language decoding and semantic processing during auditory stimulus (Kravitz et al., 2011; Forseth et al., 2018). A prior study has suggested that preoperative cortical stimulation would impair the performance of reading and hearing comprehension tasks, reflecting the important role of these brain regions for completing these tasks (Binder et al., 1997). As the severity of deafness increases, these brain regions may need to increase activity to compensate for the lack of sound stimulus.

There has been extensive literature on hearing loss and rs-fMRI methodology. For instance, a study by Xia et al. (2017) enrolled infants with CSNHL and matched normal hearing controls and analyzed rs-fMRI data. They found alterations of ReHo in brain areas for language, auditory, and visual information processing in infants with CSNHL. On the other hand, our study focused on ReHo analysis with estimates of two ReHo parameters, i.e., KCC-ReHo and Cohe-ReHo. Similar to their study, we found ReHo alterations in auditory and visual brain areas. However, we also identified additional ReHo alterations in brain regions related to motor and cognitive function in children with CSNHL. Although a large range of age in our cohort was recognized as a limitation to our study, this cohort did enable us to obtain pilot ReHo data in older children beyond 4 years of age as the Xia et al. (2017) study only enrolled children up to 4 years of age.

In addition to the rs-fMRI approach, other fMRI methods have been used to study hearing loss, which has generated promising results. For example, a study by Zhang et al. (2006) used a block-design fMRI paradigm with pure tones and found differences in brain activations in subjects with sensorineural hearing loss as compared to the controls. In addition, they also found differences in audio-evoked fields on magnetoencephalography between the patient group and the control group. It should be noted that the rs-fMRI method is robust and has been used extensively to study various disorders and conditions. A study by Ni et al. (2016) used resting-state fMRI approach and found differences in ReHo values between the subjects with mild cognitive impairment with and without lacunar infarctions. Nevertheless, our study has merits and we contributed to the hearing research through assessment of the underlying brain functional neuroplasticity in children with CSNHL.

There were several limitations to this study. First, the sample size was small, which may limit our ability to detect subtle alterations in the ReHo values in our children with CSNHL. In addition, our cohort included children with a large range of age and we did not have a sufficient sample size to separate this cohort into different age groups. We understand that brain fMRI parameters may be varied with age along the course of brain development. However, we believe that this variation should be balanced off in our cohort since there was no significant difference in age between the CSNHL group and the healthy control group. Second, our analysis of brain activity did not take into consideration the severity of deafness in this cohort with CSNHL. Third, this study was cross-sectional in design, limiting our assessment for recovery or additional alterations of ReHo parameters over time. In addition, our study was limited due to our inability to incorporate education situation as a covariate in data analysis. It was because we could not definitively gauge the educational levels for our children with CSNHL due to their various educational backgrounds and socioeconomic status. Our study was also limited by other aspects of potential differences such as emotional stress between the two groups. Lastly, sign language was not considered as a confounding variable in our data analysis. We did not include the history of using sign language in our analysis because of the discrepancy in sign language use among the participants. Some children in our cohort learned and practiced sign language, while some did not. We did not have the statistical power in this small cohort to assess the effect of sign language use on the brain changes. In the future, we will enroll a larger cohort to tease out the effect of the potential confounding variables such as the severity and duration of deafness, different age groups, sign language use, and history of treatment for hearing loss on brain function.

CONCLUSION

In summary, we found brain functional alterations as indicated by rs-fMRI ReHo values in the brain regions related to auditory, visual, motor, and cognitive function in children with CSNHL. We also observed a significant correlation between brain functional changes and age. Our study results implicated neuroplasticity and compensatory changes in children with CSNHL to adapt for hearing deprivation. Our study showed promising data for using an imaging approach to uncover the neural correlates of hearing loss and to improve the care of our vulnerable children with CSNHL.

AUTHOR CONTRIBUTIONS

MJ conceived and designed the study. PG, SL, ZW, and YL collected the data. YW, PG, and SL contributed to data analysis. MJ, PG, and SL prepared the first draft of the manuscript. BC, MJ, YW, and ZZ revised the manuscript. All authors approved the final version of the manuscript.

ACKNOWLEDGMENTS

We wish to thank Zikuan Chen, and Ebenezer Daniel, from City of Hope National Medical Center, Duarte, CA, United States for their helpful suggestions during preparation of this manuscript.

REFERENCES

Bavelier, D., Dye, M. W., and Hauser, P. C. (2006). Do deaf individuals see better? *Trends Cogn. Sci.* 10, 512–518. doi: 10.1016/j.tics.2006.09.006

Bavelier, D., and Neville, H. J. (2002). Cross-modal plasticity: where and how? *Nat. Rev. Neurosci.* 3, 443–452. doi: 10.1038/nrn848

Bedny, M., Pascual-Leone, A., Dodell-Feder, D., Fedorenko, E., and Saxe, R. (2011). Language processing in the occipital cortex of congenitally blind adults. *Proc. Natl. Acad. Sci. U.S.A.* 108, 4429–4434. doi: 10.1073/pnas.1014818108

Binder, J. R., Frost, J. A., Hammeke, T. A., Cox, R. W., Rao, S. M., and Prieto, T. (1997). Human brain language areas identified by functional magnetic resonance imaging. *J. Neurosci.* 17, 353–362. doi: 10.1523/jneurosci.17-01-00353.1997

Biswal, B., Yetkin, F. Z., Haughton, V. M., and Hyde, J. S. (1995). Functional connectivity in the motor cortex of resting human brain using echo-planar MRI. *Magn. Reson. Med.* 34, 537–541. doi: 10.1002/mrm.1910340409

Buckner, R. L. (2013). The brain's default network: origins and implications for the study of psychosis. *Dialogues Clin. Neurosci.* 15, 351–358. doi: 10.31887/dcns.2013.15.3/rbuckner

Calamante, F., Masterton, R. A., Tournier, J. D., Smith, R. E., Willats, L., Raffelt, D., et al. (2013). Track-weighted functional connectivity (TW-FC): a tool for characterizing the structural-functional connections in the brain. *Neuroimage* 70, 199–210. doi: 10.1016/j.neuroimage.2012.12.054

Chao-Gan, Y., and Yu-Feng, Z. (2010). DPARSF: a MATLAB Toolbox for "Pipeline" data analysis of resting-state fMRI. *Front. Syst. Neurosci.* 4:13. doi: 10.3389/fnsys.2010.00013

Chen, H., Nomi, J. S., Uddin, L. Q., Duan, X., and Chen, H. (2017). Intrinsic functional connectivity variance and state-specific under-connectivity in autism. *Hum. Brain Mapp.* 38, 5740–5755. doi: 10.1002/hbm.23764

Chen, H., Wang, J., Uddin, L. Q., Wang, X., Guo, X., Lu, F., et al. (2018). Aberrant functional connectivity of neural circuits associated with social and sensorimotor deficits in young children with autism spectrum disorder. *Autism Res.* 11, 1643–1652. doi: 10.1002/aur.2029

Conway, C. M., Karpicke, J., Anaya, E. M., Henning, S. C., Kronenberger, W. G., and Pisoni, D. B. (2011). Nonverbal cognition in deaf children following cochlear implantation: motor sequencing disturbances mediate language delays. *Dev. Neuropsychol.* 36, 237–254. doi: 10.1080/87565641.2010.549869

Corbetta, M., Shulman, G. L., Miezin, F. M., and Petersen, S. E. (1995). Superior parietal cortex activation during spatial attention shifts and visual feature conjunction. *Science* 270, 802–805. doi: 10.1126/science.270.5237.802

Fair, D. A., Posner, J., Nagel, B. J., Bathula, D., Dias, T. G., Mills, K. L., et al. (2010). Atypical default network connectivity in youth with attention-deficit/hyperactivity disorder. *Biol. psychiatry* 68, 1084–1091. doi: 10.1016/j.biopsych.2010.07.003

Forseth, K. J., Kadipasaoglu, C. M., Conner, C. R., Hickok, G., Knight, R. T., and Tandon, N. (2018). A lexical semantic hub for heteromodal naming in middle fusiform gyrus. *Brain* 141, 2112–2126. doi: 10.1093/brain/awy120

Greicius, M. D., Flores, B. H., Menon, V., Glover, G. H., Solvason, H. B., Kenna, H., et al. (2007). Resting-state functional connectivity in major depression: abnormally increased contributions from subgenual cingulate cortex and thalamus. *Biol. Psychiatry* 62, 429–437. doi: 10.1016/j.biopsych.2006.09.020

Guo, W. B., Liu, F., Chen, J. D., Gao, K., Xue, Z. M., Xu, X. J., et al. (2012). Abnormal neural activity of brain regions in treatment-resistant and treatment-sensitive major depressive disorder: a resting-state fMRI study. *J. Psychiatr Res.* 46, 1366–1373. doi: 10.1016/j.jpsychires.2012.07.003

Hari, R., Forss, N., Avikainen, S., Kirveskari, E., Salenius, S., and Rizzolatti, G. (1998). Activation of human primary motor cortex during action observation: a neuromagnetic study. *Proc. Natl. Acad. Sci. U.S.A.* 95, 15061–15065.

Harlor, A. D. Jr., and Bower, C. (2009). Hearing assessment in infants and children: recommendations beyond neonatal screening. *Pediatrics* 124, 1252–1263. doi: 10.1542/peds.2009-1997

Iacoboni, M., Woods, R. P., Brass, M., Bekkering, H., Mazziotta, J. C., and Rizzolatti, G. (1999). Cortical mechanisms of human imitation. *Science* 286, 2526–2528. doi: 10.1126/science.286.5449.2526

Jiang, M., Wen, Z., Long, L., Wong, C. W., Ye, N., Zee, C., et al. (2019). Assessing cerebral white matter microstructure in children with congenital sensorineural hearing loss: a tract-based spatial statistics study. *Front. Neurosci.* 13:597. doi: 10.3389/fnins.2019.00597

Klaus, J., and Schutter, D. (2018). The role of left dorsolateral prefrontal cortex in language processing. *Neuroscience* 377, 197–205. doi: 10.1016/j.neuroscience.2018.03.002

Kravitz, D. J., Peng, C. S., and Baker, C. I. (2011). Real-world scene representations in high-level visual cortex: it's the spaces more than the places. *J. Neurosci.* 31, 7322–7333. doi: 10.1523/jneurosci.4588-10.2011

Lee, D. S., Lee, J. S., Oh, S. H., Kim, S. K., Kim, J. W., Chung, J. K., et al. (2001). Cross-modal plasticity and cochlear implants. *Nature* 409, 149–150.

Lin, F. R., Yaffe, K., Xia, J., Xue, Q. L., Harris, T. B., Purchase-Helzner, E., et al. (2013). Hearing loss and cognitive decline in older adults. *JAMA Intern. Med.* 173, 293–299.

Liu, D., Yan, C., Ren, J., Yao, L., Kiviniemi, V. J., and Zang, Y. (2010). Using coherence to measure regional homogeneity of resting-state FMRI signal. *Front. Syst. Neurosci.* 4:24.

Liu, F., Guo, W., Fouche, J. P., Wang, Y., Wang, W., Ding, J., et al. (2015). Multivariate classification of social anxiety disorder using whole brain functional connectivity. *Brain Struct. Funct.* 220, 101–115. doi: 10.1007/s00429-013-0641-4

Liu, F., Hu, M., Wang, S., Guo, W., Zhao, J., Li, J., et al. (2012). Abnormal regional spontaneous neural activity in first-episode, treatment-naive patients with late-life depression: a resting-state fMRI study. *Prog. Neuropsychopharmacol. Biol. Psychiatry* 39, 326–331. doi: 10.1016/j.pnpbp.2012.07.004

Liu, F., Wang, Y., Li, M., Wang, W., Li, R., Zhang, Z., et al. (2017). Dynamic functional network connectivity in idiopathic generalized epilepsy with generalized tonic-clonic seizure. *Hum. Brain Mapp.* 38, 957–973. doi: 10.1002/hbm.23430

Liu, Y., Zhang, Y., Lv, L., Wu, R., Zhao, J., and Guo, W. (2018). Abnormal neural activity as a potential biomarker for drug-naive first- episode adolescent-onset schizophrenia with coherence regional homogeneity and support vector machine analyses. *Schizophr. Res.* 192, 408–415. doi: 10.1016/j.schres.2017.04.028

Lomber, S. G., Meredith, M. A., and Kral, A. (2010). Cross-modal plasticity in specific auditory cortices underlies visual compensations in the deaf. *Nat. Neurosci.* 13, 1421–1427. doi: 10.1038/nn.2653

Mayer, C., and Trezek, B. J. (2018). Literacy outcomes in deaf students with cochlear implants: current state of the knowledge. *J. Deaf Stud. Deaf Educ.* 23, 1–16. doi: 10.1093/deafed/enx043

Mirzaei, G., and Adeli, H. (2016). Resting state functional magnetic resonance imaging processing techniques in stroke studies. *Rev. Neurosci.* 27, 871–885. doi: 10.1515/revneuro-2016-0052

Ni, L., Liu, R., Yin, Z., Zhao, H., Nedelska, Z., Hort, J., et al. (2016). Aberrant spontaneous brain activity in patients with mild cognitive impairment and concomitant lacunar infarction: a resting-state functional MRI study. *J. Alzheimers Dis.* 50, 1243–1254. doi: 10.3233/jad-150622

Ou, Y., Liu, F., Chen, J., Pan, P., Wu, R., Su, Q., et al. (2018). Increased coherence-based regional homogeneity in resting-state patients with first-episode, drug-naive somatization disorder. *J. Affect. Disord.* 235, 150–154. doi: 10.1016/j.jad.2018.04.036

Parks, E. L., and Madden, D. J. (2013). Brain connectivity and visual attention. *Brain Connect.* 3, 317–338. doi: 10.1089/brain.2012.0139

Plichta, M. M., Vasic, N., Wolf, R. C., Lesch, K. P., Brummer, D., Jacob, C., et al. (2009). Neural hyporesponsiveness and hyperresponsiveness during immediate and delayed reward processing in adult attention-deficit/hyperactivity disorder. *Biol. Psychiatry* 65, 7–14. doi: 10.1016/j.biopsych.2008.07.008

Rivara, C. B., Sherwood, C. C., Bouras, C., and Hof, P. R. (2003). Stereologic characterization and spatial distribution patterns of Betz cells in the human primary motor cortex. *Anat. Rec. A Discov. Mol. Cell Evol. Biol.* 270, 137–151. doi: 10.1002/ar.a.10015

Rolls, E. T. (2019). The cingulate cortex and limbic systems for emotion, action, and memory. *Brain Struct. Funct.* 224, 3001–3018. doi: 10.1007/s00429-019-01945-2

Romanski, L. M., Tian, B., Fritz, J., Mishkin, M., Goldman-Rakic, P. S., and Rauschecker, J. P. (1999). Dual streams of auditory afferents target multiple domains in the primate prefrontal cortex. *Nat. Neurosci.* 2, 1131–1136. doi: 10.1038/16056

Rowe, J., Hughes, L., Eckstein, D., and Owen, A. M. (2008). Rule-selection and action-selection have a shared neuroanatomical basis in the human prefrontal and parietal cortex. *Cereb. Cortex* 18, 2275–2285. doi: 10.1093/cercor/bhm249

Shi, B., Yang, L. Z., Liu, Y., Zhao, S. L., Wang, Y., Gu, F., et al. (2016). Early-onset hearing loss reorganizes the visual and auditory network in children without cochlear implantation. *Neuroreport* 27, 197–202. doi: 10.1097/wnr.0000000000000524

Shiell, M. M., Champoux, F., and Zatorre, R. J. (2015). Reorganization of auditory cortex in early-deaf people: functional connectivity and relationship to hearing aid use. *J. Cogn. Neurosci.* 27, 150–163. doi: 10.1162/jocn_a_00683

Stanton, S. G., and Harrison, R. V. (2000). Projections from the medial geniculate body to primary auditory cortex in neonatally deafened cats. *J. Comp. Neurol.* 426, 117–129. doi: 10.1002/1096-9861(20001009)426:1<117::aid-cne8>3.0.co;2-s

Sugihara, T., Diltz, M. D., Averbeck, B. B., and Romanski, L. M. (2006). Integration of auditory and visual communication information in the primate ventrolateral prefrontal cortex. *J. Neurosci.* 26, 11138–11147. doi: 10.1523/jneurosci.3550-06.2006

Tan, L., Chen, Y., Maloney, T. C., Caré, M. M., Holland, S. K., and Lu, L. J. (2013). Combined analysis of sMRI and fMRI imaging data provides accurate disease markers for hearing impairment. *Neuroimage Clin.* 3, 416–428. doi: 10.1016/j.nicl.2013.09.008

Tanabe, H. C., and Sadato, N. (2009). Ventrolateral prefrontal cortex activity associated with individual differences in arbitrary delayed paired-association learning performance: a functional magnetic resonance imaging study. *Neuroscience* 160, 688–697. doi: 10.1016/j.neuroscience.2009.02.078

Westermann, G., and Reck Miranda, E. (2004). A new model of sensorimotor coupling in the development of speech. *Brain Lang.* 89, 393–400. doi: 10.1016/s0093-934x(03)00345-6

Wolak, T., Ciesla, K., Pluta, A., Wlodarczyk, E., Biswal, B., and Skarzynski, H. (2019). Altered functional connectivity in patients with sloping sensorineural hearing loss. *Front. Hum. Neurosci.* 13:284. doi: 10.3389/fnhum.2019.00284

Xia, S., Song, T., Che, J., Li, Q., Chai, C., Zheng, M., et al. (2017). Altered brain functional activity in infants with congenital bilateral severe sensorineural hearing loss: a resting-state functional MRI study under sedation. *Neural plast.* 2017:8986362.

Yan, C. G., Craddock, R. C., He, Y., and Milham, M. P. (2013). Addressing head motion dependencies for small-world topologies in functional connectomics. *Front. Hum. Neurosci.* 7:910. doi: 10.3389/fnhum.2013.00910

Zang, Y., Jiang, T., Lu, Y., He, Y., and Tian, L. (2004). Regional homogeneity approach to fMRI data analysis. *Neuroimage* 22, 394–400. doi: 10.1016/j.neuroimage.2003.12.030

Zhang, Y. T., Geng, Z. J., Zhang, Q., Li, W., and Zhang, J. (2006). Auditory cortical responses evoked by pure tones in healthy and sensorineural hearing loss subjects: functional MRI and magnetoencephalography. *Chin. Med. J.* 119, 1548–1554. doi: 10.1097/00029330-200609020-00008

Zhen, D., Xia, W., Yi, Z. Q., Zhao, P. W., Zhong, J. G., Shi, H. C., et al. (2018). Alterations of brain local functional connectivity in amnestic mild cognitive impairment. *Transl. Neurodegener.* 7:26.

Zhou, F., Wu, L., Guo, L., Zhang, Y., and Zeng, X. (2019). Local connectivity of the resting brain connectome in patients with low back-related leg pain: a multiscale frequency-related Kendall's coefficient of concordance and coherence-regional homogeneity study. *Neuroimage Clin.* 21, 101661. doi: 10.1016/j.nicl.2019.101661

Zuo, X. N., Xu, T., Jiang, L., Yang, Z., Cao, X. Y., He, Y., et al. (2013). Toward reliable characterization of functional homogeneity in the human brain: preprocessing, scan duration, imaging resolution and computational space. *Neuroimage* 65, 374–386.

12

Hippocampal Transcriptome-Wide Association Study Reveals Correlations between Impaired Glutamatergic Synapse Pathway and Age-Related Hearing Loss in BXD-Recombinant Inbred Mice

Tingzhi Deng[1], Jingjing Li[1,2,3], Jian Liu[4], Fuyi Xu[1,5], Xiaoya Liu[1], Jia Mi[1], Jonas Bergquist[1,6], Helen Wang[7], Chunhua Yang[1], Lu Lu[5], Xicheng Song[2], Cuifang Yao[1], Geng Tian[1]* and Qing Yin Zheng[8]*

[1] Precision Medicine Research Center, School of Pharmacy, Binzhou Medical University, Yantai, China, [2] Department of Otorhinolaryngology-Head and Neck Surgery, Yantai Yuhuangding Hospital, Qingdao University, Yantai, China, [3] Second Clinical Medical College, Binzhou Medical University, Yantai, China, [4] Department of Plastic Surgery, Shandong Provincial Qianfoshan Hospital, The First Affiliated Hospital of Shandong First Medical University, Jinan, China, [5] Department of Genetics, Genomics and Informatics, The University of Tennessee Health Science Center, Memphis, TN, United States, [6] Department of Chemistry—BMC, Analytical Chemistry and Neurochemistry, Uppsala University, Uppsala, Sweden, [7] Department of Medical Biochemistry and Microbiology, BMC, Uppsala University, Uppsala, Sweden, [8] Department of Otolaryngology-Head and Neck Surgery, Case Western Reserve University, Cleveland, OH, United States

***Correspondence:**
Cuifang Yao
yaocuifangbio@126.com
Geng Tian
tiangeng@live.se

Age-related hearing loss (ARHL) is associated with cognitive dysfunction; however, the detailed underlying mechanisms remain unclear. The aim of this study is to investigate the potential underlying mechanism with a system genetics approach. A transcriptome-wide association study was performed on aged (12–32 months old) BXD mice strains. The hippocampus gene expression was obtained from 56 BXD strains, and the hearing acuity was assessed from 54 BXD strains. Further correlation analysis identified a total of 1,435 hearing-related genes in the hippocampus ($p < 0.05$). Pathway analysis of these genes indicated that the impaired glutamatergic synapse pathway is involved in ARHL ($p = 0.0038$). Further gene co-expression analysis showed that the expression level of glutamine synthetase (*Gls*), which is significantly correlated with ARHL ($n = 26$, $r = -0.46$, $p = 0.0193$), is a crucial regulator in glutamatergic synapse pathway and associated with learning and memory behavior. In this study, we present the first systematic evaluation of hippocampus gene expression pattern associated with ARHL, learning, and memory behavior. Our results provide novel potential molecular mechanisms involved in ARHL and cognitive dysfunction association.

Keywords: hearing loss, systems genetics, cognitive dysfunction, glutamine synthetase (Gls), gene network, BXD mice strain, transcriptome-wide association study (TWAS)

INTRODUCTION

Hearing loss and cognitive impairment are two associated major concerns in aging populations. It is estimated that one-third of the aged population with hearing loss with different levels of cognitive decline and individuals with moderate-to-severe hearing loss are up to five times as likely to develop dementia (Lin et al., 2013; Stickel et al., 2021). Improving hearing with various hearing aids significantly improves cognitive functions, indicating that hearing loss may be causally related to cognitive decline (Sarant et al., 2020). Thus, understanding the molecular mechanisms between age-related hearing loss (ARHL) and cognitive impairment are essential, and may, in the long run, help prevent the development of age-related cognitive dysfunction (Uchida et al., 2019).

To illustrate the potential mechanism, studies have been conducted to reveal the association between hearing loss and central nervous system function, such as the frontal cortex and hippocampus (Yu et al., 2021). The hippocampus is the major brain region that regulates learning and memory; it is also involved in auditory working memory such as encoding and signal maintenance. Neurogenesis in the hippocampus is impaired with conductive or noise-induced hearing loss (Liu et al., 2018; Kurioka et al., 2021). Moreover, the hippocampus is known to be activated in response to recurring musical phrases while listening to music (Burunat et al., 2014). These studies suggest that auditory signals may regulate hippocampus signaling and molecular functions such as synaptic plasticity, which is chronically impaired by progressive hearing loss (Beckmann et al., 2020; Kurioka et al., 2021). These alterations can potentially be explained by the gene expression change associated with hearing loss (Christensen et al., 2009). However, to our knowledge, a systematic study of ARHL-associated hippocampal gene profiling has not yet been performed. Therefore, a gene profiling association study is in need to investigate molecular mechanisms that link ARHL and cognitive dysfunction (Hasson et al., 2013; Rasmussen et al., 2018).

Transcriptome-wide association study (TWAS) is a powerful tool to investigate the association between gene expression and traits (Civelek and Lusis, 2014; Wainberg et al., 2019). Novel susceptibility genes contributing to hearing impairment were identified with this approach (Xie et al., 2021). TWAS relies on the large-scale transcriptomic analysis from a genetic reference population (GRP). Among the current animal GRPs, the BXD mouse panel developed by the University of Tennessee Health Science Center (UTHSC) comprises more than 150 recombinant inbred (RI) strains with complementary traits. Owing to its genetic stability, the mice from the same strain can be considered as identical twins (Ashbrook et al., 2021). Thus, the data from multiple studies can be combined and used for systems genetics analysis including TWAS. In BXD strains, both ARHL and levels of cognitive decline showed significant variations (Zheng et al., 2020), which provide a unique platform to investigate the association between hearing loss and cognitive function.

The aim of this study is to identify potential mechanisms and key regulators that are involved in the association between ARHL and hippocampal gene profiles with a TWAS approach. We profiled the hippocampal gene expression and hearing acuity in aged BXD population. By comprehensive bioinformatics analysis, we identified that glutamate signaling in the hippocampal synapses is impaired with ARHL, and glutamine synthetase (Gls) is one of the key regulators involved in both hearing loss and cognitive decline with aging.

MATERIALS AND METHODS

Animals

A total of 56 BXD strains (one male and one female for most strains) and 54 BXD strains (two male and two female for most strains) plus their parental strains are used for collecting hippocampus gene expression data and hearing screening, respectively. The age of all mice except one BXD101 mouse was between 12 and 32 months. The mice were housed in groups in a temperature- and humidity-controlled vivarium with a constant 12-h light–dark cycle with *ad libitum* access to food and water. For the hippocampal profiling, the mice were anesthetized by cervical dislocation. For the hearing screening, the mice were anesthetized with an intraperitoneal injection (IP) of ketamine, xylazine, and acepromazine at doses of 40, 5, and 1 mg/kg, respectively. The present study was carried out in accordance with the Guidelines for the Care and Use of Laboratory Animals published by the National Institutes of Health and was approved by the Animal Care and Use Committee at the University of Tennessee Health Science Center (UTHSC, Memphis, TN, United States).

Hearing Acuity Assessment

Hearing acuity was assessed using an auditory-evoked brainstem response (ABR) (Intelligent Hearing Systems, Miami, FL, United States) as detailed previously (Zhou et al., 2006). Briefly, the mice were anesthetized with an intraperitoneal injection (IP) of ketamine, xylazine, and acepromazine at doses of 40, 5, and 1 mg/kg, respectively. The body temperature was maintained at 37–38°C. The ABRs were recorded using platinum subdermal needle electrodes inserted at the vertex (active electrode), ventrolateral to the right (reference electrode) and left (ground electrode) ears. The acoustic stimuli were tone-bursts (3-ms duration with a 1.5-ms cosine-gated rise/fall time) that were delivered through a high-frequency transducer. The stimuli were presented in a 5-dB step decrement from 80 dB sound pressure level (SPL) until the lowest intensity that could still evoked a reproducible ABR pattern was detected. If 80 dB could not evoke a reproducible ABR pattern, the stimuli were increased in a 5-dB step until the maximal SPL was reached. All the animals were tested with three frequencies (8, 16, and 32 kHz). For each frequency, the strain ABR is the mean value of individual ABRs, and the ABR thresholds from three frequencies were averaged and used as hearing acuity feature.

Microarray Profiling

Snap frozen hippocampi from BXD mice across 56 strains were used for RNA quantification. RNA was extracted using the RNeasy mini kit (Qiagen, CA, United States) according to the instructions of the manufacturer. The 2100 Bioanalyzer (Agilent Technologies, Santa Clara, CA, United States) was used to evaluate RNA integrity and quality. Samples with RNA Integrity Numbers (RIN values) > 8.0 were analyzed on Affy MoGene1.0 ST at the UTHSC. Raw microarray data were normalized using the Robust Multichip Array (RMA) method (Chesler et al., 2005; Geisert et al., 2009; King et al., 2015; Lu et al., 2016). The expression data were then re-normalized using a modified Z score described in a previous publication (Chesler et al., 2005). Briefly, RMAs were first transformed into log2-values. Then, the data of each single array was converted to Z-scores, multiplied by 2, and a value of 8 was added. The normalized data is available on GeneNetwork[1] under the "BXD" group and "Hippocampus mRNA" type with the identifier "UTHSC BXD Aged Hippocampus Affy MoGene1.0 ST (May 15) RMA Gene Level."

Behavioral Phenotypes Access

The published learning-related traits of the BXD mice used in this study were retrieved from our GeneNetwork. The detailed descriptions can be found in the previous publications (Graybeal et al., 2014; Delprato et al., 2015; Knoll et al., 2016; Neuner et al., 2019)]. The summary statistics and individual values are available on GeneNetwork under the "BXD" group, "trait and cofactors" type, and "BXD published phenotypes" dataset with their corresponding GN accession number listed in **Supplementary Table 1**.

Gene Function Enrichment Analysis

WEB-based Gene SeT AnaLysis Toolkit (WebGestalt) was used to perform gene set enrichment analysis with the mouse genome reference gene set as the background (Liao et al., 2019)[2]. The over-representation of Gene Ontology (GO) was determined by the hypergeometric test. KEGG Orthology-Based Annotation System (KOBAS) was used to analyze the pathways involved in the ARHL correlated genes (Bu et al., 2021).

Gene Co-expression Network Analysis

Gene co-expression network analysis has been widely used to explore the key genes in the gene sets. Therefore, we deployed this approach to identify the key genes from the gene set that correlated with hearing loss (Zhang and Horvath, 2005). Briefly, a network was constructed with Pearson's correlation coefficient matrix (**Supplementary Figure 1**). In the network, each node stands for a gene, and the correlation coefficient was set as the edge. Binomial correlation higher than 0.3 or lower than −0.3 was defined as connected. The connection weight was calculated for each node, which is the sum of the binominal correlation coefficient connected to each node. The gene with the most connectivity and connection weight in the network can be considered as the central hub gene.

[1] www.genenetwork.org

[2] http://www.webgestalt.org/

Statistics Analysis

The gene–phenotype and gene–gene correlations were performed on the GeneNetwork (see text footnote 1) online platform by using Pearson's correlation. A p-value lower than 0.05 was considered as statistically significant. A correlation coefficient higher than 0.3 or lower than −0.3 was considered as moderate correlation. To further validate the false discovery rate (FDR) of the genes-of-interest, we performed a further permutation test based on the Westfall and Young's multiple testing procedure (Chaubey, 1993), Briefly, we randomly permuted the ABR measurements 1,000 times. For each permutation, we computed the p-value of Pearson's correlation between the randomized ABR value and those transcripts that are associated with ABR. The adjusted p-value was determined by ranking the correlation coefficient.

RESULTS

The Hearing Acuity in Aged BXD Mice Is Associated With Hippocampal Glutamatergic Synapse Pathway

A total of 26 strains that overlapped between hearing and hippocampus transcriptomic data were used for association analysis. Those strains are mainly in the similar age (from 19 to 25 months), except for BXD101 (11 months), BXD55 (27 months), and BXD45 (30 months) (**Supplementary Table 2**, **Supplementary Figure 2**, and **Figure 1A**). The tested animals represent a diverse degree of hearing loss determined with ABR thresholds between 33 (BXD74) and 100 dB (BXD101). The mean ABR thresholds was 71 dB SPL (**Figure 1B**), and the median ABR thresholds was 76 dB SPL. These data were used for the association analysis with hippocampus transcriptomic profile. In total, 1,435 genes presented significant correlation with hearing acuity ($p < 0.05$, Pearson's correlation). With the FDR threshold of 0.05 determined by the Westfall and Young's multiple testing procedure, equivalent to the r-value of 0.388, all the 1,435 transcripts were achieved significance. GO analysis of this gene set showed that four of the top 10 categories were associated with synapse organization (**Figure 1C**), and these genes were abundantly enriched in cellular compartment of synapse (ratio = 0.07, $p = 6.17\text{E}{-13}$) (**Figure 1D**). Further pathway analysis indicated that the glutamatergic synapse pathway is significantly enriched (ratio = 0.08, p = 0.0038) (**Figure 1E**). Nine genes that correlated with ABR thresholds were involved in this pathway, including four genes that showed positive correlation (*Adcy4*, *Mapk3*, *Shank3*, and *Dlg4*; $n = 26$, $r > 0.4$, $p < 0.05$, Pearson's correlation), and five genes that showed negative correlation with ABR thresholds (*Adrbk2*, *Slc38a1*, *Slc38a2*, *Gria3*, and *Gls*, $n = 26$, $r < -0.4$, $p < 0.05$, Pearson's correlation) (**Figure 1F**). To better clarify the gene expression correlation to each frequency, we supplemented the gene expression of synapse pathway to each of three frequencies (**Supplementary Figure 3**), which showed that all of those genes were significantly associated with the ABR thresholds at all three frequencies.

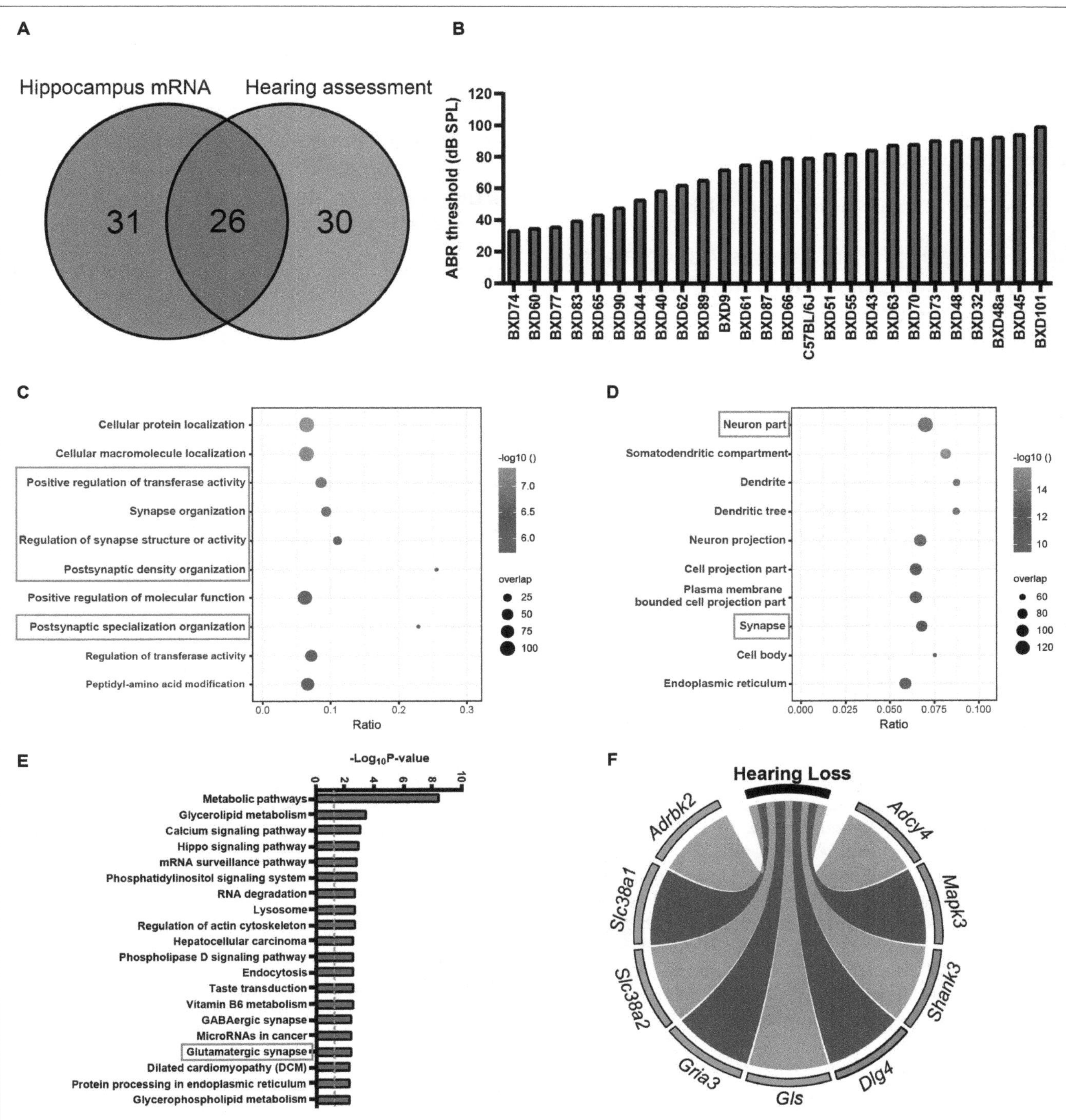

FIGURE 1 | (A) The 26 strains with both 56 strains for auditory-evoked brainstem response (ABR) thresholds and 57 strains for hippocampus mRNA transcriptomic analysis are involved in the association analysis. **(B)** The average ABR thresholds of 26 BXD mouse strains at 2 years old age. The *x*-axis shows the BXD strains and the two parental strains. The *y*-axis shows the average ABR thresholds for 8K, 16K, and 32 kHz tone bursts were averaged as hearing acuity. **(C,D)** Bubble charts of the Gene Ontology analysis enriched for age-related hearing loss (ARHL) correlated genes. Gene over-representation analysis for Gene Ontology analysis of the ARHL correlated genes (p-value < 0.05 and $r > 0.3$) were performed with WebGestalt (http://www.webgestalt.org/). The *x*-axis represents an enriched ratio, and the *y*-axis represents enriched pathways/terms. The size of the dots represents the number of genes, and the color indicates the p-values. An enriched ratio is defined as the number of observed divided by the number of expected genes from the annotation category in the gene lists. **(E)** Glutamatergic synapse is involved in ARHL correlated pathway based on the mice hippocampus transcriptome data. The ARHL correlated genes were analyzed by KEGG. The top 20 pathways associated with the network genes were tested alongside the p-values calculated using a right-tailed Fisher's exact test. **(F)** Chord-Chart of the Glutamatergic synapse pathway enriched for ARHL correlated gene. The outer color green represents negative correlation, red represents positive correlation.

The mouse strains in our study are a senile population. Even though most of the strains are in similar age, there is still age variance among the strains. To exclude potential influence of such variance on the gene expression, we performed linear regression analysis between age and various target transcripts expression. The results indicated that the transcript expression variance is dominated by strain background but not age variance. Similarly, the age variation in our senile population has little effect on ABR threshold (**Supplementary Tables 3, 4**).

Age-Related Hearing Loss Is Associated With Hippocampal Glutamate Receptors Expression Profiling

Glutamate receptors are the primary mediators of excitatory transmission in the central nervous system and play a pivotal role in learning and memory. To further investigate the glutamate receptor profiling associated with ARHL, we performed a correlation screening of ABR thresholds to 32 glutamate receptors (**Figure 2A** and **Supplementary Table 5**). Besides *Gria3*, which had the most significant correlation ($n = 26$, $r = -0.41$, $p = 0.0401$) (**Figure 2B**), six other receptors also showed moderate correlation to ABR thresholds (**Figures 2C–H**, $r < -0.3$), including *Grm7*, *Grik1*, *Gria4*, *Grm5*, *Grm8*, and *Gria2*. Notably, all these were negative correlations to ABR thresholds. These results indicated that ARHL is associated with altered glutamate receptor expression profiling in the hippocampal synapse.

Age-Related Hearing Loss Is Associated With Reduced Glutamate Synthesis in Presynaptic Neurons

Two genes involved in glutamate synthesis are significantly correlated with ABR thresholds, which are *Gls* ($n = 26$, $r = -0.46$, $p = 0.0193$) and *Slc38a2* ($n = 26$, $r = -0.49$, $p = 0.0109$) (**Figures 3A,B**). Both genes presented negative correlation to ABR thresholds. In the glutamatergic synapse pathway, the glutamine is primarily released from astroglia cells and further imported into presynaptic neurons with glutamine receptor Slc38a2. The imported glutamine is further converted to glutamate with Gls in the presynaptic neurons. The negative correlation of these two genes with ABR thresholds indicated that glutamate synthesis is impaired in ARHL.

Age-Related Hearing Loss Is Associated With Postsynaptic Glutamate Receptor Reorganization Regulation

Two glutamate receptor-interacting protein chaperones—Dlg4 and Shank3—were positively correlated with hearing loss ($n = 26$, $r = 0.39$, $p = 0.0493$); ($n = 26$, $r = 0.44$, $p = 0.0247$) (**Figures 3C,D**). Both Dlg4 and Shank3 act as chaperones to assist glutamate-receptor reorganization. Thus, we performed a further correlation screening between hearing loss and 10 known glutamate receptor chaperone proteins (**Figure 3E**). Besides *Dlg4* and *Shank3*, *Nos1* ($n = 26$, $r = 0.45$, $p = 0.0198$) (**Figure 3F**) also presented significant positive correlations with ABR thresholds. These data showed that ARHL is associated with enhanced glutamate receptor chaperone expression.

Age-Related Hearing Loss Is Associated With Hippocampus Cyclic Adenosine Monophosphate Signaling Pathway Through Adenylate Cyclase 4

The cyclic adenosine monophosphate (cAMP) signaling is a critical second messenger signaling in the glutamatergic synapse pathway. Our correlation analysis indicated that the gene expression of *Adcy4* is significantly correlated with ABR thresholds ($n = 26$, $r = 0.52$, $p = 0.0064$) (**Figure 4A**). cAMP is synthesized by adenylate cyclase (**Figure 4B**), which is a protein family including 10 different members. Thus, a correlation screen was performed between ABR thresholds and AC family members (**Figure 4C**). Among the AC family, only *Adcy4* presented a significant correlation with ABR thresholds, suggesting that ARHL is associated with cAMP signaling pathway through Adcy4.

Gene Co-expression Network Analysis Suggests That Glutamine Synthetase Is a Key Regulator Gene in Glutamate Pathway

A gene co-expression network was constructed based on nine hearing loss-associated genes in the synaptic signaling pathway. Among these genes, Gls showed the highest connectivity of eight and an average connection weight of 0.49 as a central node (**Figure 5A** and **Supplementary Tables 6, 7**). Notably, *Gls* presented a significant correlation with five other hub genes; *Gria3* ($n = 26$, $r = 0.76$, $p < 0.0001$), *Adcy4* ($n = 26$, $r = -0.55$, $p < 0.0001$), *Dlg4* ($n = 26$, $r = -0.35$, $p = 0.008$), and *Shank3* ($n = 26$, $r = -0.56$, $p < 0.0001$) (**Figures 5B–E**). Taken together, these results suggest that Gls is a central hub gene in the glutamate signaling network.

Phenotype-Wide Association Showed Glutamine Synthetase Is Associated With Learning Behavior in BXD Strains

To reveal the association between *Gls* expression and learning behavior, we performed a phenotype-wide association analysis between *Gls* and published phenotypes in BXD strains. The expression of *Gls* in the hippocampus is significantly correlated with 31 learning-related phenotypes (**Supplementary Table 1**). Briefly, the expression of *Gls* was significantly correlated to the learning latency in a touch screen test ($n = 19$, $r = 0.66$, $p = 0.0020$), the percentage of time spent freezing in contextual fear conditioning test ($n = 16$, $r = 0.52$, $p = 0.0418$), the percentage of successful alternations in the Y-maze test ($n = 22$, $r = 0.62$, $p = 0.0021$), and the number of new entries during the first 8-arm choices in an 8-arm radial maze test ($n = 41$, $r = 0.38$, $p = 0.0151$) (**Figures 6A–D**). These data collectively proved that the hippocampal *Gls* expression is associated with learning and memory behavior.

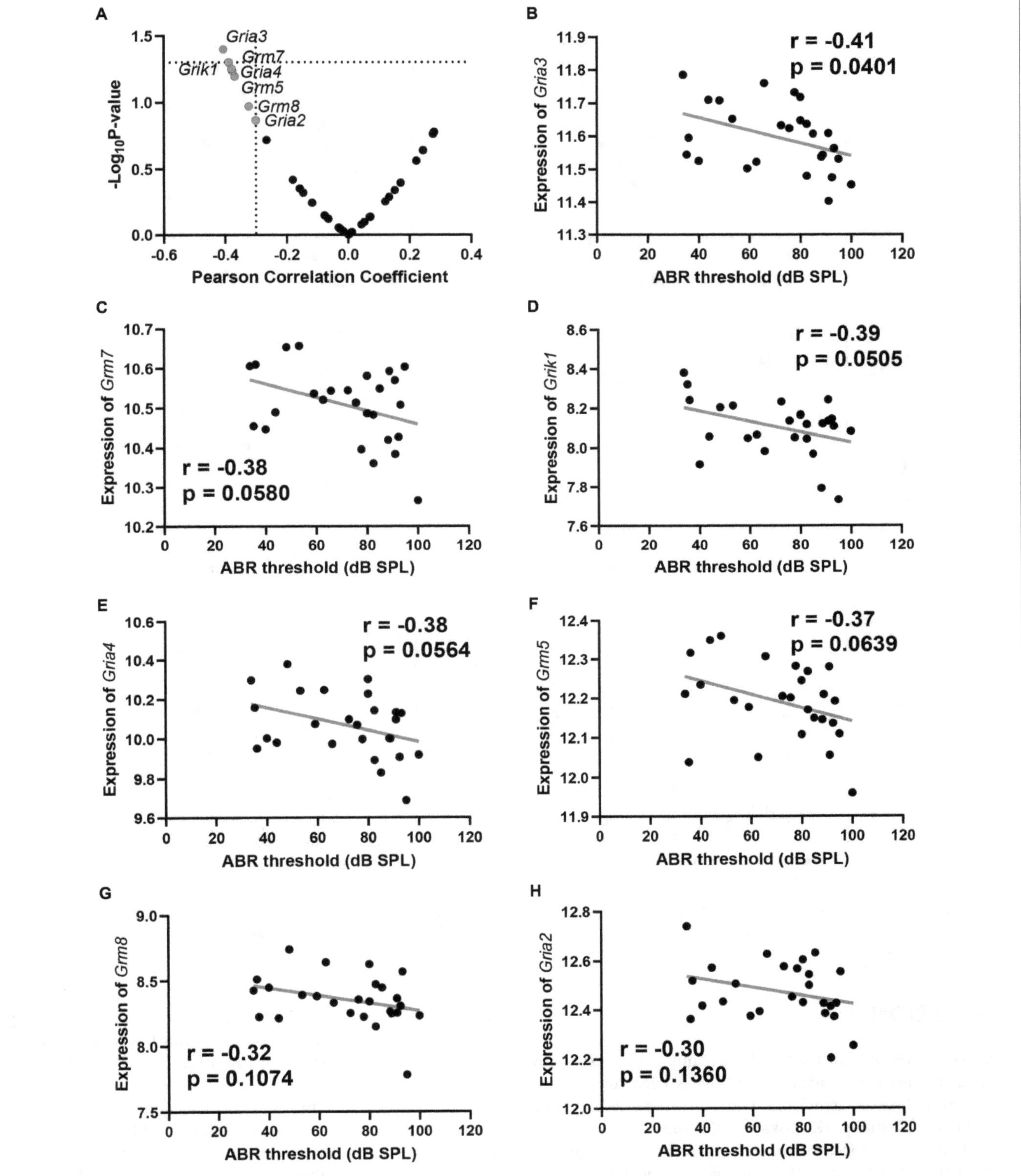

FIGURE 2 | Scatterplots of the correlations of ABR threshold [dB sound pressure level (SPL)] with all glutamate receptors expression **(A)**, *Gria3* expression **(B)**, *Grm7* expression **(C)**, *Grik1* expression **(D)**, *Gria4* expression **(E)**, *Grm5* expression **(F)**, *Grm8* expression **(G)**, and *Gria2* expression **(H)**. The Pearson correlation coefficient was used to determine the relationship. Pearson correlation and *p*-value are indicated. Gene expression levels are log2 transformed and modified with Z score.

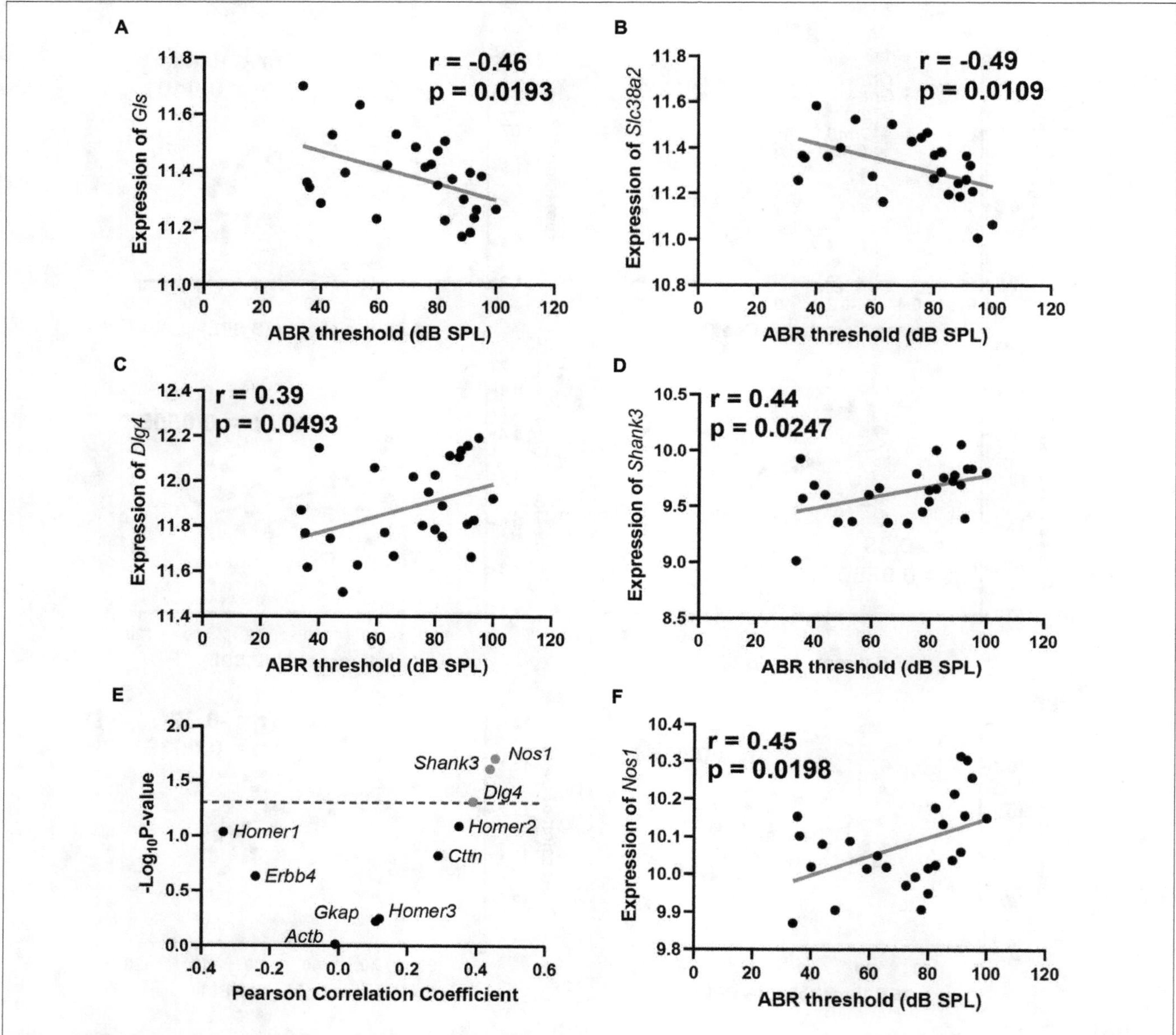

FIGURE 3 | Scatterplots of the correlations of ABR threshold (dB SPL) with glutamine synthetase (*Gls*) expression **(A)**, *Slc38a2* expression **(B)**, *Dlg4* expression **(C)**, *Shank3* expression **(D)**, 10 known glutamate receptor chaperone proteins expression **(E)**, and *Nos1* expression **(F)**. The Pearson correlation coefficient was used to determine the relationship. Pearson correlation and *p*-value are indicated. Gene expression levels are log2 transformed and modified with Z score.

DISCUSSION

In this study, we present the first hippocampal gene expression profiling that associated with ARHL. It has been hypothesized that hearing loss is associated with disturbed neurogenesis and synapse plasticity (Kurioka et al., 2021). However, the detailed molecular mechanisms remain unclear. Our analysis indicates that alternation in the glutamatergic synapse signaling is associated with ARHL, including altered glutamate receptor expression and decreased glutamate synthesis (**Figure 7**). Further gene network analysis indicates that Gls is the key node gene in the network, and Gls expression is associated with both the hearing acuity and learning, and memory behavior. The thorough examination of hippocampus gene profiling has shed light on the potential molecular mechanism of association between hearing loss and cognitive function.

We identified that the hippocampal glutamatergic synapse pathway is associated with ARHL. This is consistent with previous reports wherein the glutamatergic synaptic connectivity in the hippocampus could be altered by noise exposure (Zhang et al., 2021). Glutamate is the excitatory neurotransmitter at many synapses in the central nervous system and has been extensively studied in relation to cognition, particularly learning and memory. The impairment

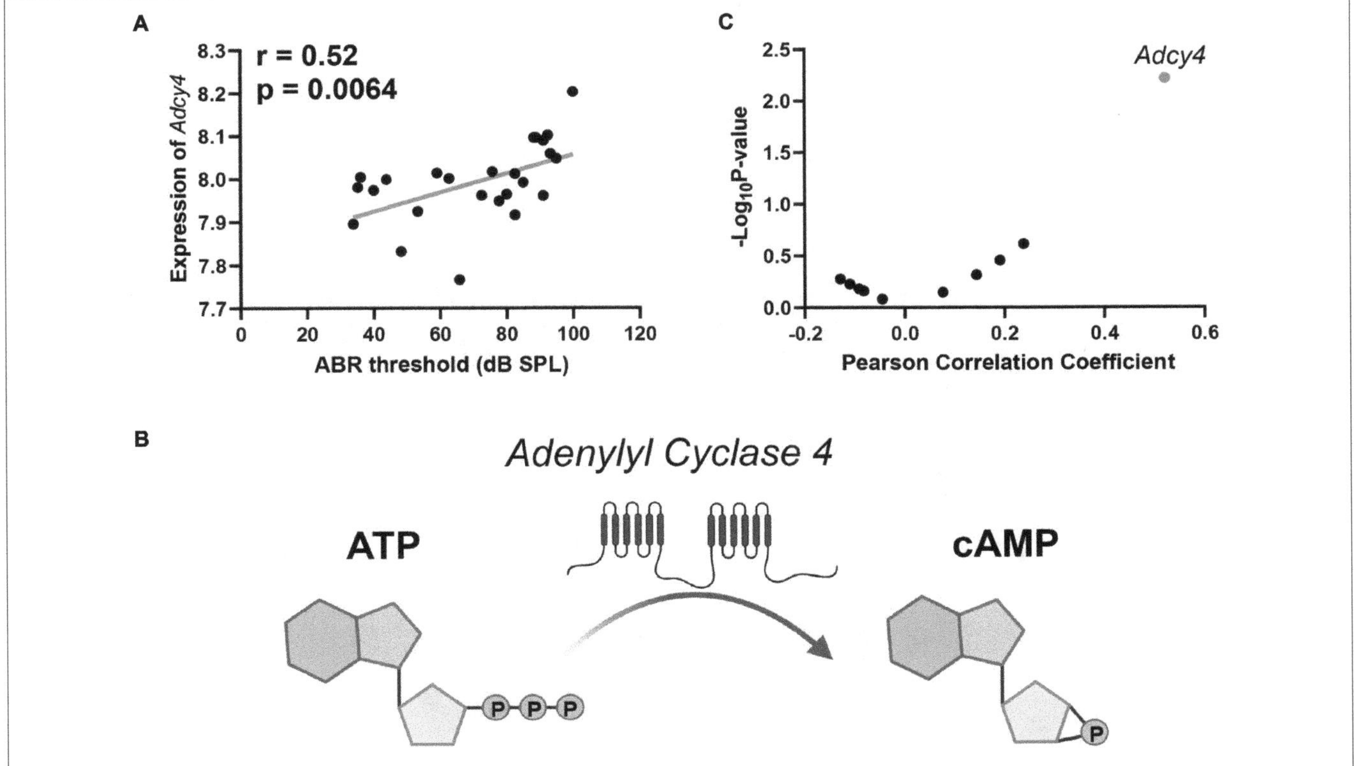

FIGURE 4 | Scatterplots of the correlations of ABR threshold (dB SPL) with *Adcy4* expression **(A)**. Adenylate cyclase 4 (Adcy4) catalyzes the conversion of ATP to cyclic adenosine monophosphate (cAMP) **(B)**. Scatterplots of the correlations of ABR threshold (dB SPL) with all Adenylate Cyclase family expression **(C)**. The Pearson correlation coefficient was used to determine the relationship. Pearson correlation and *p*-value are indicated. Gene expression levels are log2 transformed and modified with Z score.

of the glutamatergic synapse pathway is associated with neurodegenerative diseases such as Alzheimer's disease and Parkinson's disease (Findley et al., 2019). The association between glutamatergic synapse and hearing acuity provides direct support for the association between hearing loss and cognitive dysfunction.

In the hippocampal glutamatergic synapse pathway, a group of glutamate receptors showed significant correlation to hearing acuity. The expression of glutamate receptors is responsible for the excitatory drive in neuronal networks and are involved in activating downstream signaling cascades required for synaptic plasticity (Hunt and Castillo, 2012; Chater and Goda, 2014). The decreased expression of glutamate transporters was found in cognitive dysfunction diseases such as in patients with Alzheimer's disease (Benarroch, 2010). Among the glutamate receptors, Gria3 which is a component of α-amino-3-hydroxy-5-methyl-4-isoxazolepropionic acid receptors (AMPARs), showed the most negative correlation with ABR thresholds. This is consistent with a previous report in which Gria3 mediated auditory-experience plasticity at the end bulb synapse (Clarkson et al., 2016). The activation of Gria3 can directly lead to synaptic potentiation at the CA1 hippocampal synapses (Renner et al., 2017). Our results provide extra evidence that Gria3 is a critical auditory signal mediator in the hippocampus. Moreover, other AMPARs such as Gria2 also showed moderate correlation. AMPARs have fundamental roles in both basal transmission and long-term potentiation (LTP) and long-term depression (LTD), which strongly implicates ARHL associated with learning and memory defects through altering AMPARs expression profiling.

In the gene co-expression network, Gls showed most connection with other nodes and is suggested as a key regulator. We found a significant correlation between Gls in presynapse and Gria3 in postsynapse, which implies a *trans*-synapse transmission regulation in the hippocampus. The possible mechanism is the synthesized glutamate from presynapse can regulate the Gria3 expression in postsynapse. In primary mast cells, the glutamate can induce profound upregulation of a panel of glutamate receptors including both the ionotropic type and the metabotropic type (Alim et al., 2020). This hypothesis can also be explained by the negative correlation between Gls and Adcy4. In ARHL mice, the low concentration of glutamate enhances the expression of Adcy4 and provides complementary support for the feedback inhibitory circuit in glutamate synthesis and release.

Similarly, the negative correlation between Gls and Dlg4 provides a potential explanation for the positive correlation of glutamate receptor chaperones with hearing loss. Dlg4 and Shank3 are known to increase glutamate receptor organization and enhance learning and memory function (Ehrlich et al., 2007). However, we found that glutamate receptor chaperones

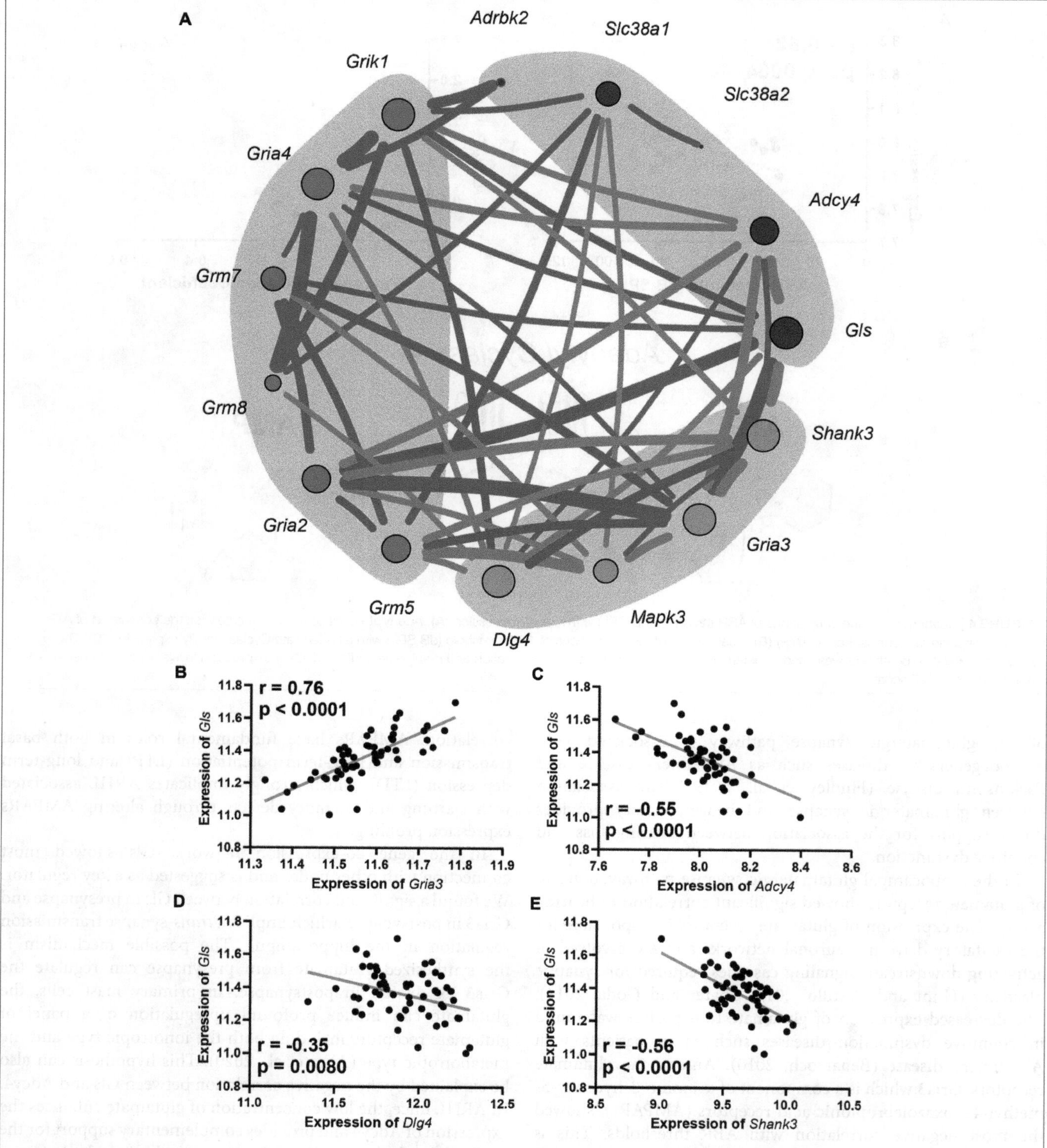

FIGURE 5 | (A) The network includes the genes enriched in the Glutamatergic pathway, as well as the glutamate receptors that were mapped. The orange dots are in postsynapse, the blue dots are the glutamate receptors with moderate correlation with ARHL, and the dark gray dots is in presynapse, the size of the point indicates its connection degree, the red line indicates a significant positive correlation, the green line indicates a significant negative correlation, and the thickness of the line indicates the value of the correlation. Scatterplots of the correlations of *Gls* expression with *Gria3* expression **(B)**, *Adcy4* expression **(C)**, *Dlg4* expression **(D)**, *Shank3* expression **(E)**. The Pearson correlation coefficient was used to determine the relationship. Pearson correlation and *p*-value are indicated. Gene expression levels are log2 transformed and modified with Z score.

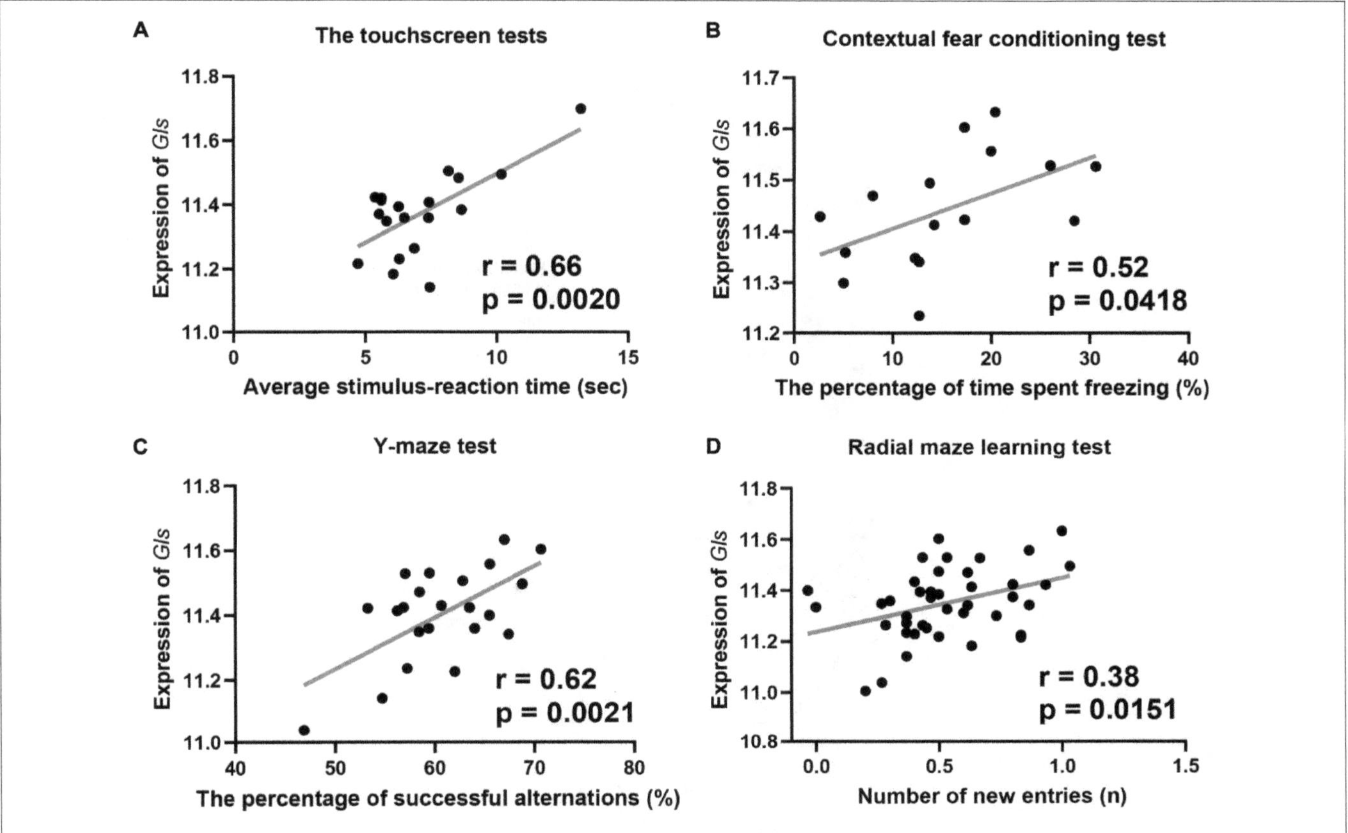

FIGURE 6 | Scatterplots of the correlations of *Gls* expression with the learning latency in a touch screen test **(A)**, the percentage of time spent freezing in Contextual fear conditioning test **(B)**, the percentage of successful alternations in Y-maze test **(C)**, the number of new entries during the first 8-arm choices in an 8-arm radial maze test **(D)**. The Pearson correlation coefficient was used to determine the relationship. Pearson correlation and *p*-value are indicated. Gene expression levels are log2 transformed and modified with Z score.

are positively correlated with hearing loss level. The potential reason for this is the existence of a glutamate receptor regulation feedback circuit, in which low-level glutamate release may enhance the expression of glutamate receptor scaffold proteins such as Dlg4 and Shank3, but further research is needed.

With a phenotype-wide association analysis, we showed that the Gls expression level is associated with various learning- and memory-related traits. This is consistent with previous animal model studies. The Gls knockout mice showed impaired glutamatergic synapse transmission (Masson et al., 2006), hippocampal hypometabolism in the hippocampus CA1 subregion, and were less sensitive to behavioral stimulating effects (Gaisler-Salomon et al., 2009). Taken together, these results proposed Gls as a key regulator in the glutamate synapse signaling pathway.

In this study, we performed a TWAS based on the BXD mouse panel. In this panel, hearing variation was found in different mice strains. The hearing loss level ranged from very mild hearing loss to nearly deafness. Such hearing loss occurs naturally, and hence BXD is considered as a unique animal model population to investigate ARHL. These mice strains together with the systems genetics approach can be a powerful tool in future studies on hearing loss. Nonetheless, so far, a systematic transcriptome profiling of inner ear tissues at a large population level is still lacking. Transcriptome profiling of inner ear tissues associated with aging at a population level would provide further knowledge about ARHL.

Although we focused on hippocampal glutamate synapse signaling in the current study, the gene profiling suggested more pathways such as GABA, calcium-signaling pathways, and several metabolic pathways are involved in the association. Given the complexity and heterogeneity of those two disorders, how those pathways involved in the ARHL associated cognitive dysfunction still need to be validated and could facilitate a better understanding of the association.

One potential limitation of this study is the ABR measurements and hippocampal transcriptomic profiling, which were generated from two independent groups of BXD mice. It may introduce potential bias in the analysis. However, due to the genetic makeup, the mice from the same strain can be considered as identical twins. Moreover, we involved relatively a large number of strains with the age range roughly aligns well between those two data sets (18–25 months old). Thus the results based on the joint analysis of those two data sets are still reliable and robust.

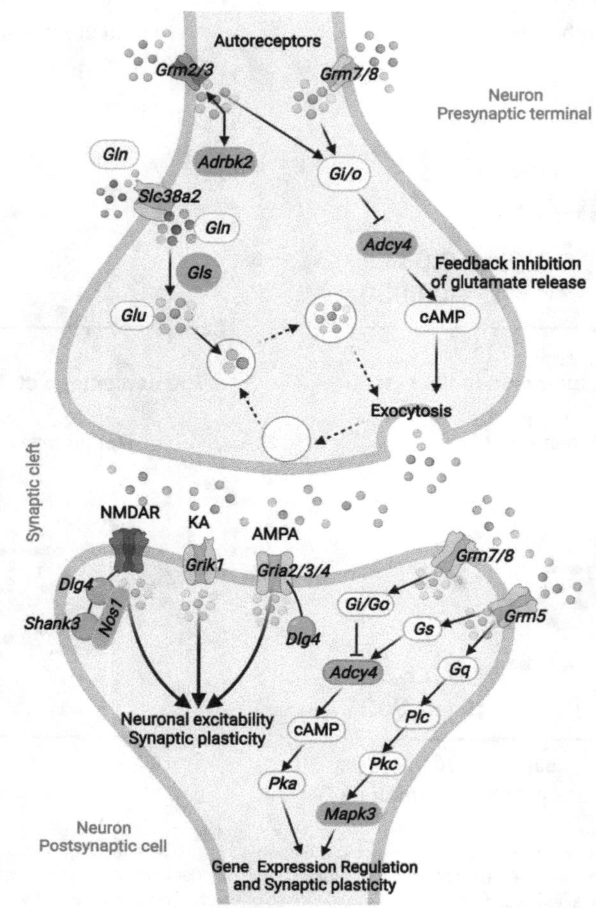

FIGURE 7 | ARHL associated Glutamatergic synapse pathway mapping. Glutamate released from presynaptic terminals acts through the activation of glutamate receptors located at the postsynaptic terminal. The interaction between glutamate and glutamate receptor favors the activation of several metabolic pathways. Glutamine is converted into glutamate by glutaminase. GLN, glutamine; GLS, Glutaminase; GLU, glutamate; Grm2, glutamate metabotropic receptor 2; Grm3, glutamate metabotropic receptor 3; Grm5, glutamate metabotropic receptor 5; Grm7, glutamate metabotropic receptor 7; Grm8, glutamate metabotropic receptor 8; Slc38a2, solute carrier family 38 member 2; Adrbk2, adrenergic, beta, receptor kinase 2; Adcy4, adenylate cyclase 4; NMDAR, N-methyl-D-aspartate receptor; KA, kainate receptors; AMPA, α-amino-3-hydroxy-5-methyl-4-isoxazolepropionic acid receptor; PSD-95, postsynaptic density protein 95; Shank3, SH3 and multiple ankyrin repeat domains 3; Grik1, glutamate ionotropic receptor kainate type subunit 1; Gria2, glutamate ionotropic receptor AMPA type subunit 2; Gria3, glutamate ionotropic receptor AMPA type subunit 3; Gria4, glutamate ionotropic receptor AMPA type subunit 4. The blue sphere indicates GLU, the purple sphere indicates GLN. Green indicates negative correlation with ABR, red indicates positive correlation with ABR. Gray indicates non-significant correlation with ABR.

In summary, our study identified that the hippocampal glutamatergic synaptic impairment is associated with ARHL using a TWAS approach. These results provide the potential molecular mechanism of the association between cognition dysfunction and ARHL. Moreover, it also provides a novel research strategy in related studies.

AUTHOR CONTRIBUTIONS

GT designed the study. QZ and TD conducted the experiment, including ABR, and performed the statistical analysis. LL, FX, and QZ organized the database. TD and JM established the network model and wrote the first draft of the manuscript. FX, JaL, JB, JnL, XL, and ChY wrote the sections of the manuscript. QZ, JB, XS, HW, CuY, and GT revised the manuscript. All authors contributed to manuscript revision, read, and approved the submitted version.

SUPPLEMENTARY MATERIAL

Supplementary Figure 1 | Pearson correlation coefficient matrix (the key genes from the gene set that correlated with hearing loss).

Supplementary Figure 2 | Violin plots of the strain ages (month) at the ABR testing and hippocampus sampling.

Supplementary Figure 3 | Heatmap of the Pearson correlation coefficient between glutamatergic synapse pathway genes and ABR thresholds.

REFERENCES

Alim, M. A., Grujic, M., Ackerman, P. W., Kristiansson, P., Eliasson, P., Peterson, M., et al. (2020). Glutamate triggers the expression of functional ionotropic and metabotropic glutamate receptors in mast cells. *Cell. Mol. Immunol.* 18, 2383–2392. doi: 10.1038/s41423-020-0421-z

Ashbrook, D. G., Arends, D., Prins, P., Mulligan, M. K., Roy, S., Williams, E. G., et al. (2021). A platform for experimental precision medicine: the extended BXD mouse family. *Cell. Syst.* 12, 235–247.e9. doi: 10.1016/j.cels.2020.12.002

Beckmann, D., Feldmann, M., Shchyglo, O., and Manahan-Vaughan, D. (2020). Hippocampal Synaptic Plasticity, Spatial Memory, and Neurotransmitter Receptor Expression Are Profoundly Altered by Gradual Loss of Hearing Ability. *Cereb. Cortex* 30, 4581–4596. doi: 10.1093/cercor/bhaa061

Benarroch, E. E. (2010). Glutamate transporters. Diversity, function, and involvement in neurologic disease. *Neurology* 74, 259–264. doi: 10.1212/WNL.0b013e3181cc89e3

Bu, D., Luo, H., Huo, P., Wang, Z., Zhang, S., He, Z., et al. (2021). KOBAS-i: intelligent prioritization and exploratory visualization of biological functions for gene enrichment analysis. *Nucleic Acids Res.* 49, W317–W325. doi: 10.1093/nar/gkab447

Burunat, I., Alluri, V., Toiviainen, P., Numminen, J., and Brattico, E. (2014). Dynamics of brain activity underlying working memory for music in a naturalistic condition. *Cortex* 57, 254–269. doi: 10.1016/j.cortex.2014.04.012

Chater, T. E., and Goda, Y. (2014). The role of AMPA receptors in postsynaptic mechanisms of synaptic plasticity. *Front. Cell. Neurosci.* 8:401. doi: 10.3389/fncel.2014.00401

Chaubey, Y. P. (1993). Resampling-Based Multiple Testing: examples and Methods for p-Value Adjustment. *Technometrics* 35, 450–451. doi: 10.1080/00401706.1993.10485360

Chesler, E. J., Lu, L., Shou, S., Qu, Y., Gu, J., Wang, J., et al. (2005). Complex trait analysis of gene expression uncovers polygenic and pleiotropic networks that modulate nervous system function. *Nat. Genet.* 37, 233–242. doi: 10.1038/ng1518

Christensen, N., D'Souza, M., Zhu, X., and Frisina, R. D. (2009). Age-related hearing loss: aquaporin 4 gene expression changes in the mouse cochlea and auditory midbrain. *Brain Res.* 1253, 27–34. doi: 10.1016/j.brainres.2008.11.070

Civelek, M., and Lusis, A. J. (2014). Systems genetics approaches to understand complex traits. *Nat. Rev. Genet.* 15, 34–48. doi: 10.1038/nrg3575

Clarkson, C., Antunes, F. M., and Rubio, M. E. (2016). Conductive Hearing Loss Has Long-Lasting Structural and Molecular Effects on Presynaptic and Postsynaptic Structures of Auditory Nerve Synapses in the Cochlear Nucleus. *J. Neurosci.* 36, 10214–10227. doi: 10.1523/jneurosci.0226-16.2016

Delprato, A., Bonheur, B., Algeo, M. P., Rosay, P., Lu, L., Williams, R. W., et al. (2015). Systems genetic analysis of hippocampal neuroanatomy and spatial learning in mice. *Genes Brain Behav.* 14, 591–606. doi: 10.1111/gbb.12259

Ehrlich, I., Klein, M., Rumpel, S., and Malinow, R. (2007). PSD-95 is required for activity-driven synapse stabilization. *Proc. Natl. Acad. Sci. U. S. A.* 104, 4176–4181. doi: 10.1073/pnas.0609307104

Findley, C. A., Bartke, A., Hascup, K. N., and Hascup, E. R. (2019). Amyloid Beta-Related Alterations to Glutamate Signaling Dynamics During Alzheimer's Disease Progression. *ASN Neuro* 11:1759091419855541. doi: 10.1177/1759091419855541

Gaisler-Salomon, I., Miller, G. M., Chuhma, N., Lee, S., Zhang, H., Ghoddoussi, F., et al. (2009). Glutaminase-Deficient Mice Display Hippocampal Hypoactivity, Insensitivity to Pro-Psychotic Drugs and Potentiated Latent Inhibition: relevance to Schizophrenia. *Neuropsychopharmacology* 34, 2305–2322. doi: 10.1038/npp.2009.58

Geisert, E. E., Lu, L., Freeman-Anderson, N. E., Templeton, J. P., Nassr, M., Wang, X., et al. (2009). Gene expression in the mouse eye: an online resource for genetics using 103 strains of mice. *Mol. Vis.* 15, 1730–1763.

Graybeal, C., Bachu, M., Mozhui, K., Saksida, L. M., Bussey, T. J., Sagalyn, E., et al. (2014). Strains and stressors: an analysis of touchscreen learning in genetically diverse mouse strains. *PLoS One* 9:e87745. doi: 10.1371/journal.pone.0087745

Hasson, D., Theorell, T., Bergquist, J., and Canlon, B. (2013). Acute Stress Induces Hyperacusis in Women with High Levels of Emotional Exhaustion. *PLoS One* 8:e52945. doi: 10.1371/journal.pone.0052945

Hunt, D. L., and Castillo, P. E. (2012). Synaptic plasticity of NMDA receptors: mechanisms and functional implications. *Curr. Opin. Neurobiol.* 22, 496–508. doi: 10.1016/j.conb.2012.01.007

King, R., Lu, L., Williams, R. W., and Geisert, E. E. (2015). Transcriptome networks in the mouse retina: an exon level BXD RI database. *Mol. Vis.* 21, 1235–1251.

Knoll, A. T., Halladay, L. R., Holmes, A. J., and Levitt, P. (2016). Quantitative Trait Loci and a Novel Genetic Candidate for Fear Learning. *J. Neurosci.* 36, 6258–6268. doi: 10.1523/JNEUROSCI.0177-16.2016

Kurioka, T., Mogi, S., and Yamashita, T. (2021). Decreasing auditory input induces neurogenesis impairment in the hippocampus. *Sci. Rep.* 11:423. doi: 10.1038/s41598-020-80218-z

Liao, Y. X., Wang, J., Jaehnig, E. J., Shi, Z. A., and Zhang, B. (2019). WebGestalt 2019: gene set analysis toolkit with revamped UIs and APIs. *Nucleic Acids Res.* 47, W199–W205. doi: 10.1093/nar/gkz401

Lin, F. R., Yaffe, K., Xia, J., Xue, Q. L., Harris, T. B., Purchase-Helzner, E., et al. (2013). Hearing loss and cognitive decline in older adults. *JAMA Intern. Med.* 173, 293–299. doi: 10.1001/jamainternmed.2013.1868

Liu, L., Xuan, C., Shen, P., He, T., Chang, Y., Shi, L., et al. (2018). Hippocampal Mechanisms Underlying Impairment in Spatial Learning Long After Establishment of Noise-Induced Hearing Loss in CBA Mice. *Front. Syst. Neurosci.* 12:35. doi: 10.3389/fnsys.2018.00035

Lu, H., Lu, L., Williams, R. W., and Jablonski, M. M. (2016). Iris transillumination defect and its gene modulators do not correlate with intraocular pressure in the BXD family of mice. *Mol. Vis.* 22, 224–233.

Masson, J., Darmon, M., Conjard, A., Chuhma, N., Ropert, N., Thoby-Brisson, M., et al. (2006). Mice Lacking Brain/Kidney Phosphate-Activated Glutaminase Have Impaired Glutamatergic Synaptic Transmission, Altered Breathing, Disorganized Goal-Directed Behavior and Die Shortly after Birth. *J. Neurosci.* 26, 4660–4671. doi: 10.1523/jneurosci.4241-05.2006

Neuner, S. M., Heuer, S. E., Huentelman, M. J., O'Connell, K. M. S., and Kaczorowski, C. C. (2019). Harnessing Genetic Complexity to Enhance Translatability of Alzheimer's Disease Mouse Models: a Path toward Precision Medicine. *Neuron* 101, 399–411.e5. doi: 10.1016/j.neuron.2018.11.040

Rasmussen, J. E., Laurell, G., Rask-Andersen, H., Bergquist, J., and Eriksson, P. O. (2018). The proteome of perilymph in patients with vestibular schwannoma. A possibility to identify biomarkers for tumor associated hearing loss? *PLoS One* 13:e0198442. doi: 10.1371/journal.pone.0198442

Renner, M. C., Albers, E. H., Gutierrez-Castellanos, N., Reinders, N. R., van Huijstee, A. N., Xiong, H., et al. (2017). Synaptic plasticity through activation of GluA3-containing AMPA-receptors. *Elife* 6:e25462. doi: 10.7554/eLife.25462

Sarant, J., Harris, D., Busby, P., Maruff, P., Schembri, A., Lemke, U., et al. (2020). The Effect of Hearing Aid Use on Cognition in Older Adults: can We Delay Decline or Even Improve Cognitive Function? *J. Clin. Med.* 9:254. doi: 10.3390/jcm9010254

Stickel, A. M., Tarraf, W., Bainbridge, K. E., Viviano, R. P., Daviglus, M., Dhar, S., et al. (2021). Hearing Sensitivity, Cardiovascular Risk, and Neurocognitive Function: the Hispanic Community Health Study/Study of Latinos (HCHS/SOL). *JAMA Otolaryngol. Head Neck Surg.* 147, 377–387. doi: 10.1001/jamaoto.2020.4835

Uchida, Y., Sugiura, S., Nishita, Y., Saji, N., Sone, M., and Ueda, H. (2019). Age-related hearing loss and cognitive decline - The potential mechanisms linking the two. *Auris Nasus Larynx* 46, 1–9. doi: 10.1016/j.anl.2018.08.010

Wainberg, M., Sinnott-Armstrong, N., Mancuso, N., Barbeira, A. N., Knowles, D. A., Golan, D., et al. (2019). Opportunities and challenges for transcriptome-wide association studies. *Nat. Genet.* 51, 592–599. doi: 10.1038/s41588-019-0385-z

Xie, C., Niu, Y., Ping, J., Zhang, Q., Zhang, Z., Wang, Y., et al. (2021). Transcriptome-wide association study identifies novel susceptibility genes contributing to hearing impairment. *Res. Sq.* [Preprint]. doi: 10.21203/rs.3.rs-465737/v1

Yu, L., Hu, J., Shi, C., Zhou, L., Tian, M., Zhang, J., et al. (2021). The causal role of auditory cortex in auditory working memory. *Elife* 10:e64457. doi: 10.7554/eLife.64457

Zhang, B., and Horvath, S. (2005). A general framework for weighted gene co-expression network analysis. *Stat. Appl. Genet. Mol. Biol.* 4:17. doi: 10.2202/1544-6115.1128

Zhang, L., Wu, C., Martel, D. T., West, M., Sutton, M. A., and Shore, S. E. (2021). Noise Exposure Alters Glutamatergic and GABAergic Synaptic Connectivity in the Hippocampus and Its Relevance to Tinnitus. *Neural Plast.* 2021:8833087. doi: 10.1155/2021/8833087

Zheng, Q. Y., Kui, L., Xu, F., Zheng, T., Li, B., McCarty, M., et al. (2020). An Age-Related Hearing Protection Locus on Chromosome 16 of BXD Strain Mice. *Neural Plast.* 2020:8889264. doi: 10.1155/2020/8889264

Zhou, X., Jen, P. H. S., Seburn, K. L., Frankel, W. N., and Zheng, Q. Y. (2006). Auditory brainstem responses in 10 inbred strains of mice. *Brain Res.* 1091, 16–26. doi: 10.1016/j.brainres.2006.01.107

Pure Tone Audiometry and Hearing Loss in Alzheimer's Disease

Susanna S. Kwok[1], *Xuan-Mai T. Nguyen*[1], *Diana D. Wu*[1], *Raksha A. Mudar*[2] and *Daniel A. Llano*[1,2,3,4,5*]

[1] Carle Illinois College of Medicine, University of Illinois Urbana-Champaign, Urbana, IL, United States, [2] Department of Speech and Hearing Sciences, University of Illinois Urbana-Champaign, Urbana, IL, United States, [3] Department of Molecular and Integrative Physiology, University of Illinois Urbana-Champaign, Urbana, IL, United States, [4] Beckman Institute for Advanced Science and Technology, University of Illinois Urbana-Champaign, Urbana, IL, United States, [5] Carle Neuroscience Institute, Carle Foundation Hospital, Urbana, IL, United States

***Correspondence:**
Daniel A. Llano
d-llano@illinois.edu

An association between age-related hearing loss (ARHL) and Alzheimer's Disease (AD) has been widely reported. However, the nature of this relationship remains poorly understood. Quantification of hearing loss as it relates to AD is imperative for the creation of reliable, hearing-related biomarkers for earlier diagnosis and development of ARHL treatments that may slow the progression of AD. Previous studies that have measured the association between peripheral hearing function and AD have yielded mixed results. Most of these studies have been small and underpowered to reveal an association. Therefore, in the current report, we sought to estimate the degree to which AD patients have impaired hearing by performing a meta-analysis to increase statistical power. We reviewed 248 published studies that quantified peripheral hearing function using pure-tone audiometry for subjects with AD. Six studies, with a combined total of 171 subjects with AD compared to 222 age-matched controls, met inclusion criteria. We found a statistically significant increase in hearing threshold as measured by pure tone audiometry for subjects with AD compared to controls. For a three-frequency pure tone average calculated for air conduction thresholds at 500–1,000–2,000 Hz (0.5–2 kHz PTA), an increase of 2.3 decibel hearing level (dB HL) was found in subjects with AD compared to controls ($p = 0.001$). Likewise, for a four-frequency pure tone average calculated at 500–1,000–2,000–4,000 (0.5–4 kHz PTA), an increase of 4.5 dB HL was measured ($p = 0.002$), and this increase was significantly greater than that seen for 0.5–2 kHz PTA. There was no difference in the average age of the control and AD subjects. These data confirm the presence of poorer hearing ability in AD subjects, provided a quantitative estimate of the magnitude of hearing loss, and suggest that the magnitude of the effect is greater at higher sound frequencies.

Systematic Review Registration: https://www.crd.york.ac.uk/prospero/, identifier: CRD42021288280.

Keywords: pure-tone audiogram, Alzheimer's disease, age-related hearing loss, dementia, peripheral hearing, pure tone audiometry

INTRODUCTION

As the sixth leading cause of death in the United States, Alzheimer's disease (AD) affects nearly 6.2 million Americans (Alzheimer's Association., 2021). Projections of the aging population show a steep increase in this number to roughly 13.8 million by the year 2060 (Alzheimer's Association., 2021). The hallmark of AD is loss of episodic memory (McKhann et al., 2011). Over time, both increasing aggregation and spread of hyper-phosphorylated tau and β-amyloid protein throughout the brain result in memory, visuospatial, executive, personality, and language deficits (Small, 2000; McKhann et al., 2011; Reed et al., 2014). Progressive debilitation caused by this neurodegeneration carries substantial burden related to direct costs (i.e., hospitalizations, skilled nursing care, home health care, and hospice) and indirect costs (i.e., caregiver burden and diminished quality of life) (Burns, 2000; Reed et al., 2014; Arijita et al., 2017). To date, no cure exists for AD (McKhann et al., 2011). However, early treatments such as cholinesterase inhibitors and memantine may be used to slow the progression of AD symptoms (Anand and Singh, 2013; Sharma, 2019). Furthermore, lifestyle modifications such as increased aerobic activity, treatment of comorbid conditions as well as modifiable risk factors such as ARHL may slow progression of AD and lessen its impact on individuals and caregivers as secondary and tertiary prevention strategies (Khalsa, 2015; Hubbard et al., 2018; Jongsiriyanyong and Limpawattana, 2018; Mattson and Arumugam, 2018; Bhatti et al., 2020; Gregory et al., 2020).

The link between age-related hearing loss (ARHL) and the subsequent development AD is increasingly well-documented; however, the nature of this relationship remains unclear (Gurgel et al., 2014; Loughrey et al., 2018; Panza et al., 2018; Ray et al., 2018; Chern and Golub, 2019; Jafari et al., 2019; Ralli et al., 2019; Mertens et al., 2020; Utoomprurkporn et al., 2020; Knopke et al., 2021). Current hypotheses postulate that hearing loss increases cognitive demand and therefore predisposes individuals to AD neurodegeneration; that hearing loss results in social isolation which is a risk factor for AD; or that ARHL is an early clinical feature of AD pathology (Loughrey et al., 2018; Chern and Golub, 2019; Jafari et al., 2019; Ralli et al., 2019; Mertens et al., 2020; Utoomprurkporn et al., 2020; Knopke et al., 2021). Regardless of etiology, diagnosis of ARHL in AD may be useful since its treatment shows potential for being a modifiable risk factor to delay disease onset or slow rate of cognitive impairment (Hubbard et al., 2018; Jafari et al., 2019; Gregory et al., 2020; Mertens et al., 2020; Utoomprurkporn et al., 2020). As AD remains incurable, promotion of healthy lifestyle and reduction of modifiable risk factors remain the most practical and cost-effective methods of addressing the disease (Khalsa, 2015; Hubbard et al., 2018; Jongsiriyanyong and Limpawattana, 2018; Mattson and Arumugam, 2018; Bhatti et al., 2020; Gregory et al., 2020). To reduce the negative impacts of ARHL on AD, determination of whether treatment of peripheral auditory processing, central auditory processing, or some combination of both, is necessary (Ralli et al., 2019; Xu et al., 2019; Jayakody et al., 2020; Johnson et al., 2021; Knopke et al., 2021). Characterization of peripheral and central hearing ability in patients with AD using a variety of assessment modalities is crucial for understanding the relationship between ARHL and AD (Xu et al., 2019; Jayakody et al., 2020). Especially as the relationship between peripheral and central auditory processing in relation to AD remains unclear (Swords et al., 2018). Additionally, this information is necessary to determine the validity of quantitative measures of hearing ability and whether these metrics are correlated to other characteristics of AD (Hubbard et al., 2018).

Despite the many epidemiological studies that suggest a link between ARHL and the later development of AD (Uhlmann et al., 1989; Strouse and Hall, 1995; Quaranta et al., 2014; Bidelman et al., 2017; Haggstrom et al., 2018; Jayakody et al., 2018, 2020; Panza et al., 2018; Ray et al., 2018; Brewster et al., 2020; Sardone et al., 2021), fewer cohort studies have found a statistically significant difference in pure tone hearing thresholds between AD and control subjects (Wang et al., 2005, 2007; Gimeno-Vilar and Cervera-Paz, 2010; Idrizbegovic et al., 2011; Lin et al., 2011, 2013; Lodeiro-Fernandez et al., 2015; Villeneuve et al., 2017; Haggstrom et al., 2018; Hardy et al., 2019). Most of these studies had small sample sizes and were underpowered when detecting a difference in hearing thresholds (Wang et al., 2005, 2007; Gimeno-Vilar and Cervera-Paz, 2010; Idrizbegovic et al., 2011; Lin et al., 2011, 2013; Lodeiro-Fernandez et al., 2015; Villeneuve et al., 2017; Haggstrom et al., 2018; Hardy et al., 2019). On the contrary, greater impairments in audiological measurements related to central auditory processing, typically assessed using dichotic hearing tasks or electrophysiologic techniques such as electroencephalography (EEG), are increasingly reported (Grimes et al., 1987; Verma et al., 1987; Uhlmann et al., 1989; Schwartz et al., 1996; Revonsuo et al., 1998; Reeves et al., 1999; Pekkonen et al., 2001; Ally et al., 2006; Muscoso et al., 2006; Gates et al., 2008; Kimiskidis and Papaliagkas, 2012; Hsiao et al., 2014; Kurt et al., 2014; Iliadou et al., 2017; Shahmiri et al., 2017; Cintra et al., 2018; Morrison et al., 2018; Swords et al., 2018; Danjou et al., 2019; Mansour et al., 2019; Jafari et al., 2020; Tarawneh et al., 2021; Wang et al., 2021). Compared to central auditory processing, peripheral hearing is less expensive and less invasive to test and treat; therefore examining pooled data from studies that measure peripheral hearing ability in AD may provide useful insights (Wang et al., 2005, 2007; Gimeno-Vilar and Cervera-Paz, 2010; Idrizbegovic et al., 2011; Lin et al., 2011, 2013; Lodeiro-Fernandez et al., 2015; Villeneuve et al., 2017; Haggstrom et al., 2018; Hardy et al., 2019). Pure-tone audiometry is a "gold standard" procedure that is universally used to objectively measure and classify hearing ability (Wang et al., 2005, 2007; Gimeno-Vilar and Cervera-Paz, 2010; Idrizbegovic et al., 2011; Lin et al., 2011, 2013; Lodeiro-Fernandez et al., 2015; Villeneuve et al., 2017; Haggstrom et al., 2018; Hardy et al., 2019). PTA uses pure tone stimuli in the range of 250 to 8000 Hz to assess air conduction hearing thresholds and measures the lowest intensity at which tones are perceived at least 50% of the time (Wang et al., 2005, 2007; Gimeno-Vilar and Cervera-Paz, 2010; Idrizbegovic et al., 2011; Lin et al., 2011, 2013; Lodeiro-Fernandez et al., 2015; Shahmiri et al., 2017; Villeneuve et al., 2017; Haggstrom et al., 2018; Hardy et al., 2019; Mansour et al., 2019). Unlike other audiologic assessments, PTA has been shown to be effective at measuring hearing ability even in those who are cognitively impaired (Liberati et al., 2009). The current meta-analysis seeks to use pooled data collected from published studies identified through PRISMA guidelines for systematic review, to characterize the peripheral hearing ability of subjects with AD measured by pure tone audiometry (Liberati et al., 2009). Quantification of the degree of hearing loss in AD subjects relative to normal hearing controls will help to understand the burden of hearing loss in these patients and to plan interventions that target ARHL.

METHODS

Search Strategy

A systematic review of literature using PRISMA guidelines was conducted on studies published prior to August 18th, 2021 using PubMed, Cochrane Library, Web of Science, and Scopus databases (Liberati et al., 2009). The search strategy was created with consultation with an expert medical and biomedicine librarian at the University Library at the University of Illinois—Urbana, Champaign. The search was implemented by one searcher (SSK). A non-MeSH search term: "pure tone" AND "(Alzheimer* OR dementia)" resulted in a total of 417 studies; no languages were excluded. All citations containing information on author, title, source, and full abstract were exported from each database as a BibTeX file and uploaded to Mendeley® citation manager for preliminary review. Once duplicates were removed, the abstracts, methods, and results of 248 studies were individually screened. Off-topic studies were removed first and the remaining studies were assessed using the inclusion/exclusion criteria set by this study. This was completed by one rater (SSK) and repeated by two raters (XMTN and DDW) for validation.

To be included for analysis, articles had to contain full-text featuring a cohort-study design that involved subjects diagnosed with AD compared against a control group, both with exclusion criteria of comorbid hearing disorders or deafness. These studies had to report pure-tone air conduction measurement pure tone average or threshold (dB) at a specified frequency (Hz). Studies that did not meet these criteria were rejected on initial review. Studies that categorized subjects based on hearing ability or studied the use of hearing aids or implants were excluded from this study using the PRISMA 2020 flow protocol for new systematic reviews of searches conducted in only databases and registers (Page et al., 2005), and this modified PRISMA flow diagram was generated using ReviewManager©5.4, a software developed by Cochrane© Reviews.

Of the 17 studies that met initial inclusion and exclusion criteria, 11 were excluded on the basis of having unclear diagnostic methods or criteria to define their AD cohort; 1 of these was excluded due to statistically significant differences in age between their AD cohort and control; and 1 study was excluded for reporting pure-tone measures in medians and not means. Diagnostic criteria for the AD cohort had to involve physician assessment of subject medical history, physical/neurological examination, and neuropsychological assessment. Studies with more specific criteria for AD cohort such as the use of NINCDS-ADRDA criteria, neuroimaging, and cerebrospinal fluid analysis were also included. 6 studies met criteria for our final analysis including 4 written in English, 1 written in Spanish, and 1 written in simplified Chinese. The non-English studies were translated into English using translation software from Google®. **Figure 1** summarizes the selection process. The methods listed above were conducted by one searcher/rater (SSK) with consultation with a medical and biomedicine librarian. These methods were repeated by two raters (XMTN and DDW) for validation.

Data Extraction

Following the identification of included studies summarized in Figure 1, full-text PDF articles were downloaded for independent, in-depth screening by three authors (SSK, RAM, and DAL). The following information was extracted from each study if available: author, year published, criteria defining subjects with AD, total number of subjects with AD, sex ratio of subjects with AD, mean age with standard deviation, pure-tone audiogram frequency and/or range of frequencies and associated hearing threshold linked to ear tested, and neurocognitive testing scores. Additional metrics were extracted (such as race, ethnicity, highest level of education attained, etc.), but due to limited reporting they could not be further analyzed. Due to variation related to the ear used for pure-tone audiometry (studies reported from left, right, combined, or better ear), mean thresholds from the "better ear" were used. These data were also collected for the control cohort of each study. Data reported as a threshold frequency (Hz) for a specific pure-tone audiogram frequency or pure-tone audiogram frequency range was extracted directly onto an Excel® spreadsheet. For studies that reported this information using a 2D graph, WebPlotDigitizer© 4.4 was used to extract thresholds (Hz) from the y-axis to their corresponding frequency from the x-axis. All graphs were uniquely calibrated using to their pre-existing scale without correction. Pure tone audiometry thresholds were averaged for 500–1,000–2,000 Hz (referred to here as 0.5–2 kHz PTA) and separately for 500–1,000–2,000–4,000 (referred to here as 0.5–4 kHz PTA).

Risk of Bias

Studies were assessed for potential bias using the Newcastle-Ottawa criteria for cohort studies by one rater (SSK) (Reeves et al., 2011; Wells et al., 2013). Each study was assessed independently in three categories: Selection, Comparability, and Outcome. Selection criteria assessed the representativeness of the AD cohort, the control cohort, certainty of diagnosis, and demonstration that hearing loss was not used to select for or against inclusion into the study. A maximum of four stars can be given in this domain. The comparability domain assesses whether a study controlled for confounding variables such as age, sex, and other factors. This domain can receive a maximum of one star. Lastly, the outcome domain, with a maximum score of three stars, measures studies based on whether independent-blinding was used and whether follow-up duration was sufficient to measure outcomes and complete follow-up for all subjects was assessed. **Table 1** summarizes the Newcastle-Ottawa scores for each study

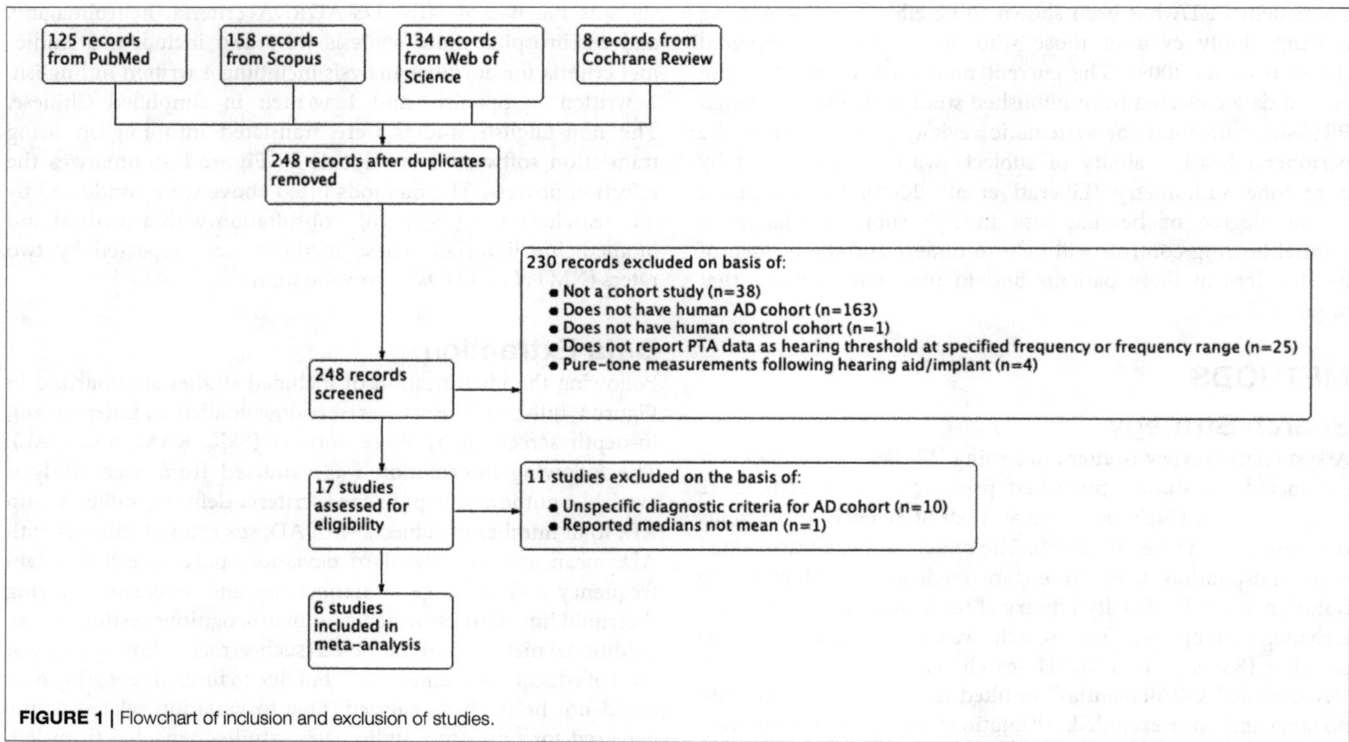

FIGURE 1 | Flowchart of inclusion and exclusion of studies.

TABLE 1 | Risk of bias scores calculated for included studies using the Newcastle Ottawa Scale for Cohort Studies.

References	Selection	Comparability	Outcome
Newcastle-Ottawa assessment of bias for cohort studies			
Gates et al. (1995)	★★★	★	★★
Gimeno-Vilar and Cervera-Paz (2010)	★★★★	★	★
Hardy et al. (2019)	★★★	★	★
Idrizbegovic et al. (2011)	★★★★	★	★
Wang et al. (2005)	★★★★	★	★
Wang et al. (2007)	★★★	★	★

that was included in the meta-analysis. These results were verified with discussion between two raters (RAM and DAL).

Statistical Analysis

Meta-analysis was conducted in Cochrane© Review's software, Review Manager 5.4, and recapitulated in R© to generate figures used in this paper. A random-effects model was applied for meta-analysis due to the heterogeneity of methods in each study. This model was selected over a fixed-effects model because our study design pooled different independent studies from a heterogeneous population. Therefore, to allow for the true effect to vary across subjects due to differences such as age, gender, race, highest and level of education achieved, we defined our combined subject populations as a random sample with a relevant distribution of effects. The combined effect estimates from our meta-analysis estimates the mean effect in this distribution instead of assuming that all of the individual study populations from each study had a single homogenous true effect size. Aggregate outcome data across the six studies were continuous in nature and only pooled study means were used for the data analysis, not individual-level data. We utilized pooled study means rather than individual level means because the latter was not publicly available in the published studies that were included in this study. The summary statistic used in this meta-analysis was the mean difference. It was assumed that the variation in standard deviation (SD) between studies reflected differences in the reliability of the outcome measurements and not differences in outcome variability in the study populations. By doing this, studies with a small SD are given relatively higher weight while studies with larger SD are given relatively smaller weights. The weight given to each of the 6 studies was determined by the inverse-variance method to assign a quantitative value to how much influence each study has on the overall results of the meta-analysis. Inverse-variance is determined by taking the inverse of the variance of the effect estimate for each study (i.e., one over the square of its standard error). Therefore, more weight is given to studies with more precision compared to those with lower precision. Subgroup analysis was conducted for frequency ranges of 500–1,000–2,000 Hz (0.5–2 kHz PTA) and 500–1,000–2,000–4,000 Hz (0.5–4 kHz PTA). Differences in means between the AD and control groups were conducted using a two-tailed *t*-test with $p < 0.05$ considered statistically significant. A t-test was used in this study to examine if hearing threshold was different among those with AD compared to controls. This analysis was completed for 0.5–2 kHz PTA and 0.5–4 kHz PTA. The mean hearing threshold difference between 0.5–2 kHz PTA and 0.5–4 kHz PTA was determined using an unpaired, two-tail t-test.

RESULTS

A total of six studies, totaling 171 (102 females) subjects with AD and 222 (135 females) control subjects (healthy aging or subjective memory complaints), were included in data analysis. Not all studies reported neurocognitive testing outcomes. For subjects with AD, only four studies reported mean Mini-Mental State Examination (MMSE) data, and these scores were combined as the summary MMSE score. For the control cohort, only three studies reported mean MMSE data which were averaged as the collective MMSE score. Average MMSE score for AD subjects = 19 ± 4.3 (SD), and average MMSE score for control subjects = 27 ± 2.1 was significantly higher ($p < 0.001$). The demographic characteristics for each study included in the meta-analysis is summarized in **Table 2**.

Due to the known positive correlation between age and hearing-loss (Loughrey et al., 2018; Panza et al., 2018; Ray et al., 2018; Chern and Golub, 2019; Jafari et al., 2019; Ralli et al., 2019; Mertens et al., 2020; Utoomprurkporn et al., 2020; Knopke et al., 2021), a pooled, standardized mean age difference was calculated. Using a random-effects model, a DerSimonian-Laird meta-analysis for mean age difference across all studies was conducted. This analysis, which weighted studies based on standard-deviation, showed that the aggregated AD cohort had a mean increase in 0.70 years compared to their respective control cohort. This difference was not statistically significant ($p = 0.292$).

Five studies reported three frequency pure tone audiometry calculated for air conduction thresholds at 500, 1,000, and 2,000 Hz (0.5–2 kHz PTA). The meta-analysis of their means showed that the AD cohort had a 2.3 decibel hearing level (dB HL) higher compared to the control cohort ($p < 0.001$). **Figure 2** summarizes the findings of the meta-analysis conducted for hearing threshold (dB HL) averaged at 0.5–2 kHz PTA.

Six studies reported pure tone audiometry calculated for air conduction thresholds at 500, 1,000, 2,000, and 4,000 Hz (0.5–4 kHz PTA). The meta-analysis of their means showed that the AD cohort had a 4.5 decibel hearing level (dB HL) higher compared to the control cohort ($p < 0.002$). **Figure 3** summarizes the findings of the meta-analysis conducted for hearing threshold (dB HL) at 0.5–24 Hz PTA. Using an unpaired t-test, the mean difference between hearing threshold for 0.5–2 kHz PTA and 0.5–4 kHz PTA was −2.66 dB (t = 22.849, df = 326, standard error of difference = 0.116, $p < 0.001$).

DISCUSSION

We observed a statistically significant increase in hearing thresholds, measured by pure tone audiometry at frequency ranges from 0.5 to 2 kHz (2.3 dB difference) and 0.5–4 kHz (4.5 dB difference), in subjects with AD compared to similar-aged controls. We found the difference in hearing thresholds at these two frequency ranges to be statistically significant where hearing threshold measured at 0.5–4 kHz PTA was greater by 2.66 dB than thresholds measured using 0.5–2 kHz PTA. These data suggest that AD is associated with an up to 4.5 dB hearing loss in frequencies associated with normal speech communication and that the loss of hearing is increased at higher frequencies.

Limitations of the Current Study

The methodology of this study was limited having a sole searcher (SSK) to identify potential studies to be included in the meta-analysis. Although the search methods were repeated by two other independent raters for verification (XMTN and DDW), having an initial search conducted by one individual may have introduced selection bias to this study. This meta-analysis was further limited by the small number of studies that met eligibility criteria. Several studies were excluded as they did not characterize AD specifically. In addition, few studies quantified peripheral hearing ability using pure tone audiometry thresholds at specific frequencies. Third, included studies were heterogeneous in their methods and reported outcomes that limited analysis to a small number of shared outcomes. Important subject characteristics such as highest level of education received, pre-retirement occupation, race, ethnicity, socio-economic status, medications taken, number and type of co-morbid conditions, number of years from initial diagnosis, and many other factors that could account for differences between groups was not reported in the majority of studies and therefore could not be analyzed in our meta-analysis. Moreover, history of noise exposure was not reported in any of the 6 studies used for this analysis. However, all 6 studies excluded subjects on the basis of hearing disorder diagnosis and deafness. Additionally, included studies varied in their definition of AD and their control population (i.e., some studies used a healthy-aging cohort while others used subjects with subjective memory complaints). However, despite these limitations which would be expected to dilute the impact of AD on hearing loss, we observed a statistically-significant increase in hearing threshold in AD subjects. Due to the aforementioned heterogeneity of reported results and lack of reported results in each individual study included in this analysis, it is possible that variables other than age and dementia impacted the difference in hearing ability of subjects with AD vs. controls. Although we sought to identify the potential for publication bias using the Newcastle Ottawa scale, we acknowledge that each study included in this meta-analysis

TABLE 2 | Demographics from each included study for subjects with Alzheimer's disease and control subjects.

References	Alzheimer's disease cohort			Control (Normal/SMC) cohort		
	Number of subjects (female)	**Mean age ± SD (years)**	**Mean MMSE ± SD**	**Number of subjects (female)**	**Mean age ± SD (years)**	**Mean MMSE ± SD**
Gates et al. (1995)	20 (10)	78.3 ± 6.5	N/A	40 (23)	76.5 ± 7.5	N/A
Gimeno-Vilar and Cervera-Paz (2010)	14 (9)	79.0 ± 6.0	N/A	14 (9)	76.0 ± 5.0	N/A
Hardy et al. (2019)	20 (9)	69.4 ± 8.1	18.6 ± 5.9	34 (15)	66.7 ± 6.3	N/A
Idrizbegovic et al. (2011)	43 (23)	64.3 ± 6.4	24.5 ± 4.8	34 (22)	64.0 ± 5.1	29.0 ± 1.0
Wang et al. (2005)	31 (10)	73.1 ± 7.5	15.0 ± 3.6	50 (33)	73.3 ± 6.6	26.2 ± 2.7
Wang et al. (2007)	43 (13)	72.7 ± 6.4	17.9 ± 3.1	50 (33)	73.3 ± 6.6	26.3 ± 2.5

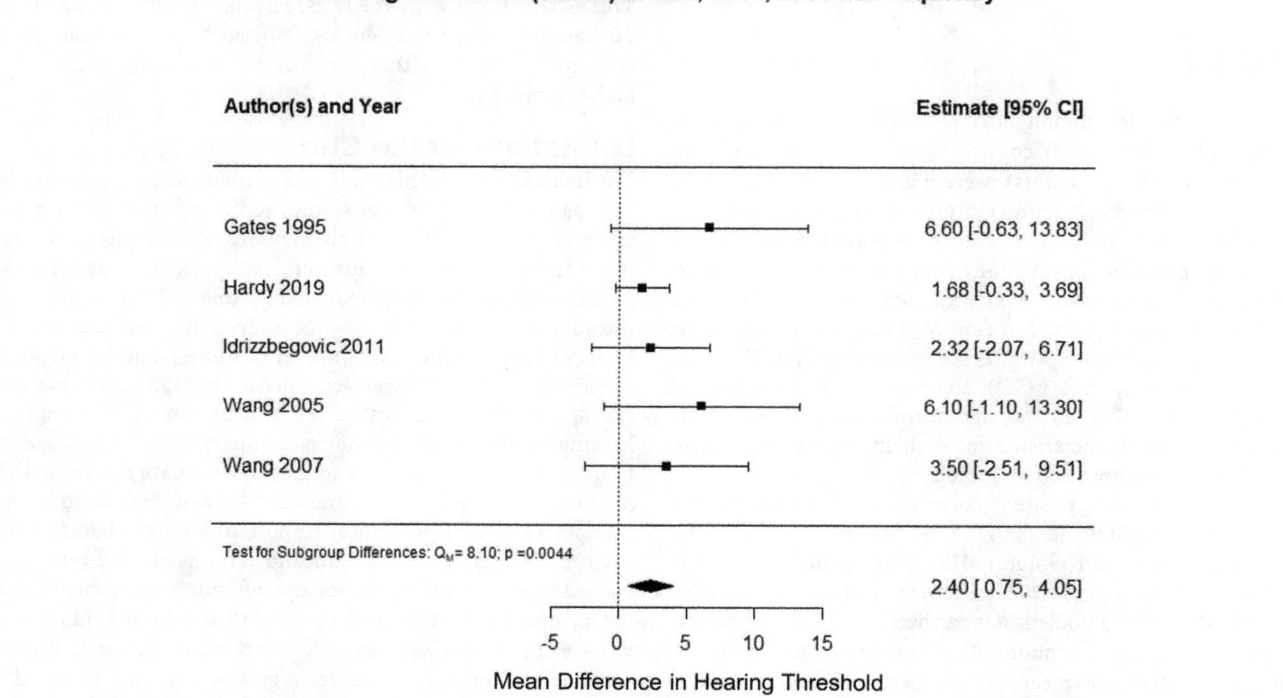

FIGURE 2 | Forest plot summarizing meta-analysis findings of hearing threshold (dB HL) difference between subjects with Alzheimer's disease and control subjects at 0.5–2 kHz PTA.

featured an individual positive correlation between hearing loss and AD, which combined provided a pooled positive correlation. We cannot ignore the propensity of studies to report only positive findings, and therefore, we acknowledge that our meta-analysis may not have captured studies with negative findings on the relationship between hearing loss and AD, as no such studies were found in our search.

There were 11 studies that were excluded from this meta-analysis due to the criteria established in the Methods section (Gates et al., 2008; Lodeiro-Fernandez et al., 2015; Bidelman et al., 2017; Villeneuve et al., 2017; Jayakody et al., 2018; Gyanwali et al., 2020; Sardone et al., 2020, 2021; Utoomprurkporn et al., 2020; Aylward et al., 2021; Jung et al., 2021). Of these, all but one demonstrated findings of subjects with dementia having increased hearing thresholds (i.e., hearing impairment) compared to controls; however, the findings of Haggstrom et al. (2018) could not be used in our analysis as they reported threshold hearing loss as median-values and not mean-values. Overall, the trend of increased hearing loss in subjects with dementia compared to controls was present in both included and excluded studies, supporting both the findings of this meta-analysis and current literature (Loughrey et al., 2018; Panza et al., 2018; Ray et al., 2018; Chern and Golub, 2019; Jafari et al., 2019; Ralli et al., 2019; Mertens et al., 2020; Utoomprurkporn et al., 2020; Knopke et al., 2021).

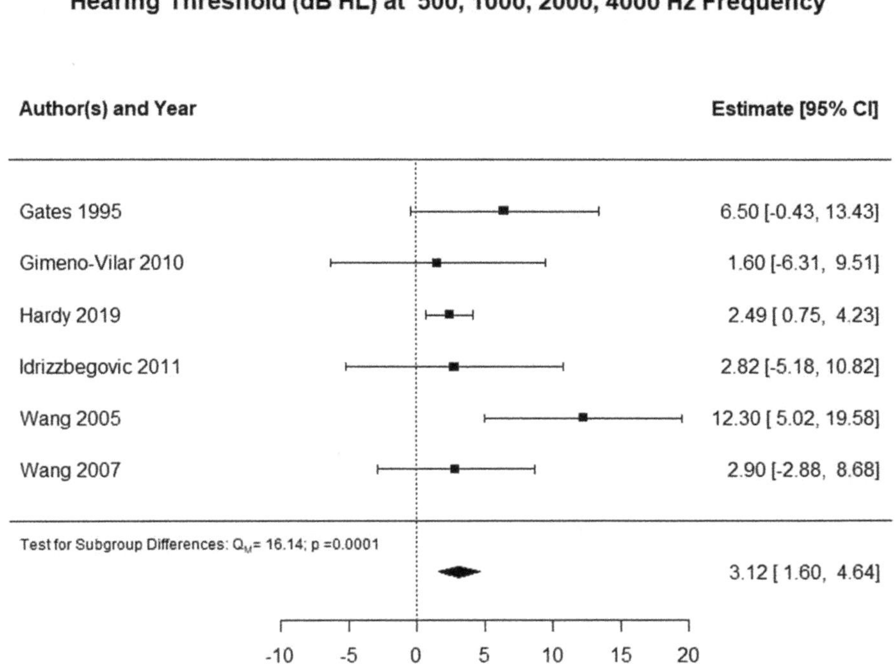

FIGURE 3 | Forest plot summarizing meta-analysis findings of hearing threshold (dB HL) difference between subjects with Alzheimer's disease and control subjects at 0.5–4 kHz PTA.

The shortcomings outlined above illustrate the importance of better characterizing peripheral hearing ability in subjects with AD compared to healthy-aging controls. Further work should characterize peripheral hearing ability using pure-tone audiometry in individuals diagnosed with clearly defined criteria for AD relative to cognitively normal age-, sex-, and education-matched controls. The findings of peripheral hearing assessment in such studies should be compared to measures of central auditory processing by carefully considering factors such as years since diagnosis, co-morbid factors, and cognitive factors such as global cognitive function, verbal language comprehension. This approach will serve to not only improve our understanding of the correlation between ARHL and AD, but also determine targets for early intervention to slow the progression of AD.

Implications of This Study in Relation to Previous Work

A large number of epidemiological studies have reported a relationship between ARHL and the later development of cognitive impairment. In a systematic review of 17 articles, Thomson et al. found pure-tone audiometry to be the most commonly reported method of quantifying ARHL in patients with dementia; in each of the studies they analyzed, all demonstrated an association between hearing loss and increased incidence of dementia (Thomson et al., 2017). Similarly, a meta-analysis conducted by Taljaard et al. (2015) showed reduced cognitive function in subjects with untreated hearing loss with the degree of cognitive function positively correlated to the degree of hearing impairment (Taljaard et al., 2015). Several prospective studies have also demonstrated risk of incident dementia increasing with worsening hearing loss measured by pure tone audiometry (Wang et al., 2005, 2007; Gimeno-Vilar and Cervera-Paz, 2010; Idrizbegovic et al., 2011; Lin et al., 2011, 2013; Lodeiro-Fernandez et al., 2015; Bidelman et al., 2017; Villeneuve et al., 2017; Haggstrom et al., 2018; Hardy et al., 2019; Chern et al., 2021). Although the underlying mechanism for this relationship remains unclear, reduction of peripheral hearing ability has been correlated to increased beta-amyloid deposition (Ray et al., 2018; Chern et al., 2021) and cortical thinning of the left frontal, right temporal, and bilateral occipital regions of the brain which suggests an important relationship between peripheral hearing and central processing in relationship to neuropathology (Uhlmann et al., 1989; Iliadou et al., 2017; Ha et al., 2020).

Conversely, some studies have not observed a correlation between ARHL and AD. For example, a meta-analysis conducted on 36 studies found that ARHL quantified by pure-tone audiometry was associated with cognitive impairment in general, but this association was not found between peripheral hearing loss and specifically for AD (Loughrey et al., 2018). The authors mention that smaller small size may have contributed to this insignificant association. Additionally, the relationship between peripheral ARHL and AD is complicated by the interactions of the peripheral and central auditory systems (Panza et al., 2018). Although the field of audiology often refers to PTA as a method of quantifying peripheral hearing ability, it is undeniable that auditory sensation, processing, and perception requires conductive, sensorineural, and central processing which is described in depth by authors of this study in their previous work (Swords et al., 2018). However, following the convention of previous audiologic studies of AD subjects, we refer to PTA as a metric of predominantly peripheral hearing. Therefore, to elucidate the relationship between peripheral and central auditory perception in relation to AD, PTA should be used to assess hearing ability alongside methods that quantify central auditory processing such as auditory evoked potentials.

In the current study a relatively small increase in threshold (2.3–4.5 dB HL) was observed in the AD cohort relative to control. Although the clinical significance of this magnitude of difference is not yet known, it is important to note that this degree of hearing loss roughly corresponds to the thresholds for detecting amplitude modulations in sounds (Scheider and Pichora-Fuller, 2001). Loss of amplitude modulation detection may lead to deficits in speech perception in AD (Page et al., 2005), which may contribute to the well-documented deficits in central auditory processing in AD (Swords et al., 2018).

CONCLUSION

To our knowledge, this is the first meta-analysis providing quantification of peripheral hearing loss measured by pure tone audiometry for subjects with AD compared to age-matched controls. Our findings suggest that subjects with AD have higher hearing thresholds at 0.5–2 kHz PTA and 0.5–4 kHz PTA compared to age-matched controls. This finding is supported by current literature from epidemiological studies on the relation of ARHL and AD. Our meta-analysis suggests that in future studies peripheral hearing should be better characterized in AD cohorts compared to age-matched controls accurately estimate the contributions of peripheral hearing loss to cognitive impairment. In addition, to use peripheral hearing loss in AD as a modifiable risk factor, assessing hearing ability using pure-tone audiometry on a routine basis would be critical. Additionally, analyses comparing pure tone audiometry measurements to other characteristics associated with AD may yield improved understanding on the effects of peripheral hearing in AD and elucidate effects of confounding variables that could not be analyzed in this study. Lastly, to characterize the pathophysiologic relationship between age-related hearing loss and AD, future studies should utilize pure-tone audiometry alongside other audiologic and neurophysiologic measures of peripheral and central hearing.

AUTHOR CONTRIBUTIONS

SK performed the systematic literature review, determined study inclusion/exclusion, extracted and analyzed data, and prepared the manuscript. X-MN validated study methods, performed data analysis, prepared the manuscript, and edited the manuscript. DW validated study methods, prepared figures, and edited the manuscript. RM determined study inclusion/exclusion criteria, validated extracted data, and prepared and edited the manuscript. DL determined study inclusion/exclusion, validated study methods, validated extracted data, and prepared and edited the manuscript. All authors contributed to the article and approved the submitted version.

ACKNOWLEDGMENTS

We would like to acknowledge the time and efforts of M. H. Burnette, PhD, medical and biomedicine librarian, who assisted us in the search process.

REFERENCES

Ally, B. A., Jones, G. E., Cole, J. A., and Budson, A. E. (2006). The P300 component in patients with Alzheimer's disease and their biological children. *Biol. Psychol.* 72, 180–187. doi: 10.1016/j.biopsycho.2005.10.004

Alzheimer's Association. (2021). 2021 Alzheimer's disease facts and figures. *Alzheimer's Dement.* 17, 327–406. doi: 10.1002/alz.12328

Anand, P., and Singh, B. (2013). A review on cholinesterase inhibitors for Alzheimer's disease. *Arch. Pharm. Res.* 36, 375–399. doi: 10.1007/s12272-013-0036-3

Arijita, D., Thornton, J. D., Sambamoorthi, U., and Innes, K. (2017). Direct and indirect cost of managing Alzheimer's disease and related dementias in the United States. *Exp. Rev. Pharmacoecon. Outcomes Res.* 17, 189–202. doi: 10.1080/14737167.2017.1313118

Aylward, A., Naidu, S. R., Mellum, C., King, J. B., Jones, K. G., Anderson, J. S., et al. (2021). Left ear hearing predicts functional activity in the brains of patients with Alzheimer's Disease Dementia. *Ann. Otol. Rhinol. Laryngol.* 130, 343–349. doi: 10.1177/0003489420952467

Bhatti, G. K., Reddy, A. P., Reddy, P. H., and Bhatti, J. S. (2020). Lifestyle modifications and nutritional interventions in aging-associated cognitive decline and Alzheimer's disease. *Front. Aging Neurosci.* 11:369. doi: 10.3389/fnagi.2019.00369

Bidelman, G. M., Lowther, J. E., Tak, S. H., and Alain, C. (2017). Mild cognitive impairment is characterized by deficient brainstem and cortical representations of speech. *J. Neurosci.* 37, 3610–3620. doi: 10.1523/JNEUROSCI.3700-16.2017

Brewster, K. K., Pavlicova, M., Stein, A., Chen, M., Chen, C., Brown, P. J., et al. (2020). A pilot randomized controlled trial of hearing aids to improve mood and cognition in older adults. *Int. J. Geriatr. Psychiatry* 35, 842–850. doi: 10.1002/gps.5311

Burns, A. (2000). The burden of Alzheimer's disease. *Int. J. Neuropsychopharmacol.* 3(Supplement 2), S31–S38. doi: 10.1017/S1461145700001905

Chern, A., and Golub, J. S. (2019). Age-related hearing loss and dementia. *Alzheimer Dis. Assoc. Disord.* 33, 285–290. doi: 10.1097/WAD.0000000000000325

Chern, A., Golub, J. S., and Lalwani, A. K. (2021). Do hearing aids help prevent cognitive decline? *Laryngoscope* 131, 2166–2168. doi: 10.1002/lary.29365

Cintra, M., Ávila, R. T., Soares, T. O., Cunha, L., and Silveira, K. D., de Moraes, E. N., et al. (2018). Increased N200 and P300 latencies in cognitively impaired elderly carrying ApoE ε-4 allele. *Int. J. Geriatr. Psychiatry* 33, e221–e227. doi: 10.1002/gps.4773

Danjou, P., Viardot, G., Maurice, D., Garcés, P., Wams, E. J., Phillips, K. G., et al. (2019). Electrophysiological assessment methodology of sensory processing dysfunction in schizophrenia and dementia of the Alzheimer type. *Neurosci. Biobehav. Rev.* 97, 70–84. doi: 10.1016/j.neubiorev.2018.09.004

Gates, G. A., Anderson, M. L., Feeney, M. P., McCurry, S. M., and Larson, E. B. (2008). Central auditory dysfunction in older persons with memory impairment or Alzheimer's dementia. *Arch. Otolaryngol. Head Neck Surg.* 134, 771–777. doi: 10.1001/archotol.134.7.771

Gates, G. A., Karzon, R. K., Garcia, P., Peterein, J., Storandt, M., Morris, J. C., et al. (1995). Auditory dysfunction in aging and senile dementia of the Alzheimer's type. *Arch. Neurol.* 52, 626–634. doi: 10.1001/archneur.1995.00540300108020

Gimeno-Vilar, C., and Cervera-Paz, F. J. (2010). Enfermedad de Alzheimer y perdida auditiva. *Rev. Neurol.* 50, 65–71. doi: 10.33588/RN.5002.2009189

Gregory, S., Billings, J., Wilson, D., Livingston, G., Schilder, A. G., and Costafreda, S. G. (2020). Experiences of hearing aid use among patients with mild cognitive impairment and Alzheimer's disease dementia: a qualitative study. *SAGE Open Med.* 8:2050312120904572. doi: 10.1177/2050312120904572

Grimes, A. M., Grady, C. L., and Pikus, A. (1987). Auditory evoked potentials in patients with dementia of the Alzheimer type. *Ear Hear.* 8, 157–161. doi: 10.1097/00003446-198706000-00005

Gurgel, R. K., Ward, P. D., Schwartz, S., Norton, M. C., Foster, N. L., and Tschanz, J. T. (2014). Relationship of hearing loss and dementia: a prospective, population-based study. *Otol. Neurotol.* 35, 775–781. doi: 10.1097/MAO.0000000000000313

Gyanwali, B., Hilal, S., Venketasubramanian, N., Chen, C., and Loo, J. (2020). Hearing handicap in Asian patients with dementia. *Am. J. Otolaryngol.* 41, 102377. doi: 10.1016/j.amjoto.2019.102377

Ha, J., Cho, Y. S., Kim, S. J., Cho, S. H., Kim, J. P., Jung, Y. H., et al. (2020). Hearing loss is associated with cortical thinning in cognitively normal older adults. *Eur. J. Neurol.* 27, 1003–1009. doi: 10.1111/ene.14195

Haggstrom, J., Rosenhall, U., Hederstierna, C., Ostberg, P., and Idrizbegovic, E. (2018). A longitudinal study of peripheral and central auditory function in Alzheimer's disease and in mild cognitive impairment. *Dement. Geriatr. Cogn. Disord.* 8: 393–401. doi: 10.1159/00493340

Hardy, C. J. D., Frost, C., Sivasathiaseelan, H., Johnson, J. C. S., Agustus, J. L., Bond, R. L., et al. (2019). Findings of impaired hearing in patients with non-fluent/agrammatic variant primary progressive aphasia. *JAMA Neurol. Brief Rep.* 76, 607–611. doi: 10.1001/jamaneurol.2018.4799

Hsiao, F. J., Chen, W. T., Wang, P. N., Cheng, C. H., and Lin, Y. Y. (2014). Temporo-frontal functional connectivity during auditory change detection is altered in Alzheimer's disease. *Hum. Brain Mapp.* 35, 5565–5577. doi: 10.1002/hbm.22570

Hubbard, H. I., Mamo, S. K., and Hopper, T. (2018). Dementia and hearing loss: interrelationships and treatment considerations. *Semin. Speech Lang.* 39, 197–210. doi: 10.1055/s-0038-1660779

Idrizbegovic, E., Hederstierna, C., Dahlquist, M., Nordstrom, C. K., Jelic, V., and Rosenhall, U. (2011). Central auditory function in early Alzheimer's disease and in mild cognitive impairment. *Age Age.* 40, 249–254. doi: 10.1093/ageing/afq168

Iliadou, V., Bamiou, D. E., Sidras, C., Moschopoulos, N., Tsolaki, P. M., Nimatoudis, I., et al. (2017). The use of gaps-in-noise test as an index of enhanced left temporal cortical thinning associated with the transition between mild cognitive impairment and Alzheimer's disease. *J. Am. Acad. Audiol.* 28, 1–9. doi: 10.3766/jaaa.16075

Jafari, Z., Kolb, B. E., and Mohajerani, M. H. (2019). Age-related hearing loss and tinnitus, dementia risk, and auditory amplification outcomes. *Ageing Res. Rev.* 56:100963. doi: 10.1016/j.arr.2019.100963

Jafari, Z., Kolb, B. E., and Mohajerani, M. H. (2020). Prepulse inhibition of the acoustic startle reflex and P50 gating in aging and alzheimer's disease. *Ageing Res. Rev.* 59:101028. doi: 10.1016/j.arr.2020.101028

Jayakody, D., Friedland, P. L., Eikelboom, R. H., Martins, R. N., and Sohrabi, H. R. (2018). A novel study on association between untreated hearing loss and cognitive functions of older adults: baseline non-verbal cognitive assessment results. *Clin. Otolaryngol.* 43, 182–191. doi: 10.1111/coa.12937

Jayakody, D., Menegola, H. K., Yiannos, J. M., Goodman-Simpson, J., Friedland, P. L., Taddei, K., et al. (2020). The peripheral hearing and central auditory processing skills of individuals with subjective memory complaints. *Front. Neurosci.* 14:888. doi: 10.3389/fnins.2020.00888

Johnson, J., Marshall, C. R., Weil, R. S., Bamiou, D. E., Hardy, C., and Warren, J. D. (2021). Hearing and dementia: from ears to brain. *Brain* 144, 391–401. doi: 10.1093/brain/awaa429

Jongsiriyanyong, S., and Limpawattana, P. (2018). Mild cognitive impairment in clinical practice: a review article. *Am. J. Alzheimer's Dis. Dement.* 33, 500–507. doi: 10.1177/1533317518791401

Jung, J., Bae, S. H., Han, J. H., Kwak, S. H., Nam, G. S., Lee, P. H., et al. (2021). Relationship between hearing loss and dementia differs according to the underlying mechanism. *J. Clin. Neurol.* 17, 290–299. doi: 10.3988/jcn.2021.17.2.290

Khalsa, D. S. (2015). Stress, meditation, and Alzheimer's disease prevention: where the evidence stands. *J. Alzheimer's Dis. JAD* 48, 1–12. doi: 10.3233/JAD-142766

Kimiskidis, V. K., and Papaliagkas, V. T. (2012). Event-related potentials for the diagnosis of mild cognitive impairment and Alzheimer's disease. *Expert Opin. Med. Diagn.* 6, 15–26. doi: 10.1517/17530059.2012.634795

Knopke, S., Schubert, A., H√§ussler, S. M., Gr√§bel, S., Szczepek, A. J., and Olze, H. (2021). Improvement of working memory and processing speed in patients over 70 with bilateral hearing impairment following unilateral cochlear implantation. *J. Clin. Med.* 10:3421. doi: 10.3390/jcm10153421

Kurt, P., Emek-Sava,ş, D. D., Batum, K., Turp, B., Güntekin, B., Karşidag, S., et al. (2014). Patients with mild cognitive impairment display reduced auditory event-related delta oscillatory responses. *Behav. Neurol.* 2014:268967. doi: 10.1155/2014/268967

Liberati, A., Altman, D. G., Tetzlaff, J., Mulrow, C., Gøtzsche, P. C., Ioannidis, J. P., et al. (2009). The PRISMA statement for reporting systematic reviews and meta-analyses of studies that evaluate healthcare interventions: explanation and elaboration. *BMJ* 339:b2700. doi: 10.1136/bmj.b2700

Lin, F. R., Metter, E. J., O'Brien, R. J., Resnick, S. M., Zonderman, A. B., and Ferrucci, L. (2011). Hearing loss and incident dementia. *Arch. Neurol.* 68, 214–222. doi: 10.1001/archneurol.2010.362

Lin, F. R., Yaffe, K., Xia, J., Xue, Q. L., Harris, T. B., Purchase-Helzner, E., et al. (2013). Hearing loss and cognitive decline in older adults. *JAMA Intern. Med.* 173, 293–299. doi: 10.1001/jamainternmed.2013.1868

Lodeiro-Fernandez, L., Lorenzo-Lopez, L., Maseda, A., Nunez-Naveira, L., Rodriguez-Villamil, J. L., and Millan-Calenti, J. C. (2015). The impact of hearing loss on language performance in older adults with different stages of cognitive function. *Clin. Interv. Aging* 10, 695–702.

Loughrey, D. G., Kelly, M. E., Kelley, G. A., Brennan, S., and Lawlor, B. A. (2018). Association of age-related hearing loss with cognitive function, cognitive impairment, and dementia: a systematic review and meta-analysis. *JAMA Otolaryngol. Head Neck Surg.* 144, 115–126. doi: 10.1001/jamaoto.2017.2513

Mansour, Y., Blackburn, K., González-González, L. O., Calderón-Garcidueñas, L., and Kulesza, R. J. (2019). Auditory brainstem dysfunction, non-invasive biomarkers for early diagnosis and monitoring of Alzheimer's disease in young urban residents exposed to air pollution. *J. Alzheimer's Dis. JAD* 67, 1147–1155. doi: 10.3233/JAD-181186

Mattson, M. P., and Arumugam, T. V. (2018). Hallmarks of brain aging: adaptive and pathological modification by metabolic states. *Cell Metab.* 27, 1176–1199. doi: 10.1016/j.cmet.2018.05.011

McKhann, G. M., Knopman, D. S., Chertkow, H., Hyman, B. T., Jack, C. R. Jr, Kawas, C. H., et al. (2011). The diagnosis of dementia due to Alzheimer's disease: recommendations from the National Institute on Aging-Alzheimer's Association workgroups on diagnostic guidelines for Alzheimer's disease. *Alzheimer's Dement.* 7, 263–269. doi: 10.1016/j.jalz.2011.03.005

Mertens, G., Andries, E., Claes, A. J., Topsakal, V., Van de Heyning, P., Van Rompaey, V., et al. (2020). Cognitive improvement after cochlear implantation in older adults with severe or profound hearing impairment: a prospective, longitudinal, controlled, multicenter study. *Ear Hear.* 42, 606–614. doi: 10.1097/AUD.0000000000000962

Morrison, C., Rabipour, S., Knoefel, F., Sheppard, C., and Taler, V. (2018). Auditory event-related potentials in mild cognitive impairment and Alzheimer's disease. *Curr. Alzheimer Res.* 15, 702–715. doi: 10.2174/1567205015666180123123209

Muscoso, E. G., Costanzo, E., Daniele, O., Maugeri, D., Natale, E., and Caravaglios, G. (2006). Auditory event-related potentials in subcortical vascular cognitive impairment and in Alzheimer's disease. *J. Neural Transm.* 113, 1779–1786. doi: 10.1007/s00702-006-0574-7

Page, M. J., McKenzie, J. E., Bossuyt, P. M., Boutron, I., Hoffmann, T. C., Mulrow, C. D., et al. (2005). The PRISMA 2020 statement: an updated guideline for reporting systematic reviews. *BMJ* 372:n71. doi: 10.1136/bmj.n71

Panza, F., Lozupone, M., Sardone, R., Battista, P., Piccininni, M., Dibello, V., et al. (2018). Sensorial frailty: age-related hearing loss and the risk of cognitive impairment and dementia in later life. *Ther. Adv. Chronic Dis.* 10:2040622318811000. doi: 10.1177/2040622318811000

Pekkonen, E., Hirvonen, J., Jääskeläinen, I. P., Kaakkola, S., and Huttunen, J. (2001). Auditory sensory memory and the cholinergic system: implications for Alzheimer's disease. *Neuroimage* 14, 376–382. doi: 10.1006/nimg.2001.0805

Quaranta, N., Coppola, F., Casulli, M., Barulli, O., Lanza, F., Tortelli, R., et al. (2014). The prevalence of peripheral and central hearing impairment and its relation to cognition in older adults. *Audiol. Neuro-otol.* 19(Suppl 1), 10–14. doi: 10.1159/000371597

Ralli, M., Gilardi, A., Stadio, A. D., Severini, C., Salzano, F. A., Greco, A., et al. (2019). Hearing loss and Alzheimer's disease: a review. *Int. Tinnitus J.* 23, 79–85. doi: 10.5935/0946-5448.20190014

Ray, J., Popli, G., and Fell, G. (2018). Association of cognition and age-related hearing impairment in the english longitudinal study of ageing. *JAMA Otolaryngol. Head Neck Surg.* 144, 876–882. doi: 10.1001/jamaoto.2018.1656

Reed, C., Belger, M., Dell'Agnello, G., Wimo, A., Argimon, J. M., Bruno, G., et al. (2014). Caregiver burden in Alzheimer's disease: differential association in adult child and spousal caregivers in the GERAS observational study. *Dement. Geriatr. Cogn. Disord.* 4, 51–64. doi: 10.1159/000358234

Reeves, B. C., Deeks, J. J., Higgins, J. P. T., and Wells, G. A. (2011). "Chapter 13: Including non-randomized studies," in *Cochrane Handbook of Systematic Reviews of Interventions, version 510*, eds J. B. T. Higgins, S. Green. Available online at: http://www.handbook.cochrane.org (accessed November 28, 2021).

Reeves, R. R., Struve, F. A., Patrick, G., Booker, J. G., and Nave, D. W. (1999). The effects of donepezil on the P300 auditory and visual cognitive evoked potentials of patients with Alzheimer's disease. *Am. J. Geriatric Psychiatry* 7, 349–352.

Revonsuo, A., Portin, R., Juottonen, K., and Rinne, J. O. (1998). Semantic processing of spoken words in Alzheimer's disease: an electrophysiological study. *J. Cogn. Neurosci.* 10, 408–420. doi: 10.1162/089892998562726

Sardone, R., Battista, P., Donghia, R., Lozupone, M., Tortelli, R., Guerra, V., et al. (2020). Age-related central auditory processing disorder, MCI, and dementia in an older population of Southern Italy. *Otolaryngol. Head Neck Surg.* 163, 348–355. doi: 10.1177/0194599820913635

Sardone, R., Castellana, F., Bortone, I., Lampignano, L., Zupo, R., Lozupone, M., et al. (2021). Association between central and peripheral age-related hearing loss and different frailty phenotypes in an older population in Southern Italy. *JAMA Otolaryngol. Head Neck Surg.* 147, 561–571. doi: 10.1001/jamaoto.2020.5334

Scheider, B. A., and Pichora-Fuller, K. M. (2001). Age-related changes in temporal processing: Speech perception. *Semin. Hear.* 22, 227–240. doi: 10.1055/s-2001-15628

Schwartz, T. J., Kutas, M., Butters, N., Paulsen, J. S., and Salmon, D. P. (1996). Electrophysiological insights into the nature of the semantic deficit in Alzheimer's disease. *Neuropsychologia* 34, 827–841. doi: 10.1016/0028-3932(95)00164-6

Shahmiri, E., Jafari, Z., Noroozian, M., Zendehbad, A., Haddadzadeh Niri, H., and Yoonessi, A. (2017). Effect of mild cognitive impairment and Alzheimer disease on auditory steady-state responses. *Basic Clin. Neurosci.* 8, 299–306.doi: 10.18869/nirp.bcn.8.4.299

Sharma, K. (2019). Cholinesterase inhibitors as Alzheimer's therapeutics (Review). *Mol. Med. Rep.* 20, 1479–1487. doi: 10.3892/mmr.2019.10374

Small, G. W. (2000). Early diagnosis of Alzheimer's disease: update on combining genetic and brain-imaging measures. *Dialogues Clin. Neurosci.* v2, 214–246. doi: 10.31887/DCNS.2000.2.3/gsmall

Strouse, A. L., Hall, J. W. 3rd, and Burger, M. C. (1995). Central auditory processing in Alzheimer's disease. *Ear Hear.* 16, 230–238. doi: 10.1097/00003446-199504000-00010

Swords, G. M., Nguyen, L. T., Mudar, R. A., and Llano, D. A. (2018). Auditory system dysfunction in Alzheimer's disease and its prodromal states: a review. *Aging Res. Rev.* 44, 49–59. doi: 10.1016/j.arr.2018.04.001

Taljaard, D. S., Olaithe, M., Brennan-Jones, C. G., Eikelboom, R. H., and Bucks, R. S. (2015). The relationship between hearing impairment and cognitive function: a meta-analysis in adults. *Clin. Otolaryngol.* 41, 718–729. doi: 10.111/coa.12607

Tarawneh, H. Y., Mulders, W., Sohrabi, H. R., Martins, R. N., and Jayakody, D. (2021). Investigating auditory electrophysiological measures of participants with mild cognitive impairment and Alzheimer's disease: a systematic review and meta-analysis of event-related potential studies. *J. Alzheimer's Dis.* doi: 10.3233/JAD-210556

Thomson, R. S., Auduong, P., Miller, A. T., and Gurgel, R. K. (2017). Hearing loss as a risk factor for dementia: a systematic review. *Laryngosc. Investig. Otolaryngol.* 2, 69–79. doi: 10.1002/lio2.65

Uhlmann, R. F., Teri, L., Rees, T. S., Mozlowski, K. J., and Larson, E. B. (1989). Impact of mild to moderate hearing loss on mental status testing. Comparability of standard and written Mini-Mental State Examinations. *J. Am. Geriatr. Soc.* 37, 223–228. doi: 10.1111/j.1532-5415.1989.tb06811.x

Utoomprurkporn, N., Hardy, C., Stott, J., Costafreda, S. G., Warren, J., and Bamiou, D. E. (2020). "The Dichotic Digit Test" as an index indicator for hearing problem in dementia: systematic review and meta-analysis. *J. Am. Acad. Audiol.* 31, 646–655. doi: 10.1055/s-0040-1718700

Verma, N. P., Greiffenstein, M. F., Verma, N., King, S. D., and Caldwell, D. L. (1987). Electrophysiologic validation of two categories of dementias—cortical and subcortical. *Clin. EEG (electroencephalography)* 18, 26–33.

Villeneuve, A., Hommet, C., Aussedat, C., Lescanne, E., Reffet, K., and Bakhos, D. (2017). Audiometric evaluation in patients with Alzheimer's disease. *Eur. Arch. Oto-rhino-laryngol.* 274, 151–157. doi: 10.1007/s00405-016-4257-1

Wang, C., Wang, Z., Xie, B., Shi, X., Yang, P., Liu, L., et al. (2021). Binaural processing deficit and cognitive impairment in Alzheimer's disease. *Alzheimer's Dementia.* 2021, 1–15. doi: 10.1002/alz.12464

Wang, N. Y., Su, J. F., Dong, H. Q., Jia, J. P., and Han, D. M. (2005). Hearing impairment in patients with mild cognitive impairment and Alzheimer's disease. *Chin. J. Otorhinolaryngol. Head Neck Surg.* 40, 279–282.

Wang, N. Y., Yang, H. J., Su, J. F., Kong, F., Zhang, M. X., Dong, H. Q., et al. (2007). Hearing impairment in senile dementia of Alzheimer's type. *J. Otol.* 2, 14–17. doi: 10.1016/S1672-2930(07)50003-6

Wells, G., Shea, B., O'Connell, D., Peterson, J., Welch, V., Losos, M., et al. (2013). *The Newcastle-Ottawa Scale (NOS) for Assessing the Quality of Nonrandomised Studies in Meta-analyses.* Available online at: http://www.ohri.ca/programs/clinical_epidemiology/oxford.asp (accessed November 28, 2021).

Xu, W., Zhang, C., Li, J. Q., Tan, C. C., Cao, X. P., Alzheimer's Disease Neuroimaging Initiative, et al. (2019). Age-related hearing loss accelerates cerebrospinal fluid tau levels and brain atrophy: a longitudinal study. *Aging* 11, 3156–3169. doi: 10.18632/aging.101971

14

Complete Elimination of Peripheral Auditory Input before Onset of Hearing Causes Long-Lasting Impaired Social Memory in Mice

Rui Guo[†]*, Yang Li*[†]*, Jiao Liu, Shusheng Gong** *and Ke Liu**

Department of Otolaryngology Head and Neck Surgery, Beijing Friendship Hospital, Capital Medical University, Beijing, China

***Correspondence:**
Shusheng Gong
gongss@ccmu.edu.cn
Ke Liu
liuke@ccmu.edu.cn

[†]*These authors have contributed equally to this work and share first authorship*

Hearing is one of the most important senses needed for survival, and its loss is an independent risk factor for dementia. Hearing loss (HL) can lead to communication difficulties, social isolation, and cognitive dysfunction. The hippocampus is a critical brain region being greatly involved in the formation of learning and memory and is critical not only for declarative memory but also for social memory. However, until today, whether HL can affect learning and memory is poorly understood. This study aimed to identify the relationship between HL and hippocampal-associated cognitive function. Mice with complete auditory input elimination before the onset of hearing were used as the animal model. They were first examined via auditory brainstem response (ABR) to confirm hearing elimination, and behavior estimations were applied to detect social memory capacity. We found significant impairment of social memory in mice with HL compared with the controls ($p < 0.05$); however, no significant differences were seen in the tests of novel object recognition, Morris water maze (MWM), and locomotion in the open field ($p > 0.05$). Therefore, our study firstly demonstrates that hearing input is required for the formation of social memory, and hearing stimuli play an important role in the development of normal cognitive ability.

Keywords: hearing, hearing loss, congenital, learning memory, social memory, hippocampus

INTRODUCTION

Hearing is one of the most important senses needed for survival, and its loss is a highly prevalent sensory deficit in humans. Approximately 1.57 billion people in the world have hearing loss (HL), with increasing prevalence over the years (Haile et al., 2021). HL can lead to communication difficulties, social isolation, and cognitive dysfunction. A series of epidemiological studies have shown that HL may be an independent risk factor for dementia (Taljaard et al., 2016; Livingston et al., 2017; Loughrey et al., 2018; Griffiths et al., 2020). However, the underlying mechanism is still unclear.

The hippocampus serves as a critical brain region in the formation and maturation of learning and memory. A recent human study proposed that midlife HL can lead to atrophy of the hippocampus and entorhinal cortex (Armstrong et al., 2019), suggesting that HL may have negative effects on the hippocampus. Previous animal studies also showed that HL is able to disrupt the function of the hippocampus and lead to memory decline. The hippocampus is involved not only in declarative memory but also in social memory, which is the ability to remember and discriminate novel conspecifics from familiar ones in social activities (Barbara and Contreras, 1985). Although HL has been reported to negatively affect the quality of social interactions in patients (Hughes et al., 2018), these types of studies are usually limited because the patient samples are not quite uniform for precise analyses. Therefore, an animal model with diminished peripheral hearing input is necessary to verify the association between HL and social memory.

In this study, we created *Otof* mutation mice which are functionally equivalent to the otoferlin knockout mice (Otof$^{-/-}$) via genetic manipulations. In this congenital deaf mouse model, the peripheral hearing input has been totally eliminated before hearing onset due to the complete loss of exocytosis in the cochlear ribbon synapses (Roux et al., 2006). Auditory brainstem response (ABR) examinations were used to confirm elimination of hearing, and the behavior estimations including three-chamber social interaction assay, novel object recognition, open field, and Morris water maze (MWM) were applied to detect the cognition and locomotion in this mouse model. We also found that mice with auditory input elimination before hearing onset have impaired social novelty memory, coupling with unimpaired locomotor activity and sociability. Thus, our study may firstly demonstrate that hearing input is required to establish social memory in mice.

MATERIALS AND METHODS

Animals

Otof knockout mice were constructed by the CRISPR–Cas9 system. In brief, a frameshift mutation was introduced into the conserved domain (14 exon) of otoferlin using the AAV loading Cas9 protein and sgRNA (GTGAAAATTTACCGAGCAGA), respectively. The mutation site was identified by Sanger sequencing. The heterozygous animals were interbred to generate Otof$^{+/+\backslash u0001}$, Otof$^{\pm}$, and Otof$^{-/-}$ mice. C57BL/6J mice served as the control group and were purchased from the Vital River Laboratory (Beijing, China). All mice were bred in the Experimental Animal Department of the Capital Medical University at 22–25°C, 50% humidity, and 12 h light–dark cycle, with food and water available *ad libitum*. Only male mice were used in this study. The animal study was reviewed and approved by the Animal Ethics Committee of the Capital Medical University.

Assessment of Auditory Function

Auditory brainstem response detection was performed at the ages of P14, P56, and P168. Mice were anesthetized with an intraperitoneal injection of ketamine (100 mg/kg, Sigma, Saint Louis, MO, United States) plus xylazine (10 mg/kg, Sigma), and then placed in an electrically shielded and soundproofed audiometric chamber (Shanghai Shengnuo Acoustic Equipment, Shanghai, China). Meanwhile, body temperature was maintained with a constant temperature heating pad. The needle electrodes were placed subcutaneously, with a reference electrode beneath the pinna of the tested ear, a recording electrode (+) at the junction of anterior edges of both auricles and the midline of the cranial apex, and a ground electrode in the contralateral ear. Acoustic stimuli were delivered monaurally by an earphone attached to a customized plastic speculum inserted into the ear canal. Calibrated tone bursts with 5 ms duration and 0.5 ms rise–fall time were synthesized and presented using TDT System 3 hardware and SigGen/BioSig software (Tucker-Davis Technologies, Alachua, FL, United States). ABRs were measured at click and tong burst. A total of 1,024 responses were averaged near the threshold at various intensities with 5 dB intervals. The lowest level at which ABR waves could be clearly detected was defined as the threshold.

Immunostaining and Confocal Microscopy

Cochleas of the mice were perfused with 4% paraformaldehyde (PFA) in PBS (pH 7.4) and incubated in the same fixative at 4°C, overnight. The cochleas were rinsed three times with PBS and decalcified by incubation with 10% ethylenediamine tetraacetic acid (EDTA) for 4–6 h. The organ of Corti was dissected into a surface preparation, preincubated in 0.3% Triton X-100 and 5% normal goat serum in PBS at room temperature for 1 h, and incubated overnight at 4°C, with the primary antibody:mouse anti-otoferlin antibody (1:300, Abcam, Cambridge, MA, United States, ab53233). The samples were rinsed three times in PBS buffer and incubated at room temperature for 2 h with the appropriate secondary antibody:goat anti-mouse Alexa Fluor 488. The samples were washed three times in PBS and mounted on a glass slide using a fluorescent mounting medium with DAPI (ZSGB-BIO, ZLI-9557). Fluorescence confocal z stacks of the organ of Corti were obtained with a Leica scanning laser confocal microscope (model TCS SP8 II, Leica, Wetzlar, Germany), equipped with a high-resolution objective (numerical aperture of 1.18, × 63 oil-immersion objective). Images were acquired in a 1,024 × 512 (pixel size = 0.036 μm in *x* and *y*) from top to bottom with an interval of 0.5 μm/layer.

For otoferlin staining on hippocampal slices, after anesthesia and cardiac perfusion with precooling PBS, the mouse brain was quickly removed and fixed in 4% PFA at 4°C, for 24 h, and then transferred into 30% sucrose for cryoprotection. After that, the brain was subjected to OCT embedding (Tissue-Tek, Torrance, CA, United States, 4853) and sliced into 40 μm coronal sections by a cryostat microtome (Leica CM3050S, Wetzlar, Germany) at −20°C,. The floating brain sections were washed in PBS three times for 10 min and blocked in 10% goat serum diluted in 0.3% Triton X-100 for 1 h at room temperature. After the block, the brain sections were incubated with primary antibody overnight at 4°C, and then incubated with secondary antibody for 2 h at room temperature. After three times washing with PBS, the sections were mounted on the glass slides with mounting medium with DAPI. Primary antibodies used in this study were rabbit anti-MAP2 (1:500, Abcam, ab32454) and mouse anti-otoferlin (1:100, Abcam, ab53233). Secondary antibodies used were goat anti-mouse Alexa Fluor 488 (1:500, Invitrogen, Waltham, MA, United States, A11029) and goat anti-rabbit Alexa Fluor 594 (1:500, Invitrogen, A11037). Images were taken by a confocal microscope (Leica TCS SP8).

Three-Chamber Social Interaction Experiment

The three-chamber social interaction test was adapted from previous research (Wang et al., 2018). The three-chamber apparatus (Xinruan, Shanghai, China) was divided into three compartments (each compartment $L \times W \times H$: 20 cm × 40 cm × 22 cm). Mice can freely explore the three chambers through two doors (W × H: 5 cm × 8 cm). Briefly, the social interaction experiment included three continuous phases with two small wire cages (15 cm height with a diameter of 7 cm) in the left and right chamber. In the first phase, two empty wire cages were placed in the left and right chamber, respectively, and the WT or Otof$^{-/-}$ mouse was introduced into the middle chamber and allowed to explore the apparatus freely for 10 min. In the second phase (social interaction test), an age-matched C57BL/6J male mouse (stranger 1, S1) was restricted into one of the wire cages randomly. The WT or Otof$^{-/-}$ mouse was allowed to explore the apparatus freely for 10 min. After the second 10 min, in the third phase (social novelty test), another age-matched C57BL/6J male mouse (stranger 2, S2) was restricted into the previously empty wire cage, and the subject mouse was allowed to explore for 10 min. The close interaction area was defined as the surrounding area (20 cm × 17.5 cm) containing the wire cage. Time spent in each chamber by the subject mouse was recorded by SuperMaze software (Xinruan).

Morris Water Maze

The MWM test was adapted from previous research (Hunt et al., 2013). The core device for MWM is a circular pool (120 cm in diameter) filled with non-toxic paint mixed with water. A circular platform (10 cm in diameter) was located in one quadrant of the pool above or beneath the water surface. Briefly, mice were trained to find and land a visible platform on day 1, and the escape latency (first time to land the platform) and swimming speed were evaluated to exclude those mice with visual impairment or dyskinesia. Then, the platform was fixed in another quadrant and beneath the water surface 0.5–1 cm. Mice were trained to learn and remember the location of the platform according to spatial cues around the pool for five sessions (days 2–4). Two daily sessions were ~3.5 h interval. Each session included four trials, and mice were introduced into the water from four different start points and were allowed to swim for 60 s. Once the mouse landed the platform or did not find the platform within 60 s, it was allowed to stay on the platform for 30 s to remember the platform position. The probe was performed 24 h after the last training in session 5. The platform was removed and the mice were allowed to swim in the pool for 60 s. The percent time (%) in the platform quadrant and the first time to the platform by subject mice were recorded and used in the statistical analysis. The software used in this test was Smart v3.0 (Panlab Harvard Apparatus, Barcelona, Spain).

Novel Object Recognition

Novel object recognition (Wang et al., 2020) was performed in the open arena ($L \times W \times H$: 50 cm × 50 cm × 50 cm). The task included two phases: acquisition phase and retrieval phase. In the acquisition phase, two similar objects (object A and A′) were placed in two corners of the arena; the mouse was gently placed into the open field and was allowed to explore for 10 min, and then the mouse came back to its home cage. Four hours later, in the retrieval phase, one of the objects (A) was replaced by a novel object (object B). The mouse was put back to the arena for another 10 min. The exploration time of each object in the retrieval phase was recorded by the SuperMaze software (Xinruan). The discrimination index (DI) was time with (object B - object A)/(object B + object A).

Open Field

The open field test was performed as described previously (Wang et al., 2020) to test the spontaneous motor activity. The mouse was placed in the open field ($L \times W \times H$: 50 cm × 50 cm × 50 cm) for 5 min. The speed and distance of the test mouse was recorded by the SuperMaze software (Xinruan).

Statistical Analysis

Statistical analysis was performed by GraphPad Prism 8.0.1 software. For two groups, data were analyzed by unpaired *t*-test. One-/two-way ANOVA was used for the comparison of more than two groups.

RESULTS

Auditory Detection Confirms Complete Elimination of Hearing Input in Mice

To confirm the complete elimination of hearing function in Otof$^{-/-}$ mice in this study, we then detected the ABR thresholds at ages of P14, 56, and 168, respectively. No visible ABR waveforms were detected at any point (Otof$^{-/-}$, **Figure 1A**), and normal waveforms were detected in the control mice (WT, **Figure 1A**). This shows that peripheral hearing input was eliminated, and no hearing information was being delivered from the ear to the brain in these deaf mice. In addition, we estimated the ABR threshold across frequencies in both Otof$^{-/-}$ and WT mice. No ABR thresholds could be identified in Otof$^{-/-}$ mice across all frequencies, whereas normal thresholds were observed in the control ones (**Table 1**). Otof$^{-/-}$ mice can serve as complete deaf models without peripheral hearing input, similar to those previously reported (Roux et al., 2006). Furthermore, we detected otoferlin expression in the cochlear hair cells of Otof$^{-/-}$

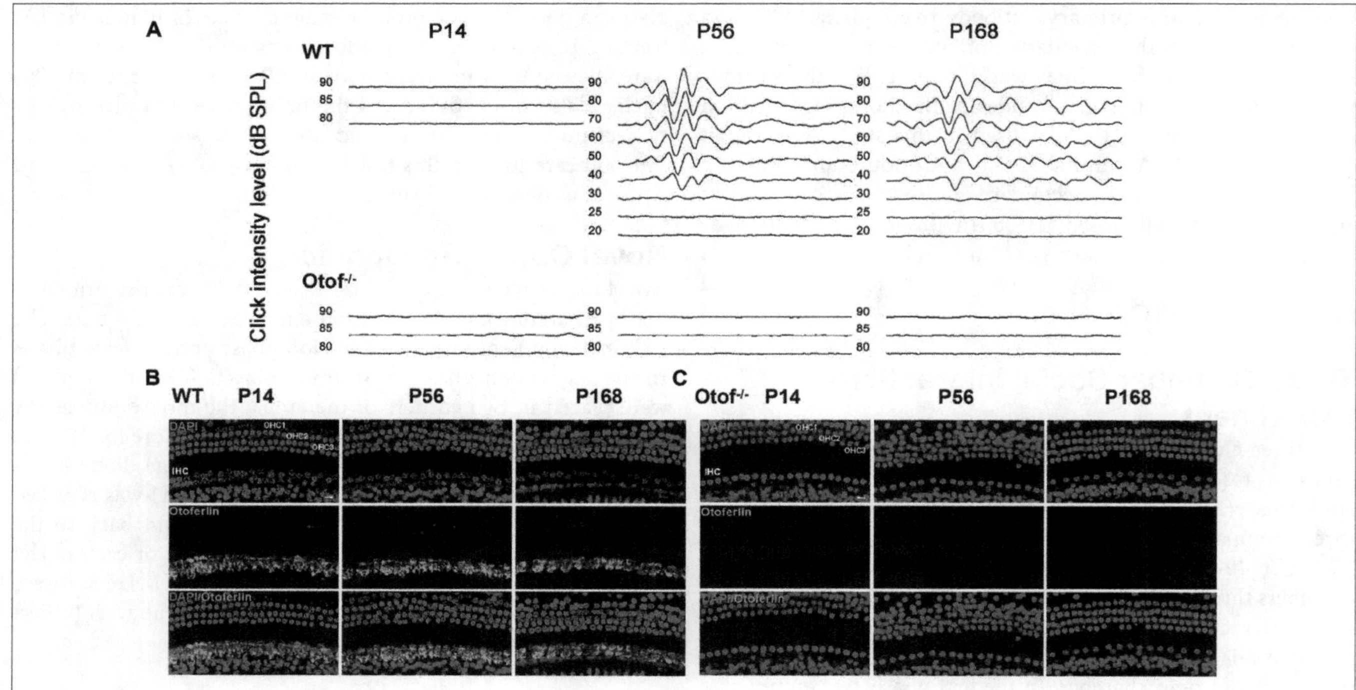

FIGURE 1 | Complete elimination of hearing input presented before and after hearing onset in Otof$^{-/-}$ mice. **(A)** No visible ABR waveforms (click) were found at P14, P56, and P168 in Otof$^{-/-}$ mice, respectively; also, no ABR waveforms (click) were seen at P14 in WT mice. However, there are normal ABR waveforms (click) at P56 and P168 in WT mice. **(B)** Normal otoferlin expressions were seen in cochlear inner hair cells (IHCs) at P14, P56, and P168 in WT mice (green). **(C)** No positive immunostaining signals were found at P14, P56, and P168 in Otof$^{-/-}$ mice. Bar = 10 μm; WT, wild-type mice; Otof$^{-/-}$, otoferlin knockout mice; dB, decibel.

and WT mice at P14, P56, and P168. There were no positive immunostaining signals in Otof$^{-/-}$ mice (**Figure 1C**), whereas normal expression was observed in the control ones (**Figure 1B**), confirming complete hearing elimination.

Elimination of Hearing Input Causes Impaired Social Memory

To explore whether HL can alter the hippocampal-dependent social interaction, a three-chamber social interaction experiment was used to sequentially test sociability and social novelty (**Figure 2A**). In this test, 2-month-old mice were allowed to explore either a chamber containing a stranger mouse (stranger 1, S1) restrained in a wire cage or the other chamber with an empty wire cage for 10 min. Both WT and deaf mice spent more time interacting with the S1 than the empty cage according to bilateral chambers (WT: 313.189 ± 22.303 vs. 91.147 ± 13.700 s, $n = 20$, $^{****}p < 0.0001$, t-test; Otof$^{-/-}$: 268.093 ± 17.306 vs. 147.071 ± 16.959 s, $n = 21$, $^{****}p < 0.0001$, t-test; **Figures 2B, C**) and close interaction measurements (WT: 281.170 ± 24.467 vs. 55.398 ± 7.569 s, $n = 20$, $^{****}p < 0.0001$, t-test; Otof$^{-/-}$: 191.996 ± 15.949 vs. 100.990 ± 16.590 s, $n = 21$, $^{***}p < 0.001$, t-test; **Figures 2B, C**), indicating that deaf mice also have similar sociability as WT mice. Immediately after the social interaction test, we placed another novel mouse (stranger 2, S2) into the previously empty cage. The subject mouse was allowed to explore the three chambers for another 10 min. Taking advantage of the natural novelty instincts in rodents, both in bilateral chambers and close interaction measurements, WT mice spent more time exploring the S2 than S1 (time in compartment: 244.259 ± 13.968 vs. 163.984 ± 13.008 s, $^{***}p < 0.001$, t-test; time in close interaction: 202.713 ± 15.540 vs. 123.043 ± 9.475 s,

TABLE 1 | Click and tone burst examinations in both WT and Otof$^{-/-}$ mice.

Intensity level (dB SPL)	Click	4 kHz	8 kHz	16 kHz	24 kHz
		WT			
90	Y	Y	Y	Y	Y
80	Y	Y	Y	Y	Y
70	Y	Y	Y	Y	Y
60	Y	Y	Y	Y	Y
50	Y	Y	Y	Y	Y
40	Y	Y	Y	Y	Y
30	Y	Y	Y	Y	Y
25	**Y**	**Y**	Y	Y	Y
20	N	N	Y	Y	Y
15			Y	Y	Y
10			**Y**	**Y**	**Y**
		Otof$^{-/-}$			
90	N	N	N	N	N
85	N	N	N	N	N
80	N	N	N	N	N

In WT mice, the thresholds of click and 4, 8, 16, and 32 kHz are 25, 25, 10, 10, and 10 dB SPL, respectively. In Otof$^{-/-}$ mice, no detectable thresholds are found at click, 4, 8, 16, and 32 kHz. Y means "Yes"; N means "No."

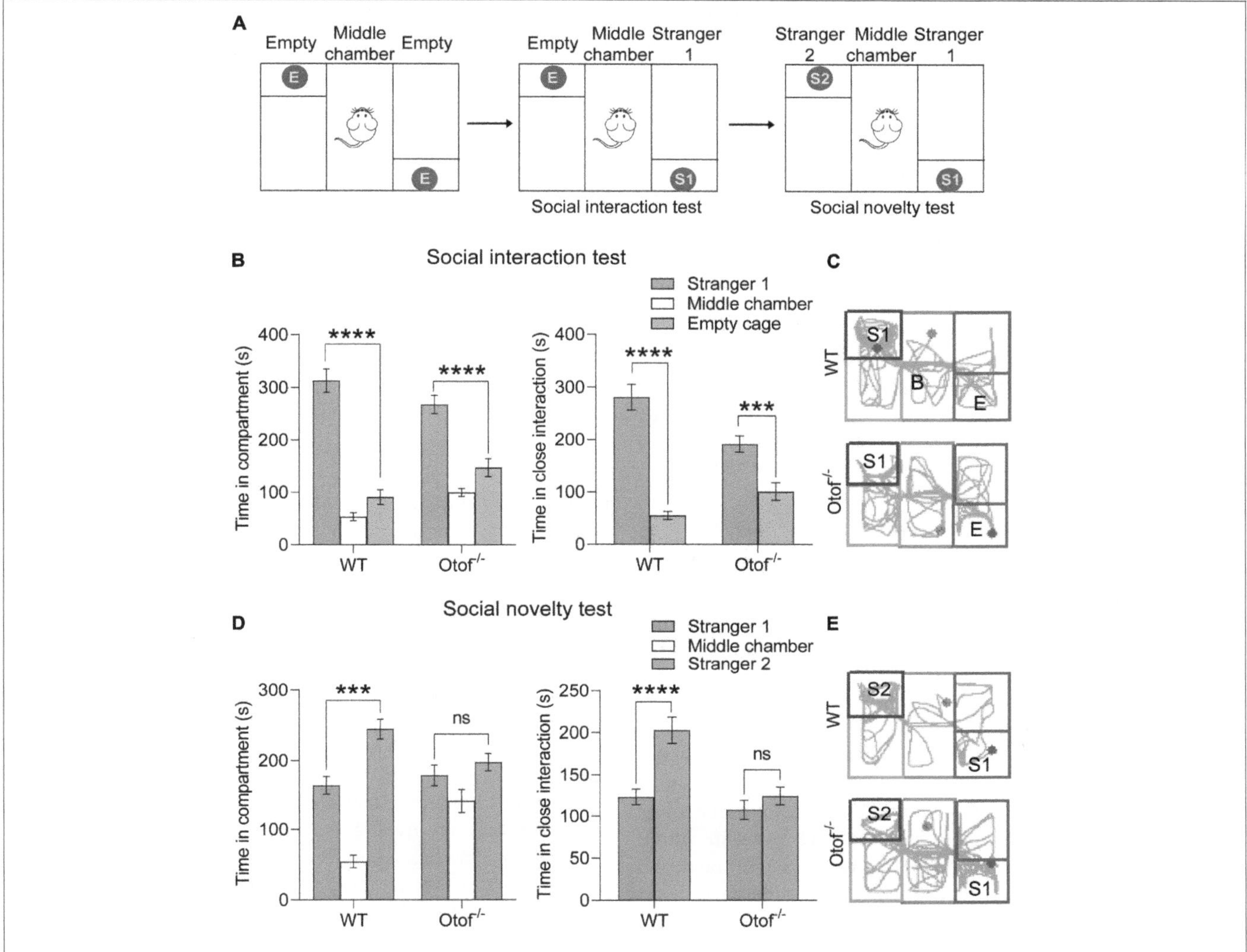

FIGURE 2 | Otof$^{-/-}$ mice showed impaired social memory in a three-chamber social interaction experiment at 2 months old. **(A)** The schematic diagram of a three-chamber social interaction experiment. **(B)** Both WT and Otof$^{-/-}$ mice showed normal sociability in the social interaction test: the subject mouse spent more time interacting with stranger 1 (S1) than the empty wire cage E. **(C)** Representative tracks of WT and Otof$^{-/-}$ mice in the social interaction test. **(D)** Otof$^{-/-}$ mice showed impaired social memory in the social novelty test compared with WT mice. **(E)** Representative tracks of WT and Otof$^{-/-}$ mice in the social novelty test. The starting point and the ending point of tracks in **(C,E)** were represented by a red dot and a green dot, respectively. All values are presented as mean ± SEM and analyzed by unpaired *t*-test for **(B)** and **(D)**. $^{***}p < 0.001$, $^{****}p < 0.0001$ vs. WT. WT: $n = 20$; Otof$^{-/-}$: $n = 21$. WT, wild-type mice; Otof$^{-/-}$, otoferlin knockout mice; E, empty; S1, stranger 1; S2, stranger 2; ns, not significant.

$^{****}p < 0.0001$, *t*-test; $n = 20$, **Figures 2D, E**). However, deaf mice spent comparable time between S1 and S2 without significant differences (time in compartment: 197.645 ± 12.500 vs. 178.459 ± 15.198 s, $p > 0.05$, *t*-test; time in close interaction: 124.299 ± 10.728 vs. 107.609 ± 11.491 s, $p > 0.05$, *t*-test; $n = 21$, **Figures 2D, E**). Thus, our study indicated that the social memory in deaf mice was significantly impaired.

Elimination of Hearing Input Causes Long-Lasting Impaired Social Memory

Although we have found the impaired social memory in this study, however, we still do not know whether the impairment of social memory is transient or long-lasting. We then performed a three-chamber test in both deaf and control mice at 6 months of age. Consistent with the previous results at 2 months, the deaf mice showed normal sociability in bilateral chambers (WT: 250.302 ± 6.883 vs. 160.178 ± 6.490 s, $n = 10$, $^{****}p < 0.0001$, *t*-test; Otof$^{-/-}$: 261.633 ± 17.249 vs. 143.451 ± 13.093 s, $n = 10$, $^{****}p < 0.0001$, *t*-test; **Figures 3A, B**) and close interaction (WT: 160.269 ± 9.927 vs. 88.121 ± 4.935 s, $n = 10$, $^{****}p < 0.0001$, *t*-test; Otof$^{-/-}$: 202.845 ± 19.163 vs. 74.424 ± 8.319 s, $n = 10$, $^{****}p < 0.0001$, *t*-test; **Figures 3A, B**). In the social novelty test, although WT mice were unable to display a time preference in bilateral chambers (time in compartment: 216.517 ± 16.661 vs. 177.134 ± 11.296 s, $n = 10$, $p > 0.05$, *t*-test; **Figures 3C, D**), they had a distinct preference for close social interaction (time in close interaction: 124.593 ± 12.547 vs. 89.195 ± 11.004 s, $n = 10$,

$^{*}p < 0.05$, t-test; **Figures 3C, D**). However, in this study, the deaf mice (age: 6 months) were still unable to distinguish the S2 from S1 in bilateral chambers (time in compartment: 202.872 ± 10.463 vs. 205.414 ± 18.567 s, $n = 10$, $p > 0.05$, t-test; **Figures 3C, D**) and close interaction (time in close interaction: 123.763 ± 11.396 vs. 128.570 ± 15.194 s, $n = 10$, $p > 0.05$, t-test; **Figures 3C,D**), suggesting a long-lasting impaired social memory in deaf mice.

Elimination of Hearing Input Is Unable to Affect Novel Object Recognition

To examine whether the HL affects the ability of object novelty, we carried out a novel object recognition test in both deaf and control mice at 2 months of age (**Figure 4A**). In this study, the DI showed that there is no significant difference between the groups. Deaf mice exhibited normal hippocampal-dependent object recognition capacity (5.771 ± 4.702 vs. 14.09 ± 6.346%, $p > 0.05$, t-test, WT: $n = 10$, Otof$^{-/-}$: $n = 14$; **Figure 4B**).

Elimination of Hearing Input Does Not Disrupt Spatial Learning and Memory

To explore whether the HL affects the capacity of spatial learning and memory, here, we use classic assessment of the MWM to estimate hippocampal-dependent spatial learning and memory in both deaf and control mice at 2 months of age. No significant differences in the visible platform test of escape latency (44.27 ± 2.868 vs. 41.42 ± 3.518 s, $p > 0.05$, t-test, WT: $n = 12$, Otof$^{-/-}$: $n = 17$; **Figure 5E**) and swimming speed (17.91 ± 0.3840 vs. 19.13 ± 0.5327 cm/s, $p > 0.05$, t-test, WT: $n = 12$, Otof$^{-/-}$: $n = 17$; **Figure 5F**) were found between both groups. Furthermore, no differences were found in escape latency in hidden platform training (**Figures 5A,B**). In the probe test after withdrawing platform, no significant differences were identified in the first-time arriving platform (31.03 ± 3.989 vs. 26.32 ± 5.092 s, $p > 0.05$, t-test, WT: $n = 12$, Otof$^{-/-}$: $n = 17$; **Figure 5C**) and the percentage of platform quadrant (22.01 ± 1.150 vs. 22.74 ± 1.409%, $p > 0.05$, t-test, WT: $n = 12$, Otof$^{-/-}$: $n = 17$; **Figure 5D**) between the two groups.

Elimination of Hearing Input Is Unable to Disrupt Locomotion in the Open Field

To exclude the possibility of motor alteration between the deaf and control mice groups, in this study, the open field testing was carried out to detect the locomotion distance (cm) and speed (cm/s) during a 5-min free exploration (**Figure 6**). No significant differences were found in the distance between the two groups, irrespective of age (2 months: 2,692 ± 163.2 vs. 2,597 ± 103.0 cm, $p > 0.05$, t-test, WT: $n = 15$, Otof$^{-/-}$: $n = 17$; 6 months: 2,672 ± 197.1 vs. 2,169 ± 159.8 cm, $p > 0.05$, t-test, WT: $n = 10$, Otof$^{-/-}$: $n = 10$; **Figures 6A, D**). Similarly, there was no significant difference in the mean speed (2 months: 9.897 ± 0.6342 vs. 10.44 ± 0.4822 cm/s, $p > 0.05$, t-test, WT: $n = 15$, Otof$^{-/-}$: $n = 17$; 6 months: 9.446 ± 0.7823 vs. 7.871 ± 0.4931 cm/s, $p > 0.05$, t-test, WT: $n = 10$, Otof$^{-/-}$: $n = 10$; **Figures 6B, E**), suggesting that HL is unable to affect spontaneous locomotor activity.

Otoferlin Expression Is Nearly Undetectable in the Hippocampus of WT Mouse Brain

It has been once reported that otoferlin could be expressed in the brain (Wu et al., 2015). In order to exclude the possible effects on the cognitive function that otoferlin may have, we then investigated the expression level of otoferlin in the hippocampus. We performed otoferlin staining on hippocampal slices, and we did not identify clear positive signals of otoferlin expression in both WT and Otof$^{-/-}$ mice (**Figure 7**), suggesting an excluded effect of hippocampal otoferlin expression on social memory.

DISCUSSION

In this study, we found that mice with auditory input elimination before hearing onset have impaired social memory and unimpaired sociability, novel object recognition, spatial learning, memory, and locomotor activity. This result shows that hearing input might be necessary to establish social memory in mice.

A significant number of studies have proposed that HL can lead to cognitive impairment, especially in the aspects of learning and memory (Beckmann et al., 2020; Griffiths et al., 2020; Slade et al., 2020). Under the impoverished auditory environments, HL patients have fewer chances to access normal social interactions. In addition, poor long-term social interactions are also risk factors for dementia (Kuiper et al., 2015). However, an investigation has been carried out to explore the relationships between HL and social memory; particularly, until today, no study has investigated the potential links between them using animal models. Therefore, to the best of our knowledge, this is the first study that focused on the relationship between the two via a congenital deaf mouse model, in which the peripheral hearing input was eliminated before its onset.

It has been fully reported that otoferlin is a critical synaptic protein, which specifically expresses in the inner hair cells (IHCs) of a mature cochlea (Roux et al., 2006). It interacts with SNARE to form a functional complex to account for neurotransmitter exocytosis at the ribbon synapses (Roux et al., 2006). Otof knockout or equivalent genetic manipulations can completely abolish neurotransmitter exocytosis, leading to profound HL (Yasunaga et al., 1999). In this study, we created a mouse strain with profound HL (the equivalent of Otof$^{-/-}$) through a point mutation approach (frameshift mutation). The Otof$^{-/-}$ mice were detected by ABR testing at the ages of P14, P56, and P168, respectively, and there were no visual ABR waveforms at any checking points. On the other hand, normal waveforms were seen in the control mice (**Figure 1A**). It is consistent with the hearing detection above; there are no positive immunostaining signals of otoferlin in the cochlear hair cells of Otof$^{-/-}$ mice (**Figure 1C**), compared with normal expression in control mice (**Figure 1B**), indicating that we obtained a suitable mice model for eliminating peripheral sound signal input before the onset of hearing. It has been reported that otoferlin could have an expression in the brain (Wu et al., 2015); however, we performed otoferlin immunostaining on hippocampal slices of WT mice, and we

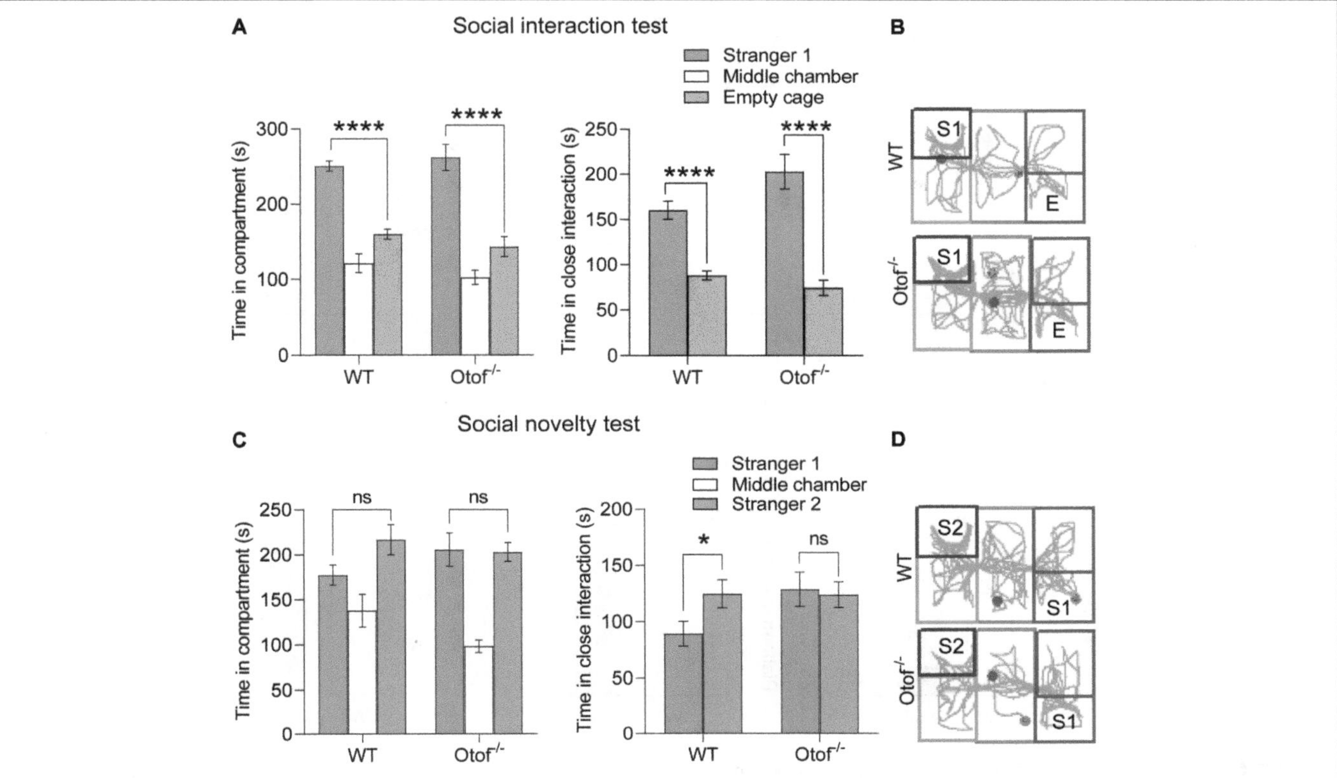

FIGURE 3 | Otof$^{-/-}$ mice showed impaired social memory in a three-chamber social interaction experiment at 6 months old. **(A)** WT and Otof$^{-/-}$ mice showed normal sociability in the social interaction test. **(B)** Representative tracks of WT and Otof$^{-/-}$ mice in the social interaction test. **(C)** Otof$^{-/-}$ mice showed impaired social memory in the social novelty test. **(D)** Representative tracks of WT and Otof$^{-/-}$ mice in the social novelty test. The starting point and the ending point of tracks in **(B,D)** were represented by a red dot and a green dot, respectively. All values are presented as mean ± SEM and analyzed by unpaired *t*-test for panels **(A,C)**. $^{*}p < 0.05$, $^{****}p < 0.0001$ vs. WT. WT: $n = 10$; Otof$^{-/-}$: $n = 10$. WT, wild-type mice; Otof$^{-/-}$, otoferlin knockout mice; E, empty; S1, stranger 1; S2, stranger 2; ns, not significant.

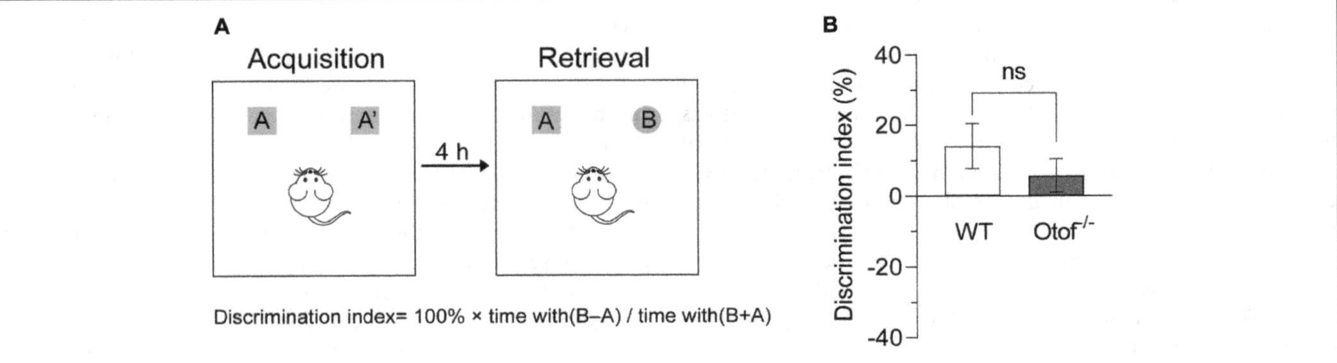

FIGURE 4 | Otof$^{-/-}$ mice showed unimpaired novel object recognition. **(A)** Experiment diagram of the novel object recognition test. **(B)** Compared with WT mice, Otof$^{-/-}$ mice showed a comparable object discrimination index (DI). All values are presented as mean ± SEM and analyzed by unpaired *t*-test. WT: $n = 11$; Otof$^{-/-}$: $n = 14$. WT, wild-type mice; Otof$^{-/-}$, otoferlin knockout mice; ns, not significant.

did not identify clear positive signals of otoferlin expression. In addition, it was reported that in an *in vitro* experiment, a deficiency of otoferlin in hippocampal neurons does not impair its presynaptic exocytosis function (Reisinger et al., 2011). Thus, our study excluded the possible effect that otof knockout in hippocampal neurons could disrupt social memory.

Social communication in rodents primarily depends on auditory, olfactory, and tactile feedback. Deprivation of sound information reduces the communication capacity and attenuates social memory. Somatosensory experiences can reorganize the cortical neural plasticity; similarly, cortical plasticity could be disrupted by long-term sensory deprivation

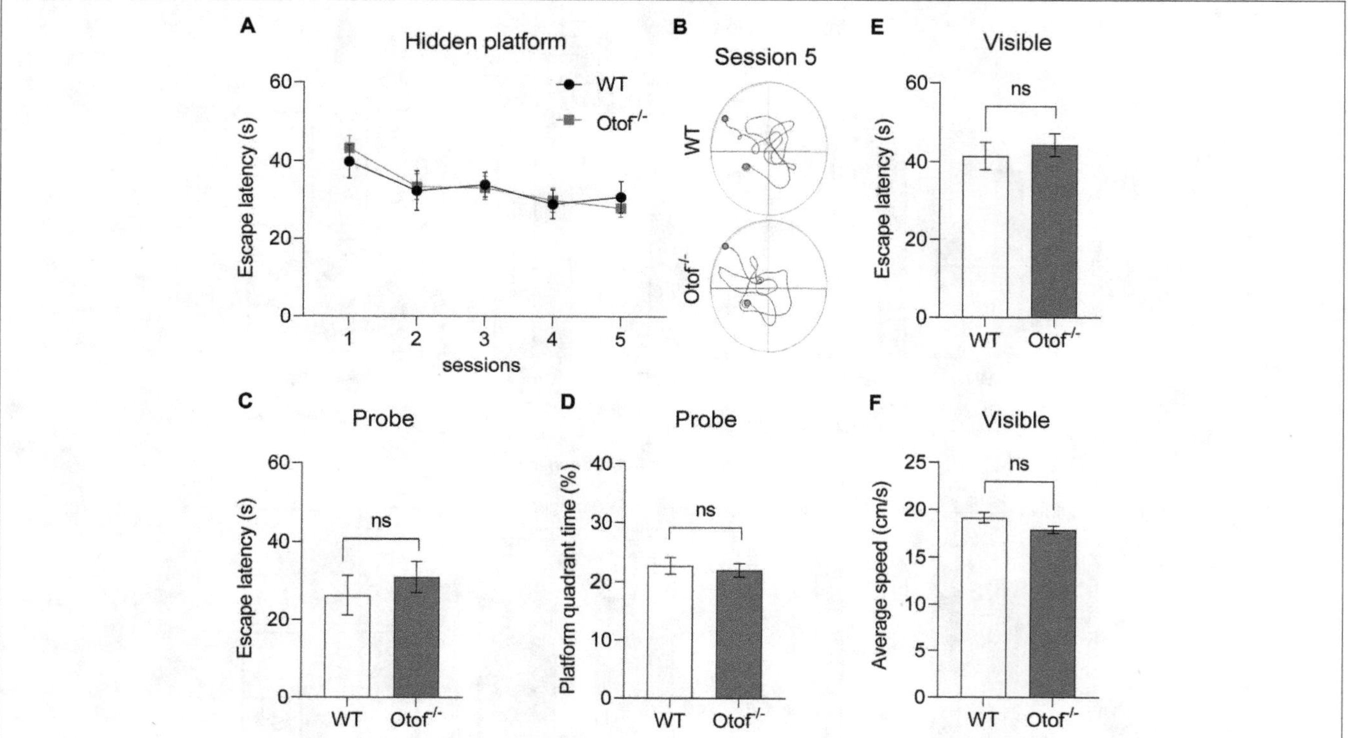

FIGURE 5 | Otof$^{-/-}$ mice showed normal spatial learning and memory in the Morris water maze (MWM). **(A)** The escape latency (time to find the hidden platform) recorded in training sessions. **(B)** Representative swimming trace of WT and Otof$^{-/-}$ mice in session 5. **(C)** The escape latency (s) in the probe. **(D)** The percent time (%) in the platform quadrant in the probe. **(E)** The escape latency (s) in the visible platform period. **(F)** The average swimming speed (cm/s) in the visible platform period. All values are presented as mean ± SEM and analyzed by unpaired *t*-test for **(C–F)** and two-way ANOVA for panel **(A)** vs. WT. WT: $n = 12$; Otof$^{-/-}$: $n = 17$. WT, wild-type mice; Otof$^{-/-}$, otoferlin knockout mice; ns, not significant.

(Merabet and Pascual-Leone, 2010). Our previous study showed that aberrant neural activity in the central auditory pathway is often accompanied by abnormal neural activity in the limbic system, especially in the hippocampus and amygdala. Therefore, it could have a functional connectivity between the central auditory pathway and the limbic system (Qu et al., 2019). It has been proposed that neuropsychiatric disorders may have social memory deficits, such as schizophrenia and autism (Meltzer et al., 1996). Thus, HL can induce alterations in social circuit neuroplasticity.

The hippocampal dorsal CA2 (dCA2) has been proved as an essential subfield in social memory (Hitti and Siegelbaum, 2014). The CA2 is highly expressed with the vasopressin 1b (Avpr1b) receptor (Young et al., 2006), and the knockout of Avpr1b results in social memory impairment (Wersinger et al., 2002; DeVito et al., 2009), whereas targeted activation of CA2 Avpr 1b during the acquisition period could enhance social memory (Smith et al., 2016), demonstrating their association. Dorsal CA2 projects to ventral CA1 (vCA1) (Meira et al., 2018), which then projects to the nucleus accumbens (NAc) also contributing to social memory storage, and vCA1 neurons greatly respond to familiar conspecifics than a novel mouse in the social memory test (Okuyama et al., 2016). Social isolation was shown to decrease the number of parvalbumin interneurons in the vCA1 and then disrupt social memory retrieval in mice (Deng et al., 2019). vCA1 projection to the medial prefrontal cortex (mPFC) and the NAc also play a critical role in social memory recall (Phillips et al., 2019; Xing et al., 2021). However, little is known about the underlying mechanism of how hearing deprivation disrupts neural circuits engaged in social memory. In this study, we completely eliminated hearing input from the cochlea to the brain and demonstrated that hearing input is truly necessary for the development of social memory. We hypothesize that hearing deprivation may reorganize functional connectivity between the auditory pathway and social memory circuit, resulting in negative effects on associated brain regions, such as the hippocampus (dCA2, vCA1), mPFC, NAc, and amygdala (Kwon et al., 2021). Also, HL can partially induce chronic inactivation of social memory-related networks, which in turn leads to discrimination failure between familiar and novel conspecifics in deaf mice. However, the underlying mechanism requires further investigation.

In our study, the deaf mice showed normal hippocampal-dependent spatial memory and novel object recognition, indicating that HL may have no significant effects on these targeted functions. However, some studies have shown that hearing impairment in adult rodents, induced by noise exposure, can impair hippocampal-dependent spatial learning and memory through decreased neurogenesis (Kraus et al., 2010; Liu et al., 2016, 2018; Zhuang et al., 2020). A possible explanation is

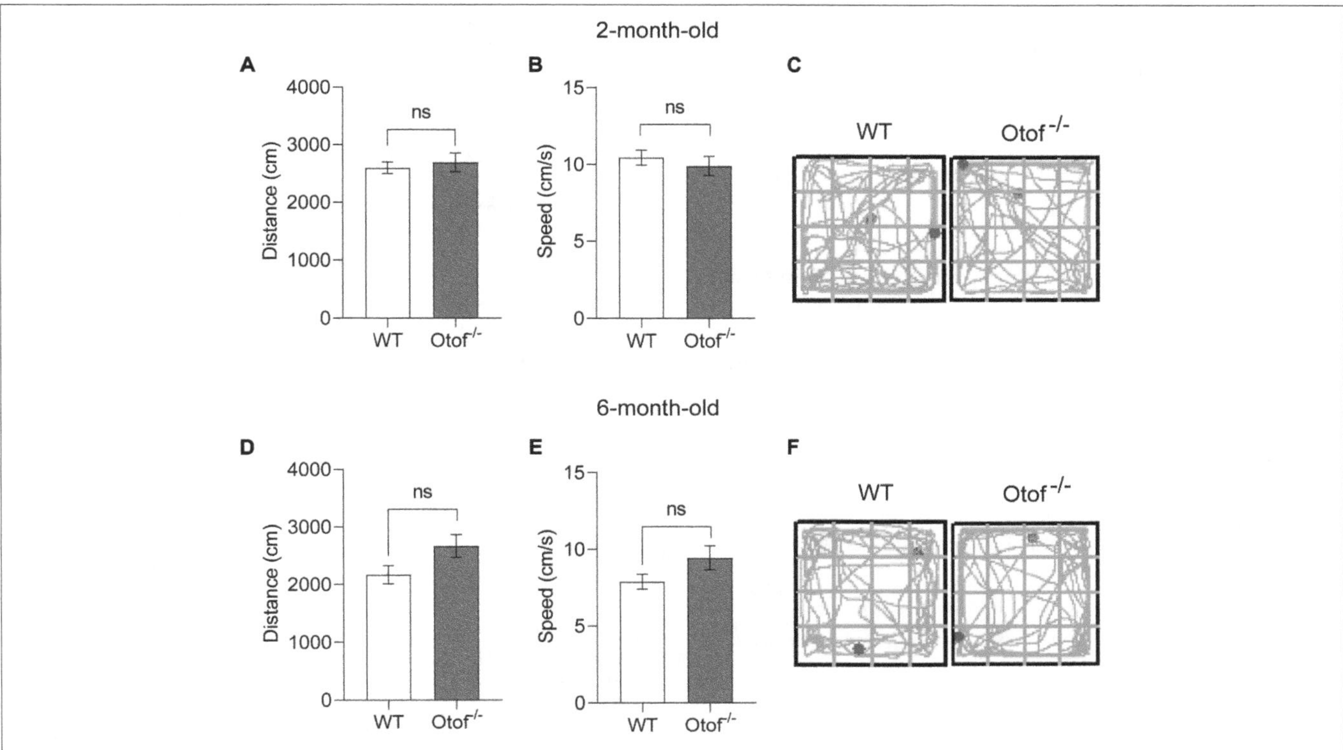

FIGURE 6 | Otof$^{-/-}$ mice showed normal motor ability in the open field ($L \times W$: 50 × 50 cm) at the ages of 2 and 6 months. **(A,D)** In the open field, there was no significant difference in the exploration distance (cm) between WT and Otof$^{-/-}$ mice group. **(B,E)** WT and Otof$^{-/-}$ mice showed no significant difference of speed (cm/s). **(C,F)** Representative exploration traces of WT mice and Otof$^{-/-}$ mice. The starting point and ending point of tracks in panels **(C,F)** were represented by a red dot and a green dot, respectively. All values are presented as mean ± SEM and analyzed by unpaired t-test for panels **(A,B,D,E)**. 2-month-old: WT, n = 15; Otof$^{-/-}$, n = 17. 6-month-old: WT, n = 10; Otof$^{-/-}$, n = 10. WT, wild-type mice; Otof$^{-/-}$, otoferlin knockout mice; ns, not significant.

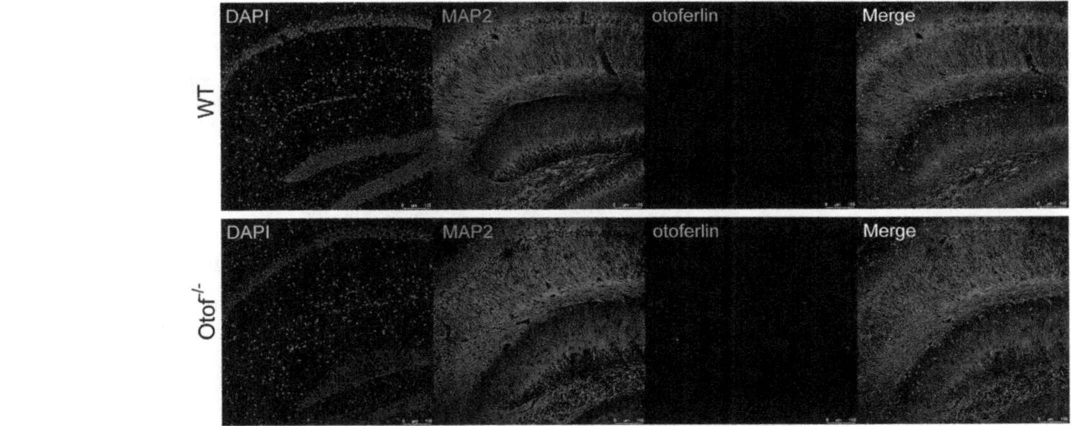

FIGURE 7 | Otoferlin staining in the hippocampus of WT and Otof$^{-/-}$ mice. Immunofluorescence of WT and Otof$^{-/-}$ hippocampus slices with otoferlin (green), MAP2 (red), and DAPI (blue). WT, wild-type mice; Otof$^{-/-}$, otoferlin knockout mice. Scale bars: 100 μm.

that, in our study, auditory input has been entirely eliminated before the onset of hearing through genetic manipulation, and the reorganization of neural circuits occurred in its critical period in early development and thus exhibited normal general hippocampus functions by employing more cognitive resources during development. By contrast, noise trauma only reduced or destroyed hearing function in adult mice, which could have greatly disrupted the development of hippocampal-dependent spatial learning and memory in mice. Moreover, before the noise exposure, these mice still had the capacity to sense and deliver hearing input from the cochlea to the brain. Nonetheless, our results are consistent with those of a previous study indicating that HL in middle age is more likely to induce dementia (Griffiths et al., 2020). Our study has a significant limitation of not identifying the neural mechanism that is responsible for the association between HL and social memory impairment, and further studies addressing this issue need to be conducted.

CONCLUSION

Our study found through a three-chamber social interaction assay that deprivation of peripheral auditory input before the onset of hearing can lead to social memory impairment in mice. Furthermore, we verified the relationship between hearing stimuli and hippocampal-associated cognitive function. Taken together, our findings demonstrated that hearing input is required for social memory since the initial development of hearing function in mice. In this study, we have established a mouse model with complete elimination of hearing input in the early stage of development. Prospectively, different types of mouse model with a distinct degree of HL might be applied to investigate the mechanisms underlying the associations of hearing input and memory.

AUTHOR CONTRIBUTIONS

YL and KL contributed to the design of the study, analyzed and interpreted the result, and wrote the manuscript. SG contributed to the design of the study. YL and RG performed the experiments and analyzed the data. JL contributed to the data collection. All authors reviewed and approved the final version of the manuscript.

ACKNOWLEDGMENTS

We thank Jingjing Wang as well as Shuang Zhang for providing the public laboratory platform for behavioral experiments.

REFERENCES

Armstrong, N. M., An, Y., Doshi, J., Erus, G., Ferrucci, L., Davatzikos, C., et al. (2019). Association of Midlife Hearing Impairment With Late-Life Temporal Lobe Volume Loss. *JAMA Otolaryngol. Head Neck Surg.* 145, 794–802. doi: 10.1001/jamaoto.2019.1610

Barbara, J. A., and Contreras, M. (1985). Mortality of HBsAg positive blood donors. *Lancet* 1:641. doi: 10.1016/s0140-6736(85)92178-6

Beckmann, D., Feldmann, M., Shchyglo, O., and Manahan-Vaughan, D. (2020). Hippocampal Synaptic Plasticity, Spatial Memory, and Neurotransmitter Receptor Expression Are Profoundly Altered by Gradual Loss of Hearing Ability. *Cereb. Cortex* 30, 4581–4596. doi: 10.1093/cercor/bhaa061

Deng, X., Gu, L., Sui, N., Guo, J., and Liang, J. (2019). Parvalbumin interneuron in the ventral hippocampus functions as a discriminator in social memory. *Proc. Natl. Acad. Sci. U. S. A.* 116, 16583–16592. doi: 10.1073/pnas.1819133116

DeVito, L. M., Konigsberg, R., Lykken, C., Sauvage, M., Young, W. S. III., and Eichenbaum, H. (2009). Vasopressin 1b receptor knock-out impairs memory for temporal order. *J. Neurosci.* 29, 2676–2683. doi: 10.1523/JNEUROSCI.5488-08.2009

Griffiths, T., Lad, M., Kumar, S., Holmes, E., McMurray, B., Maguire, E., et al. (2020). How Can Hearing Loss Cause Dementia? *Neuron* 108, 401–412. doi: 10.1016/j.neuron.2020.08.003

Haile, L. M., Kamenov, K., Briant, P. S., Orji, A. U., Steinmetz, J. D., Abdoli, A., et al. (2021). Hearing loss prevalence and years lived with disability, 1990-2019: findings from the Global Burden of Disease Study 2019. *Lancet* 397, 996–1009. doi: 10.1016/s0140-6736(21)00516-x

Hitti, F. L., and Siegelbaum, S. A. (2014). The hippocampal CA2 region is essential for social memory. *Nature* 508, 88–92. doi: 10.1038/nature13028

Hughes, S. E., Hutchings, H. A., Rapport, F. L., McMahon, C. M., and Boisvert, I. (2018). Social Connectedness and perceived listening effort in adult cochlear implant users: a grounded theory to establish content validity for a new patient-reported outcome measure. *Ear Hear* 39, 922–934. doi: 10.1097/AUD.0000000000000553

Hunt, R., Girskis, K., Rubenstein, J., Alvarez-Buylla, A., and Baraban, S. (2013). GABA progenitors grafted into the adult epileptic brain control seizures and abnormal behavior. *Nat. Neurosci.* 16, 692–697. doi: 10.1038/nn.3392

Kraus, K. S., Mitra, S., Jimenez, Z., Hinduja, S., Ding, D., Jiang, H., et al. (2010). Noise trauma impairs neurogenesis in the rat hippocampus. *Neuroscience* 167, 1216–1226. doi: 10.1016/j.neuroscience.2010.02.071

Kuiper, J. S., Zuidersma, M., Oude Voshaar, R. C., Zuidema, S. U., van den Heuvel, E. R., Stolk, R. P., et al. (2015). Social relationships and risk of dementia: a systematic review and meta-analysis of longitudinal cohort studies. *Ageing Res. Rev.* 22, 39–57. doi: 10.1016/j.arr.2015.04.006

Kwon, J. T., Ryu, C., Lee, H., Sheffield, A., Fan, J., Cho, D. H., et al. (2021). An amygdala circuit that suppresses social engagement. *Nature* 593, 114–118. doi: 10.1038/s41586-021-03413-6

Liu, L., Shen, P., He, T., Chang, Y., Shi, L., Tao, S., et al. (2016). Noise induced hearing loss impairs spatial learning/memory and hippocampal neurogenesis in mice. *Sci. Rep.* 6:20374. doi: 10.1038/srep20374

Liu, L., Xuan, C., Shen, P., He, T., Chang, Y., Shi, L., et al. (2018). Hippocampal Mechanisms Underlying Impairment in Spatial Learning Long After Establishment of Noise-Induced Hearing Loss in CBA Mice. *Front. Syst. Neurosci.* 12:35. doi: 10.3389/fnsys.2018.00035

Livingston, G., Sommerlad, A., Orgeta, V., Costafreda, S., Huntley, J., Ames, D., et al. (2017). Dementia prevention, intervention, and care. *Lancet* 390, 2673–2734. doi: 10.1016/s0140-6736(17)31363-6

Loughrey, D., Kelly, M., Kelley, G., Brennan, S., and Lawlor, B. (2018). Association of Age-Related hearing loss with cognitive function, cognitive impairment, and dementia: a Systematic review and meta-analysis. *JAMA otolaryngol. Head Neck Surg.* 144, 115–126. doi: 10.1001/jamaoto.2017.2513

Meira, T., Leroy, F., Buss, E. W., Oliva, A., Park, J., and Siegelbaum, S. A. (2018). A hippocampal circuit linking dorsal CA2 to ventral CA1 critical for social memory dynamics. *Nat. Commun.* 9:4163. doi: 10.1038/s41467-018-06501-w

Meltzer, H. Y., Thompson, P. A., Lee, M. A., and Ranjan, R. (1996). Neuropsychologic deficits in schizophrenia: relation to social function and effect of antipsychotic drug treatment. *Neuropsychopharmacology* 14, 27S–33S. doi: 10.1016/0893-133X(95)00202-O

Merabet, L. B., and Pascual-Leone, A. (2010). Neural reorganization following sensory loss: the opportunity of change. *Nat. Rev. Neurosci.* 11, 44–52. doi: 10.1038/nrn2758

Okuyama, T., Kitamura, T., Roy, D. S., Itohara, S., and Tonegawa, S. (2016). Ventral CA1 neurons store social memory. *Science* 353, 1536–1541. doi: 10.1126/science.aaf7003

Phillips, M. L., Robinson, H. A., and Pozzo-Miller, L. (2019). Ventral hippocampal projections to the medial prefrontal cortex regulate social memory. *Elife* 8:e44182. doi: 10.7554/eLife.44182

Qu, T., Qi, Y., Yu, S., Du, Z., Wei, W., Cai, A., et al. (2019). Dynamic Changes of Functional Neuronal Activities Between the Auditory Pathway and Limbic Systems Contribute to Noise-Induced Tinnitus with a Normal Audiogram. *Neuroscience* 408, 31–45. doi: 10.1016/j.neuroscience.2019.03.054

Reisinger, E., Bresee, C., Neef, J., Nair, R., Reuter, K., Bulankina, A., et al. (2011). Probing the functional equivalence of otoferlin and synaptotagmin 1 in exocytosis. *J. Neurosci.* 31, 4886–4895. doi: 10.1523/jneurosci.5122-10.2011

Roux, I., Safieddine, S., Nouvian, R., Grati, M., Simmler, M. C., Bahloul, A., et al. (2006). Otoferlin, defective in a human deafness form, is essential for exocytosis at the auditory ribbon synapse. *Cell* 127, 277–289. doi: 10.1016/j.cell.2006.08.040

Slade, K., Plack, C. J., and Nuttall, H. E. (2020). The Effects of Age-Related Hearing Loss on the Brain and Cognitive Function. *Trends Neurosci.* 43, 810–821. doi: 10.1016/j.tins.2020.07.005

Smith, A. S., Williams Avram, S. K., Cymerblit-Sabba, A., Song, J., and Young, W. S. (2016). Targeted activation of the hippocampal CA2 area strongly enhances social memory. *Mol. Psychiatry* 21, 1137–1144. doi: 10.1038/mp.2015.189

Taljaard, D., Olaithe, M., Brennan-Jones, C., Eikelboom, R., and Bucks, R. (2016). The relationship between hearing impairment and cognitive function: a meta-analysis in adults. *Clin. Otolaryngol.* 41, 718–729. doi: 10.1111/coa.12607

Wang, C., Liu, H., Li, K., Wu, Z., Wu, C., Yu, J., et al. (2020). Tactile modulation of memory and anxiety requires dentate granule cells along the dorsoventral axis. *Nat. Commun.* 11:6045. doi: 10.1038/s41467-020-19874-8

Wang, S., Tan, N., Zhu, X., Yao, M., Wang, Y., Zhang, X., et al. (2018). Sh3rf2 haploinsufficiency leads to unilateral neuronal development deficits and autistic-like behaviors in mice. *Cell Reports* 25, 2963–2971.e2966. doi: 10.1016/j.celrep.2018.11.044

Wersinger, S. R., Ginns, E. I., O'Carroll, A. M., Lolait, S. J., and Young, W. S. III. (2002). Vasopressin V1b receptor knockout reduces aggressive behavior in male mice. *Mol. Psychiatry* 7, 975–984. doi: 10.1038/sj.mp.4001195

Wu, W., Rahman, M., Guo, J., Roy, N., Xue, L., Cahill, C., et al. (2015). Function coupling of otoferlin with GAD65 acts to modulate GABAergic activity. *J. Mol. Cell Biol.* 7, 168–179. doi: 10.1093/jmcb/mjv011

Xing, B., Mack, N. R., Guo, K. M., Zhang, Y. X., Ramirez, B., Yang, S. S., et al. (2021). A Subpopulation of Prefrontal Cortical Neurons Is Required for Social Memory. *Biol. Psychiatry* 89, 521–531. doi: 10.1016/j.biopsych.2020.08.023

Yasunaga, S., Grati, M., Cohen-Salmon, M., El-Amraoui, A., Mustapha, M., Salem, N., et al. (1999). A mutation in OTOF, encoding otoferlin, a FER-1-like protein, causes DFNB9, a nonsyndromic form of deafness. *Nat. Genet.* 21, 363–369. doi: 10.1038/7693

Young, W. S., Li, J., Wersinger, S. R., and Palkovits, M. (2006). The vasopressin 1b receptor is prominent in the hippocampal area CA2 where it is unaffected by restraint stress or adrenalectomy. *Neuroscience* 143, 1031–1039. doi: 10.1016/j.neuroscience.2006.08.040

Zhuang, H., Yang, J., Huang, Z., Liu, H., Li, X., Zhang, H., et al. (2020). Accelerated age-related decline in hippocampal neurogenesis in mice with noise-induced hearing loss is associated with hippocampal microglial degeneration. *Aging* 12, 19493–19519. doi: 10.18632/aging.103898

15

Unilateral Conductive Hearing Loss Disrupts the Developmental Refinement of Binaural Processing in the Rat Primary Auditory Cortex

*Jing Liu, Xinyi Huang and Jiping Zhang**

Key Laboratory of Brain Functional Genomics, Ministry of Education, NYU-ECNU Institute of Brain and Cognitive Science at NYU Shanghai, School of Life Sciences, East China Normal University, Shanghai, China

Correspondence:
Jiping Zhang
jpzhang@bio.ecnu.edu.cn

Binaural hearing is critically important for the perception of sound spatial locations. The primary auditory cortex (AI) has been demonstrated to be necessary for sound localization. However, after hearing onset, how the processing of binaural cues by AI neurons develops, and how the binaural processing of AI neurons is affected by reversible unilateral conductive hearing loss (RUCHL), are not fully elucidated. Here, we determined the binaural processing of AI neurons in four groups of rats: postnatal day (P) 14–18 rats, P19–30 rats, P57–70 adult rats, and RUCHL rats (P57–70) with RUCHL during P14–30. We recorded the responses of AI neurons to both monaural and binaural stimuli with variations in interaural level differences (ILDs) and average binaural levels. We found that the monaural response types, the binaural interaction types, and the distributions of the best ILDs of AI neurons in P14–18 rats are already adult-like. However, after hearing onset, there exist developmental refinements in the binaural processing of AI neurons, which are exhibited by the increase in the degree of binaural interaction, and the increase in the sensitivity and selectivity to ILDs. RUCHL during early hearing development affects monaural response types, decreases the degree of binaural interactions, and decreases both the selectivity and sensitivity to ILDs of AI neurons in adulthood. These new evidences help us to understand the refinements and plasticity in the binaural processing of AI neurons during hearing development, and might enhance our understanding in the neuronal mechanism of developmental changes in auditory spatial perception.

Keywords: unilateral conductive hearing loss, binaural processing, binaural interaction, auditory cortex, interaural level differences, rats

---

Abbreviations: UCHL, unilateral conductive hearing loss; RUCHL, reversible unilateral conductive hearing loss; AI, primary auditory cortex; ABL, average binaural level; ILD, interaural level difference; ITD, interaural time difference; CF, characteristic frequency; P, postnatal day; PILDR, preferred ILD range; PILDR75, the PILDR over which the normalized response strength was 0.75; PILDR50, the PILDR over which the normalized response strength was 0.5; ABR, auditory brainstem response.

INTRODUCTION

The central auditory system receives, integrates, and analyses inputs from the two ears. This binaural processing contributes to localizing the sound source (Middlebrooks, 2015), separating the target sound from competing noisy background (Middlebrooks and Waters, 2020), and improving speech perception in noise (Hawley et al., 2004). The perception of acoustic space in humans exhibits developmental changes in sound localization accuracy and auditory spatial discrimination (Van Deun et al., 2009; Kuhnle et al., 2013), and it develops from an initially imprecise representation of spatial positions in infants and young children to a concise representation in young adults (Kuhnle et al., 2013; Freigang et al., 2015). In addition, the sensitivity to binaural cues in human is evident early in life (Bundy, 1980) and reaches adult-like behavior by 4–5 years of age (Van Deun et al., 2009). It is generally believed that the binaural cues for the perception of the sound-source location in horizontal plane are the interaural time differences (ITDs) and interaural level differences (ILDs), and the ILDs provide the major cue for the horizontal location of high-frequency sounds (Middlebrooks, 2015). Animal studies have shown the importance of binaural processing in sound localization, e.g., the sound localization accuracy can be disrupted when one ear was occluded with an earplug (Potash and Kelly, 1980; Keating et al., 2015). However, the neural mechanism for the normal development of binaural processing is still not fully understood.

The primary auditory cortex (AI) has been demonstrated to be necessary for binaural processing. Lesion or inactivation of AI leads to sound localization deficits (Malhotra and Lomber, 2007; Nodal et al., 2010). AI neurons have been shown to be sensitivity to sound-source azimuth in cats (Samson et al., 1994), monkeys (Woods et al., 2006), bats (Razak, 2011), ferrets (Wood et al., 2019), and rats (Yao et al., 2013; Gao et al., 2018; Wang et al., 2019). The spatial sensitivity of AI neurons to sound-source azimuth largely depends on binaural processing. Abnormal inputs from the two ears disrupt the tuning of AI neurons to sound-source azimuth (Samson et al., 1994; Wang et al., 2019). The binaural cues are first computed in the superior olive complex (Grothe et al., 2010), and the ILDs are further processed in the inferior colliculus (Semple and Kitzes, 1987) and auditory cortex (Zhang et al., 2004). Based on the spiking responses of AI neurons to monaural and binaural stimuli at corresponding stimulus levels, the integrations of the inputs from both ears are often categorized into facilitatory, inhibitory, and mixed binaural interactions (Irvine et al., 1996; Zhang et al., 2004). These studies on the binaural processing in AI focused on the adult animals. Studies using auditory evoked potentials to measure the binaural interaction of newborn infants have demonstrated immature binaural interactions at brainstem (Cone-Wesson et al., 1997) and auditory cortex (Nemeth et al., 2015). However, at single neuron level, how the binaural processing in AI develops after hearing onset is not fully elucidated.

After the onset of hearing, the auditory cortex undergoes developmental refinements in the tonotopic map of sound frequency (Zhang et al., 2001), and in the spectral and temporal response selectivity (Chang et al., 2005; Zhao et al., 2015; Cai et al., 2018). The role of inhibition contributes to the progressive maturation in frequency tuning (Chang et al., 2005) and temporal processing (Cai et al., 2018). The pace of cortical synaptic receptive field development is set by progressive, experience-dependent refinement of intracortical inhibition (Dorrn et al., 2010) or a fine adjustment of excitatory input strength (Sun et al., 2010). As the sound localization ability improves from infants to young adults, we hypothesize that the binaural processing which contributes to sound localization might also undergo a progressive refinement in AI at single neuron level after hearing onset.

Humans with unilateral conductive hearing loss (UCHL), such as congenital UCHL and otitis media with effusion in early childhood, show persistent binaural hearing deficits after corrective surgery (Pillsbury et al., 1991; Wilmington et al., 1994). Neurophysiology studies have shown that chronic UCHL in rats from early onset of hearing disrupts the normal spatial azimuth tuning of AI neurons in adulthood (Wang et al., 2019). Monaural deprivation in young rats enhances the responsiveness of inputs from the developmentally opened ipsilateral ear in AI and disrupts the binaural integration of ILD (Popescu and Polley, 2010). In addition, brief UCHL at young age disrupts the normal coregistration of interaural frequency tuning and ILD sensitivity in the mice AI (Polley et al., 2013). These studies have enhanced our understanding of how UCHL at young age induces the experience-dependent plasticity in AI. Otitis media with effusion often induces UCHL in human infants (Hogan et al., 1997), and the binaural hearing abilities was not completely restored even if the hearing threshold returned to normal after corrective surgery for the UCHL (Pillsbury et al., 1991). Until now, whether and how the reversible UCHL (RUCHL) at young age affects the developmental refinement of binaural processing in the adult AI is not fully understood.

In the present study, we first investigated the developmental refinement of binaural processing in AI by determining and comparing the monaural response types and the binaural processing properties (i.e., the binaural interaction types, the degree of binaural interactions, the sensitivity and selectivity to ILDs) of AI neurons among different age groups of rats with normal hearing development. We then studied the effects of RUCHL at young age on the binaural processing of AI neurons in adulthood by comparing the binaural response properties of AI neurons between the normal developing adult rats and the RUCHL rats in adulthood. We have demonstrated that there exists a developmental refinement of binaural processing in AI after hearing onset, and that RUCHL at young age disrupts the developmental refinement of binaural processing in AI.

MATERIALS AND METHODS

Animals and Animal Groups

Four groups of Sprague–Dawley rats were used: (1) group 1, postnatal day (P) 14–18 rats (n = 45), the ages of these rats were within 1 week after hearing onset (usually at P12); (2) group 2, P19–P30 rats (n = 53); (3) group 3, P57–P70 adult rats (n = 47); (4) group 4, RUCHL rats (n = 60, P57–70) with UCHL only during P14–30. Rats in groups 1–3 had normal binaural hearing development. For convenience, we randomly picked the rats with different ages and assigned them to the four groups from P14, i.e., the P14–18 group, the P19–30 group, the adult group, and the RUCHL group, respectively. The adult group was also used as the control to study the effects of RUCHL at young age on the binaural processing of AI neurons in adulthood. The rats were bred in-house from Sprague–Dawley breeding pairs purchased from Shanghai Jie Si Jie Laboratory Animal Co., Ltd., (Shanghai, China). The rat pups were raised with their parents until P26. All rats had free access to food and water, and were reared in the housing environments (20–24°C temperature) with 12-h light-dark cycles.

For the rats in the RUCHL group, unilateral middle ear poloxamer hydrogel injections adapted from a previous study were made to induce RUCHL at young age (Polley et al., 2013). Briefly, after the P14 rats were anesthetized by Nembutal (50 mg/kg, i.p.), a slit in the right tragus was made to better visualize the tympanic membrane in the right ear. A small hole was made in the pars flaccid to allow the injection of poloxamer 407 solutions through a glass capillary with about 15 μm tip in diameter. The blunt end of the glass capillary was attached to the syringe infusion set, and the syringe was filled with a 30% (w/w) solutions of poloxamer 407 and blue dye. About 10 μl poloxamer solutions (around 4°C) were injected to the middle ear to fill the middle-ear cavity under an operating microscope. Additional two injections of 5 μl poloxamer 407 solutions were done at P16 and P18, respectively. The poloxamer 407 solutions rapidly transitioned to gels in the middle ear cavity at body temperature after injection, which induced a conductive hearing loss at the injected ear. The poloxamer 407 gels spontaneously dissolved through hydrolysis several days later, and the thresholds of auditory brainstem response (ABR) were fully resolved 14–15 days after the initial poloxamer injection (Polley et al., 2013). In this way, this method provides us a convenient way to induce RUCHL in rats. We determined the hearing threshold of each ear by measuring the ABR wave I threshold. For a small number of rats (n = 11), ABR measurements were conducted for each ear at P14–P30 with an interval of 2 days. For all the rats in the RUCHL group, ABR measurements were conducted for each ear on the days of injection and P30. At P30, the hearing threshold of the injected ear was considered to be recovered to normal levels if the ABR threshold difference between the injected ear and the normal control ear of a rat was less than 5 dB. These rats were raised until adulthood, and they constituted the RUCHL group of rats.

Acoustical Stimulus Presentation System

Acoustic stimulus presentation were performed through TDT System 3 hardware and software (Tucker-Davis Technologies, United States) controlled by a PC. The hardware for acoustic stimulus presentation includes a multifunction processor (RX6-A5), a stereo power amplifier (SA1), and two multi-field magnetic speakers (MF1). All acoustic stimuli were delivered to ears via a close-field system. The speakers (MF1) were incorporated internal parabolic cones and coupled to the ears through 9.5-cm-long PVC plastic tubes (1/16 inch ID, 1/8 inch OD, and 1/32 inch wall thickness) leading to the ear canal. Adaptable plastic tubes were used to couple the ear canals of infant rats when necessary. The end of each tube was about 5 mm from the tympanic membrane. The output of each MF1 speaker was calibrated from 2.0 to 44.0 kHz (sampling rate, 100 kHz) using a 1/4-in. condenser microphone (model 7016; ACO Pacific Inc.). The calibration data were stored in a computer for obtaining the desired sound pressure levels in decibel (dB SPLs, re: 20 μPa) within the calibrated frequency range.

Auditory Brainstem Response Measurement

The procedure for ABR measurement was similar to that described in our previous study (Wang et al., 2019). Briefly, rats were anesthetized with Nembutal (50 mg/kg, i.p.) and then placed in a stereotaxic frame in a double-walled sound-proof room. The acoustic signal was present from the MF1 speaker coupled to the ear. The subdermal needle electrodes (Rochester Electro-Medical, Inc., United States), headstage (RA4LI), preamplifier (RA4PA), and RX5A2 processor were used to record ABR signals. The electrodes were placed subcutaneously at the vertex (active), the mastoid ipsilateral to the acoustic signal source (reference), and the tail of the rats (ground). The ABR thresholds were measured independently for both ears with tone bursts (5 ms duration, 0.5 ms cosine ramps, 21 Hz repetition rate). The tone bursts were 4.0–36.0 kHz in frequency with 4.0-kHz increments and were 80 to 15 dB SPL in level with 5-dB decrements (or 2-dB steps at near ABR wave I threshold by visual inspections). The ABR signals were bandpass filtered (0.3–3 kHz), averaged from 512 stimulus pairs, and analyzed in BioSigRP software. The ABR Wave I threshold was defined as the lowest sound level that could reliably produce an acoustic stimulus-evoked peak which followed the progressive trend for decreasing amplitude and increasing latency obtained over the range of tested sound levels (Popescu and Polley, 2010). We determined the ABR Wave I threshold by visual inspections of ABR wave data, and by using a statistical measure, i.e., the lowest sound level that evoked a wave I with the peak-to-peak amplitude greater than 2 SDs of the background activity.

Animal Surgery and Single-Unit Recording in Primary Auditory Cortex

Rats were anesthetized by urethane (1.5 g/kg, i.p.) before surgery and were given an injection of atropine sulfate subcutaneously (0.01 mg/kg) to reduce bronchial secretions. Body temperature was monitored and maintained at 37.5°C by an animal temperature regulator. The surgical procedures were similar to that described in our previous studies (Wang et al., 2019). Briefly, the trachea of the rat was cannulated to allow unobstructed respiration, and then a midline skin incision was made on the rat head to allow the exposure of the dorsal and temporal skull. A nail (4 cm long) was attached to the dorsal surface of the skulls with 502 super glue and dental cement. The rat was then fixed to a head holder through the nail. A small hole was made over the left auditory cortex. The dura was removed, and the exposed cortex was kept moist by warm saline.

The neurophysiologic recording was conducted in a sound-proof room. Glass electrodes (filled with 2 M NaCl, 1.0–2.0 MΩ impedance) were advanced orthogonally to the pial surface of AI by a remotely controlled microdrive (SM-21; Narishige, Japan). The recording depth of AI neurons was within the range of 300–900 μm under the pial surface. Action potentials were recorded, amplified (× 1,000), and band pass filtered (0.3–3.0 kHz) by a DAM80 amplifier (WPI, United States), and then fed into a pre-amplifier RA8GA, a RX5A2, and a PC for online and offline data processing. The signal was also monitored on an oscilloscope (TDS 2024, United States) and an audio monitor.

The responses of rat AI neurons were determined by presenting tone bursts varied with frequencies and levels. The frequencies were varied within the range of 4.0–44.0 kHz with 1-kHz increments, and the levels were varied within the range of 0–80 dB SPL with 10-dB steps. The tonal stimuli (50 ms duration including 1.5 ms rise/fall time) were monaurally presented to either ear or binaurally presented to the two ears in dichotic conditions. Absolute stimulus levels (dB SPL) and ILDs (dB) were set by computer through OpenEX software (TDT system 3). The interstimulus interval was 800 ms. The searching stimuli were presented monaurally to either ear and binaurally with equal levels at both ears. Single units were identified by the criteria of equal spike height, constant wave form, and significant signal-to-noise ratio.

Data Analysis and Binaural Interaction Classification

Once a single neuron was identified, the characteristic frequency (CF; the frequency at which the neuron showed the lowest response threshold) was determined by presenting various frequency-level combinations in the audiovisually determined frequency-level response range. The rat AI was identified based on the unique rostral-to-caudal tonotopy (Doron et al., 2002) and short-latency responses to sound stimuli in the auditory cortex. The monaural rate-level functions were determined by presenting CF tonal stimuli (repeated 30 times) to the contralateral ear or the ipsilateral ear from 0 to 80 dB SPL in 10 dB increments (**Figure 1A**, filled circles). Then a matrix of binaural stimuli at CF was presented in which the ILDs and the average binaural levels (ABLs) were varied systematically in dichotic conditions (**Figure 1A**, filled diamonds). The ILDs were varied from −20 to + 20 dB in 10-dB steps, and the positive ILDs indicate greater sound levels in the contralateral (right) ear. The ABL was defined as the sum (in dB) of the contralateral and ipsilateral sound levels divided by 2. At each ILD, ABLs were varied from 20 to 70 in 10-dB steps. A binaural stimulus can be described in terms of its ILD and ABL, or in terms of the levels at the contralateral and the ipsilateral ears (**Figure 1A**). The binaural stimulus matrix included 30 binaural level combinations (repeated 30 times each).

The sensitivity and selectivity of AI neurons to ILDs were evaluated from the ILD response functions, i.e., spike counts versus ILD functions at various ABLs (**Figure 1B**), and averaged ILD response functions across ABLs (**Figure 1C**). A linear curve fitting was performed to the averaged ILD response function (**Figure 1C**, dotted line), and the slope value of this linear function was used as a measure of neuronal sensitivity to ILDs. A greater absolute slope value indicates greater sensitivity to ILD. We then normalized the response strength relative to the maximum spike counts in the averaged ILD response function, and the maximum response strength was 1.0. In the normalized ILD response functions (**Figures 1D–F**), the best ILD was defined as the ILD at which the normalized response strength was 1.0, and the modulation depth was defined as the differences in the normalized response strength between the maximum value and the minimum value (**Figures 1D–F**, vertical lines with double arrow head). A greater modulation depth indicates a greater sensitivity to ILDs. The selectivity of AI neurons to ILDs was assessed from normalized ILD response functions by determining the preferred ILD range (PILDR) over which the normalized response strength was 0.75 (PILDR75) and 0.50 (PILDR50) (**Figures 1D–F**). In the bottom row of **Figure 1**, the dotted lines show the normalized responses strength at 0.75 and 0.5, respectively, and the horizontal line with the double arrow show the PILDR75 and PILDR50 (**Figures 1D–F**). If the dotted line intersects with only one side of the normalized ILD response function, the PILDR was defined as the ILD range from the intersect of the dotted line with the normalized ILD response function to the contralateral limit (i.e., + 20 dB ILD, **Figure 1D**) or the ipsilateral limit (i.e., −20 dB ILD, **Figure 1E**). If the dotted line intersects with both sides of the normalized ILD response function, the PILDR was the ILD range between the two intersects (**Figure 1F**, PILDR75). In contrast, if the dotted line did not intersect with either side of the normalized ILD response function, the PILDR was defined as the ILD range from −20 to + 20 dB (**Figure 1F**, PILDR50). For the few instances where the ILD function has multiple PILDR75s or PILDR50s, the PILDR was defined as the sum of the extent of the PILDRs. The location of the PILDR indicates ILD preference, and the width of the PILDR was used as a measure of ILD selectivity. A narrower PILDR indicates a greater ILD selectivity. Using the same idea, for each neuron, we also analyzed the PILDR75 and PILDR50 from the ILD response function at each ABL to determine the ILD selectivity at different ABLs.

We categorized the binaural interaction of rat AI neurons following a previous classification scheme (Zhang et al., 2004). Rat AI neurons were first classified as EE, EO, OE, and PB types according to their monaural response properties (**Figures 2–4**): EO if the neuron was responsive to monaural stimulation in the contralateral ear but not in the ipsilateral ear (**Figure 2**); EE if it was driven by monaural stimulation of either ear (**Figure 3**); OE if the neuron responded to monaural stimulation in the ipsilateral ear but not in the contralateral ear (**Figure 4**); and PB (i.e., predominantly binaural) if the neuron did not respond or responded very weakly to monaural stimulation of either ear,

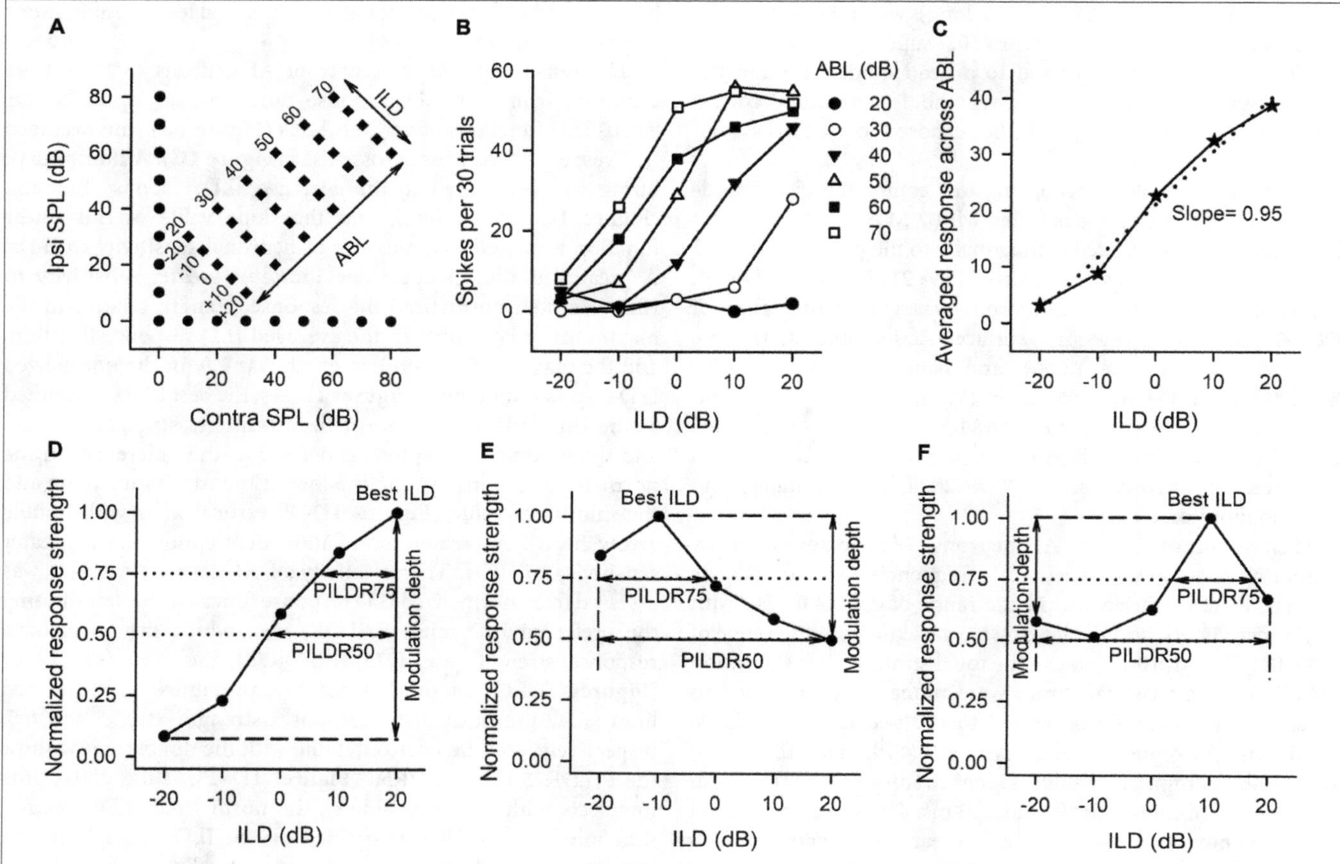

FIGURE 1 | The sound stimulus paradigm and the method to determine the neuronal sensitivity and selectivity to ILDs from the ILD response functions of AI neurons. **(A)** The sound stimulus paradigm. The monaural stimuli (filled circles) and the binaural stimuli (filled diamonds) are designated in terms of contralateral (contra) and ipsilateral (ipsi) sound pressure levels in dB (dB SPL). The binaural stimulus can also be shown in terms of interaural level difference (ILD) and average binaural level (ABL). Positive ILDs favor the contralateral ear and negative ILDs favor the ipsilateral ear. **(B)** The ILD response functions of an AI neuron determined at different ABLs. **(C)** The averaged ILD response function across ABLs from the data in panel **(B)** (solid line) and the linear curve fitting function (dotted line). The slope value of this linear function was used as a measure of neuronal sensitivity to ILDs. **(D–F)** The method to determine the modulation depth, the preferred ILD range (PILDR75, PILDR50), and the best ILDs from the normalized ILD response functions. See texts in section "MATERIALS AND METHODS" for details.

but did respond strongly to binaural stimulation (**Figure 4**). Neurons within the category of each monaural response type were further classified according to their binaural interaction behavior within the binaural stimulus matrix. To quantify the degree of binaural interactions, we computed a binaural interaction index by dividing the response in spike counts to a binaural stimulus by the sum of the monaural responses in spike counts at corresponding monaural stimulus levels. In the present study, all of the recorded neurons showed onset responses. The responses to sound stimuli in spike counts were determined over the sound duration. Similar to the scheme used to classify the binaural interaction type (Zhang et al., 2004), a binaural interaction evoked by a binaural stimulus in the matrix was considered as facilitatory (F) if the binaural interaction index was greater than 1.2, inhibitory (I) if the binaural interaction index was less than 0.8, or no interaction (N) if the binaural interaction index was within the ranges of 0.8–1.2 (**Figures 2–4**, bottom row). Due to low number of spikes sometimes evoked by the stimuli in the binaural stimulus matrix, if both the binaural responses to a binaural combination (repeated 30 times each) and the monaural responses to monaural stimuli at corresponding levels (repeated 30 times each) were < 6 spikes, this binaural combination was excluded from the binaural interaction classification analysis (e.g., **Figure 2A4**, the stimulus combination at ILD −20 dB and ABL 20 dB; **Figure 2B4**, the stimulus combinations at ILD -20 dB and ABL 20 dB, ILD −10 dB and ABL 20 dB; **Figure 4C4**, the binaural combinations at the ILD −20 dB and ABL 20 dB, the ILD −20 dB and ABL 30 dB, the ILD −10 dB and ABL 20 dB). The binaural interaction type of a neuron was then classified according to the kinds of binaural interaction behavior within the binaural stimulus matrix (**Figures 2–4**). To reduce the number of binaural interaction categories for a neuron, designation of no interaction (N) was not included in the binaural interaction classification scheme unless no other type of binaural interaction occurred in the matrix. The binaural interaction type of a neuron was considered to be F, I, or N if it demonstrated predominately facilitatory (F), inhibitory (I), or completely no binaural interaction (N) in the binaural stimulus

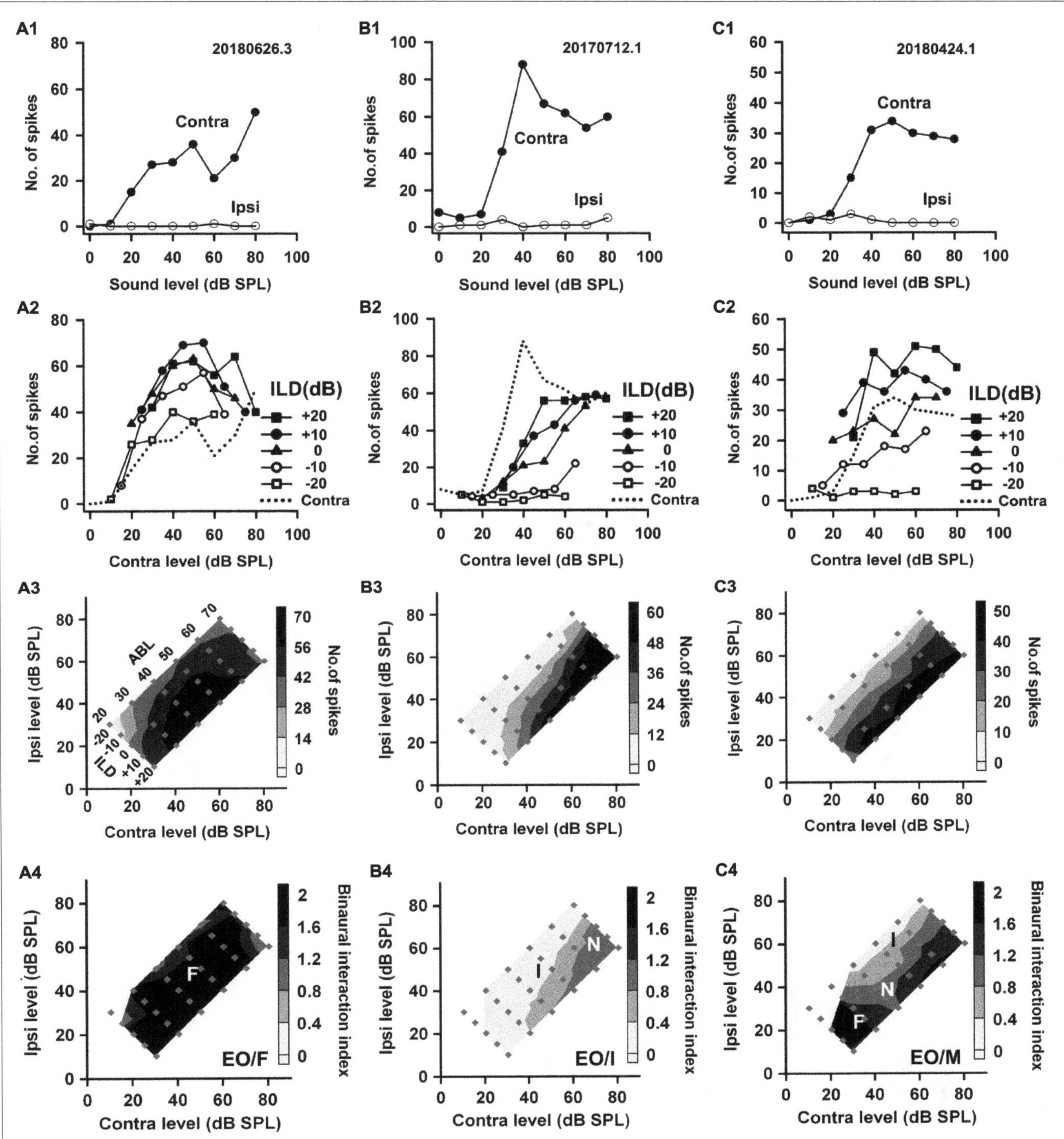

FIGURE 2 | The responses of three EO neurons to both monaural and binaural stimuli. The data shown in each column are from one neuron. **(A1–C1)** The monaural responses of the neurons to stimuli from the contralateral (contra) ear and the ipsilateral (ipsi) ear. **(A2–C2)** The binaural responses of the neurons to stimuli in the binaural stimulus matrix plotted as a function of contralateral levels and at different ILDs. For comparison, the monaural contralateral response functions are shown in dotted lines. **(A3–C3)** The binaural response contours plotted at different contralateral and ipsilateral levels within the binaural stimulus matrix. Filled diamonds represent binaural stimulus conditions, and the stimuli are also shown in ABL vs. ILD in panel **(A3)**. **(A4–C4)** The contour plots of the binaural interaction index within the binaural stimulus matrix. F, I, and N: facilitatory, inhibitory, and no binaural interaction in the contour plots, respectively. The binaural response type of a neuron was classified as mixed (M) if both facilitatory and inhibitory binaural interactions occurred within the binaural stimulus matrix (e.g., neuron C). The three neurons were categorized as EO/F, EO/I, and EO/M, respectively.

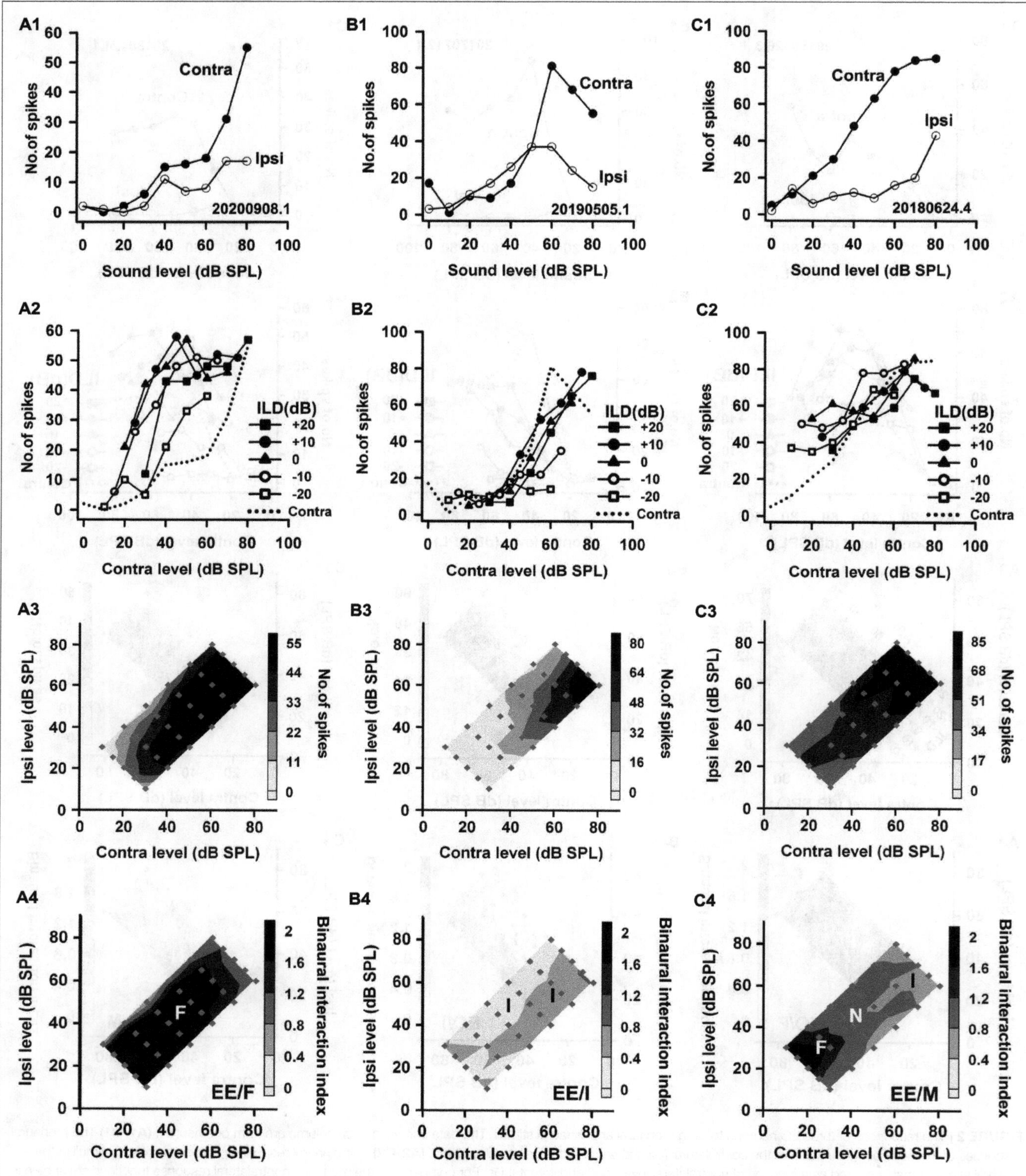

FIGURE 3 | The responses of three EE neurons to both monaural and binaural stimuli. The data shown in each column are from one neuron. The legends for the panels in the four rows are similar to those in **Figure 2**. According to monaural responses and the binaural interaction behaviors in the binaural stimulus matrix, the three neurons were categorized as EE/F, EE/I, and EE/M, respectively.

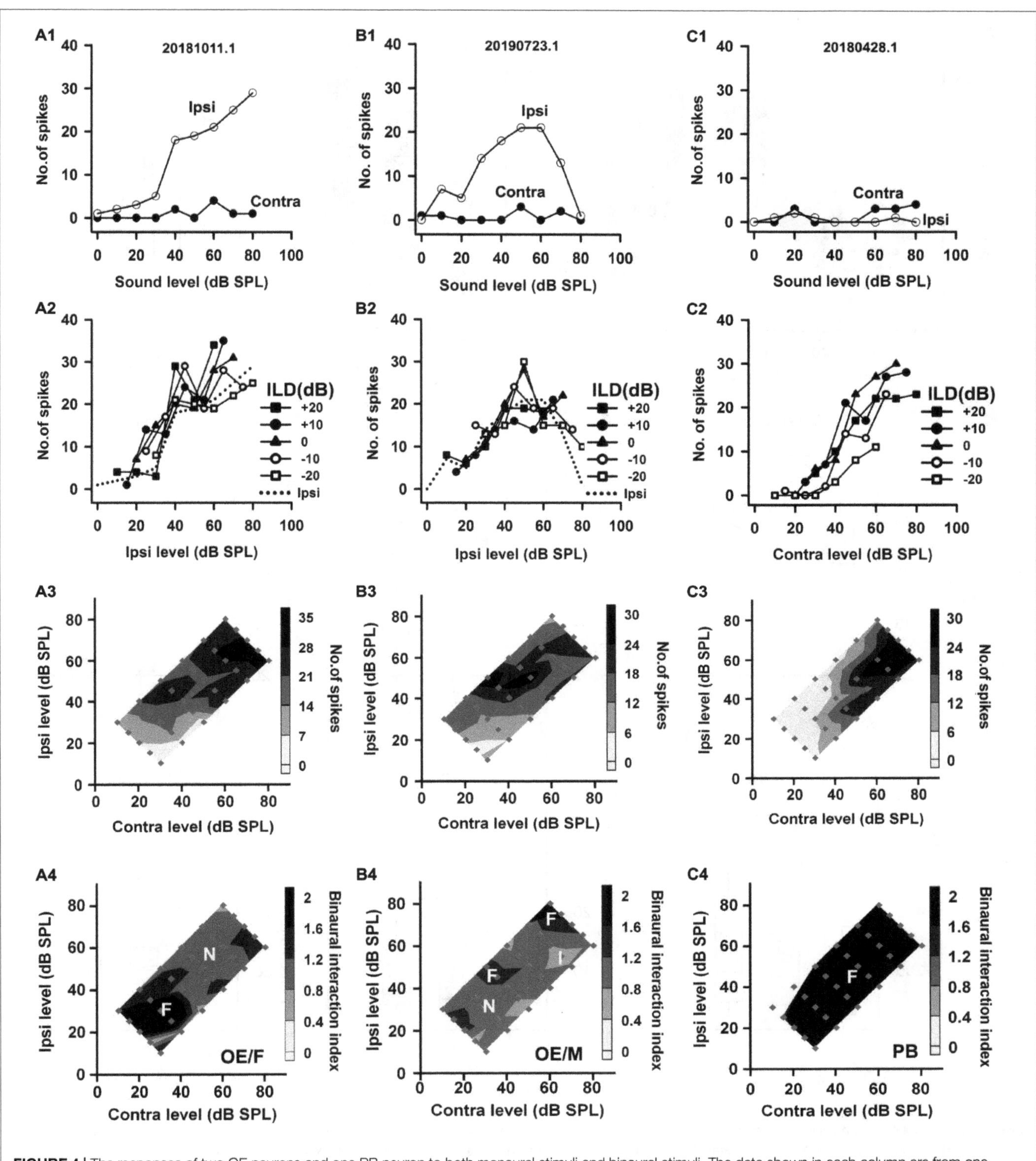

FIGURE 4 | The responses of two OE neurons and one PB neuron to both monaural stimuli and binaural stimuli. The data shown in each column are from one neuron. The legends for the four rows are similar to those in **Figure 2**. The three neurons were categorized as OE/F, OE/M, and PB, respectively.

matrix; the binaural response type was classified as mixed (M) if both facilitatory and inhibitory binaural interactions occurred within the binaural stimulus matrix (**Figures 2–4**, bottom row). Therefore, the binaural interaction type of an AI neuron was designated into one of the following: EE/F, EE/I, EE/N, EE/M, EO/F, EO/I, EO/N, EO/M, OE/F, OE/I, OE/N, OE/M, and PB.

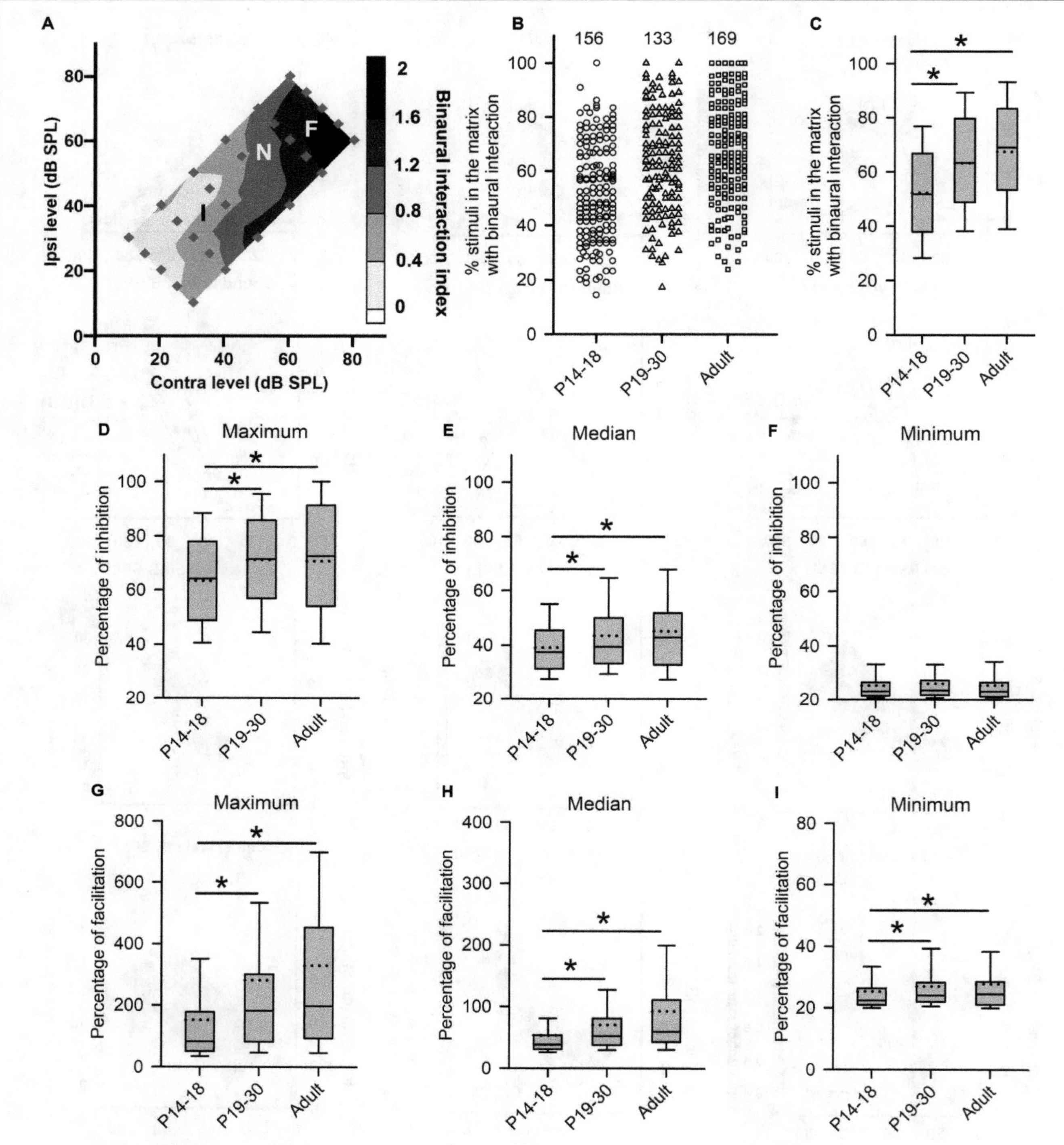

FIGURE 5 | Age-related changes in the degree of binaural interactions of rat AI neurons. **(A)** Contour plot of the binaural interaction index of a representative AI neuron in responding to the binaural stimulus matrix. F, I, and N: facilitatory, inhibitory, and no binaural interaction evoked by a binaural stimulus in the matrix, respectively. **(B,C)** The scatter plot **(B)** and box plot **(C)** showing the distributions in the percentages of stimuli that evoked binaural interaction in the binaural matrix. Each symbol in panel B represents the data from one neuron. The numbers indicate the number of neurons in each group. **(D–F)** Box plots showing age-related changes in the degree of inhibitory binaural interaction. The population data for the percentages of inhibition in maximum **(D)**, median **(E)**, and minimum **(F)** are determined from each AI neuron in each group of rats. **(G–I)** Box plots showing the comparison in the degree of facilitatory binaural interaction among the three groups of AI neurons. The population data for the percentages of facilitation in maximum **(G)**, media **(H)**, and minimum **(I)** are determined from each AI neuron in each group of rats. Box plots indicate the median (solid line in the boxes), mean (dotted line in the boxes), quartiles (box extremities), and 10th/90th percentiles (error bars). * indicates significant difference between two groups (Mann–Whitney *U*-test, $p < 0.05$).

For each AI neuron, the degree of binaural interaction was determined by three aspects of analysis (**Figure 5**): (1) the percentage of stimuli in the binaural matrix that evoked binaural interactions, i.e., [the total number of stimulus points that evoked binaural interactions (I and F) in the binaural matrix]/[the total number of stimulus points with binaural interaction assessment (I, F, and N) in the binaural matrix] × 100%; (2) the percentage of inhibition for each inhibitory binaural interaction in the binaural matrix. This was calculated from the binaural response to a binaural stimulus and the monaural responses to monaural stimuli at corresponding monaural levels, i.e., (the sum of the monaural responses − the binaural response)/(the sum of monaural responses) × 100%. For each AI neuron, we then analyzed the maximum, median, mean, and minimum among the percentages of inhibition in the binaural matrix. (3) The percentage of facilitation for each facilitatory binaural interaction, i.e., (the binaural response to a binaural stimulus - the sum of the monaural responses at corresponding monaural levels)/(the sum of the monaural responses) × 100%. We then analyzed the maximum, median, mean, and minimum among the percentages of facilitation in the binaural matrix for each AI neuron.

Statistical analyses were performed in SPSS, and a criterion of $p < 0.05$ was considered as significantly different between groups.

RESULTS

The neuronal responses to both monaural stimuli and binaural stimuli were collected from 601 neurons in the AI of four groups of rats. We analyzed the population data from AI neurons in the three age groups of rats with normal hearing development [i.e., the P14–18 group (n = 156), the P19–30 group (n = 136), and the adult group (n = 171)] to investigate the developmental changes of the monaural response types and the binaural processing of AI neurons. We then compared the data of AI neurons between the RUCHL group (n = 138) and the adult group to investigate the effects of RUCHL at young age on the monaural response types and the binaural processing of AI neurons in adulthood.

Based on the monaural response properties of the 601 neurons collected in the rat AI, we classified the monaural response types of these neurons as EO, EE, OE, and PB (see example neurons in **Figures 2–4**). The monaural and binaural responses of the three EO neurons shown in **Figure 2** demonstrated various binaural interactions. Neuron A showed predominantly facilitatory binaural interaction whereas neuron B showed predominantly inhibitory binaural interaction in the binaural stimulus matrix. Therefore, the two neurons were categorized as EO/F (**Figure 2A4**) and EO/I (**Figure 2B4**), respectively. Neuron C was categorized as EO/M because it showed predominantly facilitatory binaural interaction at ILDs + 10 to + 20 dB, and predominantly inhibitory binaural interaction at ILDs −20 to −10 dB (**Figure 2C4**). **Figure 3** shows the responses of three EE neurons to both monaural and binaural stimuli. These EE neurons responded to monaural stimulation at either ear (**Figures 3A1–C1**). Their binaural responses varied with binaural stimuli in the binaural matrix (**Figures 3A2–C2, A3–C3**). According to the monaural response type and the binaural interaction behavior in the binaural matrix, the three EE neurons were categorized as EE/F (**Figure 3A4**), EE/I (**Figure 3B4**), and EE/M (**Figure 3C4**), respectively. **Figure 4** shows the responses of two OE neurons (**Figure 4**, the first and the second columns) and one PB neuron (**Figure 4**, the third column) to both monaural stimuli and binaural stimuli. The two OE neurons were classified as OE/F (**Figure 4A4**) and OE/M (**Figure 4B4**). The neuron C in **Figure 4** exhibited the property of predominant binaural response. By definition, this neuron was categorized as PB (**Figure 4C4**).

Developmental Refinement of Binaural Processing in Primary Auditory Cortex After Hearing Onset

We first analyzed the age-related changes in both the monaural response type and the binaural interaction type of AI neurons in the three age groups of rats with normal hearing development. The proportions of neurons within each monaural response type were as follows (**Figure 6A**): the P14–18 group, 86.54% for EO and 13.46% for EE; the P19–30 group, 88.97% for EO, 8.82% for EE, and 2.21% for PB; the adult group, 92.40% for EO, 6.43% for EE, and 1.17% for PB. In each age group, the proportion of EO neurons was the largest, and most neurons were categorized as EO and EE types. Because the proportions of PB neurons are very small in the three age groups, in the following data analysis, we focus on the age-related changes of binaural processing in the population of EO and EE neurons.

The population data analysis from AI neurons including both EO and EE types showed no significant differences in the distributions of binaural interaction types among the three age groups (**Figures 6B–D**). The majority AI neurons were categorized as mixed binaural interaction type (**Figure 6B**), i.e., 69.23% in the P14–18 group, 64.66% in the P19–30 group, and 60.95% in the adult group, respectively. The proportions of neurons categorized as inhibitory binaural interaction type were 21.25% in the P14–18 group, 19.55% in the P19–30 group, and 17.16% in the adult group, respectively. In addition, the proportions of neurons categorized as facilitatory binaural interaction type were 9.62% in the P14–18 group, 15.79% in the P19–30 group, and 21.89% in the adult group, respectively. We did not find significant differences in the distributions of binaural interaction types among the three age groups of A1 neurons (χ^2-test, df = 4, χ^2 = 9.219, p = 0.056). Within the population of EO neurons in each age group, the proportions of neurons with various binaural interaction types were as follows: the P14–18 group, 11.11% for EO/F, 19.26% for EO/I, and 69.63% for EO/M; the P19–30 group, 17.36% for EO/F, 18.18% for EO/I, and 64.46% for EO/M; the adult group, 21.52% for EO/F, 17.09% for EO/I, and 61.39% for EO/M, respectively (**Figure 6C**). Chi-square test did not show significant differences in the distributions of binaural interaction types among the three age groups of EO neurons (df = 4, χ^2 = 5.641, p = 0.228). Moreover, the proportions of EE neurons with various binaural interaction types in each age group were as follows: the P14–18 group, 33.33% for EE/I and

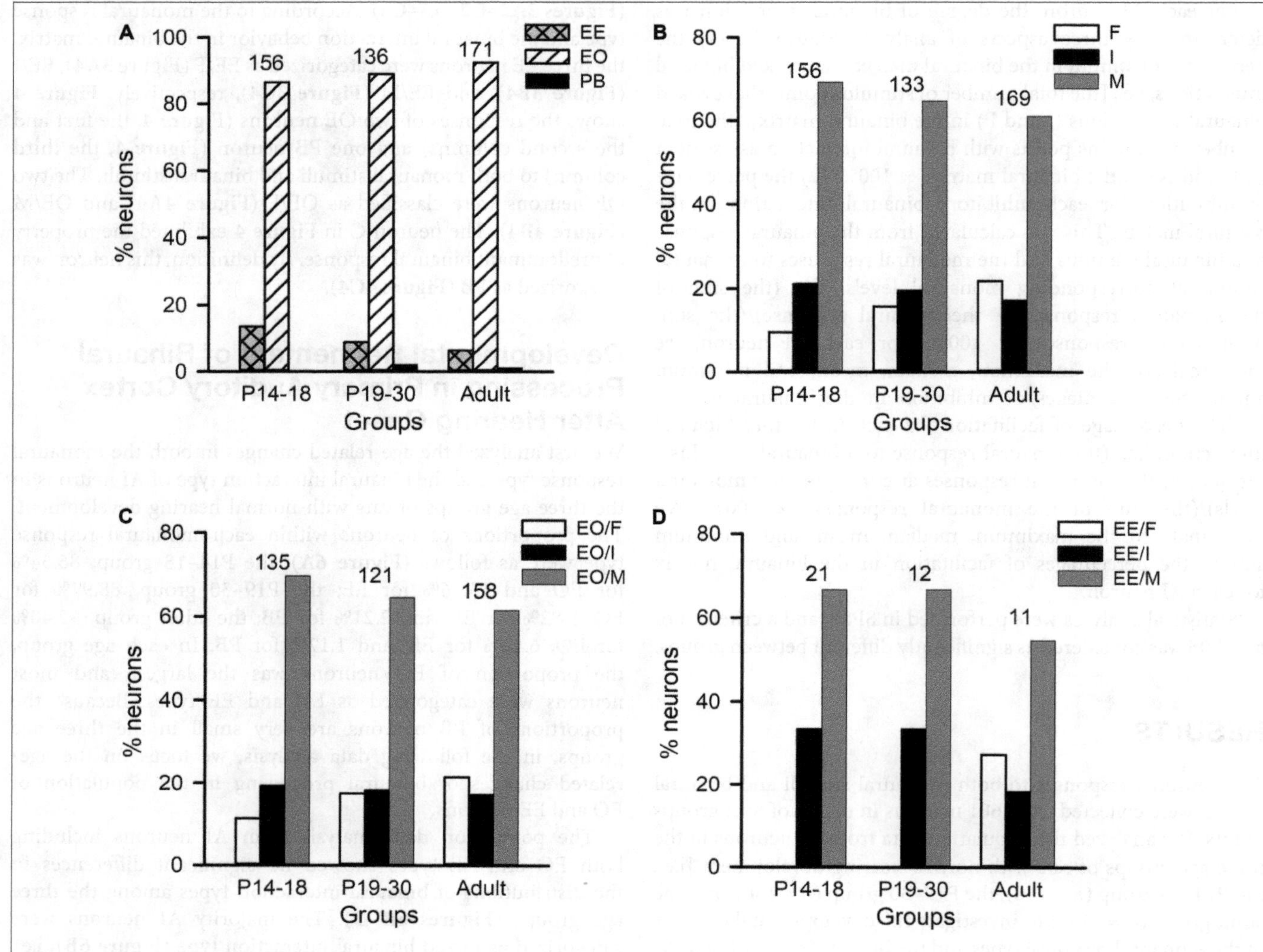

FIGURE 6 | Distributions of the monaural response types and the binaural interaction types of AI neurons in the three age groups of rats. The three age groups are P14–18 group, P19–30 group, and adult group, respectively. **(A)** The distributions of the monaural response types (i.e., EE, EO, and PB) of AI neurons. **(B)** The distributions of the binaural interaction types for the population including both EO and EE neurons. The binaural interaction of each neuron was classified into one of the three categories: inhibitory (I), facilitatory (F), and mixed (M). **(C,D)** The distributions of the binaural interaction types in the population of EO neurons **(C)** and EE neurons **(D)**. Numbers shown on the top of the bars indicate the number of neurons in each age group.

66.67% for EE/M; the P19–30 group, 33.33% for EE/I and 66.67% for EE/M; the adult group, 27.27% for EE/F, 18.18% for EE/I, and 54.54% for EE/M (**Figure 6D**). We did not encounter EE/F type in the AI in both the P14–18 group and the P19–30 group. No significant differences were found in the distributions of EE/I and EE/M types among the three age groups of EE neurons (χ^2-test, $df = 2$, $\chi^2 = 0.207$, $p = 0.902$).

We next determined whether there are age-related changes in the degree of binaural interactions in AI after hearing onset. One measure for the degree of binaural interaction was the percentages of the number of stimuli that evoked binaural interactions in the binaural stimulus matrix. A greater percentage from this measure implies a higher degree of binaural interaction. For each neuron, we determined the number of stimulus points with facilitatory (F), inhibitory (I), or no interactions (N) in the binaural stimulus matrix according to the binaural interaction index (**Figure 5A**). For the example neuron in **Figure 5A**, the numbers of stimulus points with facilitatory, inhibitory, or no binaural interactions were 10, 15, and 5, respectively. Consequentially, the percentage of stimulus points with binaural interactions in the binaural stimulus matrix was 83.33% (25/30) (see texts in the Methods section for detailed calculations in this measure). The population data analysis showed age-related changes in the percentages of stimuli with binaural interactions in the binaural stimulus matrix. The degree of binaural interactions in this measure was lowest in the P14–18 group than in both the P19–30 group and the adult group, and was very similar between the P19–30 group and the adult group (**Figures 5B,C**, Kruskal–Wallis test, $\chi^2 = 47.111$, $df = 2$, $p < 0.001$; Mann–Whitney U-test, P14–18 group vs. P19–30 group, $z = -4.463$, $p < 0.001$; P14–18 group vs. adult group, $z = -6.638$, $p < 0.001$; P19–30 group vs. adult group, $z = -1.867$, $p = 0.062$). These data demonstrated a developmental increase in the degree of binaural interaction at early postnatal age after hearing onset.

Another measure for the degree of binaural interaction is the degree of inhibition (or facilitation) when a binaural stimulus evoked the inhibitory (or facilitatory) binaural interaction. The detail method for this analysis is introduced in the materials and methods. For each AI neuron, we determined the maximum, median, and minimum of the percentage of inhibition (or facilitation) in the binaural matrix. If only one stimulus in the binaural matrix evoked an inhibitory (or facilitatory) interaction, the data were excluded from the degree of inhibition (or facilitation) analysis. For the neuron in **Figure 5A**, the maximum, median, and minimum percentages of inhibition in the whole binaural matrix were 91.67, 53.66, and 25.00%, respectively. In addition, the maximum, median, and minimum percentages of facilitation in the whole binaural matrix were 188.89, 42.48, 62.97, and 24.00%, respectively. The population data analysis for this measure indicates that the maximum percentages of inhibition were significantly smaller in the P14–18 group than in both the P19–30 group and the adult group; in contrast, no significant differences in the maximum percentages of inhibition were found between the P19–30 group and the adult group (**Figure 5D**, Kruskal–Wallis test, $\chi^2 = 11.914$, $df = 2$, $p = 0.003$; Mann-Whitney U-test, P14–18 group vs. P19–30 group, $z = -3.023$, $p = 0.003$; P14–18 group vs. adult group, $z = -2.897$, $p = 0.004$; P19–30 group vs. adult group, $z = -0.208$, $p = 0.835$). A similar trend was found in the median percentages of inhibition among groups (**Figure 5E**, Kruskal–Wallis test, $\chi^2 = 9.949$, $df = 2$, $p = 0.007$; Mann-Whitney U-test, P14–18 group vs. P19–30 group, $z = -2.276$, $p = 0.023$; P14–18 group vs. adult group, $z = -2.960$, $p = 0.003$; P19–30 group vs. adult group, $z = -0.30$, $p = 0.976$). However, no significant differences in the minimum percentages of inhibition were found among the three age groups of AI neurons (**Figure 5F**, Kruskal–Wallis test, $df = 2$, $\chi^2 = 1.2149$, $p = 0.545$). Using the same idea, we compared the maximum, median, and minimum percentages of facilitation in the binaural stimulus matrix among the three age groups of AI neurons. We found that the maximum percentages of facilitation were significantly smaller in the P14–18 group than in both the P19–30 group and the adult group; however, no significant differences were found in the maximum percentages of facilitation between the P19–30 group and the adult group (**Figure 5G**, Kruskal–Wallis test, $\chi^2 = 34.397$, $df = 2$, $p < 0.001$; Mann-Whitney U-test, P14–18 group vs. P19–30 group, $z = -4.390$, $p < 0.001$; P14–18 group vs. adult group, $z = -5.483$, $p < 0.001$; P19–30 group vs. adult group, $z = -1.249$, $p = 0.212$). A similar trend was found for the median and minimum percentages of facilitation when the population data of AI neurons were compared among the three age groups (**Figure 5H**, for the median percentage of facilitation, Kruskal–Wallis test, $\chi^2 = 40.672$, $df = 2$, $p < 0.001$; Mann-Whitney U-test, P14–18 group vs. P19–30 group, $z = -4.373$, $p < 0.001$; P14–18 group vs. adult group, $z = -6.101$, $p < 0.001$; P19–30 group vs. adult group, $z = -1.883$, $p = 0.060$; **Figure 5I**, for the minimum percentage of facilitation, Kruskal–Wallis test, $\chi^2 = 10.462$, $df = 2$, $p = 0.005$; Mann-Whitney U-test, P14–18 group vs. P19–30 group, $z = -2.324$, $p = 0.020$; P14–18 group vs. adult group, $z = -3.066$, $p = 0.002$; P19–30 group vs. adult group, $z = -0.800$, $p = 0.424$). The data in **Figure 5** demonstrate that rat AI neurons undergo refinement in the degree of binaural interactions during early postnatal hearing development after hearing onset.

To further determine the age-related changes of binaural processing after hearing onset, for each AI neuron, we determined the sensitivity of the neuron to ILD by measuring the modulation depth and the slope value from the averaged ILD response functions (see **Figure 1** for methods). A greater modulation depth or a greater absolute slope value indicates a greater sensitivity to the variations of ILDs. The population data analysis showed that the values of the modulation depth were significantly smaller in the P14–18 group than in both the P19–30 group and the adult group; however, no significant differences in the modulation depth were found between the P19–30 group and the adult group (**Figures 7A,B**, Kruskal–Wallis test, $\chi^2 = 46.927$, $df = 2$, $p < 0.001$; Mann-Whitney U-test, P14–18 group vs. P19–30 group, $z = -4.643$, $p < 0.001$; P14–18 group vs. adult group, $z = -6.655$, $p < 0.001$; P19–30 group vs. adult group, $z = -1.676$, $p = 0.094$). The distributions of the slope values in the three groups of AI neurons indicated that the absolute slope values in the P14–18 group were smaller than those in both the P19–30 group and the adult group, and that no significant differences in the absolute slope values were found between the P19–30 group and the adult group (**Figures 7C,D**, Kruskal–Wallis test, $\chi^2 = 11.214$, $df = 2$, $p < 0.001$; Mann-Whitney U-test, P14–18 group vs. P19–30 group, $z = -2.068$, $p = 0.0391$; P14–18 group vs. adult group, $z = -3.306$, $p = 0.001$; P19–30 group vs. adult group, $z = -1.676$, $p = 0.094$). These data demonstrated a developmental refinement in the ILD sensitivity of AI neurons after hearing onset.

The selectivity of AI neurons to ILD was determined from the two measures: PILDR50 and PILDR75 (see methods in **Figure 1**). A smaller PILDR value indicates a greater selectivity for ILD. The data analysis showed that the values of PILDR50s in the P14–18 group were greater than those in both the P19–30 group and the adult group (**Figures 7E,F**, Kruskal–Wallis test, $\chi^2 = 35.09$, $df = 2$, $p < 0.001$; Mann-Whitney U-test, P14–18 group vs. P19–30 group, $z = -3.8918$, $p < 0.001$; P14–18 group vs. adult group, $z = -5.845$, $p < 0.001$). However, no significant differences in the values of PILDR50s were found between the P19–30 group and the adult group (**Figures 7E,F**, P19–30 group vs. adult group, $z = -1.7716$, $p = 0.077$). In contrast, the distributions of the PILDR75s determined from the averaged ILD response functions across ABLs in the three age groups of AI neurons were very similar (**Figures 7G,H**, Kruskal–Wallis test, $df = 2$, $\chi^2 = 2.693$, $p = 0.260$). It is possible that the PILDRs determined from the averaged ILD response functions across ABLs underestimate the ILD selectivity of the AI neurons. We further determined the PILDR75 for each neuron from the ILD response function at each ABL. The data analysis for PILDR75s at each ABL within 40–70 dB indicated that the PILDR75s of AI neurons were significantly larger in the P14–18 group than in the adult

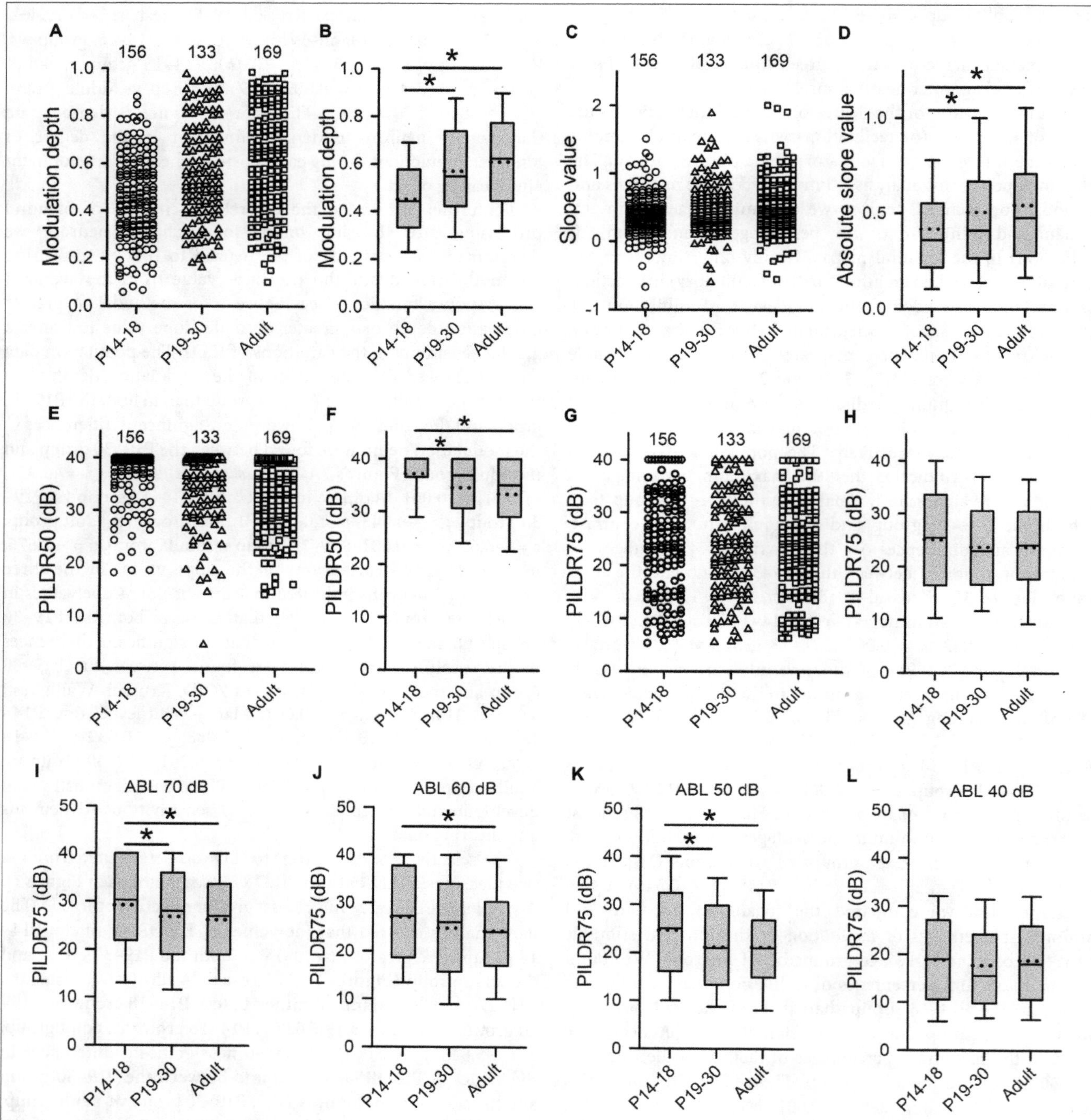

FIGURE 7 | Age-related changes in both the sensitivity and the selectivity of AI neurons to ILDs determined from the ILD response functions in the three age groups. **(A–H)** Population data showing the distributions of modulation depth **(A,B)**, slope value **(C,D)**, PILDR50 **(E,F)**, and PILDR75 **(G,H)** in both scatter plots and box plots, respectively. In the scatter plots, each symbol represents the data from one neuron. The PILDR50 and the PILDR75 data shown in the second row are determined from the averaged ILD response functions across ABL. **(I–L)** Box plots showing the distributions of PILDR75 determined from the ILD response functions at ABL 40–70 dB. * indicates significant difference between two groups (Mann–Whitney *U*-test, $p < 0.05$). The greater values in the modulation depth and the absolute slope value indicate greater sensitivity to ILDs. Moreover, the smaller values in the PILDR50 and the PILDR75 indicate greater selectivity to ILDs.

group at ABLs 50–70 dB, but not at ABL 40 dB (**Figures 7I–L**, Mann–Whitney *U*-test,P14–18 group vs. adult group, at ABL 70 dB, $z = -3.034$, $p = 0.002$; at ABL 60 dB, $z = -2.598$, $p = 0.009$; at ABL 50 dB, $z = -3.004$, $p = 0.002$; at ABL 40 dB, $z = -0.120$, $p = 0.905$). Moreover, the PILDR75s were significant larger in the P14–18 group than those in the P19–30 group at ABL 50 and ABL 70 dB, but not at ABL 40 dB and ABL 60 dB (**Figures 7I–L**, Mann–Whitney U-test, P14–18 group vs. the P19–30 group, at ABL 70 dB, $z = -2.087$, $p = 0.037$; at ABL 50 dB, $z = -2.766$, $p = 0.006$; at ABL 60 dB, $z = -1.951$, $p = 0.051$; at ABL 40 dB, $z = -1.019$, $p = 0.308$). In addition, we did not find significant differences in the PILDR75s between P19–30 group and adult group at ABL 40–70 dB (**Figures 7I–L**, Mann–Whitney U-test, P19–30 group vs. adult group, at ABL 70 dB, $z = -0.778$, $p = 0.437$; at ABL 60 dB, $z = -0.665$, $p = 0.506$; at ABL 50 dB, $z = -0.109$, $p = 0.913$; at ABL 40 dB, $z = -0.963$, $p = 0.336$). We also determined the PILDR50 for each neuron from the ILD response function at each ABL. The PILDR50s were significant larger in the P14–18 group than in both the P19–30 group and the adult group at ABL 40–70 dB (Mann–Whitney U-test, P14–18 group vs. P19–30 group: at ABL 70 dB, $z = -3.254$, $p = 0.001$; at ABL 60 dB, $z = -4.332$, $p < 0.001$; at ABL 50 dB, $z = -3.390$, $p = 0.001$; at ABL 40 dB, $z = -2.717$, $p = 0.007$. For P14–18 group vs. adult group, at ABL 70 dB, $z = -4.833$, $p < 0.001$; at ABL 60 dB, $z = -6.740$, $p < 0.001$; at ABL 50 dB, $z = -4.879$, $p < 0.001$; at ABL 40 dB, $z = -2.708$, $p = 0.007$). We did not find significant differences in the PILDR50s between P19–30 group and adult group at ABL40–70 dB (Mann–Whitney U-test, at ABL 70 dB, $z = -1.154$, $p = 0.248$; at ABL 60 dB, $z = -1.729$, $p = 0.084$; at ABL 50 dB, $z = -1.3019$, $p = 0.193$; at ABL 40 dB, $z = -0.057$, $p = 0.955$). These results demonstrated a developmental refinement in the selectivity of AI neurons to ILD after hearing onset.

The best ILD of AI neurons in the three age groups mainly distributed at ILDs 0 dB, 10 dB, and 20 dB, and only few neurons had their best ILDs at −10 dB and −20 dB (**Figure 8A**). We did not find significant differences in the distribution of the best ILDs of AI neurons among the three age groups (from ILD −10 to + 20 dB, χ^2-test, $df = 6$, $\chi^2 = 6.91$, $p = 0.329$). We classified the ILD preference of AI neurons from the averaged ILD response functions into the following categories: contra, midline, ipsi, insensitive, and multipeak. The ILD preference was considered as "contra" if the best ILD was at + 10 dB or + 20 dB, and the PILDR75 was restrictively or predominantly distributed within the range of 0 to + 20 dB. The neuron was classified as "ipsi" ILD preference if the best ILD was at −10 dB or −20 dB, and the PILDR75 was restrictively or predominantly distributed within the range of 0 to −20 dB. The neuron was assigned as "midline" ILD preference if the best ILD was at 0 dB and the PILDR75 was restrictively distributed within the range of −10 to + 10 dB. The ILD preference was considered as "insensitive" if the continuous width of the PILDR75 was greater than 30 dB. The neuron was classified as "multipeak" if there were two or more separated PILDR75. The distributions in the ILD preferences of AI neurons in each age group demonstrate that most neurons preferred contralateral ILDs, and only few neurons preferred ipsilateral ILDs or midline ILDs (**Figure 8B**). With increasing ages, the AI neurons with contralateral ILD preference showed a weak trend of increase in percentages, and the largest difference in the percentages was 10.39% between the P14–18 group and the adult group; in contrast, the AI neurons that were insensitive to ILD showed a weak trend of decrease in percentages with increasing ages, and the largest difference in the percentages was 10.16% between the P14–18 group and the adult group (**Figure 8B**). However, no significant differences were found in the distribution of ILD preferences among the three age groups (**Figure 8B**, χ^2-test, $df = 8$, $p = 0.379$).

The Effect of Reversible Unilateral Conductive Hearing Loss at Young Age on Binaural Processing of Primary Auditory Cortex Neurons in Adulthood

We injected a thermoreversible poloxamer hydrogel into the middle ear cavity of one ear in rats on P14, and did additional injections at both P16 and P18 to induce RUCHL at young age. We tracked the changes of hearing thresholds determined from both the injected ear and the control ear (non-injected ear) based on the ABR wave I thresholds in a portion of rats ($n = 11$) with a 2-day interval. The data in **Figure 9** indicate that intratympanic poloxamer injections elevated the ABR wave I thresholds at different tested frequencies, and the threshold differences between the injected ear and the control ear varied with postnatal days after poloxamer injection (**Figures 9A–F**, Wilcoxon signed-rank test, injected ear vs. control ear, $p < 0.05$ at all tested frequencies on each day). The average threshold differences were within the range of 5–25 dB until P28 (**Figure 9F**). At P30, we determined the ABR wave I thresholds at both the control ear and the injected ear for the 60 rats in the RUCHL group. Although the ABR thresholds at the injected ear were still higher than those at the control ear (**Figure 9G**, Wilcoxon signed-rank test, injected ear vs. control ear, $p < 0.05$ at all tested frequencies), the ABR threshold differences between the injected ear and the control ear at P30 were less than 5 dB (**Figure 9H**). We consider that the hearing thresholds at the injected ear already recovered to normal hearing at P30.

To determine the effects of RUCHL at young age on the monaural response type and the binaural processing of AI neurons in adulthood, we used the data from the adult group as control. We found that RUCHL at young age decreased the proportion of EO neuron but increased the proportion of EE neurons in the AI of RUCHL rats in adulthood (**Figure 10A**, RUCHL group, 70.29% for EO type and 24.64% for EE type; adult group, 93.40% for EO type and 6.43% for EE type; χ^2-test, RUCHL group vs. adult group, $\chi^2 = 20.387$, $df = 1$, $p < 0.001$). In addition, we encountered few OE neurons in the RUCHL group but not in the adult group (**Figure 10A**). Because the proportions of OE neurons (3.63%) and PB neurons (1.45%) in the RUCHL group are very small, in the following data analysis, we only focus on the data from the EO and EE neurons.

For the population of AI neurons including both EO and EE neuron in the RUCHL group ($n = 131$) and in the adult group ($n = 169$), the data showed that RUCHL at young age did not significantly change the proportions of AI neurons within each binaural interaction category or within each type of ILD preference in adulthood. The proportions of neurons categorized into different binaural interaction types are as follows

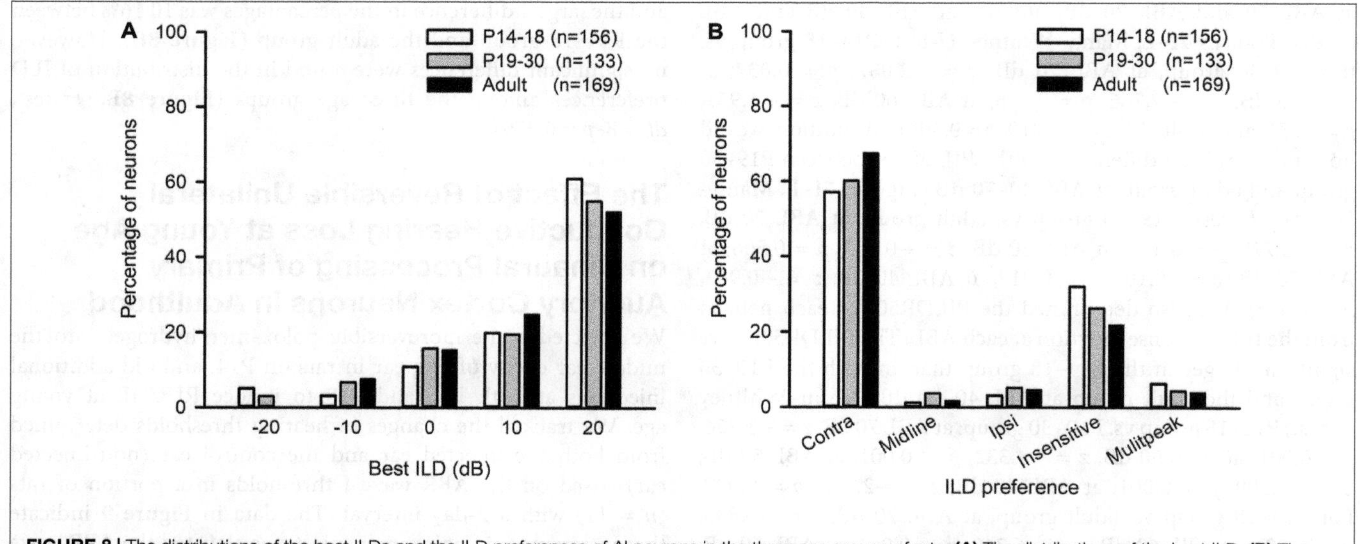

FIGURE 8 | The distributions of the best ILDs and the ILD preferences of AI neurons in the three age groups of rats. **(A)** The distributions of the best ILD. **(B)** The distributions of the ILD preference. "*n*" indicates the number of neurons in each group.

(**Figure 10B**): RUCHL group versus adult group, 66.41% vs. 60.95% for mixed binaural interaction type, 21.37% vs. 21.89% for facilitatory binaural interaction type, and 12.21% vs. 17.16% for inhibitory binaural interaction type. No significant differences are found in the distributions of various binaural interaction types between the RUCHL group and the adult group (χ^2-test, $\chi^2 = 1.561$, $df = 2$, $p = 0.458$). Similar to the distributions in the best ILDs of AI neurons in the adult group, the best ILDs of majority AI neurons in the RUCHL group are distributed in the contralateral ILDs (i.e., + 10 dB and + 20 dB), and RUCHL at young age did not significantly affect the distributions of the best ILDs of AI neurons in adulthood (**Figure 10C**, Fisher's exact test, RUCHL vs. adult, $p = 0.134$). For the ILD preference, majority of AI neurons in both the RUCHL group and the adult group showed contralateral ILD preference or insensitive to the change of ILD. Fisher's exact test showed a significant difference in the distributions of ILD preferences between the adult group and the RUCHL group (**Figure 10D**, $p = 0.002$). However, the proportions of AI neurons within the categories of both "contra" and "insensitive" in the RUCHL group were not significantly different from those in the adult group, respectively (**Figure 10D**, χ^2-test, RUCHL vs. adult, $\chi^2 = 1.913$, $df = 1$, $p = 0.167$).

We next determined the effects of RUCHL at young age on the degrees in binaural interactions of AI neurons in adulthood. The data in **Figure 11** demonstrated that RUCHL at young age decreased the degree of binaural interactions of AI neurons in adulthood. We used Mann–Whitney *U*-test to compare the data between the RUCHL group and the adult group, and found that the percentages in the number of stimuli evoking binaural interactions in the binaural matrix were significantly lower in the AI neurons of the RUCHL group than in the AI neurons of the adult group (**Figures 11A,B**, RUCHL vs. adult, $z = -3.585$, $p < 0.001$). We also found that, for the population of AI neurons, the maximum and the median percentages of inhibition in the binaural matrix in the RUCHL group were significantly smaller than those in the adult group, respectively (**Figure 11C**, maximum, $z = -2.007$, $p = 0.045$; **Figure 11D**, median, $z = -2.059$, $p = 0.040$). However, no significant differences in the minimum percentages of inhibition were found between the RUCHL group and the adult group (**Figure 11E**, $z = -1.087$, $p = 0.277$). In addition, the maximum, median, and minimum percentages of facilitation in the binaural matrix for the AI neurons in the RUCHL group were significantly smaller than those in the adult group, respectively (**Figure 11F**, maximum, $z = -2.009$, $p = 0.045$; **Figure 11G**, median, $z = -3.140$, $p = 0.002$; **Figure 11H**, minimum, $z = -2.099$, $p = 0.036$).

To determine whether RUCHL at young age affects the tuning of AI neurons to ILDs in adulthood, we compared both the sensitivity and the selectivity of AI neurons to ILDs between the RUCHL group and the adult group by Mann–Whitney *U*-test. The results demonstrated that RUCHL at young age decreased both the selectivity and the sensitivity of AI neurons to ILDs in adulthood. For the sensitivity of AI neurons to ILDs, both the values of the modulation depth and the absolute slope values of the averaged ILD response functions were significantly smaller in the RUCHL group than in the adult group, respectively (**Figure 12A**, $z = -3.576$, $p < 0.001$; **Figure 12B**, $z = -1.988$, $p = 0.047$). For the selectivity of AI neurons to ILDs, our data showed that the preferred ILD ranges of AI neurons determined from the averaged ILD response functions were significantly larger in the RUCHL group than in the adult group (**Figure 12C**, PILDR50, $z = -2.985$, $p = 0.003$; **Figure 12D**, PILDR75, $z = -2.090$, $p = 0.037$). We further analyzed the PILDR50 and PILDR75 of AI neurons determined from the ILD response functions at ABLs 40–70 dB. We found that the PILDR75s of AI neurons were larger in the RUCHL group than in the adult group at ABLs 50–70 dB but not at ABL 40 dB (RUCHL group vs. adult group, at ABL 70 dB, $z = -3.029$, $p = 0.002$; at ABL 60 dB, $z = -3.029$, $p = 0.002$; at ABL 50 dB, $z = -2.994$, $p = 0.003$; at ABL 40 dB, $z = -1.674$, $p = 0.094$). Moreover, the PILDR50s

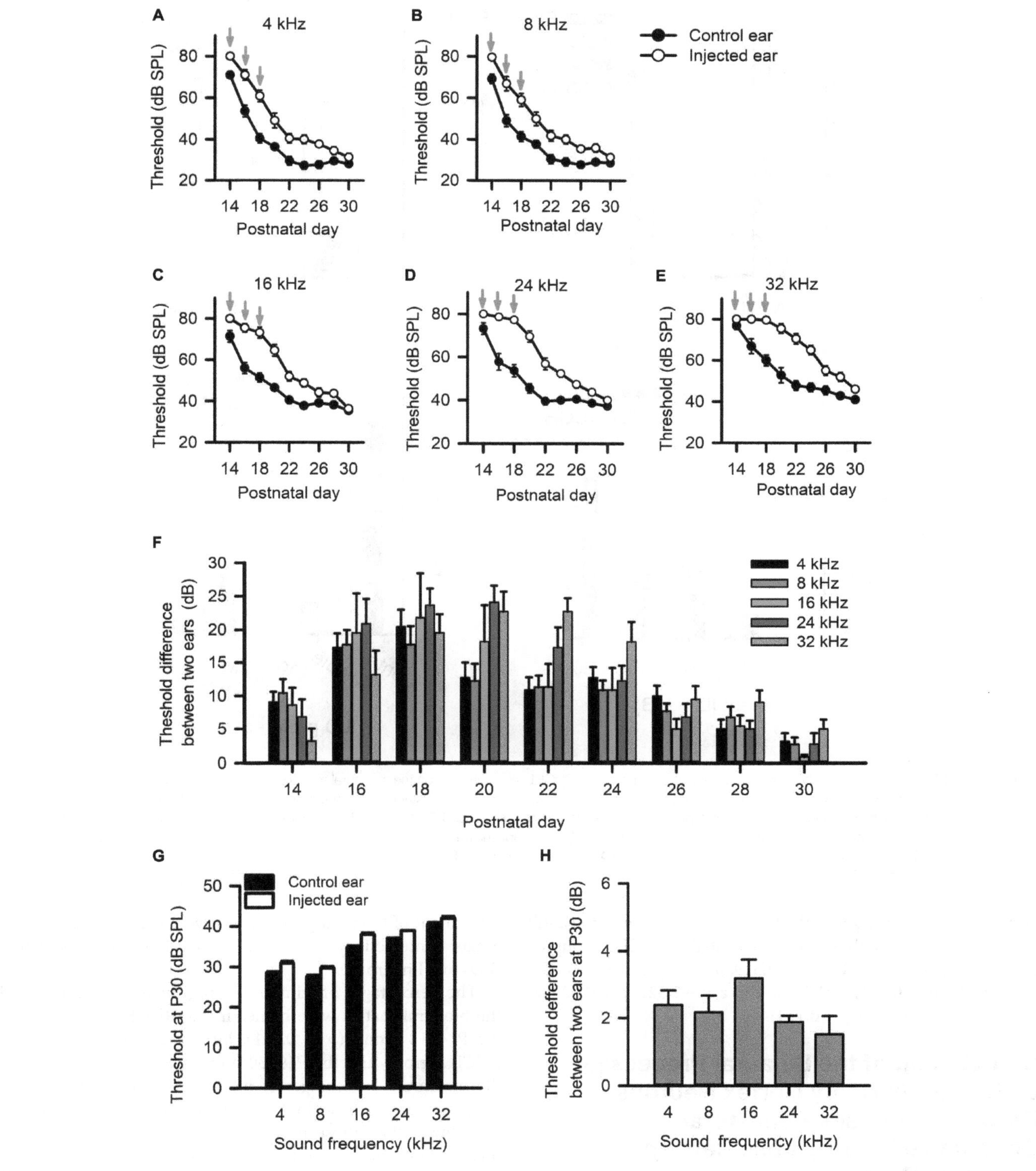

FIGURE 9 | The effects of intratympanic poloxamer injections on the hearing threshold of the injected ear determined from the wave I of auditory brainstem response (ABR). **(A–E)** The response thresholds for ABR wave I elicited with tone bursts at the frequencies of 4 kHz **(A)**, 8 kHz **(B)**, 16 kHz **(C)**, 24 kHz **(D)**, and 32 kHz **(E)**, respectively. The intratympanic poloxamer injections (red arrows) were made on P14, P16, and P18 in the right ear (the injected ear). The control ear was the intact left ear. **(F)** The differences in ABR wave I threshold, i.e., the threshold of the injected ear minus the threshold of the control ear. These data are determined from 11 rats. **(G)** The ABR wave I thresholds for both the injected ear and the control ear determined at P30 (n = 60 rats). **(H)** The differences in ABR wave I threshold between the injected ear and the control ear determined at P30 (n = 60 rats).

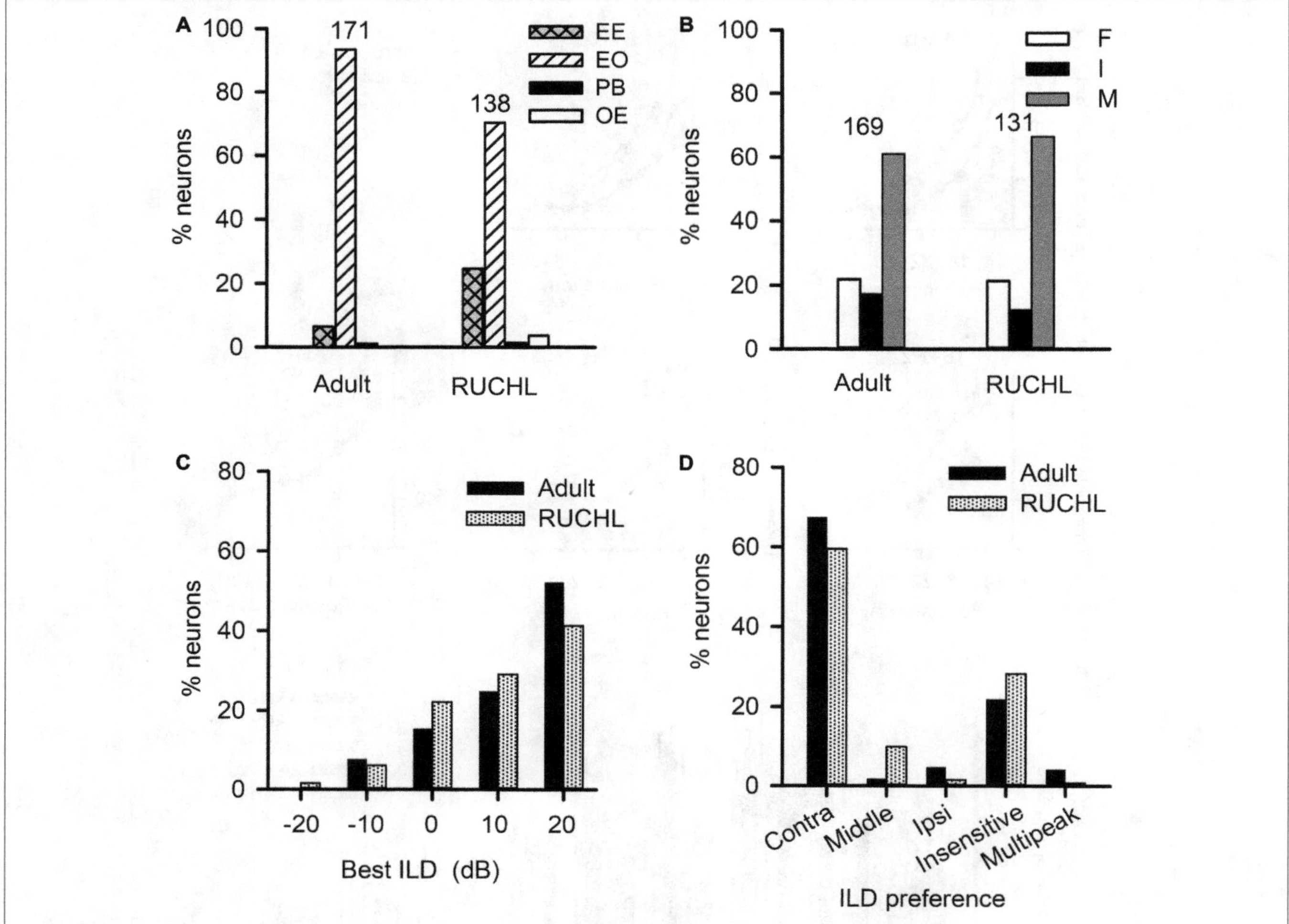

FIGURE 10 | The effects of reversible unilateral conductive hearing loss (RUCHL) at young age on the monaural response types and the binaural processing of rat AI neurons in adulthood. Data from the adult group were used as control for comparison. **(A)** The distributions in the monaural response types (i.e., EE, EO, OE, and PB). **(B)** The distributions of the binaural interaction types of AI neurons including both EE and EO neurons. The binaural interaction of each neuron was classified into one of the three categories: inhibitory (I), facilitatory (F), and mixed (M). Numbers shown on the top of the bars in panels A and B indicate the number of neurons in each group. **(C)** The distribution of the best ILDs of AI neurons. **(D)** The distributions of ILD preferences of AI neurons.

of AI neurons were larger in the RUCHL group than in the adult group at ABLs 50–70 dB but not at ABL 40 dB (RUCHL group vs. adult group, at ABL 70 dB, $z = -4.529$, $p < 0.001$; at ABL 60 dB, $z = -4.642$, $p < 0.001$; at ABL 50 dB, $z = -2.322$, $p = 0.020$; at ABL 40 dB, $z = -1.359$, $p = 0.174$).

Comparison of the Binaural Processing of Primary Auditory Cortex Neurons Between Reversible Unilateral Conductive Hearing Loss Rats and Immature Rats

To determine whether the RUCHL halt the development of binaural processing, we compared the data from the RUCHL rats and the data from two groups of immature rats by Kruskal–Wallis test and Mann–Whitney U-test. The results indicate that, to some extent, brief RUCHL at early age seems to retard the refinement of binaural processing at young age in the degree of binaural interaction, and in both the selectivity and sensitivity to ILDs of AI neurons.

The percentages of stimuli evoking binaural interactions in the binaural matrix were higher in the RUCHL group than in the P14–18 group ($p < 0.001$), but were similar between the RUCHL group and the P19–30 group ($p = 0.178$). In addition, the maximum percentages of inhibition in the RUCHL group were similar to those in the P14–18 group ($p = 0.476$), but were lower than those in the P19–30 group ($p = 0.049$). The median (and the minimum) percentages of inhibition were not significantly different among the three groups (Kruskal–Wallis test, for the median, $p = 0.068$; for the minimum, $p = 0.332$). The maximum and the median percentages of facilitation in the RUCHL group were higher than those in the P14–18 group (both $p = 0.001$), but were not significantly different from those in the P19–30 group, respectively (for maximum, $p = 0.346$; for

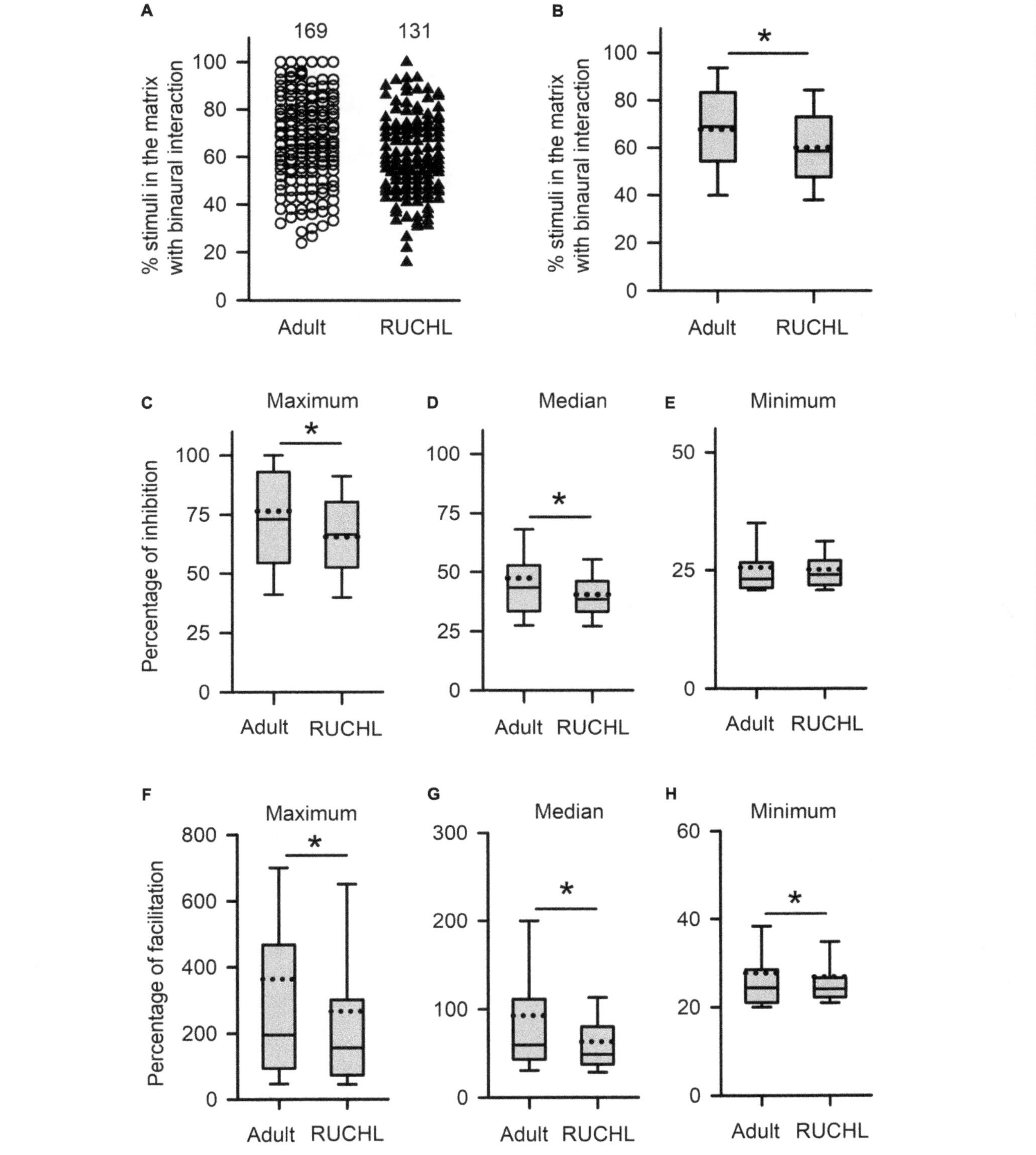

FIGURE 11 | The effects of RUCHL at young age on the degree of binaural interactions of AI neurons in adulthood. **(A,B)** Scatter plot **(A)** and box plot **(B)** showing the distributions in the percentages of stimuli that evoked binaural interactions in the binaural matrix. Each symbol in panel A represents the data from one neuron. The numbers indicate the number of neurons in each group. **(C–E)** Box plots showing the comparison in the degree of inhibitory binaural interaction between the two groups of AI neurons. The population data for the percentages of inhibition in maximum **(C)**, media **(D)**, and minimum **(E)** are determined from each AI neuron in each group of rats. **(F–H)** Box plots showing the comparison in the degree of facilitatory binaural interaction between the two groups of AI neurons. The population data for the percentages of facilitation in maximum **(F)**, media **(G)**, and minimum **(H)** are determined from each AI neuron in each group of rats. * indicates significant difference between two groups (Mann–Whitney *U*-test, $p < 0.05$).

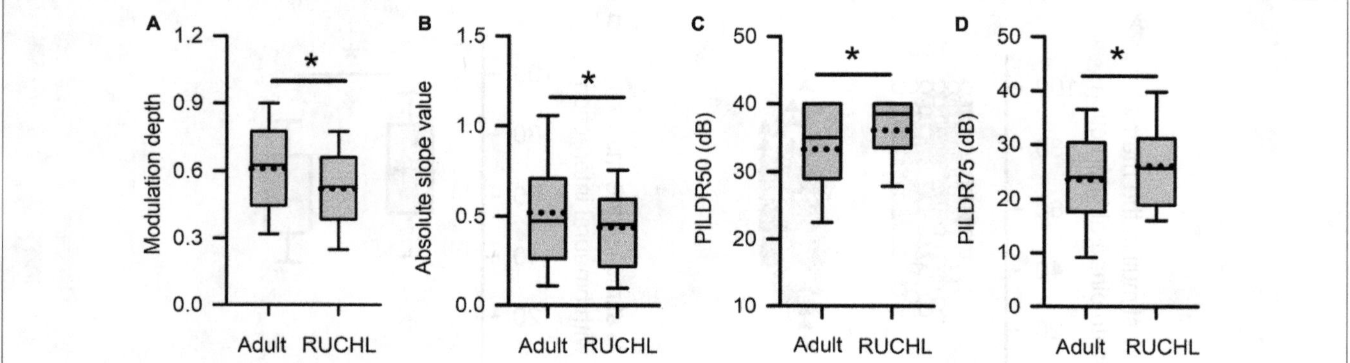

FIGURE 12 | Box plots showing the effects of RUCHL at young age on the sensitivity and the selectivity to ILDs of AI neurons in adulthood. **(A)** Modulation depth; **(B)** absolute slope value; **(C)** PILDR50; **(D)** PILDR75. The data for the PILDR50 the PILDR75 were determined from the averaged ILD response functions across ABL. * indicates significant difference between two groups (Mann–Whitney *U*-test, $p < 0.05$).

median, $p = 0.246$). No significant differences were found in the minimum percentages of facilitation among the three groups (Kruskal–Wallis test, $p = 0.082$).

The absolute slope values were not significantly different among the three groups (Kruskal–Wallis test, $p = 0.100$). However, the modulation depths in the RUCHL group were larger than those in the P14–18 group ($p = 0.001$) and were similar to those in the P19–30 group ($p = 0.119$). Kruskal–Wallis tests showed that the PILDR75s were not significantly different among the three groups at ABL 70 dB ($p = 0.069$), ABL 60 dB ($p = 0.082$), and ABL 40 dB ($p = 0.061$) except at ABL 50 dB ($p = 0.007$). At ABL 50, the PILDR75s in the RUCHL group were similar to those in the P14–18 group ($p = 0.721$), but were larger than those in the P19–30 group ($p = 0.002$). Moreover, the PILDR50s in the RUCHL group were significantly larger than those in the P19–30 group at ABL 70 dB ($p = 0.002$) and ABL 60 dB ($p = 0.018$), but not at ABL 50 dB ($p = 0.426$) and ABL 40 dB ($p = 0.138$); the PILDR50s in the RUCHL group were significantly smaller than those in the P14–18 group at ABL 60 dB ($p = 0.024$) and ABL 50 dB ($p = 0.002$), but not at ABL 70 dB ($p = 0.636$) and ABL 40 dB ($p = 0.121$), respectively.

The Basic Response Properties of Primary Auditory Cortex Neurons in the Four Groups of Rats

The CFs of AI neurons in the four groups of rats are shown in **Table 1**. Whereas the CFs of AI neurons in the P14–18 group were significantly different from those both in the P19–30 group and in the adult group, the CFs of AI neurons showed no significant differences between the P19-30 group and the adult group (Mann–Whitney *U*-test, P14–18 group vs. P19–30 group, $z = -3.780$, $p < 0.001$; P14–18 group vs. adult group, $z = -2.543$, $p = 0.011$; P19–30 group vs. adult group, $z = -1.059$, $p = 0.289$). In addition, we did not find significant differences in the CFs of AI neurons between the RUCHL group and the adult group (Mann–Whitney *U*-test, $z = -0.530$, $p = 0.596$). For the neurons categorized into inhibitory, facilitatory, and mixed binaural interactions, we did not find specific CF bands that contributed to one of three binaural interaction categories.

TABLE 1 | The basic response properties of primary auditory cortex (AI) neurons in the four groups of rats.

	P14–18 group	P19–30 group	Adult group	RUCHL group
CF (kHz)	21.08 ± 10.05*#	25.63 ± 10.69	24.06 ± 11.04	23.59 ± 11.60
MT (dB)	29.42 ± 10.24*	28.16 ± 7.81	26.60 ± 7.68&	28.99 ± 7.67
Latency (ms)	24.23 ± 5.31*#	16.73 ± 3.47$	15.05 ± 3.18	14.29 ± 3.54

*Data are shown in mean and SD. CF, characteristic frequency; MT, minimum threshold. *, #, $, and & indicate p < 0.05 (Mann–Whitney U-test) at P14–18 group vs. adult group, P14–P18 group vs. P19–30 group, P19–30 group vs. adult group, and UCHL group vs. adult group, respectively.*

We used CF stimuli to determine the minimum threshold of each neuron at 0 dB ILD (i.e., equal levels at both ears) with ABL varying from 0 to 80 dB at 10-dB steps. The minimum threshold was defined as the ABL that elicited 20% of the maximum response in the rate versus ABL function. The minimum thresholds of AI neurons in the four groups of rats are shown in **Table 1**. The minimum thresholds of AI neurons were higher in the P14–18 group than in the adult group; however, the minimum thresholds of AI neurons in the P19–30 group were not significantly different from those both in the P14–18 group and in the adult group (Mann–Whitney *U*-test, P14–18 group vs. adult group, $z = -2.987$, $p = 0.003$; P14–18 group vs. P19–30 group, $z = -1.418$, $p = 0.156$; P19–30 group vs. adult group, $z = -1.647$, $p = 0.099$). In addition, the minimum thresholds of AI neurons were significantly different between the RUCHL group and the adult group (Mann–Whitney *U*-test, $z = -2.732$, $p = 0.006$).

We analyzed the response latencies (i.e., first spike latencies) of AI neurons to the sound stimulus with 70 dB SPL at both ears. The response latencies of AI neurons in the four groups of rats are shown in **Table 1**. Mann–Whitney *U*-test showed that the response latencies were significantly different among AI neurons in the three age groups of rats with normal hearing development (P14–18 group vs. P19–30 group, $z = -11.522$, $p < 0.001$; P14–18 group vs. adult group, $z = -13.888$, $p < 0.001$; P19–30 group vs. adult group, $z = -4.454$, $p < 0.001$); however, the response latencies of AI neurons were not significantly different between the RUCHL group and the adult group ($z = -1.866$, $p = 0.062$).

Our data analysis did not find a specific range in CFs, minimum thresholds, and response latencies that contributes to a specific binaural interaction type; therefore, we did not find any specific relationships between the basic response properties and the binaural interaction types. Due to the time-consuming nature of the data collection for each neuron in our experimental design, it was difficult to get at a complete tonotopic map in one rat, and consequentially we could not determine the relationship between the basic response properties and the tonotopic maps.

DISCUSSION

During postnatal hearing development, the perception of sound spatial locations undergoes age-related changes (Freigang et al., 2015), experience-dependent plasticity (Keating and King, 2013; Keating et al., 2015), and training-induced plasticity in both behavior performance and auditory cortical spatial tuning (Zhang et al., 2013; Keating et al., 2016; Cheng et al., 2020). Whereas early age bilateral conductive hearing loss impairs sound loudness perception (Sun et al., 2011) and spatial memory (Zhao et al., 2018), UCHL during development impair performance on tasks such as sound localization and spatial release from masking that rely on binaural processing (Kumpik and King, 2019). The effects of hearing loss on the cognitive function depend on both the type of hearing loss and the time period of hearing loss during development. In the present study, we used CF tones to determine the age-related changes of binaural processing after the onset of hearing in the rat AI and investigated the effects of RUCHL at young age on the binaural processing of AI neurons in adulthood.

The results in the present study show that the EO and EE types are the two dominant monaural response types, and that the neurons in the rat AI exhibit inhibitory, facilitatory, and mixed binaural interactions. Our data have demonstrated that (1) the monaural response type, the binaural interaction type, and the distributions of the best ILDs in the rat AI are already adult-like shortly after hearing onset; (2) there exist developmental refinements in binaural processing, which were exhibited by an increase in the degree of binaural interaction, and the increase in the sensitivity and selectivity to ILDs during early period after hearing onset. (3) RCUHL at young age disrupts the developmental refinement of binaural processing of AI neurons in adulthood, i.e., decreases the degree of binaural interactions, and decreases both the selectivity and sensitivity to ILDs of AI neurons in adulthood. These results might help us to understand the neuronal mechanism of the refinement and plasticity in the perception of sound spatial locations during hearing development.

Postnatal Development in the Binaural Interactions in Primary Auditory Cortex

Our data indicate that the degree of binaural interactions in rat AI is relative weak at early ages after hearing onset and then progressively strengthens to maturity. In the binaural stimulus matrix, the percentages of stimuli evoking binaural interactions increase with age during the early period after hearing onset. Whereas the degrees of inhibitory/facilitatory binaural interactions in rat AI neurons are the lowest in the P14–18 group, they showed no significant differences between the P19–30 group and the adult group (**Figure 5**). To our knowledge, this is the first study to determine the developmental refinements in the degree of binaural interactions of AI neurons.

The auditory responses to binaural stimuli at early period after hearing onset have been reported in several previous studies. Evoked potential studies have demonstrated that human newborn infants show detectable although immature binaural interactions in the brainstem (Cone-Wesson et al., 1997) and auditory cortex (Nemeth et al., 2015). At single neuron level, the responses of cat AI neurons are influenced by binaural stimuli as early as at P8 before the hearing thresholds have declined below 100 dB SPL, and the binaural interaction types determined by P44 were similar in kind to those recorded in adult cats (Brugge et al., 1988). The hearing onset of rats occurs normally at P12, and the sound-evoked neuronal responses with high thresholds and poor frequency selectivity could be recorded in the rat auditory cortex as early as P13 (Zhang et al., 2001). In the present study, we determined the binaural interactions of rat AI neurons using CF tones from P14 because the response thresholds and frequency selectivity of rat AI neurons at P12–13 are not suitable for us to evaluate the binaural processing in our experiment paradigm. Our results show that both the monaural response types and the binaural interaction types in the P14–18 group are similar to those in the P19–30 group and the adult group. In the auditory cortex of pallid bats, the adult-like clustered organization of binaural properties is present at P15 before the morphological development of external ears and head is complete; however, the binaural facilitation was not observed in bats younger than 25 days (Razak and Fuzessery, 2007). Therefore, previous studies from cats and bats, and the present study from rats have demonstrated that the binaural interaction types observed immediately after hearing onset are largely adult-like. Furthermore, the present study demonstrates that the degree of binaural interactions undergoes developmental increase after hearing onset.

In the adult cat AI, purely monaural neurons are rare (Zhang et al., 2004). Consistent with this result, we found that all of the recorded rat AI neurons showed some sort of binaural interactions. For those stimuli that evoked binaural interactions in the binaural stimulus matrix, the responses to the sound stimuli in one ear can be facilitated and/or suppressed by presenting the stimuli at the other ear. Even in the AI of RUCHL rats that experienced asymmetric binaural hearing, we did not encounter purely monaural neurons. Although we cannot rule out the possibility of monaural neurons in the rat AI, the data in the present study suggest that purely monaural neurons are rare in the rat AI.

Postnatal Development of Interaural Level Differences Processing in the Auditory Cortex

The ability to perceive the acoustic space changes during postnatal hearing development (Freigang et al., 2015). In the central auditory system, the encoding of sound spatial information undergoes maturational changes after hearing onset. For example, the rudimentary ILD coding in the lateral superior olive (Sanes and Rubel, 1988), inferior colliculus (Blatchley and Brugge, 1990), and auditory cortex (Brugge et al., 1988; Mrsic-Flogel et al., 2003) is evident soon after the onset of hearing and further matures with age (Moore and Irvine, 1981). The ILD responses in the lateral superior olive of young gerbils show smaller dynamic range and shallower slope than that of adult gerbils (Sanes and Rubel, 1988). Moreover, EEG studies in 4–7 years age of normal hearing children have demonstrated that adult-like ILD coding patterns are evident in the immature cortical responses of children at this age (Easwar et al., 2018).

In the present study, we found that AI neurons in the P14–18 group had larger values in PILDRs and smaller values in the slope and the modulation depth of the ILD response functions than the AI neurons in both the P19–30 group and the adult group (**Figure 7**). The results indicate that both the sensitivity and the selectivity of rat AI neurons to ILD are immature during 1 week after the onset of hearing. Moreover, the sensitivity and the selectivity to ILD for AI neurons in the P19–30 group were similar to those in the adult group. Therefore, both the sensitivity and the selectivity of rat AI neurons to ILD undergo a developmental refinement after hearing onset, which might contribute to the development of auditory spatial tuning in rat AI.

The factors that influence the development of ILD processing in AI could be from auditory peripheral and/or central neural circuits. During postnatal hearing development, the binaural cues (ITD and ILD) vary as the head and the external ears grow. The auditory periphery has been demonstrated to be critically involved in limiting the maturation of spatial selectivity in the ferret auditory cortex (Mrsic-Flogel et al., 2003). In the present study, we determined the binaural responses of high-frequency (> 4 kHz) AI neurons to stimuli varying in ILDs. The age-related changes in ILDs from auditory peripheral could be one factor contributing to the observed refinement of ILD processing in AI. Previous studies have shown that binaural interaction shapes the virtual space receptive field and changes the spatial selectivity of AI neurons (Brugge et al., 1994). In the present study, the age-related changes in the degree of binaural interactions in rat AI might be another factor in the central circuits contributing to the developmental refinement of ILD processing. However, how the age-related changes in binaural interactions directly refine the ILD processing during hearing development is still not clear.

Our data show that majority of AI neurons preferred ILDs favoring contralateral spatial azimuth in both the adult and developing rats (**Figure 8**). Studies in the adult animals in a variety of species have demonstrated the dominant preference of AI neurons to contralateral spatial locations, e.g., in cats (Irvine et al., 1996; Zhang et al., 2004), bats (Razak, 2011), monkeys (Zhou and Wang, 2012; Lui et al., 2015), rats (Yao et al., 2013; Gao et al., 2018; Wang et al., 2019), and mice (Panniello et al., 2018). The results in the immature rats suggest that the dominant contralateral preference of AI neurons is already present immediately after the onset of hearing and is adult-like.

The Effect of Reversible Unilateral Conductive Hearing Loss at Young Age on the Binaural Processing in Adult Primary Auditory Cortex

In the present study, we injected the poloxamer into the right ear of rats to induce a short-term UCHL in the RUCHL group. This manipulation induced an asymmetric binaural hearing because UCHL degraded the excitatory input from the injected ear whereas the excitatory input from the non-injected ear remained normal. Even if the hearing threshold of the injected ear returned to normal at P30 (**Figure 9**), the AI neurons in the RUCHL group showed a lower degree of binaural interaction and lower sensitivity and selectivity to ILDs compared with the AI neurons in adult group (**Figure 10**). We have shown the developmental refinement in the binaural processing of AI neurons during postnatal hearing development; the data from the RUCHL group indicated that the short-term asymmetric binaural hearing at young age disrupted the developmental refinement of binaural processing in the rat AI in adulthood, and the effects lasted at least 1 month after the hearing threshold of the injected ear recovered.

Reversible Unilateral Conductive Hearing Loss at young age did not significantly affect the distributions in both the ILD preferences and the best ILDs of AI neurons (**Figure 10**). Previous studies have shown that a stronger and longer period of UCHL (by removing the tympanic membrane and malleus in the right ear from P14) greatly reduced the proportion of rat AI neurons with contralateral azimuth preference and increased the proportion of AI neurons with ipsilateral azimuth preference when determined in adulthood (Wang et al., 2019). In addition, monaural deprivation in rats by ear canal ligation from P14 weakened the deprived ear's representation, strengthened the open ear's representation, and disrupted binaural integration of ILD in AI (Popescu and Polley, 2010). It is very likely that the short-term and moderate UCHL used in the present study was not strong enough to change the distributions in both the ILD preferences and the best ILD of AI neurons in the RUCHL group.

For the monaural response types in rat AI, RUCHL at young age decreased the proportion of EO neurons and increased the proportion of EE neurons in the RUCHL group; in addition, we observed few OE neurons in the RUCHL group but not in the adult group with normal hearing development (**Figure 10A**). Although the differences in the proportions of neurons within the same monaural response type category between the RUCHL group and the adult group are not large, the data from our study indicated that, for a small proportion of AI neurons in the RUCHL group, the RUCHL at young age indeed increased representation of ipsilateral normal hearing ear, and consequentially increased the proportions of EE neurons and OE neurons in the rat AI of RUCHL group. Furthermore, the results suggest that the adult-like distributions in monaural response types of AI neurons immediately after hearing onset can be modified by abnormal hearing experience during the early period of hearing development.

Possible Mechanisms for the Developmental Plasticity of Binaural Processing

During postnatal hearing development, the auditory system undergoes developmental changes in synaptic responses and synaptic receptor components. The synaptic responses in the lateral superior olive of P12–14 gerbils indicate that both the amplitude and temporal processing remain compromised (Sanes, 1993). In the mouse auditory cortex, both the intrinsic and synaptic properties undergo a transitional period between P10 and P18 prior to reaching steady state at P19–P29 (Oswald and Reyes, 2008). Immediately after hearing onset, the excitatory and the inhibitory synaptic responses in rat AI to sound stimuli are equally strong; however, the excitation and inhibition are not matched and correlated until during the third postnatal week (Dorrn et al., 2010). In addition, the inhibitory synaptic inputs in developing AI are longer in duration than those in adult AI (Cai et al., 2018). The refinement of binaural processing found in the present study might depend on the changes of the inhibitory and excitatory synaptic responses in AI (Dorrn et al., 2010; Sun et al., 2010; Cai et al., 2018), or the changes of the strength of inhibitory and excitatory intracortical connections in AI (Chang et al., 2005). During postnatal hearing development, the synaptic receptor components in AI also undergo age-related changes. In the rat auditory cortex, AMPA receptor subunit GluR2 protein expression increases with age after hearing onset (Xu et al., 2007), and the expression of NMDA receptor subunit NR1 mRNA increases from birth to P35 (Lu et al., 2008). In addition, the NR2A and NR2B mRNA expression in the rat auditory cortex peaks about 1 week after the onset of hearing before declining slightly into adulthood (Hsieh et al., 2002). Moreover, the GABAA receptor subunit (α1 and α3) expression in the rat auditory cortex also exhibits age-related changes (Xu et al., 2010). These age-related changes in the subunits of AMPA, NMDA, and GABA receptors might play an important role in the auditory functional development. However, whether these changes are directly related to the developmental refinements of binaural processing observed in the present study needs to be further studied.

Acoustic experience can induce plasticity in the neuronal connections and aural dominance in the central auditory system. During the critical period of hearing development, the neuronal connections in the mouse auditory cortex are shaped by hearing experience (Meng et al., 2020). Early onset of unilateral deafening cats leads to a massive reorganization of aural preference in the auditory cortex in favor of the hearing ear (Kral et al., 2013). Moreover, UCHL in young rats induced a significant shift of the aural dominance from contralateral preference to ipsilateral preference in AI but not in the inferior colliculus (Popescu and Polley, 2010), and this result suggests that the effect of RUCHL exerts stronger plasticity in the auditory cortex than in the inferior colliculus. Consistently, a 2-deoxyglucose uptake study in gerbils demonstrated that RUCHL at young age could restore balanced afferent activity on both sides of the anteroventral cochlear nucleus, the medial superior olive, and the inferior colliculus 1 week after restoring binaural hearing from P28 (Hutson et al., 2009). Based on these findings, we postulate that the observed RUCHL effects in the present study most likely occurred above the inferior colliculus. In the present study, the RUCHL at young age did not significantly change the CF distributions and the response latencies of AI neurons in adulthood. Our data showed that, to some extent, RUCHL at young age might retard the refinement of binaural processing in the degree of binaural interaction, and in both the selectivity and sensitivity to ILDs of AI neurons. It is possible that the RUCHL at young age might induce abnormal development changes in the excitatory/inhibitory synaptic responses and the synaptic receptor components in the auditory cortex, and therefore disrupt normal developmental refinement of binaural processing.

The present study was conducted in urethane-anesthetized rats. Because the data collection in the experimental design was time consuming, it is difficult to perform this study in awaking rats. If urethane has any effects on the neuronal responses in AI, it would affect both the monaural and binaural responses. As we determined the binaural interactions of AI neurons by comparing the binaural responses with monaural responses, this possible effect should not have great influences on our conclusions.

AUTHOR CONTRIBUTIONS

JZ and JL designed this study, analyzed the data, and drafted the article. JL and XH engaged in data collection. All authors contributed to the final version of the article and approved the submitted version.

ACKNOWLEDGMENTS

We acknowledge the support by the NYU-ECNU Institute of Brain and Cognitive Science at NYU Shanghai, and the support by the open project of Key Laboratory of Brain Functional Genomics, Ministry of Education. We also acknowledge the support by the Instruments Sharing Platform of School of Life Sciences, East China Normal University.

REFERENCES

Blatchley, B. J., and Brugge, J. F. (1990). Sensitivity to binaural intensity and phase difference cues in kitten inferior colliculus. *J. Neurophysiol.* 64, 582–597. doi: 10.1152/jn.1990.64.2.582

Brugge, J. F., Reale, R. A., Hind, J. E., Chan, J. C., Musicant, A. D., and Poon, P. W. (1994). Simulation of free-field sound sources and its application to studies of cortical mechanisms of sound localization in the cat. *Hear. Res.* 73, 67–84. doi: 10.1016/0378-5955(94)90284-4

Brugge, J. F., Reale, R. A., and Wilson, G. F. (1988). Sensitivity of auditory cortical neurons of kittens to monaural and binaural high frequency sound. *Hear. Res.* 34, 127–140. doi: 10.1016/0378-5955(88)90100-1

Bundy, R. S. (1980). Discrimination of sound localization cues in young infants. *Child Dev.* 51, 292–294. doi: 10.2307/1129627

Cai, D., Han, R., Liu, M., Xie, F., You, L., Zheng, Y., et al. (2018). A Critical Role of Inhibition in Temporal Processing Maturation in the Primary Auditory Cortex. *Cereb. Cortex* 28, 1610–1624. doi: 10.1093/cercor/bhx057

Chang, E. F., Bao, S., Imaizumi, K., Schreiner, C. E., and Merzenich, M. M. (2005). Development of spectral and temporal response selectivity in the auditory cortex. *Proc. Natl. Acad. Sci. U. S. A.* 102, 16460–16465. doi: 10.1073/pnas.0508239102

Cheng, Y., Zhang, Y., Wang, F., Jia, G., Zhou, J., Shan, Y., et al. (2020). Reversal of Age-Related Changes in Cortical Sound-Azimuth Selectivity with Training. *Cereb. Cortex* 30, 1768–1778. doi: 10.1093/cercor/bhz201

Cone-Wesson, B., Ma, E., and Fowler, C. G. (1997). Effect of stimulus level and frequency on ABR and MLR binaural interaction in human neonates. *Hear. Res.* 106, 163–178. doi: 10.1016/s0378-5955(97)00016-6

Doron, N. N., Ledoux, J. E., and Semple, M. N. (2002). Redefining the tonotopic core of rat auditory cortex: physiological evidence for a posterior field. *J. Comp. Neurol.* 453, 345–360. doi: 10.1002/cne.10412

Dorrn, A. L., Yuan, K., Barker, A. J., Schreiner, C. E., and Froemke, R. C. (2010). Developmental sensory experience balances cortical excitation and inhibition. *Nature* 465, 932–936. doi: 10.1038/nature09119

Easwar, V., Yamazaki, H., Deighton, M., Papsin, B., and Gordon, K. (2018). Cortical Processing of Level Cues for Spatial Hearing is Impaired in Children with Prelingual Deafness Despite Early Bilateral Access to Sound. *Brain Topogr.* 31, 270–287. doi: 10.1007/s10548-017-0596-5

Freigang, C., Richter, N., Rubsamen, R., and Ludwig, A. A. (2015). Age-related changes in sound localisation ability. *Cell Tissue Res.* 361, 371–386. doi: 10.1007/s00441-015-2230-8

Gao, F., Chen, L., and Zhang, J. (2018). Nonuniform impacts of forward suppression on neural responses to preferred stimuli and nonpreferred stimuli in the rat auditory cortex. *Eur. J. Neurosci.* 47, 1320–1338. doi: 10.1111/ejn.13943

Grothe, B., Pecka, M., and McAlpine, D. (2010). Mechanisms of sound localization in mammals. *Physiol. Rev.* 90, 983–1012. doi: 10.1152/physrev.00026.2009

Hawley, M. L., Litovsky, R. Y., and Culling, J. F. (2004). The benefit of binaural hearing in a cocktail party: effect of location and type of interferer. *J. Acoust. Soc. Am.* 115, 833–843. doi: 10.1121/1.1639908

Hogan, S. C., Stratford, K. J., and Moore, D. R. (1997). Duration and recurrence of otitis media with effusion in children from birth to 3 years: prospective study using monthly otoscopy and tympanometry. *BMJ* 314, 350–353. doi: 10.1136/bmj.314.7077.350

Hsieh, C. Y., Chen, Y., Leslie, F. M., and Metherate, R. (2002). Postnatal development of NR2A and NR2B mRNA expression in rat auditory cortex and thalamus. *J. Assoc. Res. Otolaryngol.* 3, 479–487. doi: 10.1007/s10162-002-2052-8

Hutson, K. A., Durham, D., and Tucci, D. L. (2009). Reversible conductive hearing loss: restored activity in the central auditory system. *Audiol. Neurootol.* 14, 69–77. doi: 10.1159/000158535

Irvine, D. R., Rajan, R., and Aitkin, L. M. (1996). Sensitivity to interaural intensity differences of neurons in primary auditory cortex of the cat. I. types of sensitivity and effects of variations in sound pressure level. *J. Neurophysiol.* 75, 75–96. doi: 10.1152/jn.1996.75.1.75

Keating, P., Dahmen, J. C., and King, A. J. (2015). Complementary adaptive processes contribute to the developmental plasticity of spatial hearing. *Nat. Neurosci.* 18, 185–187. doi: 10.1038/nn.3914

Keating, P., and King, A. J. (2013). Developmental plasticity of spatial hearing following asymmetric hearing loss: context-dependent cue integration and its clinical implications. *Front. Syst. Neurosci.* 7:123. doi: 10.3389/fnsys.2013.00123

Keating, P., Rosenior-Patten, O., Dahmen, J. C., Bell, O., and King, A. J. (2016). Behavioral training promotes multiple adaptive processes following acute hearing loss. *Elife* 5:e12264. doi: 10.7554/eLife.12264

Kral, A., Hubka, P., Heid, S., and Tillein, J. (2013). Single-sided deafness leads to unilateral aural preference within an early sensitive period. *Brain* 136, 180–193. doi: 10.1093/brain/aws305

Kuhnle, S., Ludwig, A. A., Meuret, S., Kuttner, C., Witte, C., Scholbach, J., et al. (2013). Development of auditory localization accuracy and auditory spatial discrimination in children and adolescents. *Audiol. Neurootol.* 18, 48–62. doi: 10.1159/000342904

Kumpik, D. P., and King, A. J. (2019). A review of the effects of unilateral hearing loss on spatial hearing. *Hear. Res.* 372, 17–28. doi: 10.1016/j.heares.2018.08.003

Lu, J., Cui, Y., Cai, R., Mao, Y., Zhang, J., and Sun, X. (2008). Early auditory deprivation alters expression of NMDA receptor subunit NR1 mRNA in the rat auditory cortex. *J. Neurosci. Res.* 86, 1290–1296. doi: 10.1002/jnr.21577

Lui, L. L., Mokri, Y., Reser, D. H., Rosa, M. G., and Rajan, R. (2015). Responses of neurons in the marmoset primary auditory cortex to interaural level differences: comparison of pure tones and vocalizations. *Front. Neurosci.* 9:132. doi: 10.3389/fnins.2015.00132

Malhotra, S., and Lomber, S. G. (2007). Sound localization during homotopic and heterotopic bilateral cooling deactivation of primary and nonprimary auditory cortical areas in the cat. *J. Neurophysiol.* 97, 26–43. doi: 10.1152/jn.00720.2006

Meng, X., Solarana, K., Bowen, Z., Liu, J., Nagode, D. A., Sheikh, A., et al. (2020). Transient Subgranular Hyperconnectivity to L2/3 and Enhanced Pairwise Correlations During the Critical Period in the Mouse Auditory Cortex. *Cereb. Cortex* 30, 1914–1930. doi: 10.1093/cercor/bhz213

Middlebrooks, J. C. (2015). Sound localization. *Handb. Clin. Neurol.* 129, 99–116.

Middlebrooks, J. C., and Waters, M. F. (2020). Spatial Mechanisms for Segregation of Competing Sounds, and a Breakdown in Spatial Hearing. *Front. Neurosci.* 14:571095. doi: 10.3389/fnins.2020.571095

Moore, D. R., and Irvine, D. R. (1981). Development of responses to acoustic interaural intensity differences in the car inferior colliculus. *Exp. Brain Res.* 41, 301–309. doi: 10.1007/BF00238887

Mrsic-Flogel, T. D., Schnupp, J. W., and King, A. J. (2003). Acoustic factors govern developmental sharpening of spatial tuning in the auditory cortex. *Nat. Neurosci.* 6, 981–988. doi: 10.1038/nn1108

Nemeth, R., Haden, G. P., Torok, M., and Winkler, I. (2015). Processing of Horizontal Sound Localization Cues in Newborn Infants. *Ear Hear.* 36, 550–556. doi: 10.1097/AUD.0000000000000160

Nodal, F. R., Kacelnik, O., Bajo, V. M., Bizley, J. K., Moore, D. R., and King, A. J. (2010). Lesions of the auditory cortex impair azimuthal sound localization and its recalibration in ferrets. *J. Neurophysiol.* 103, 1209–1225. doi: 10.1152/jn.00991.2009

Oswald, A. M., and Reyes, A. D. (2008). Maturation of intrinsic and synaptic properties of layer 2/3 pyramidal neurons in mouse auditory cortex. *J. Neurophysiol.* 99, 2998–3008. doi: 10.1152/jn.01160.2007

Panniello, M., King, A. J., Dahmen, J. C., and Walker, K. M. M. (2018). Local and Global Spatial Organization of Interaural Level Difference and Frequency Preferences in Auditory Cortex. *Cereb. Cortex* 28, 350–369. doi: 10.1093/cercor/bhx295

Pillsbury, H. C., Grose, J. H., and Hall, J. W. III (1991). Otitis media with effusion in children. Binaural hearing before and after corrective surgery. *Arch. Otolaryngol. Head Neck Surg.* 117, 718–723. doi: 10.1001/archotol.1991.01870190030008

Polley, D. B., Thompson, J. H., and Guo, W. (2013). Brief hearing loss disrupts binaural integration during two early critical periods of auditory cortex development. *Nat. Commun.* 4:2547. doi: 10.1038/ncomms3547

Popescu, M. V., and Polley, D. B. (2010). Monaural deprivation disrupts development of binaural selectivity in auditory midbrain and cortex. *Neuron* 65, 718–731. doi: 10.1016/j.neuron.2010.02.019

Potash, M., and Kelly, J. (1980). Development of directional responses to sounds in the rat (*Rattus norvegicus*). *J. Comp. Physiol. Psychol.* 94, 864–877. doi: 10.1037/h0077819

Razak, K. A. (2011). Systematic representation of sound locations in the primary auditory cortex. *J. Neurosci.* 31, 13848–13859. doi: 10.1523/jneurosci.1937-11.2011

Razak, K. A., and Fuzessery, Z. M. (2007). Development of functional organization of the pallid bat auditory cortex. *Hear. Res.* 228, 69–81. doi: 10.1016/j.heares.2007.01.020

Samson, F. K., Barone, P., Clarey, J. C., and Imig, T. J. (1994). Effects of ear plugging on single-unit azimuth sensitivity in cat primary auditory cortex. II. Azimuth tuning dependent upon binaural stimulation. *J. Neurophysiol.* 71, 2194–2216. doi: 10.1152/jn.1994.71.6.2194

Sanes, D. H. (1993). The development of synaptic function and integration in the central auditory system. *J. Neurosci.* 13, 2627–2637. doi: 10.1523/jneurosci.13-06-02627.1993

Sanes, D. H., and Rubel, E. W. (1988). The ontogeny of inhibition and excitation in the gerbil lateral superior olive. *J. Neurosci.* 8, 682–700. doi: 10.1523/jneurosci.08-02-00682.1988

Semple, M. N., and Kitzes, L. M. (1987). Binaural processing of sound pressure level in the inferior colliculus. *J. Neurophysiol.* 57, 1130–1147. doi: 10.1152/jn.1987.57.4.1130

Sun, W., Manohar, S., Jayaram, A., Kumaraguru, A., Fu, Q., Li, J., et al. (2011). Early age conductive hearing loss causes audiogenic seizure and hyperacusis behavior. *Hear. Res.* 282, 178–183. doi: 10.1016/j.heares.2011.08.004

Sun, Y. J., Wu, G. K., Liu, B. H., Li, P., Zhou, M., Xiao, Z., et al. (2010). Fine-tuning of pre-balanced excitation and inhibition during auditory cortical development. *Nature* 465, 927–931. doi: 10.1038/nature09079

Van Deun, L., van Wieringen, A., Van den Bogaert, T., Scherf, F., Offeciers, F. E., Van de Heyning, P. H., et al. (2009). Sound localization, sound lateralization, and binaural masking level differences in young children with normal hearing. *Ear Hear.* 30, 178–190. doi: 10.1097/AUD.0b013e318194256b

Wang, X., Liu, J., and Zhang, J. (2019). Chronic Unilateral Hearing Loss Disrupts Neural Tuning to Sound-Source Azimuth in the Rat Primary Auditory Cortex. *Front. Neurosci.* 13:477. doi: 10.3389/fnins.2019.00477

Wilmington, D., Gray, L., and Jahrsdoerfer, R. (1994). Binaural processing after corrected congenital unilateral conductive hearing loss. *Hear. Res.* 74, 99–114. doi: 10.1016/0378-5955(94)90179-1

Wood, K. C., Town, S. M., and Bizley, J. K. (2019). Neurons in primary auditory cortex represent sound source location in a cue-invariant manner. *Nat. Commun.* 10:3019. doi: 10.1038/s41467-019-10868-9

Woods, T. M., Lopez, S. E., Long, J. H., Rahman, J. E., and Recanzone, G. H. (2006). Effects of stimulus azimuth and intensity on the single-neuron activity in the auditory cortex of the alert macaque monkey. *J. Neurophysiol.* 96, 3323–3337. doi: 10.1152/jn.00392.2006

Xu, F., Cai, R., Xu, J., Zhang, J., and Sun, X. (2007). Early music exposure modifies GluR2 protein expression in rat auditory cortex and anterior cingulate cortex. *Neurosci. Lett.* 420, 179–183. doi: 10.1016/j.neulet.2007.05.005

Xu, J., Yu, L., Cai, R., Zhang, J., and Sun, X. (2010). Early continuous white noise exposure alters auditory spatial sensitivity and expression of GAD65 and GABAA receptor subunits in rat auditory cortex. *Cereb. Cortex* 20, 804–812. doi: 10.1093/cercor/bhp143

Yao, J. D., Bremen, P., and Middlebrooks, J. C. (2013). Rat primary auditory cortex is tuned exclusively to the contralateral hemifield. *J. Neurophysiol.* 110, 2140–2151. doi: 10.1152/jn.00219.2013

Zhang, J., Nakamoto, K. T., and Kitzes, L. M. (2004). Binaural interaction revisited in the cat primary auditory cortex. *J. Neurophysiol.* 91, 101–117. doi: 10.1152/jn.00166.2003

Zhang, L. I., Bao, S., and Merzenich, M. M. (2001). Persistent and specific influences of early acoustic environments on primary auditory cortex. *Nat. Neurosci.* 4, 1123–1130. doi: 10.1038/nn745

Zhang, Y., Zhao, Y., Zhu, X., Sun, X., and Zhou, X. (2013). Refining cortical representation of sound azimuths by auditory discrimination training. *J. Neurosci.* 33, 9693–9698. doi: 10.1523/JNEUROSCI.0158-13.2013

Zhao, H., Wang, L., Chen, L., Zhang, J., Sun, W., Salvi, R. J., et al. (2018). Temporary conductive hearing loss in early life impairs spatial memory of rats in adulthood. *Brain Behav.* 8:e01004. doi: 10.1002/brb3.1004

Zhao, Y., Xu, X., He, J., Xu, J., and Zhang, J. (2015). Age-related changes in neural gap detection thresholds in the rat auditory cortex. *Eur. J. Neurosci.* 41, 285–292. doi: 10.1111/ejn.12791

Zhou, Y., and Wang, X. (2012). Level dependence of spatial processing in the primate auditory cortex. *J. Neurophysiol.* 108, 810–826. doi: 10.1152/jn.00500.2011

16

Mirror Mechanism Behind Visual–Auditory Interaction: Evidence from Event-Related Potentials in Children with Cochlear Implants

Junbo Wang[1†], Jiahao Liu[1†], Kaiyin Lai[2], Qi Zhang[3], Yiqing Zheng[1], Suiping Wang[2] and Maojin Liang[1*]*

[1] Department of Otolaryngology, Sun Yat-sen Memorial Hospital, Guangzhou, China, [2] South China Normal University, Guangzhou, China, [3] School of Foreign Languages, Shenzhen University, Shenzhen, China

***Correspondence:**
Suiping Wang
wangsuiping@m.scnu.edu.cn
Maojin Liang
liangmj3@mail.sysu.edu.cn

† These authors have contributed equally to this work

The mechanism underlying visual-induced auditory interaction is still under discussion. Here, we provide evidence that the mirror mechanism underlies visual–auditory interactions. In this study, visual stimuli were divided into two major groups—mirror stimuli that were able to activate mirror neurons and non-mirror stimuli that were not able to activate mirror neurons. The two groups were further divided into six subgroups as follows: visual speech-related mirror stimuli, visual speech-irrelevant mirror stimuli, and non-mirror stimuli with four different luminance levels. Participants were 25 children with cochlear implants (CIs) who underwent an event-related potential (ERP) and speech recognition task. The main results were as follows: (1) there were significant differences in P1, N1, and P2 ERPs between mirror stimuli and non-mirror stimuli; (2) these ERP differences between mirror and non-mirror stimuli were partly driven by Brodmann areas 41 and 42 in the superior temporal gyrus; (3) ERP component differences between visual speech-related mirror and non-mirror stimuli were partly driven by Brodmann area 39 (visual speech area), which was not observed when comparing the visual speech-irrelevant stimulus and non-mirror groups; and (4) ERPs evoked by visual speech-related mirror stimuli had more components correlated with speech recognition than ERPs evoked by non-mirror stimuli, while ERPs evoked by speech-irrelevant mirror stimuli were not significantly different to those induced by the non-mirror stimuli. These results indicate the following: (1) mirror and non-mirror stimuli differ in their associated neural activation; (2) the visual–auditory interaction possibly led to ERP differences, as Brodmann areas 41 and 42 constitute the primary auditory cortex; (3) mirror neurons could be responsible for the ERP differences, considering that Brodmann area 39 is associated with processing information about speech-related mirror stimuli; and (4) ERPs evoked by visual speech-related mirror stimuli could better reflect speech recognition ability. These results support the hypothesis that a mirror mechanism underlies visual–auditory interactions.

Keywords: mirror mechanism, event-related potential, cochlear implant, hearing loss, speech performance, visual auditory

INTRODUCTION

Visual–auditory interactions represent the interference between the visual system and the auditory system (Bulkin and Groh, 2006). A classic example of a visual–auditory interaction is the McGurk effect, in which video lip movements for [ga], dubbed by syllable sound [ba], lead to the auditory illusion of the fused syllable [da] (McGurk and MacDonald, 1976). This indicates that the visual system interferes with the auditory system. Another example is that pictures containing auditory information, such as "playing the violin" or "welding," can activate the primary auditory cortex Brodmann area 41, while other pictures without auditory information do not (Proverbio et al., 2011). Furthermore, people with hearing loss show greater activation in the auditory cortex than normal-hearing controls during these kinds of stimuli; this suggests that the visual cortex compensates for hearing loss and could explain the basis of visual–auditory interactions (Finney et al., 2001; Liang et al., 2017).

Neuroimaging evidence has suggested that cross-modal plasticity might underlie visual–auditory interactions in patients with hearing loss (Finney et al., 2001; Mao and Pallas, 2013; Stropahl and Debener, 2017). This could indicate that a loss of auditory input causes the visual cortex to "take up" the auditory cortex *via* cross-modal plasticity and causes an interference of the visual system on the auditory system.

However, there are still some questions under discussion. For example, the McGurk effect is seen not only in patients with hearing loss but also in normal-hearing people, whose sensory tendency (a preference for visual or auditory interference) is no different to patients with hearing loss (Rosemann et al., 2020). Considering that cross-modal plasticity differs between these two groups while they showed no difference in visual–auditory interaction, there might be other mechanisms underlying visual–auditory interactions. We hypothesized that the mirror mechanism is one such mechanism underlying this visual–auditory interaction.

First, neurons that discharge in response to both observation and execution are called mirror neurons, and the theory to explain their functions is called mirror mechanism. For example, it has been reported that a large proportion of a monkey's premotor cortical neurons discharge not only while performing specific actions but also when hearing associated sounds or observing the same actions (Keysers et al., 2002); thus, in observational processes, mirror neurons imitate what they do in executional processes. Incidentally, visual–auditory interactions are associated with a similar phenomenon, whereby the auditory cortex imitates what it does in response to auditory stimuli during the presentation of visual stimuli.

Second, mirror mechanism allows "hearing" to be an executional process. One ongoing issue is that hearing is a feeling rather an executable action and thus cannot be classified as a "motor action," which refers to the executional process of the mirror mechanism. However, some researchers have argued that "motor actions" encoded by the mirror mechanism are actually "action goals" rather than muscle contractions or joint displacement (Rizzolatti et al., 2001; Rizzolatti and Sinigaglia, 2016). For example, mirror mechanism has been related with empathy (Gazzola et al., 2006) and animal sounds that were mistakenly recognized as tool sounds, thus activating similar cortical areas as the tool sounds (Brefczynski et al., 2005); empathy and sound recognition are not muscle contractions or joint displacement. Currently, mirror mechanism has been defined as "a basic brain mechanism that transforms sensory representations of others' behavior into one's own motor or visceromotor representations concerning that behavior and, depending on the location, can fulfill a range of cognitive functions, including action and emotion understanding"; furthermore, "motor actions" usually refer to the outcomes induced by actions rather than the actions themselves (Rizzolatti and Sinigaglia, 2016). Thus, mirror mechanism might allow "hearing" to be an executional process.

Third, we have consistency of activated nerve localization in visual–auditory interaction and mirror neurons. One experiment reported that visual–auditory stimuli can activate mirror neurons (Proverbio et al., 2011), but has not been further discussed. This might be due to limitations that are inherent to the study design, whereby pictures with no auditory information are complex and may therefore cause activation of mirror neurons.

To conclude, it is reasonable to suspect that the mirror mechanism might underlie visual–auditory interactions. In this study, we measured event-related potentials (ERPs) and speech recognition ability in children with cochlear implants (CIs) during mirror neuron-activated and mirror neuron-silent visual–auditory interaction tasks. We aimed to determine the role of this mirror mechanism in visual–auditory interactions.

MATERIALS AND METHODS

Participants

Twenty-five prelingually deaf children fitted with a CI for at least 4 years were recruited. These included 12 boys and 13 girls aged between 5 and 18 years (mean: 9.86; SD: 3.80). **Table 1** presents the detailed demographic information. All participants were right-handed and had normal or corrected-to-normal vision. Ethical approval was obtained from the Institutional Review Board at Sun Yat-sen Memorial Hospital at Sun Yat-sen University. Detailed information was provided to the parents, and written consent was obtained before proceeding with the study.

Speech-Related Behavioral Tests

Of the 25 participants, 11 took part in the behavioral experiment. The behavioral experiment comprised six tasks as follows: easy tone, difficult tone, easy vowel, difficult vowel, easy consonant, and difficult consonant. For the experimental materials and classification standards, we referred to *Research on the Spectrogram Similarity Standardization of Phonetic Stimulus for Children* (Xibin, 2006). Vowels were classified according to the opening characteristics and internal structural characteristics of the first sound. As a result, vowel recognition can be divided into four groups according to these two dimensions, namely, the same structure with different openings, the same opening with

TABLE 1 | Information of all participants in this study.

Number	Gender	Age at experiment(y)	CI side	Age at CI(y)	Age at hearing loss(y)	Speech test
1	Male	7	Right	1	0	No
2	Male	8	Left	3	2	No
3	Male	13	Right	5	0	No
4	Female	16	Right	3	0	No
5	Male	11	Right	2	0	Yes
6	Female	9	Right	5	4	Yes
7	Male	13	Right	10	1	No
8	Female	7	Right	3	0	Yes
9	Female	8	Right	4	2	Yes
10	Male	7	Right	2	0	Yes
11	Male	7	Right	2	0	Yes
12	Female	10	Both	4	1	No
13	Male	7	Right	1	0	Yes
14	Female	18	Right	6	1.5	No
15	Male	7	Right	2	6	No
16	Female	6	Right	1	0	No
17	Female	9	Right	3	1.4	No
18	Female	9	Right	3	2	No
19	Male	10	Right	2	0	No
20	Female	17	Right	3	0	Yes
21	Female	6	Right	2	0	No
22	Female	18	Right	13	4	Yes
23	Male	9	Left	2	1	Yes
24	Male	9	Right	2	Unknown	No
25	Female	7	Right	1	0	Yes

different structures, the same opening with the same structure, and the compound vowels of the front nose and the rear nose. Consonants can be classified into six groups according to the two dimensions of pronunciation position and pronunciation mode, namely, fricative/non-fricative recognition, voiced consonant/clear consonant recognition, aspirated/non-aspirated consonant recognition, same position/different consonant recognition, rolled tongue/non-rolled tongue sound recognition, and same position/different consonant recognition (Note: The recognition of/z/zh/,/c/ch/, and/s/sh/fall under the recognition groups of flat tongue sound and crooked tongue sound. Given that the stimulation is very close to the pronunciation part, it is also very difficult for the normal-hearing population, so it is classified as a separate group as the most difficult content.).

Using the syllable as the task unit, recognition difficulty was defined to control for its different effects between consonants and vowels, in the tone discrimination task, and consonants within syllables of the same category, and pure in the plosives. Vowels only included the monophonies of/a/,/e/,/i/,/o/, and/u/. In the easy tone task, subjects were asked to distinguish between the first tone and the fourth tone, which are evidently different; in the difficult tone task, subjects were asked to distinguish between the third tone and the fourth tone, which are more similar to each other. There were 80 syllable pairs presented in the easy and difficult tone discrimination conditions, and the task contained 32 "same" and 48 "different" trials.

In the consonant recognition task, as mentioned above, we divided consonants into six groups according to the two dimensions. To reduce the effect of the syllable and vowel, the syllables in each group contained four tones, and the vowels in each group were monosyllabic. The difficulty of a consonant discrimination task was determined by the similarity of the two consonants. Those with a large difference in consonant type were classified as easy, while those with a small difference were classified as difficult. For example,/h/and/m/are different in pronunciation position and pronunciation mode, while/h/and/k/are only different in pronunciation mode; thus,/h/and/m/are classified as belonging to the easy recognition group, while/h/and/k/are classified as belonging to the difficult recognition group. There were a total of 100 syllable pairs in the consonant recognition task, with 40 "same" and 60 "different" trials.

In the vowel recognition task, vowels were divided into four groups according to the two dimensions. The syllables of each group contained four tones. Easy vowel recognition trials contained vowels from different vowel groups, and difficult vowel recognition trials included compound vowels with more similarity, thus making it harder to distinguish syllables. The vowel discrimination task included 60 easy trials, namely, 36 different stimulus pairs and 24 same stimulus pairs. There were 100 trials, which included 40 "same" stimulus pairs and 60 "different" stimulus pairs.

ERP Measurement

Non-mirror Stimuli

All children underwent ERP measurements. We adopted visual stimuli consisting of reversing displays of circular checkerboard patterns created by Sandmann et al. (2012), which have been used to examine cross-modal reorganization in the auditory cortex of CI users. There were four different pairs of checkerboard patterns, which systematically varied by the luminance ratio. The proportions of white pixels in the stimulus patterns were 12.5% (Level 1), 25% (Level 2), 37.5% (Level 3), and 50% (Level 4) (**Supplementary Figure 1**). The contrast between white and black pixels was identical in all images used.

Subjects were seated comfortably in front of a high-resolution 19-inch VGA computer monitor at a viewing distance of approximately 1 m, in a soundproof and electromagnetically shielded room. All stimuli were presented *via* E-prime 2.0, and stimulus software was compatible with Net Station 4 (Electrical Geodesics, Inc.). The checkerboard stimulus remained on the monitor for 500 ms and was immediately followed by blank-screen with an inter-stimulus interval of 500 ms. Each presented blank stimulus image included a fixation point (a white cross) at the center of the screen. Participants performed four experimental blocks (i.e., conditions), in which they were presented with one of the four image pairs. The block order was counterbalanced across participants. During the experimental session, each checkerboard image was repeated 60 times, resulting in a total of 480 stimuli (4 conditions × 2 images × 60 repetitions). Participants were instructed to keep their eyes on the pictures before each condition and could rest for over 1 min between blocks.

Mirror Stimuli

In this study, the mirror stimulus is a visual stimulus with certain behavioral information, thus they are able to active mirror neurons. Based on the relationship of behavioral information to speech, mirror stimulus could be further divided into speech-related mirror stimulus (i.e., a photograph of the action of reading) and speech-irrelevant stimulus (i.e., a photograph of the action of singing). Considering that current CIs cannot faithfully relay musical rhythm (Kong et al., 2004; Galvin et al., 2007; Limb and Roy, 2014), the picture of singing might just mean the movement of mouth to CI children. However, we will still use the term "singing" to describe the action in this paper. Visual stimuli were presented in a similar way to those in the study by Proverbio (Proverbio et al., 2011). These stimuli have been found to induce visual–auditory interactions in a previous study (Liang et al., 2017). Photographs that most of the children were familiar with and the content of which was understood were chosen. **Supplementary Figure 2** shows the experimental block design, which consisted of an intermittent stimulus mode using speech-related mirror stimuli and speech-irrelevant mirror stimuli. To measure ERPs elicited by speech-related mirror stimuli, the experiment consisted of 85 trials of the "reading" photo stimuli and 15 trials of the "singing" photo stimuli as deviant stimuli. In contrast, to measure ERPs elicited by speech-irrelevant mirror stimuli, the experiment consisted of 85 trials of the "singing" photo stimuli and 15 trials of the "reading" photo stimuli as deviant stimuli. As shown in **Supplementary Figure 2**, each stimulus was presented for 1 s, followed by a blank screen (1.7–1.9 s in duration) as the inter-stimulus. To ensure that participants remained focused on the stimuli, one novel trial of 15 photographs was presented after 5–10 trials, in response to which children were asked to press a button when they saw the deviant photograph.

EEG Recording

Electroencephalography (EEG) data were continuously recorded using a 128-channel EEG electrode recording system (Electrical Geodesics, Inc.). The sampling rate for the EEG recording was 1 kHz, and electrode impedances were kept below 50 kΩ. For ERP analyses, the data of individual participants were band-pass filtered offline at 0.3–30 Hz and segmented into epochs of 100 ms pre-stimulus and 600 ms post-stimulus. Artifact rejection set at 200 mV was applied to visual EEG, and epochs were rejected if they contained any eye blinking (eye channel exceeded 140 mV) or eye movement (eye channel exceeded 55 mV). Bad channels were removed from the recording. Data were then re-referenced using a common average reference. The data were baseline-corrected to the pre-stimulus time of −100 to 0 ms.

Amplitudes and latencies of the P1–N1–P2 complex on the 75(Oz) electrode for individual participants were analyzed. The time window was set to 90–180 ms for the P1, 110–320 ms for the N1, and 220–400 ms for the P2. The amplitudes of the P1, N1, and P2 were measured as the baseline to peak value. Individual subject latencies were defined using the highest peak amplitude for each visually evoked potential. Individual waveform averages were averaged together for each group to compute a grand-average waveform.

Statistical Analysis

For statistical analysis, groups were divided by the various types of stimuli as follows: speech-related mirror stimuli, speech-irrelevant mirror stimuli, non-mirror stimuli level 1, non-mirror stimuli level 2, non-mirror stimuli level 3, and non-mirror stimuli level 4. An ANOVA was applied to examine between-group differences in ERP components. The Least Significant Difference test was then used to determine from which group–group comparison the significant difference originated.

Applying standardized low-resolution brain electromagnetic tomography (sLORETA) (Fuchs et al., 2002; Pascual-Marqui, 2002; Jurcak et al., 2007), a source location analysis was performed for the ERP components (P1, N1, and P2). The point in ERP (such as group A vs. group B) we chose to measure the difference in latency was calculated from the mean of group A and group B {[Latency (A) + Latency (B)]/2}. The top five brain regions in which there was a difference were revealed.

The assumption of a normal distribution was not satisfied, and so Spearman's correlation coefficient was used to test the correlations between ERP components (amplitude and latency included) and speech behavior. For all tests, a p-value < 0.05 was taken to indicate significance.

RESULTS

Event-Related Potentials

Between-Group Differences

Event-Related Potentials results are summarized in **Figure 1**. Significant differences were observed in the P1, N1, and P2 components between ERPs evoked by mirror stimuli and those evoked by non-mirror stimuli (**Figure 1C**). The data from normal-hearing controls are shown in **Supplementary Figure 1**. In a word, in the two major stimulus groups, ERPs elicited by the mirror stimuli differed significantly to the non-mirror stimuli. However, in subgroups, no significant difference in ERPs was found between the speech-related mirror stimuli and speech-irrelevant mirror stimuli, nor between the four types of non-mirror stimuli. Data for the normal-hearing control group are shown in **Supplementary Data**.

Source Location of ERP Differences

An sLORETA analysis was applied to the ERP data to assess between-group differences, and the results are shown in **Figure 2**.

On comparing ERPs between the non-mirror and mirror stimuli groups, the primary auditory cortex in the superior temporal gyrus, including Brodmann area 41 (B41) and BA42, was strongly activated for the mirror stimuli, which indicates the presence of a visual–auditory interaction. Furthermore, the precentral gyrus, including BA4 and BA6, was more strongly activated in the mirror stimuli vs. the non-mirror stimuli groups. Moreover, compared with ERPs elicited by the non-mirror stimuli, BA39, the visual speech area in the angular gyrus was strongly activated only for the speech-related mirror group. This was not observed when comparing ERPs between the non-mirror stimuli and speech-irrelevant mirror groups.

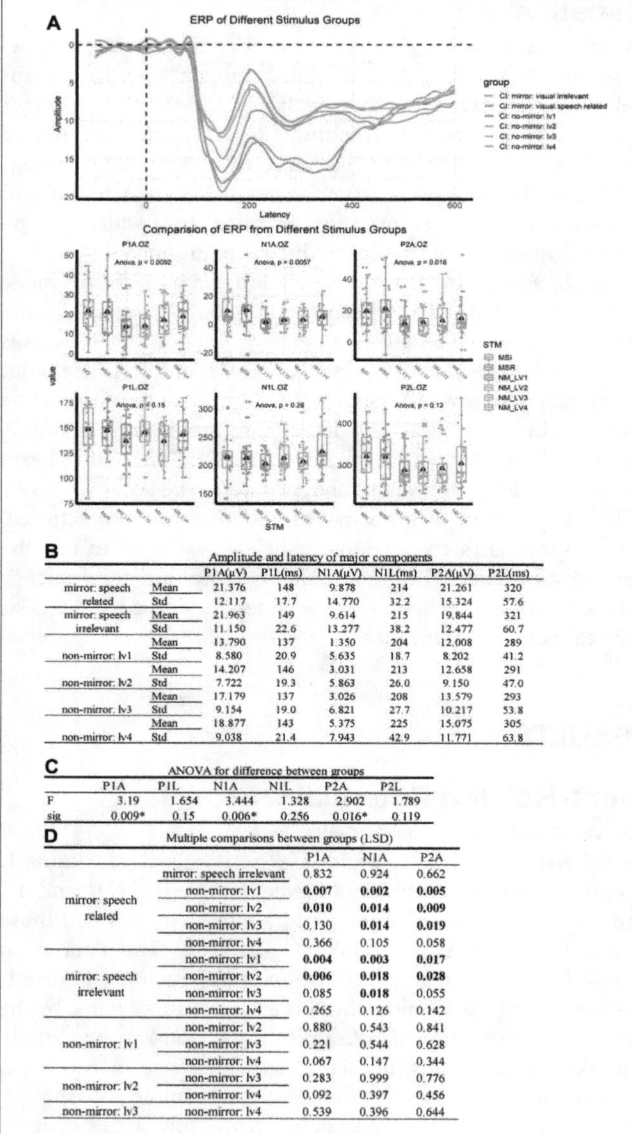

B

Amplitude and latency of major components

		P1A(μV)	P1L(ms)	N1A(μV)	N1L(ms)	P2A(μV)	P2L(ms)
mirror: speech related	Mean	21.376	148	9.878	214	21.261	320
	Std	12.117	17.7	14.770	32.2	15.324	57.6
mirror: speech irrelevant	Mean	21.963	149	9.614	215	19.844	321
	Std	11.150	22.6	13.277	38.2	12.477	60.7
non-mirror: lv1	Mean	13.790	137	1.350	204	12.008	289
	Std	8.580	20.9	5.635	18.7	8.202	41.2
non-mirror: lv2	Mean	14.207	146	3.031	213	12.658	291
	Std	7.722	19.3	5.863	26.0	9.150	47.0
non-mirror: lv3	Mean	17.179	137	3.026	208	13.579	293
	Std	9.154	19.0	6.821	27.7	10.217	53.8
non-mirror: lv4	Mean	18.877	143	5.375	225	15.075	305
	Std	9.038	21.4	7.943	42.9	11.771	63.8

C

ANOVA for difference between groups

	P1A	P1L	N1A	N1L	P2A	P2L
F	3.19	1.654	3.444	1.328	2.902	1.789
sig	0.009*	0.15	0.006*	0.256	0.016*	0.119

D

Multiple comparisons between groups (LSD)

		P1A	N1A	P2A
mirror: speech related	mirror: speech irrelevant	0.832	0.924	0.662
	non-mirror: lv1	**0.007**	**0.002**	**0.005**
	non-mirror: lv2	**0.010**	**0.014**	**0.009**
	non-mirror: lv3	0.130	**0.014**	**0.019**
	non-mirror: lv4	0.366	0.105	0.058
mirror: speech irrelevant	non-mirror: lv1	**0.004**	**0.003**	**0.017**
	non-mirror: lv2	**0.006**	**0.018**	**0.028**
	non-mirror: lv3	0.085	**0.018**	0.055
	non-mirror: lv4	0.265	0.126	0.142
non-mirror: lv1	non-mirror: lv2	0.880	0.543	0.841
	non-mirror: lv3	0.221	0.544	0.628
	non-mirror: lv4	0.067	0.147	0.344
non-mirror: lv2	non-mirror: lv3	0.283	0.999	0.776
	non-mirror: lv4	0.092	0.397	0.456
non-mirror: lv3	non-mirror: lv4	0.539	0.396	0.644

FIGURE 1 | ERP results. **(A)** ERP traces for the different groups. Stimuli were delivered at 0 ms, and a P1–N1–P2 complex was observed after 100 ms. MVSR: mirror and visual speech-related, MVSI: mirror and visual speech-irrelevant, NM: no-mirror. Delta: mean value. **(B)** Values used to describe ERP components. **(C)** An ANOVA showed that the difference between groups was mainly caused by differences in ERP amplitudes. *$p < 0.05$. **(D)** Multiple comparisons post-ANOVA. "Boldface number" means $p < 0.05$, indicating that significant differences in the ANOVA were mainly caused by the difference between the mirror stimulus group (including speech-related mirror stimuli and speech-irrelevant stimuli) and the non-mirror stimulus group (including the four types of non-mirror stimuli).

Correlation Between ERP Component and Speech Recognition

Correlation analysis showed that the combination of stimulus ERP peak–task RT performance enriches most significant correlations (**Figures 3A,B**, left). Further crosstab analysis revealed that the combination of ERP peak in mirror and visual speech-related (MVSR)–task reaction time performance includes most significant correlations within the combination of ERP peak–task RT performance. This indicates that, compared with the "mirror: visual speech-irrelevant" and "no-mirror" stimuli, the "mirror: visual speech-irrelevant" stimuli induced ERPs that better reflected speech task performance.

DISCUSSION

Explanation for the Results

We hypothesized that the mirror mechanism underlies visual–auditory interactions. Concerning the visual–auditory interaction element, mirror stimuli denoting reading and singing actions were able to induce visual–auditory interactions, while the non-mirror stimuli did not. People with hearing loss tend to receive speech-related information indirectly, such as *via* lip reading (Geers et al., 2003; Burden and Campbell, 2011). Also, rehabilitation training in those with hearing loss encourages reading loudly; while the sounds may not be accurate, this may activate the auditory cortex. Singing is obviously sound-related, while a black–white checkerboard is not related to sound. This could explain why the two major stimulus groups (mirror vs. non-mirror groups) induced different ERPs, which was driven by the primary auditory cortex (BA41and BA42).

Concerning the element of the mirror mechanism, mirror stimuli showing reading and singing might activate mirror neurons, unlike non-mirror stimuli. Since mirror stimuli that evoke this mirror mechanism should have the same action goal while both observing and executing the process, stimuli with an imitable action are likely to activate mirror neurons; this interpretation is consistent with previous studies (Kohler et al., 2002; Vogt et al., 2004; Michael et al., 2014). In contrast, a checkerboard image is much less likely to activate mirror neurons, as the function of mirror mechanism is to benefit the individual by imitating actions, comprehending actions, and understanding feelings; a meaningless geometric figure fits none of these functions. This could explain why the two major stimulus groups evoked different neural activities, reflected in ERP differences.

Spatial source of ERP difference is located in mirror neurons. According to the mirror mechanism theory, a mirror neuron can be activated during both execution and observation of an action. In this context, both the action and perception of reading will activate the visual speech area (BA39). To be classified as a mirror neuron, the neuron needs to be activated in both the observation and execution of reading. For singing, our region of interest was the motor cortex, including BA4 and BA6.

Previous works have noted that visual–auditory interactions differ between normal-hearing people and those with hearing loss (Stropahl and Debener, 2017; Rosemann et al., 2020), and that visual–auditory interactions might be related to speech performance in children with a CI (Liang et al., 2017). This indicates that visual–auditory interactions are related to speech comprehension in people with hearing loss. Considering the ability of mirror neurons to encode motor actions (di Pellegrino et al., 1992; Gallese et al., 1996;

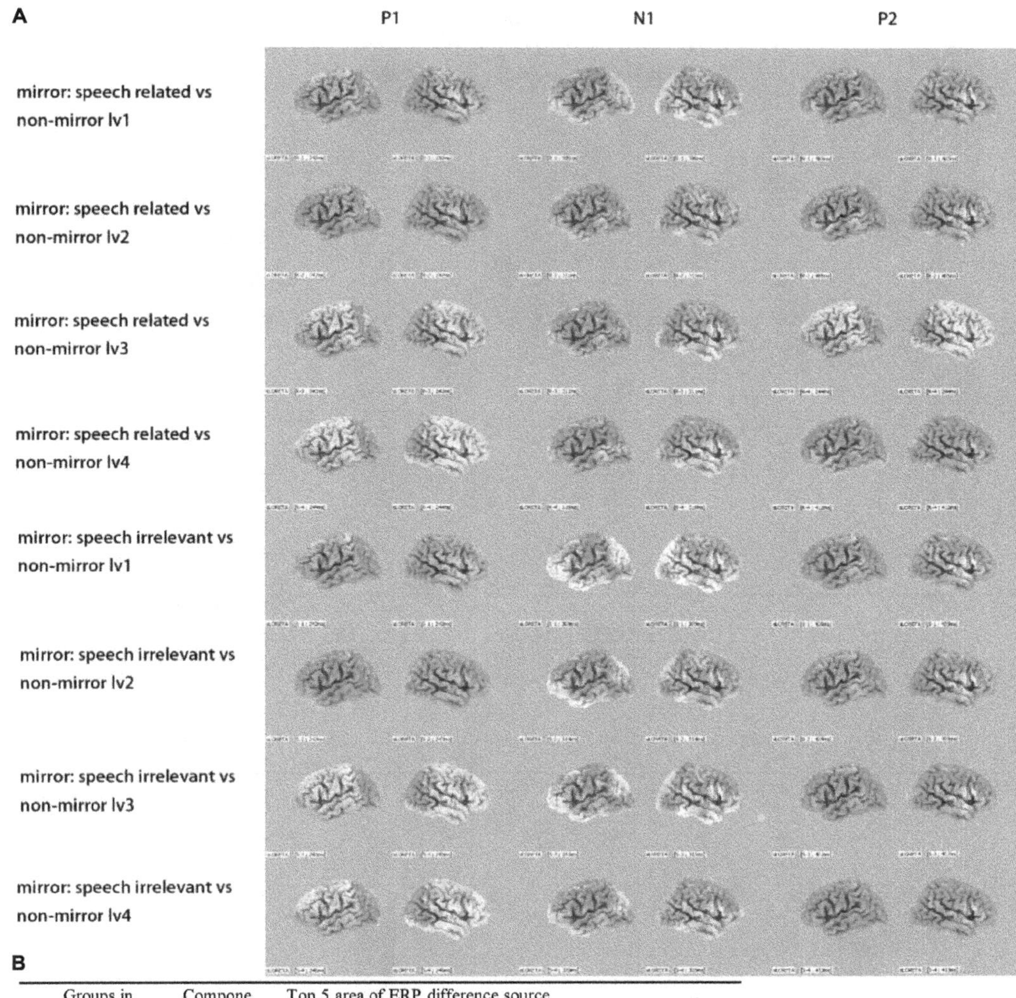

B

Groups in comparison		Component	Top 5 area of ERP difference source (Number of Brodmann area)					Side
mirror: speech related	lv1	P1	36	20	35	37	13	Left
		N1	40	13	2	41	42	Left
		P2	9	45	44	6	8	Right
	lv2	P1	39	19	22	40	37	Left
		N1	4	3	6	1	2	Right
		P2	22	21	44	38	13	Left
	lv3	P1	7	19	39	40	31	Left
		N1	40	2	13	3	41	Left
		P2	47	45	46	10	11	Left
	lv4	P1	7	19	39	31	18	Left
		N1	13	41	22	2	39	Left
		P2	47	45	46	10	11	Left
mirror: speech irrelevant	lv1	P1	17	18	19	23	30	Right
		N1	40	13	2	41	42	Left
		P2	20	21	22	38	13	Right
	lv2	P1	30	31	23	18	29	Right
		N1	4	3	6	1	2	Right
		P2	22	21	41	42	40	Right
	lv3	P1	23	30	31	29	18	Middle
		N1	31	3	5	6	24	Left
		P2	17	18	23	31	30	Right
	lv4	P1	23	30	31	29	18	Middle
		N1	21	20	22	38	13	Right
		P2	18	30	23	17	31	Right

FIGURE 2 | Source location of ERP differences. **(A)** sLORETA for ERP differences between groups. Colorful regions indicate the source of ERP differences. **(B)** Red: BA39 (left), which is the visual speech cortex. Green: BA41 and BA42, which make up the primary auditory cortex. Yellow: BA4 and BA6, which make up the precentral gyrus. Only speech-related stimuli activated BA39 differently, compared with non-mirror stimuli.

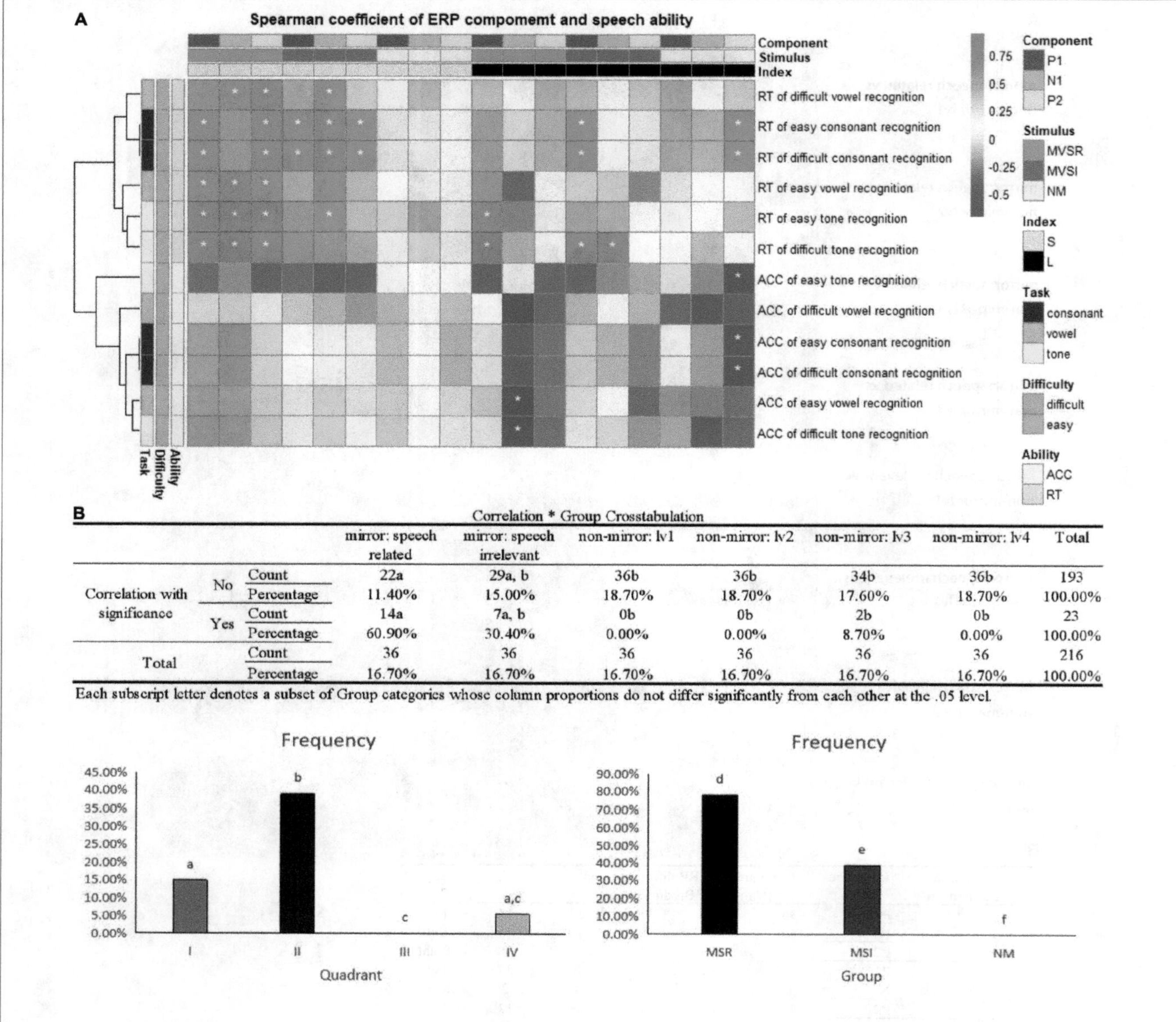

Correlation * Group Crosstabulation

			mirror: speech related	mirror: speech irrelevant	non-mirror: lv1	non-mirror: lv2	non-mirror: lv3	non-mirror: lv4	Total
Correlation with significance	No	Count	22a	29a, b	36b	36b	34b	36b	193
		Percentage	11.40%	15.00%	18.70%	18.70%	17.60%	18.70%	100.00%
	Yes	Count	14a	7a, b	0b	0b	2b	0b	23
		Percentage	60.90%	30.40%	0.00%	0.00%	8.70%	0.00%	100.00%
Total		Count	36	36	36	36	36	36	216
		Percentage	16.70%	16.70%	16.70%	16.70%	16.70%	16.70%	100.00%

Each subscript letter denotes a subset of Group categories whose column proportions do not differ significantly from each other at the .05 level.

FIGURE 3 | Correlation between ERP component and speech recognition. **(A)** Heatmaps of Spearman's correlation coefficient (–1, +1). ACC, accuracy; RT, reaction time; MVSR, mirror and visual speech-related; MVSI, mirror and visual speech-irrelevant; S, stimulus peak; L, latency; **p* < 0.05. **(B)** As the heatmap is a combination of ERP components and speech measures, we tried to find which type of combination (for example: ERP latency–task RT performance vs. ERP peak–task RT performance) resulted in stronger correlations by calculating the percentage of cells with "*" in all cells of specific combination. Left: four quadrants as four combinations; right: in II quadrant, MSR/MSI/NM peak–RT performance as three combinations. (I, II, III, IV: quadrant of the heatmap, I: latency–task RT performance, II: peak–task RT performance, III: peak–task ACC performance, IV: latency–task ACC performance. a, b, c, d, e, f: in analysis of crosstab, the same character indicates no significant difference, while a different character indicates a significant difference).

Rizzolatti et al., 1996), the relationship between visual–auditory interactions and speech recognition ability might be related to this ability. This could explain why the speech-related stimuli evoked stronger visual–auditory interactions that are reflected by speech recognition ability.

ERP Results

First, ERP results revealed that visual–auditory interactions were induced in the mirror stimuli groups, whether the stimuli were speech-related or irrelevant, with the strongest activation in the primary auditory cortex (**Figure 2**). Our finding of the primary auditory cortex activation is consistent with those of a previous study, in which the primary auditory cortex (BA41) was activated by sound-related photos at around 200 ms after stimulus presentation (Proverbio et al., 2011).

Second, on comparing the ERPs elicited by the mirror stimuli and non-mirror stimuli, the results indicated that the mirror neurons were more strongly activated in the "motor action" condition than in the functional cortex. More precisely, an image of reading evoked a stronger activation in the visual speech area (left BA39; **Figure 2**), while the image of singing induced a stronger activation in the precentral gyrus (BA4 and BA6), where the mouth and hand areas are located (**Figure 2**).

Third, we found that that difference in the degree of checkerboard lightness did not significantly affect ERPs. However, a trend was found in the effect of luminance on ERPs, which is consistent with a previous study (Sandmann et al., 2012). Given that we only used four luminance (lightness-value of the ERP component), a correlation analysis was not possible. Even if differences in ERPs between mirror and non-mirror stimuli partly originated from other differences between stimuli, such as lightness or color, these differences do not convincingly explain the activation in response to a "motor action" corresponding to activity of the functional cortex.

Finally, the activated BA39, BA41, and BA42 regions are spatially close to each other and may be involved in the function of the left inferior parietal lobe in social cognition, language, and other comprehension tasks (Hauk et al., 2005; Jefferies and Lambon, 2006; Binder and Desai, 2011; Ishibashi et al., 2011; Bzdok et al., 2016). This finding supports the idea that the mirror mechanism is one of the mechanisms underlying visual–auditory interactions.

Behavioral Results and Correlation Analysis

The significant correlation found between ERP features and speech recognition ability indicates that visual speech-related mirror stimuli better reflect the ability of speech recognition than non-mirror stimuli and visual speech-irrelevant mirror stimuli. Considering that the function of the mirror mechanism is to comprehend motor actions, this indicates that the function of visual–auditory interactions to reflect speech behavior is one function of the mirror mechanism.

Above all, the behavioral results and correlation analysis indicate that the function of visual–auditory interactions to reflect speech behavior is one function of the mirror mechanism, but that the primary cortex also participates in this function of visual–auditory interaction.

Cross-Modal Plasticity and the Mirror Mechanism

Cross-modal plasticity is a double-edged sword in the auditory cortex regeneration of post-CI deaf people who regain auditory input. On the one hand, in the early period, cross-modal plasticity allows the visual cortex to take over the auditory cortex for functional compensation, which weakens auditory function (Finney et al., 2001; Hauk et al., 2005). On the other hand, cross-modal plasticity allows the occupied auditory cortex to regain its auditory function under auditory input *via* a CI (Anderson et al., 2017; Liang et al., 2017). Thus, it is controversial to include speech-related visual stimuli into rehabilitation training of post-CI children.

In the context of the mirror mechanism, we can also give an explanation to the dual effect to auditory function of cross-modal plasticity. In normal-hearing people, there is a balance between the executing and observing processes of a visual–auditory interaction, since they can verify whether executing (such as reading/speaking) and observing processes (such as seeing/hearing) share the same outcome of action goal (Rizzolatti et al., 2001), and auditory information benefits this process.

However, in people with hearing loss, especially those with prelingual deafness, the observing process (hearing) is absent, which causes an imbalance between executing and observing processes. This means that the patient uses the visual input (such as reading lips) as the observing process to compensate for the imbalance, which changes the outcome of the action goal into certain movements of a muscle or joint (such as lip movement). Some mirror neurons in the auditory cortex change the input of the observing process from auditory input into visual input to compensate for the absence of the observing process, which leads to a "takeover" or "inhibition" phenomenon, according to the theory of cross-modal plasticity (Finney et al., 2001; Rizzolatti et al., 2001).

Considering that the mirror mechanism is also sensitive to mastery, whereby skilled individuals have greater mirror neuron activation (Glaser et al., 2005; Calvo-Merino et al., 2006; Cross et al., 2006), the departure of auditory information and body movement (such as lip language) will be strengthened in the hearing loss period of prelingually deaf patients through repeated "training" of "comprehending" the meaning of some speech-related movements, such as lip movement (Geers et al., 2003; Burden and Campbell, 2011), for survival. Even when they regain auditory input after cochlear implantation (Giraud et al., 2001), the misleading departure is still strong. Considering the mirror mechanism sensitivity to mastery, proper rehabilitation training may change input mirror neurons to the auditory cortex from those sensitive to the observing process into an auditory input. Learning allows the auditory cortex to regain its auditory function, which leads to the phenomenon of auditory cortex recovery (weakened activation of cross-modal regions is related to improved speech performance) (Sandmann et al., 2012; Liang et al., 2017), according to cross-modal plasticity theory.

Implications for Rehabilitation Training

For post-CI children, in the observing process, body movements to produce speech that are related to sound, such as lip reading, should be limited, since they will strengthen the misleading departure of action goal as mentioned above (Cooper and Craddock, 2006; Oba et al., 2013). However, abstract visual input to produce speech-related sound, such as words and sentences, should be promoted, since associating words or text with speech for speech comprehension is an ability of normal-hearing people and mirror neurons contribute to the comprehension of motor actions.

In the executing process, children should be trained to verify whether what they say is consistent with what they hear, which calls for the cochlear to promote the quality of auditory input and the correct of speech from others.

CONCLUSION

Compared with non-mirror stimuli, mirror stimuli activated the primary auditory cortex, including BA41 and BA42, which prompted a visual–auditory interaction. Speech-related mirror stimuli (reading) activated BA39, the visual speech area, which implies the activation of mirror neurons. ERPs of the speech-related mirror stimuli group could best reflect the speech recognition ability of participants. Cross-modal plasticity is considered to underlie the correlation between visual–auditory interactions and speech recognition performance, and we hypothesized that the mirror mechanism is related to cross-modal plasticity and underlies visual–auditory interactions.

AUTHOR CONTRIBUTIONS

All authors listed have made a substantial, direct and intellectual contribution to the work, and approved it for publication.

REFERENCES

Anderson, C. A., Wiggins, I. M., Kitterick, P. T., and Hartley, D. E. H. (2017). Adaptive benefit of cross-modal plasticity following cochlear implantation in deaf adults. *Proc. Natl. Acad. Sci. U S A* 114, 10256–10261. doi: 10.1073/pnas.1704785114

Binder, J. R., and Desai, R. H. (2011). The neurobiology of semantic memory. *Trends Cogn. Sci.* 15, 527–536. doi: 10.1016/j.tics.2011.10.001

Brefczynski, J. A., Phinney, R. E., Janik, J. J., and DeYoe, E. A. (2005). Distinct cortical pathways for processing tool versus animal sounds. *J. Neurosci.* 25, 5148–5158. doi: 10.1523/jneurosci.0419-05.2005

Bulkin, D. A., and Groh, J. M. (2006). Seeing sounds: visual and auditory interactions in the brain. *Curr. Opin. Neurobiol.* 16, 415–419. doi: 10.1016/j.conb.2006.06.008

Burden, V., and Campbell, R. (2011). The development of word-coding skills in the born deaf: An experimental study of deaf school-leavers. *Br. J. Dev. Psychol.* 12, 331–349. doi: 10.1111/j.2044-835x.1994.tb00638.x

Bzdok, D., Hartwigsen, G., Reid, A., Laird, A. R., Fox, P. T., and Eickhoff, S. B. (2016). Left inferior parietal lobe engagement in social cognition and language. *Neurosci. Biobehav. Rev.* 68, 319–334. doi: 10.1016/j.neubiorev.2016.02.024

Calvo-Merino, B., Grèzes, J., Glaser, D. E., Passingham, R. E., and Haggard, P. (2006). Seeing or doing? Influence of visual and motor familiarity in action observation. *Curr. Biol.* 16, 1905–1910. doi: 10.1016/j.cub.2006.07.065

Cooper, H., and Craddock, L. (2006). *Cochlear Implants: A Practical Guide, 2nd Edition. Practical Aspects of Audiology.* Hoboken, NJ: Wiley.

Cross, E. S., Hamilton, A. F., and Grafton, S. T. (2006). Building a motor simulation de novo: observation of dance by dancers. *Neuroimage* 31, 1257–1267. doi: 10.1016/j.neuroimage.2006.01.033

di Pellegrino, G., Fadiga, L., Fogassi, L., Gallese, V., and Rizzolatti, G. (1992). Understanding motor events: a neurophysiological study. *Exp. Brain Res.* 91, 176–180. doi: 10.1007/bf00230027

Finney, E. M., Fine, I., and Dobkins, K. R. (2001). Visual stimuli activate auditory cortex in the deaf. *Nat. Neurosci.* 4, 1171–1173. doi: 10.1038/nn763

Fuchs, M., Kastner, J., Wagner, M., Hawes, S., and Ebersole, J. S. (2002). A standardized boundary element method volume conductor model. *Clin. Neurophysiol.* 113, 702–712. doi: 10.1016/s1388-2457(02)00030-5

Gallese, V., Fadiga, L., Fogassi, L., and Rizzolatti, G. (1996). Action recognition in the premotor cortex. *Brain* 119(Pt 2), 593–609. doi: 10.1093/brain/119.2.593

Galvin, J. R., Fu, Q. J., and Nogaki, G. (2007). Melodic contour identification by cochlear implant listeners. *Ear. Hear* 28, 302–319. doi: 10.1097/01.aud.0000261689.35445.20

Gazzola, V., Aziz-Zadeh, L., and Keysers, C. (2006). Empathy and the somatotopic auditory mirror system in humans. *Curr. Biol.* 16, 1824–1829. doi: 10.1016/j.cub.2006.07.072

Geers, A., Brenner, C., and Davidson, L. (2003). Factors associated with development of speech perception skills in children implanted by age five. *Ear. Hear* 24(1 Suppl.), 24S–35S.

Giraud, A. L., Price, C. J., Graham, J. M., Truy, E., and Frackowiak, R. S. (2001). Cross-modal plasticity underpins language recovery after cochlear implantation. *Neuron* 30, 657–663. doi: 10.1016/s0896-6273(01)00318-x

Glaser, D. E., Grèzes, J., Passingham, R. E., and Haggard, P. (2005). Action observation and acquired motor skills: an FMRI study with expert dancers. *Cereb Cortex* 15, 1243–1249. doi: 10.1093/cercor/bhi007

Hauk, O., Nikulin, V. V., and Ilmoniemi, R. J. (2005). Functional links between motor and language systems. *Eur. J. Neurosci.* 21, 793–797. doi: 10.1111/j.1460-9568.2005.03900.x

Ishibashi, R., Lambon Ralph, M. A., Saito, S., and Pobric, G. (2011). Different roles of lateral anterior temporal lobe and inferior parietal lobule in coding function and manipulation tool knowledge: evidence from an rTMS study. *Neuropsychologia* 49, 1128–1135. doi: 10.1016/j.neuropsychologia.2011.01.004

Jefferies, E., and Lambon, R. M. (2006). Semantic impairment in stroke aphasia versus semantic dementia: a case-series comparison. *Brain* 129(Pt 8), 2132–2147. doi: 10.1093/brain/awl153

Jurcak, V., Tsuzuki, D., and Dan, I. (2007). 10/20, 10/10, and 10/5 systems revisited: their validity as relative head-surface-based positioning systems. *Neuroimage* 34, 1600–1611. doi: 10.1016/j.neuroimage.2006.09.024

Keysers, C., Umiltà, M. A., Fogassi, L., Gallese, V., and Rizzolatti, G. (2002). Hearing sounds, understanding actions: action representation in mirror neurons. *Science* 297, 846–848.

Kohler, E., Keysers, C., Umiltà, M. A., Fogassi, L., Gallese, V., and Rizzolatti, G. (2002). Hearing sounds, understanding actions: action representation in mirror neurons. *Science* 297, 846–848. doi: 10.1126/science.1070311

Kong, Y. Y., Cruz, R., Jones, J. A., and Zeng, F. G. (2004). Music perception with temporal cues in acoustic and electric hearing. *Ear Hear* 25, 173–185. doi: 10.1097/01.aud.0000120365.97792.2f

Liang, M., Zhang, J., Liu, J., Chen, Y., Cai, Y., Wang, X., et al. (2017). Visually Evoked Visual-Auditory Changes Associated with Auditory Performance in Children with Cochlear Implants. *Front. Hum. Neurosci.* 11:510.

Limb, C. J., and Roy, A. T. (2014). Technological, biological, and acoustical constraints to music perception in cochlear implant users. *Hear Res.* 308, 13–26. doi: 10.1016/j.heares.2013.04.009

Mao, Y. T., and Pallas, S. L. (2013). Cross-modal plasticity results in increased inhibition in primary auditory cortical areas. *Neural. Plast* 2013:530651.

McGurk, H., and MacDonald, J. (1976). Hearing lips and seeing voices. *Nature* 264, 746–748. doi: 10.1038/264746a0

Michael, J., Sandberg, K., Skewes, J., Wolf, T., Blicher, J., Overgaard, M., et al. (2014). Continuous theta-burst stimulation demonstrates a causal role of premotor homunculus in action understanding. *Psychol. Sci.* 25, 963–972. doi: 10.1177/0956797613520608

Oba, S. I., Galvin, J. R., and Fu, Q. J. (2013). Minimal effects of visual memory training on auditory performance of adult cochlear implant users. *J. Rehabil. Res. Dev.* 50, 99–110. doi: 10.1682/jrrd.2011.12.0229

Pascual-Marqui, R. D. (2002). Standardized low-resolution brain electromagnetic tomography (sLORETA): technical details. *Methods Find Exp. Clin. Pharmacol.* 2002(24 Suppl. D), 5–12.

Proverbio, A. M., D'Aniello, G. E., Adorni, R., and Zani, A. (2011). When a photograph can be heard: vision activates the auditory cortex within 110 ms. *Sci. Rep.* 1:54.

Rizzolatti, G., and Sinigaglia, C. (2016). The mirror mechanism: a basic principle of brain function. *Nat. Rev. Neurosci.* 17, 757–765. doi: 10.1038/nrn.2016.135

Rizzolatti, G., Fadiga, L., Gallese, V., and Fogassi, L. (1996). Premotor cortex and the recognition of motor actions. *Brain Res. Cogn. Brain Res.* 3, 131–141. doi: 10.1016/0926-6410(95)00038-0

Rizzolatti, G., Fogassi, L., and Gallese, V. (2001). Neurophysiological mechanisms underlying the understanding and imitation of action. *Nat. Rev. Neurosci.* 2, 661–670. doi: 10.1038/35090060

Rosemann, S., Smith, D., and Dewenter, M. (2020). Thiel, Age-related hearing loss influences functional connectivity of auditory cortex for the McGurk illusion. *Cortex* 129, 266–280. doi: 10.1016/j.cortex.2020.04.022

Sandmann, P., Dillier, N., Eichele, T., Meyer, M., Kegel, A., Pascual-Marqui, R. D., et al. (2012). Visual activation of auditory cortex reflects maladaptive plasticity in cochlear implant users. *Brain* 135(Pt 2), 555–568. doi: 10.1093/brain/awr329

Stropahl, M., and Debener, S. (2017). Auditory cross-modal reorganization in cochlear implant users indicates audio-visual integration. *Neuroimage Clin.* 16, 514–523. doi: 10.1016/j.nicl.2017.09.001

Vogt, S., Ritzl, A., Fink, G. R., Zilles, K., Freund, H. J., and Rizzolatti, G. (2004). Neural circuits underlying imitation learning of hand actions: an event-related fMRI study. *Neuron* 42, 323–334. doi: 10.1016/s0896-6273(04)00181-3

Xibin, S., Zhang, L., Huang, Z., Du, X., and Chen, X.. (2006). Standardization of lexical and spectral similarity in children's Chinese speech recognition. *Chinese Entific J.Hear. Speech Rehabilit.* 1, 16–20. doi: CNKI:Sun:tlkf.0.2006-01-004

17

Stress Response and Hearing Loss Differentially Contribute to Dynamic Alterations in Hippocampal Neurogenesis and Microglial Reactivity in Mice Exposed to Acute Noise Exposure

Qian Li[1], Hong Li[1], Xiuting Yao[2], Conghui Wang[2], Haiqing Liu[1], Dan Xu[3], Chenxi Yang[2], Hong Zhuang[2], Yu Xiao[2], Rui Liu[2], Sinuo Shen[2], Shaoyang Zhou[2], Chenge Fu[2], Yifan Wang[2], Gaojun Teng[4]* and Lijie Liu[2]*

[1] School of Life Science and Technology, Southeast University, Nanjing, China, [2] Medical College, Southeast University, Nanjing, China, [3] School of Public Health, Southeast University, Nanjing, China, [4] Jiangsu Key Laboratory of Molecular Imaging and Functional Imaging, Department of Radiology, Medical School, Zhongda Hospital, Southeast University, Nanjing, China

***Correspondence:**
Gaojun Teng
gjteng@seu.edu.cn
Lijie Liu
liulijie@seu.edu.cn;
Liulijie1973@163.com

Noise-induced hearing loss (NIHL) is one of the most prevalent forms of acquired hearing loss, and it is associated with aberrant microglial status and reduced hippocampal neurogenesis; however, the nature of these associations is far from being elucidated. Beyond its direct effects on the auditory system, exposure to intense noise has previously been shown to acutely activate the stress response, which has increasingly been linked to both microglial activity and adult hippocampal neurogenesis in recent years. Given the pervasiveness of noise pollution in modern society and the important implications of either microglial activity or hippocampal neurogenesis for cognitive and emotional function, this study was designed to investigate how microglial status and hippocampal neurogenesis change over time following acoustic exposure and to analyze the possible roles of the noise exposure-induced stress response and hearing loss in these changes. To accomplish this, adult male C57BL/6J mice were randomly assigned to either a control or noise exposure (NE) group. Auditory function was assessed by measuring ABR thresholds at 20 days post noise exposure. The time-course profile of serum corticosterone levels, microglial status, and hippocampal neurogenesis during the 28 days following noise exposure were quantified by ELISA or immunofluorescence staining. Our results illustrated a permanent moderate-to-severe degree of hearing loss, an early but transient increase in serum corticosterone levels, and time-dependent dynamic alterations in microglial activation status and hippocampal neurogenesis, which both present an early but transient change and a late but enduring change. These findings provide evidence that both the stress response and hearing loss contribute to the dynamic alterations of microglia and hippocampal neurogenesis following noise exposure; moreover, noise-induced permanent hearing loss rather than noise-induced transient stress is more likely to be responsible for perpetuating the neurodegenerative process associated with many neurological diseases.

Keywords: noise exposure, noise-induced hearing loss, stress, hippocampal neurogenesis, microglia

INTRODUCTION

In recent decades, a massive shift has been observed in the global burden of disease from communicable causes (e.g., diarrheal and other infectious diseases) to non-communicable causes (e.g., dementia) (Benziger et al., 2016). Dementia is among the most common chronic non-communicable neurodegenerative diseases (Collaborators, 2019; Bazargan-Hejazi et al., 2020). Given the substantial social and economic implications of dementia as well as the lack of curative treatment, an identification and understanding of risk factors associated with dementia are needed to accelerate disease prevention and realize morbidity improvements (Livingston et al., 2017).

Convergent lines of evidence from epidemiological and experimental studies indicate that acquired peripheral hearing loss (HL) is a significant risk factor for dementia (Lin et al., 2011; Liu et al., 2016a; Livingston et al., 2017, 2020; Thomson et al., 2017; Loughrey et al., 2018; Nixon et al., 2019; Orgeta et al., 2019; Uchida et al., 2019). Excessive exposure to environmental noise, a pervasive pollutant that directly affects the health and well-being of exposed subjects (Stansfeld and Matheson, 2003; Uran et al., 2010; Basner et al., 2014; Liu et al., 2016b; Hahad et al., 2019; Zhuang et al., 2020) is the most common contributing factor leading to acquired peripheral HL (Nelson et al., 2005; Jeschke et al., 2020). According to the World Health Organization (WHO), one-third of all cases of HL can be attributed to noise exposure (No authors listed, 1990; Nelson et al., 2005; Le et al., 2017). In our previous study using animals with noise-induced hearing loss (NIHL), impaired cognitive behavior and hippocampal neurogenesis as well as abnormal microglia were observed months after noise exposure (Tao et al., 2015; Liu et al., 2016a, 2018; Zhuang et al., 2020), which not only provided supportive evidence for the causative role of acquired peripheral HL in the development of dementia but also suggested the mediating roles of hippocampal neurogenesis impairment and microglial dysfunction in this causative relationship. However, beyond its direct effects on the auditory system, exposure to intense noise has previously been shown to acutely activate the stress response (Samson et al., 2007; Liu et al., 2016b; Hahad et al., 2019), which has increasingly been linked to both microglial activity (Frank et al., 2019) and adult hippocampal neurogenesis in recent years (Surget and Belzung, 2021). Given the pervasiveness of noise pollution in modern society (Goines and Hagler, 2007), the potential vulnerability of the hippocampus to intense noise exposure (Kraus et al., 2010; Cui et al., 2012; Cheng et al., 2016; Hayes et al., 2019), and the well-known important implications of either microglial activity or hippocampal neurogenesis for cognitive function (De Lucia et al., 2016; Hansen et al., 2018; Rodriguez-Iglesias et al., 2019; Suss and Schlachetzki, 2020), simultaneously analyzing the time course for changes in the stress response, hearing threshold, microglial status, and hippocampal neurogenesis after cessation of brief intensive noise exposure is essential for better comprehending the deleterious effects of noise on brain function.

Therefore, the main purpose of this study was to investigate how microglial status and hippocampal neurogenesis change over time following acoustic exposure and to analyze the possible roles of noise exposure-induced stress responses and HL in these changes. To accomplish this, adult male C57BL/6J mice were randomly assigned to either a control or noise exposure (NE) group. Auditory function was assessed by measuring auditory brainstem response (ABR) thresholds at 20 days post NE. The dynamic profile of serum corticosterone levels, microglial status, and hippocampal neurogenesis over the time span from immediately after to 28 days after the cessation of NE were analyzed by ELISA or immunofluorescence staining. Our results illustrated a permanent moderate-to-severe degree of NIHL, an early but transient increase in serum corticosterone levels, and dynamic alterations in microglial activation status and hippocampal neurogenesis, which both consist of an early but transient change and a late but enduring change. These findings corroborate previous observations demonstrating the association between NIHL and hippocampal neurodegenerative changes (Liu et al., 2016a, 2018; Zhuang et al., 2020) and provide further insights into the potential mechanisms underlying the adverse effect of NE on the brain.

MATERIALS AND METHODS

Animals

Young adult (aged 2 months) male C57BL/6J mice were purchased from SPF Biotechnology Co., Ltd. (Beijing, China; No. SCXK 2019-0010). In total, 64 mice that passed the Preyer reflex test were used in the study. The mice were housed four per cage under standard conditions (8 a.m.–8 p.m. light cycle, 22°C, 55% humidity, and *ad libitum* access to food and water) provided by the University Committee for Laboratory Animals of Southeast University, China (SCXK2011-0003). One week after arrival, the mice were randomly assigned to a control group and seven NE groups (n = 8/group). Animals in each NE group were separately exposed to broadband noise for 2 h at a sound pressure level (SPL) of 123 dB. The subgroups of NE animals were separately sacrificed immediately after or at 12 h, 1, 3, 7, 14, and 28 days after NE (0HPN, 12HPN, 1DPN, 3DPN, 7DPN, 14DPN, and 28DPN, respectively).

Noise Exposure

The animals in the NE groups were exposed to a single dose of broadband noise at 123 dB SPL for 2 h during the light phase as previously described (Liu et al., 2016a, 2018; Zhuang et al., 2020). The awake and unrestrained animals were kept individually in a metal wire mesh cage (cage size: 11 cm × 11 cm × 23 cm) located 40 cm below the horns of two loudspeakers (an NJ speaker YD380-8bH and a BM professional speaker HG10044XT, nominal bandwidth 1–20 kHz). The noise signal was generated by a System III processor from Tucker–Davis Technologies (TDT, Alachua, FL, United States) and amplified by a Yamaha P9500S power amplifier. Animals were acclimatized for 30 min in the exposure chamber before the loudspeakers were turned on. During the exposure, which began at 06:00 p.m., the noise level was monitored and controlled within the range of 123 dB SPL ± 1 dB by using a 1/4-inch microphone linked to a sound level meter (Larson Davis, Depew, NY, United States; 2,520 microphone and 824 sound level meter, Larson Davis, Depew, NY, United States). For the control group, all operations were the same as those in the 0 HPN group except that the animals were treated with sham exposure, in which the loudspeaker was not turned on.

Auditory Brainstem Response Assessment

A number of studies in animal models have demonstrated that, after NEs that are intense enough to produce permanent effects, hearing thresholds recover exponentially for periods extending up to 2~3 weeks and finally reach a steady state (Kujawa and Liberman, 2006; Ryan et al., 2016). Thus, the ABRs of 28DPN and control mice were assessed 8 days before their sacrifice (i.e., 20 days after NE) in a sound-attenuating chamber to determine the hearing thresholds of mice. The animals were anesthetized by intraperitoneal injection of pentobarbital (50 mg/kg body weight), and their body temperature was maintained at approximately 37.5 ± 0.5°C by placing them on a thermostatic heating pad during testing and recovery from anesthesia. Three subdermal needles were inserted ventrolateral to the left pinna (active), vertex (reference), and right hind limb (ground) of the testing mice, and they served as electrodes for ABR recording. TDT hardware (RZ6, System III) and software (BioSig and SigGen) were used for signal generation and ABR acquisition. Tone bursts of 2, 4, 8, 16, and 32 kHz (10-ms duration with $\cos^2$ gating and 0.5-ms rise/fall time, at the rate of 21.1/s) were presented monaurally in an open field using a broadband speaker (MF1; TDT) located 10 cm in front of the animal's head. The evoked responses were amplified 20 times *via* an RA16PA preamplifier (TDT) and filtered between 100 and 3,000Hz. The responses were averaged 1,000 times. At each frequency, the test was performed in a degressive sequence starting from 90 dB SPL, which was weakened in 5-dB steps until no ABR response was detected. The ABR threshold at each frequency was defined as the lowest sound level at which a repeatable wave III in ABR was detected. If a repeatable wave III was not detected at an SPL of 90 dB, then a threshold of 95dB was assigned to the mouse.

Tissue and Blood Harvest

Sample collections of each group except the 12 HPN group were performed between 08:00 and 09:00 a.m. to avoid potential variations related to the circadian rhythm; for the 12 HPN group, the collections were performed between 08:00 p.m. and 09:00 p.m. At the defined time of sacrifice, mice were deeply anesthetized with pentobarbital (100 mg/kg, i.p.) and blood was rapidly collected by cardiac puncture into centrifugal tubes and allowed to clot. After blood collection, the animals were perfused transcardially with 20 ml 0.9% saline followed by 20 ml of 4% paraformaldehyde (PFA) in 0.1 M PBS, and whole brains were quickly excised, postfixed in 4% PFA for 6–8 h at 4°C, cryoprotected in 30% sucrose in PBS until the organ sank, embedded in OCT compound, and then stored at −80°C until ready for sectioning.

Measurement of Corticosterone Levels

The clotted blood samples were centrifuged to separate the cells from the serum. The resulting serum was collected and stored at −80°C until use. The amount of corticosterone in serum was analyzed by enzyme-linked immunosorbent assay (ELISA) using a commercial mouse corticosterone quantification kit (CSB-E07969 m; Cusabio, Houston, TX 77054, United States).

Immunohistochemistry

Hippocampal neurogenesis and the microglia status in each region of interest (ROI) were determined by immunohistochemistry as previously described (Zhuang et al., 2020). The frozen brain blocks were cut into 40-μm-thick sections using a cryostat (Leica Cryostat Microtome 1900, Heidelberger, Germany). All sections were collected and stored in cryoprotectant solution (30% ethylene glycol and 25% glycerin in 0.1 M phosphate buffer) at −20°C until needed. For each animal, five to six sections (320 μm apart) across the hippocampus were included for the study of neurogenesis or microglia status. For the ventral cochlear nucleus (VCN), dorsal cochlear nucleus (DCN), inferior colliculus (IC), and auditory cortex (AC), two to three coronal sections per ROI (sections 120 μm apart for the VCN and DCN and 320 μm apart for the IC and AC) per animal were used for microglial analysis.

Staining was performed using selected free-floating sections. The selected sections were permeabilized with 0.1% Triton X-100 in PBS for 30 min. After blocking with blocking solution for 2 h, the following primary antibodies were incubated overnight at 4°C: rabbit anti-Ki67 (for proliferating cells; Abcam, 1:500, ab16667), guinea pig anti-DCX (doublecortin, for newly generated neurons; Millipore, 1:1,000, AB2253), rabbit anti-Iba1 (ionized calcium-binding adaptor molecule 1, for microglia; Wako, 1:1,500, 019-19741), and rat anti-CD68 (cluster of differentiation 68, for phagocytic microglia; Bio-Rad, 1:1,500, MCA1957). After extensive washing, the sections were incubated with the appropriate secondary antibody for 2 h at room temperature: Alexa-488 goat anti-rabbit (Abcam, Cambridge, CB2 0AX, United Kingdom, 1:1,000, ab150077), Alexa-568 goat anti-guinea pig (Abcam, 1:1,000, ab175714), Alexa-568 goat anti-rabbit (Abcam, 1:1,000, ab175471), and Alexa-488 goat anti-rat (Thermo Fisher Scientific, 1:1,000, A11006). All sections were counterstained with DAPI (Beyotime, Shanghai, China, 1:750, C1027) at room temperature for 15 min to visualize the cell nuclei.

Image Analysis

Images were captured using a fluorescence microscope (Olympus BX53, Japan) or a confocal microscope (Olympus FV3000, Japan). Samples were analyzed by an observer blinded to the experimental treatment using ImageJ software (US National Institutes of Health, Bethesda, MD, United States). Maximum intensity projections of confocal z-series stacks at an interval of 1.0 μm were created and aligned in the x–y plane to create two-dimensional images. The target brain regions of interest (ROIs) were confirmed according to the Allen Mouse Brain Atlas (Allen Institute for Brain Science, 2008). The number of DCX- or Ki67-positive cells in each image was manually counted using the cell counter function of ImageJ in an area of the subgranular zone (SGZ), which is defined as the SGZ length in the image multiplied by an SGZ height of 20 μm [a layer of cells expanding 5 μm into the hilus and 15 μm into the granular cell layer (GCL)] (Sierra et al., 2010; Zhuang et al., 2020).

Microglial cells were identified by immunofluorescence staining using Iba1-specific antibodies, enabling an analysis of the morphology of individual microglial cells (Kreisel et al., 2014; Young and Morrison, 2018). The following parameters were employed to characterize the microglial phenotypic profile (Gebara et al., 2015; Hong et al., 2016; Fernandez-Mendivil et al., 2021) in the defined brain ROIs: (1) microglial density, which was defined as the number of Iba1-positive ($Iba1^+$) cells per brain area; (2) average microglial soma area, which was defined as the area of the spherical part of $Iba1^+$ cells that contains the nucleus; (3) average microglial territory area, which was defined as the two-dimensional area formed by connecting the outermost points of an $Iba1^+$ cell's dendritic processes; and (4) microglial CD68 score, which was determined by the CD68 occupancy within $Iba1^+$ microglia, ranging from 0 (low CD68 occupancy) to 3 (high CD68 occupancy), where a higher score corresponded to higher microglial phagocytic activity.

Statistical Analysis

The data were analyzed using GraphPad Prism 5 (GraphPad Software). All values are expressed as the mean ± standard error (SE). The level of statistical significance between groups was determined using one- or two-way analysis of variance (ANOVA) followed by Tukey's or Dunnett's *post hoc* test or Student's two-tailed *t*-test as appropriate. Relationships between parameters were assessed by Pearson's coefficient analysis. Values of $p < 0.05$ were accepted as statistically significant.

RESULTS

Permanent Hearing Loss Induced by Noise Exposure

Because auditory thresholds caused by NE recover exponentially with increasing post exposure time and reach a steady state within 2~3 weeks (Kujawa and Liberman, 2006; Ryan et al., 2016), ABR audiograms of the 28DPN group were obtained at 20 days post exposure and compared with the time-matched value from the control group to evaluate the extent of permanent NIHL (**Figure 1A**). **Figure 1B** shows that the ABR threshold was significantly higher in 28DPN mice than in control mice at every tested frequency [two-way ANOVA, effect of noise: $F_{(1, 75)} = 498.5, p < 0.0001$]. The frequency-averaged threshold (**Figure 1C**) of the 28DPN group was significantly higher than that of the control group (88.75 ± 0.8814 dB SPL vs. 48.33 ± 2.571 dB SPL, $p < 0.0001$). These results indicated that a moderate-to-severe degree of permanent hearing loss was induced by the NE experiments.

Early but Transient Stress Response Induced by Noise Exposure

The serum corticosterone (CORT) concentration of each group is shown in **Figure 2**. One-way ANOVA followed by Dunnett's multiple-comparison test revealed that only the 0 HPN group exhibited significantly elevated serum CORT levels compared with the control group ($p = 0.0044$), indicating that an immediate but transient stress response was induced by the NE experiments.

Dynamic Changes in Hippocampal Neurogenesis After Noise Exposure

To evaluate the impact of acute high-intensity NE on hippocampal neurogenesis, we stained the hippocampal sections for Ki67 (an endogenous proliferative marker of adult neurogenesis) and DCX (an endogenous marker of newly generated neurons expressed for a duration of 20–30 days after cell division) and counted the number of immunopositive cells.

Figures 3A–F shows representative images of DCX and Ki67 immunostaining in the SGZ from each group. One-way ANOVA followed by Dunnett's multiple-comparison test revealed that the noise-exposed mice exhibited significantly fewer Ki67 + cells than the control mice at 1DPN, 7DPN, and 28DPN (**Figure 3G**) and clearly fewer DCX^+ cells than the control mice at 28DPN (**Figure 3H**, $p = 0.0602$).

Dynamic Alterations of Microglia in Auditory Brain Regions After Acute Noise Exposure

Figures 4A1–F4 show representative confocal images of microglial cells stained for Iba-1 and CD68 from each group across auditory brain ROIs. Similar to previous observations (Olah et al., 2011; Zhuang et al., 2020), microglia in the control mice exhibited ramified morphologies that differed in cell density and process ramification at distinct anatomical regions of the brain (**Figures 4A1–4**). Compared with the control group, the noise-exposed groups showed comparable microglial density in each ROI. Microglia with larger somas, fewer branches, thicker processes, and increased CD68 occupancy were more frequently observed in noise-exposed groups, indicating microglial activation caused by NE (Hong et al., 2016; Zhuang et al., 2020).

Consistent with previous studies (Campos Torres et al., 1999; Baizer et al., 2015; Zhuang et al., 2020), quantification of the morphological features of microglia (**Figures 4G,I1–L4**) revealed that the microglia in the VCN, DCN, IC, and AC assumed an activated phenotype at 28DPN characterized by increased soma area (**Figures 4J1,J4**), decreased microglial territory area (**Figures 4K1–3**), increased percentage of microglia with high CD68 score, but decreased percentage of microglia with lower CD68 score (**Figures 4L1–4**). Microglia in the VCN were persistently activated from 3DPN to 28DPN (**Figures 4J1,K1,L1**). Although few signs of microglial activation were observed in the DCN and IC at 3DPN (**Figures 4L2,L3**) and the AC at 7DPN (**Figures 4J4,L4**), no signs of microglial activation were observed in the auditory ROIs at 14DPN except for the VCN.

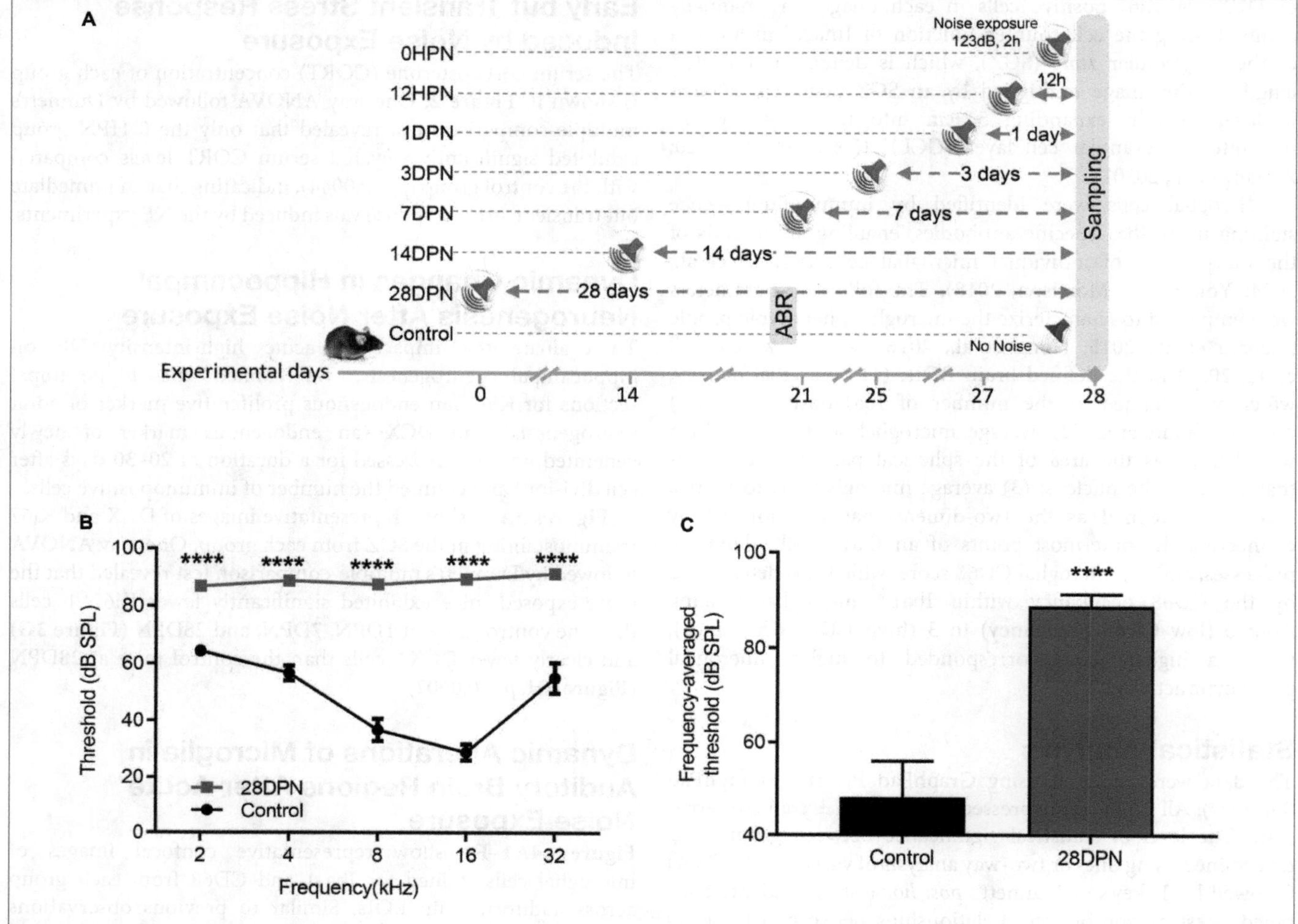

FIGURE 1 | Noise-induced ABR threshold shift measured at 20 days post noise exposure. **(A)** Experimental design for noise exposure and sampling. **(B)** ABR frequency-threshold curves of the 28DPN and control groups obtained at 20 days after noise exposure. **(C)** ABR frequency-averaged thresholds for the 28DPN and control groups obtained at 20 days after noise exposure. The values are presented as the mean ± SEM of eight mice per group. $^{****}p < 0.0001$ in the *post hoc* comparisons between the 28DPN group and the control group using two-way repeated-measure ANOVA **(B)** or *t*-test **(C)**.

Dynamic Alterations in Hippocampal Microglia After Acute Noise Exposure

As shown in **Figure 5**, Iba1$^+$ microglial cells were widely distributed in the DG, CA3, and CA1 of both the control and noise-exposed mice. Similar to our previous study (Zhuang et al., 2020), microglia in the control mice exhibited ramified morphologies that differed in cell density and process ramification at distinct anatomical regions of the hippocampus (**Figures 5A1–3**). Microglial density in the ROIs was comparable between the groups. However, microglia with enlarged soma, decreased territory area, and increased CD68 occupancy were more frequently observed in the noise-exposed mice (**Figures 5B1–F3**), suggesting that an abnormal hippocampal microglial reaction developed in the noise-exposed mice.

The time-course profile of hippocampal microglial parameters following NE is shown in **Figures 5G1–J3**. *Post hoc* comparisons using Dunnett's test indicated microglial overactivation in the DG and CA3 at 28DPN, as evidenced by a significant increase in the soma area (**Figures 5H1,H2**), decrease in the territory area (**Figures 5I1,I2**), increase in the percentage of microglia with higher CD68 score (**Figure 5J1**), and/or decrease in the percentage of microglia with lower CD68 score (**Figures 5J1,J2**). Signs of microglial activation (i.e., significantly larger than the control soma area, smaller than the control territory area, and enhanced CD68 expression reflected by the CD68 score) were observed in the DG and CA3 at 3DPN and 7DPN but disappeared at 14DPN. Except for the decreased percentage of microglia with lower CD68 scores exhibited at 7DPN and 28DPN (**Figure 5J3**), no sign of abnormal microglial status was observed in CA1.

DISCUSSION

Acquired peripheral HL has been ranked as the largest potentially modifiable health and lifestyle factor for the development of dementia (Lin et al., 2011; Livingston et al., 2017, 2020;

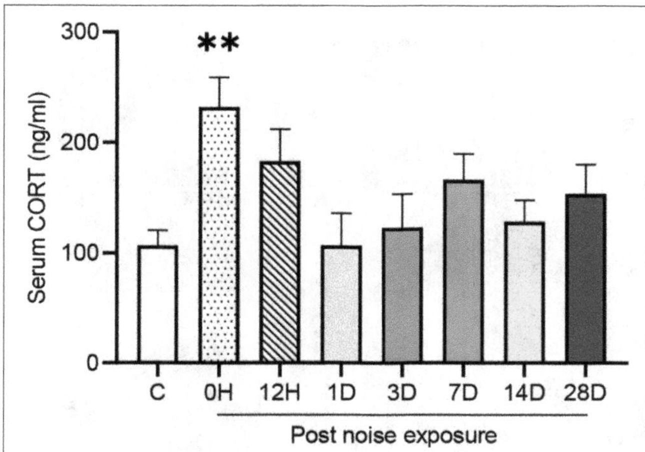

FIGURE 2 | Noise-exposed mice exhibited an early but transient increase in serum corticosterone (CORT). The values are presented as the mean ± SEM of 6–8 mice per group. $^{**}p < 0.01$ in the *post hoc* comparisons between the noise group and the controls after one-way ANOVA.

Thomson et al., 2017; Nixon et al., 2019; Orgeta et al., 2019; Uchida et al., 2019). Environmental noise represents the most common preventable cause of acquired sensorineural hearing loss, and it is increasingly encountered in many aspects of day-to-day modern life (Rabinowitz, 2000; Le et al., 2017). Worldwide, 16% of the disabling hearing loss in adults is attributed to occupational noise including construction, agriculture, mining, manufacturing, utilities, transportation, and the military (Chepesiuk, 2005; Nelson et al., 2005). NIHL resulting from hazardous recreational noise (e.g., sporting events, concerts, nightclubs, firearms, and personal stereos) is increasing in modern society (Meinke et al., 2017; Feder et al., 2019; Gopal et al., 2019). Popular "boom cars" equipped with powerful stereo systems that are usually played with the volume and bass turned up abnormally high, and the car windows rolled down can hit 140–150 dBA (Chepesiuk, 2005). It is estimated that 12% or more of the global population is at risk of hearing loss due to unsafe levels of sound exposure (Le et al., 2017). According to WHO reports, one-third of all cases of hearing loss can be attributed to NE No authors listed (1990), and the prevalence of NIHL is still increasing (Imam and Hannan, 2017). Considering the tremendous disability weight and the expanding healthcare burden posed by dementia (Livingston et al., 2020) as well as the increasing pervasiveness of noise (Goines and Hagler, 2007), the animal model of NIHL is undoubtedly optimal for studying the underlying mechanisms linking dementia and acquired peripheral HL.

The hippocampus, a kernel cognition- and emotion-related brain region embedded deep into the temporal lobe, is generally considered one of the earliest affected brain regions in patients with dementia (Braak and Braak, 1997; Xue et al., 2019). Adult hippocampal neurogenesis is a unique form of neural circuit plasticity that results in the generation of new neurons in the dentate gyrus (DG) throughout life and plays a vital role in hippocampus-dependent learning and memory (Sahay et al., 2011; Lazarov and Hollands, 2016). Adult hippocampal neurogenesis generates only granule cells, the principal neuron in the DG (Kempermann et al., 2015). The first relay in the hippocampal trisynaptic circuit is composed of granule cells, which extend dendrites into the molecular layer and present axons that form the mossy fiber tract that extends to CA3, and these cells are thought to be essential to cognitive function (GoodSmith et al., 2017). Emerging evidence has indicated that altered hippocampal neurogenesis represents an early critical event in the course of dementia (Mu and Gage, 2011; Tobin et al., 2019; Disouky and Lazarov, 2021).

Adult neurogenesis is a complex multistage and multiweek process involving cell proliferation, neuronal differentiation, and, ultimately, survival, and integration into functional circuits (Lagace et al., 2010; Kempermann et al., 2015). This dynamic process is regulated both positively and negatively by a variety of growth factors and environmental experiences (Zhao et al., 2008). Microglia, the resident macrophages and primary immune cells of the brain, can orchestrate their highly plastic, context-specific adaptive responses to remodel neuronal circuit structures and functions (Wake et al., 2013; Delpech et al., 2015). They play integral roles in both the healthy and injured brain, from surveillance and monitoring to sculpting neuronal circuits and guiding plasticity (Sierra et al., 2010; Gemma and Bachstetter, 2013; Sato, 2015; Chugh and Ekdahl, 2016). Increasing evidence indicates that microglial cells indeed exert vital roles in the maintenance of the functional neurogenic niche and are actively involved in crucial steps of adult neurogenesis, including the proliferation, differentiation, and survival of newborn cells (Gemma and Bachstetter, 2013; Kohman and Rhodes, 2013; Sato, 2015; Mosser et al., 2017).

Microglial cells are heterogeneous and dynamically pleomorphic. It is well established that the morphology of microglia is inextricably linked to their functional status (Ajami et al., 2007; Angelova and Brown, 2019). Surveillance microglia display a ramified phenotype marked by a stable number, small soma, and numerous long, thin, motile processes with delicate arborization that constantly monitor their immediate surroundings by extending and retracting their processes (also called ramified microglia) (Davalos et al., 2005). If signs of damage are detected, the microglia convert to an activated or reactive state and assume an amoeboid-like phenotype, characterized by shorter, thicker processes and a larger soma, with increased expression of phagocytic markers, such as CD68 (Nimmerjahn et al., 2005; Olah et al., 2011; Tejera and Heneka, 2016; Angelova and Brown, 2019). Many neurodegenerative diseases, such as Parkinson's disease and Alzheimer's disease, are associated with abnormal functional phenotypes of microglia (Sarlus and Heneka, 2017; Subramaniam and Federoff, 2017; Baik et al., 2019).

In our previous studies (Liu et al., 2016a, 2018; Zhuang et al., 2020), a single noise (identical to the present noise setting) was used to create permanent HL in CBA mice, a mouse strain that has been demonstrated to maintain good hearing threshold sensitivity well into old age (Spongr et al., 1997; Kujawa and Liberman, 2006). Cognitive function was evaluated by the Morris water maze (MWM) task at 3 months

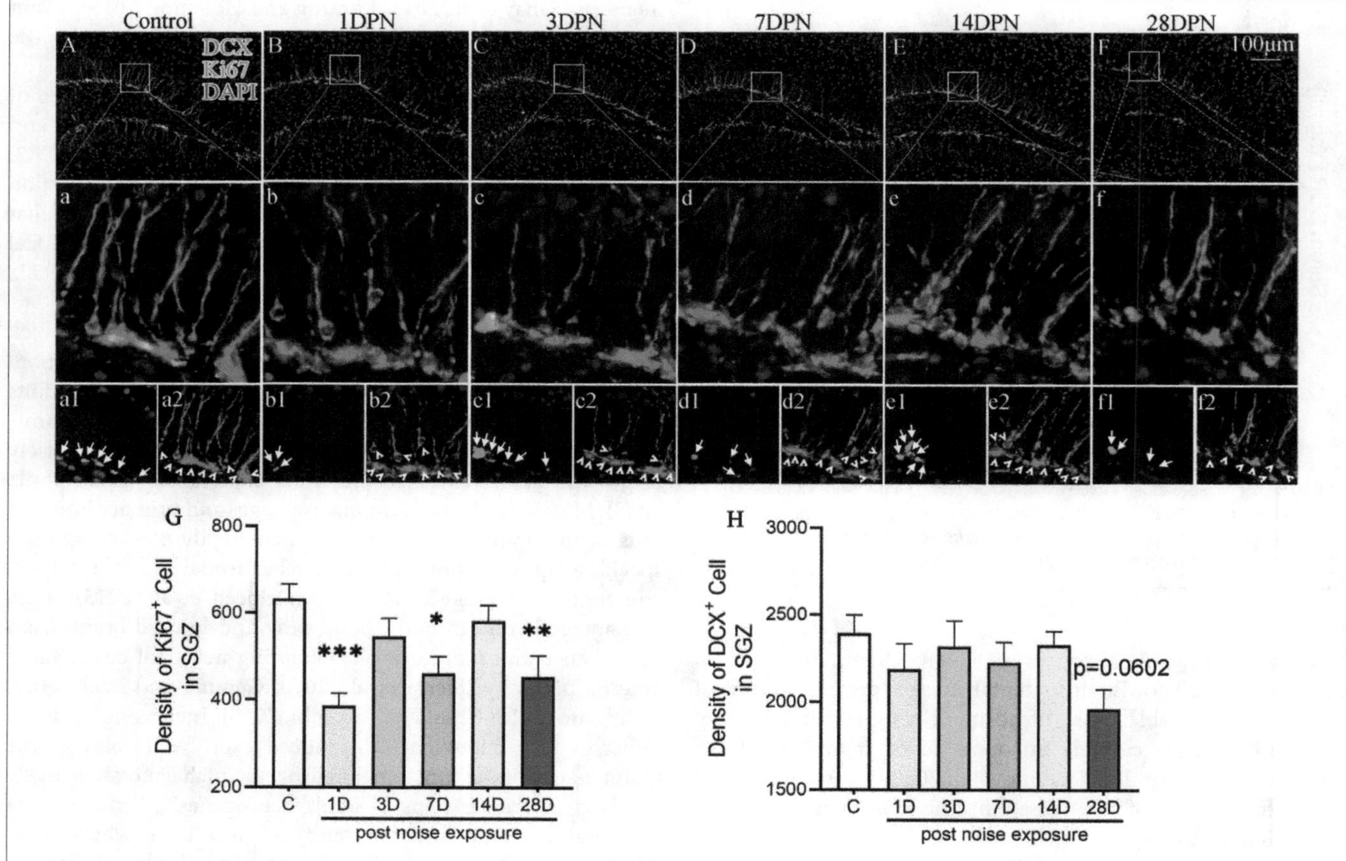

FIGURE 3 | Noise-exposed mice exhibited dynamic changes in hippocampal neurogenesis. **(A–F)** Representative images of DCX$^+$ (red) and Ki67$^+$ (green) cells in the DG of control and noise-exposed mice. Scale bar: 100 μm. The white rectangle shows the field of view that is shown in the row **(a–f)** below in higher magnification and the third row **(a1–f2)** for Ki67$^+$ cells (green, indicated by arrows in **a1–f1**) and DCX$^+$ cells (red, indicated by arrowheads in **a2–f2**). **(G,H)** Quantitative analyses of Ki67$^+$ cells **(G)** and DCX$^+$ cells **(H)** in the SGZ of each group. The values are presented as the mean ± SEM of 8 mice per group. *$p < 0.05$, **$p < 0.01$, ***$p < 0.001$ in *post hoc* comparisons between the noise-exposed group and the control group following one-way ANOVA.

post exposure (Liu et al., 2016a, 2018), and hippocampal neurogenesis and microglial status were monitored for up to 12 months following NE by quantitative immunohistochemical analysis of Ki67 (a proliferating cell marker), doublecortin (DCX; an immature progenitor cell marker), Iba1 (a microglia marker), and CD68 (a lysosomal marker indicative of phagocytic activity of microglia) (Liu et al., 2016a, 2018; Zhuang et al., 2020). We observed that CBA mice with NIHL exhibited prolonged significant cognitive impairment accompanied by marked hippocampal neurogenesis decline (Liu et al., 2016a, 2018). Our observations not only provide compelling evidence for the causal role of HL in the development of cognitive impairment (Liu et al., 2016a, 2018) but also suggest that the accelerated age-related hippocampal neurogenesis decline and persistent microglial dysfunction may contribute to the cognitive deficiency that occurs in animals with NIHL (Zhuang et al., 2020). However, the exact mechanisms leading to alterations in hippocampal neurogenesis and microglial status in NIHL mice remain largely mysterious.

Microglia are versatile modulators of neurogenesis, and their influence is dependent on their activation status. Recent findings in human and animal studies indicated that microglial activation inversely correlates with hippocampal volume in neurodegenerative diseases with dementia, providing compelling evidence for the central role of microglial activation in neurodegenerative diseases (Femminella et al., 2016; Salter and Stevens, 2017; Suss and Schlachetzki, 2020). Consistent with our previous observation in CBA mice (Zhuang et al., 2020), C57BL/6J mice subjected to brief NE at high intensity developed permanent hearing loss and exhibited decreased hippocampal neurogenesis and aberrant microglial activation at 28DPN, thus providing further support for the assumption that hippocampal microglial dysfunction might contribute to acquired hearing loss-related hippocampal neurogenesis (Zhuang et al., 2020).

The brain is a finely tuned machine that has a fascinating capacity to continually undergo structural and functional changes in response to environmental inputs and organism needs; that is, it exhibits neural plasticity (Kleim and Jones, 2008; Sale et al., 2014). Neural circuits that are frequently used have strong connections, while those not actively engaged in task performance for an extended period of time begin to degrade, i.e., they present a "use-it-or-lose-it" characteristic

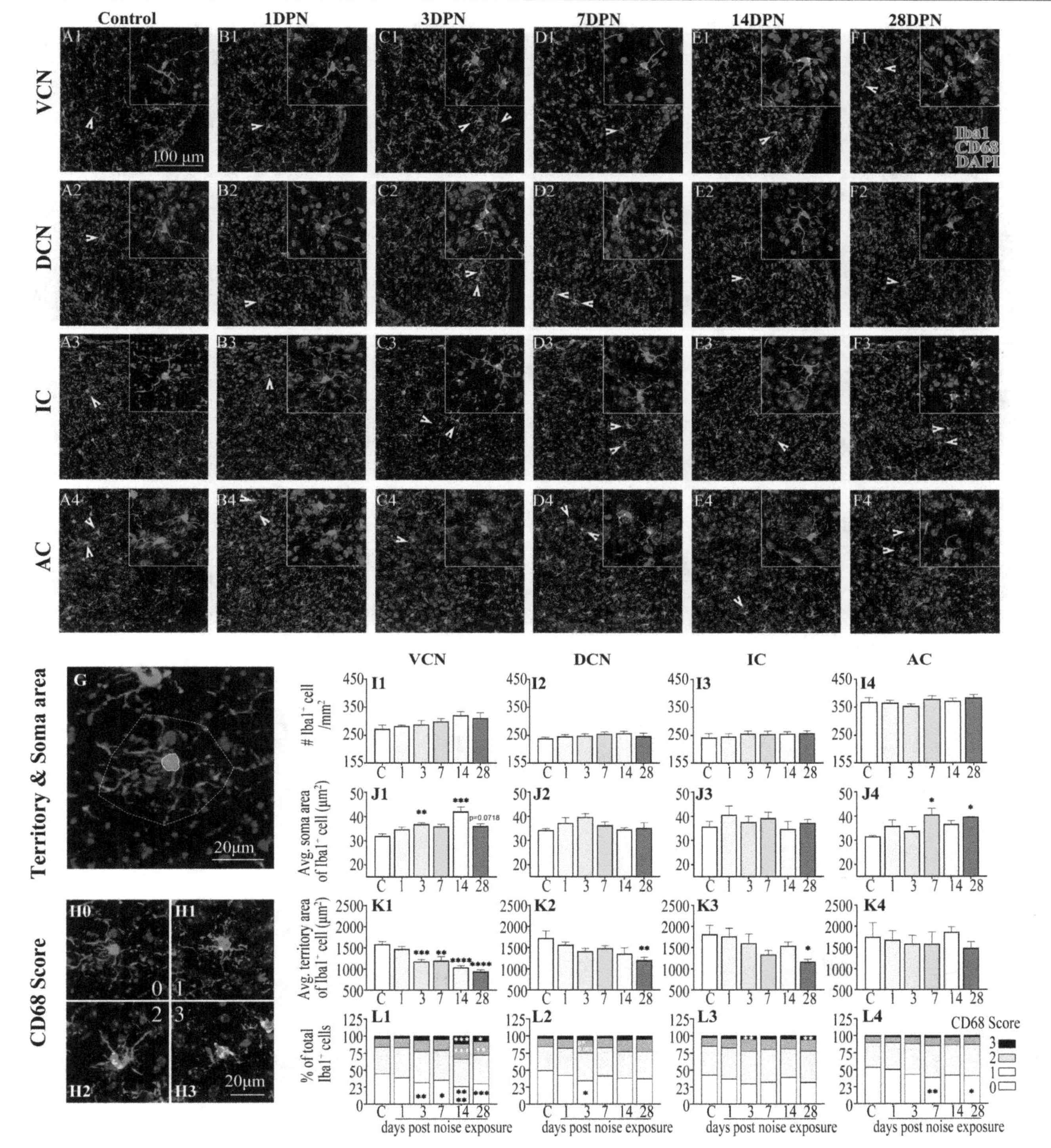

FIGURE 4 | Noise-exposed mice exhibited dynamic microglial alterations in auditory brain regions. **(A1–F4)** Representative images of Iba1 (red)-, CD68 (green)- and DAPI (blue)-stained brain sections of the control and noise-exposed mice. Scale bar: 100 μm. The insets show higher magnifications of the corresponding microglia signified by arrowheads. **(G)** Soma area and territory area of microglia delineated by a solid (soma area) line and a dotted (territory area) line, respectively. **(H0–H3)** Representative images of the scoring of CD68 levels within Iba1^{+} cells. A score of 0 indicates no/scarce expression **(H0)**; 1 signifies only patchy positivity **(H1)**; 2 represents punctate expression roughly covering one-third to two-thirds of cells **(H2)**; and 3 represents greater than two-thirds occupancy **(H3)**. **(I1–L4)** Quantification of the impact of NE on each individual parameter of microglia in the VCN, DCN, IC, and AC. The values are presented as the mean ± SEM of 3–6 mice per group. *$p < 0.05$, **$p < 0.01$, ***$p < 0.001$, ****$p < 0.0001$ in *post hoc* comparisons between the noise-exposed group and the control group following one-way ANOVA.

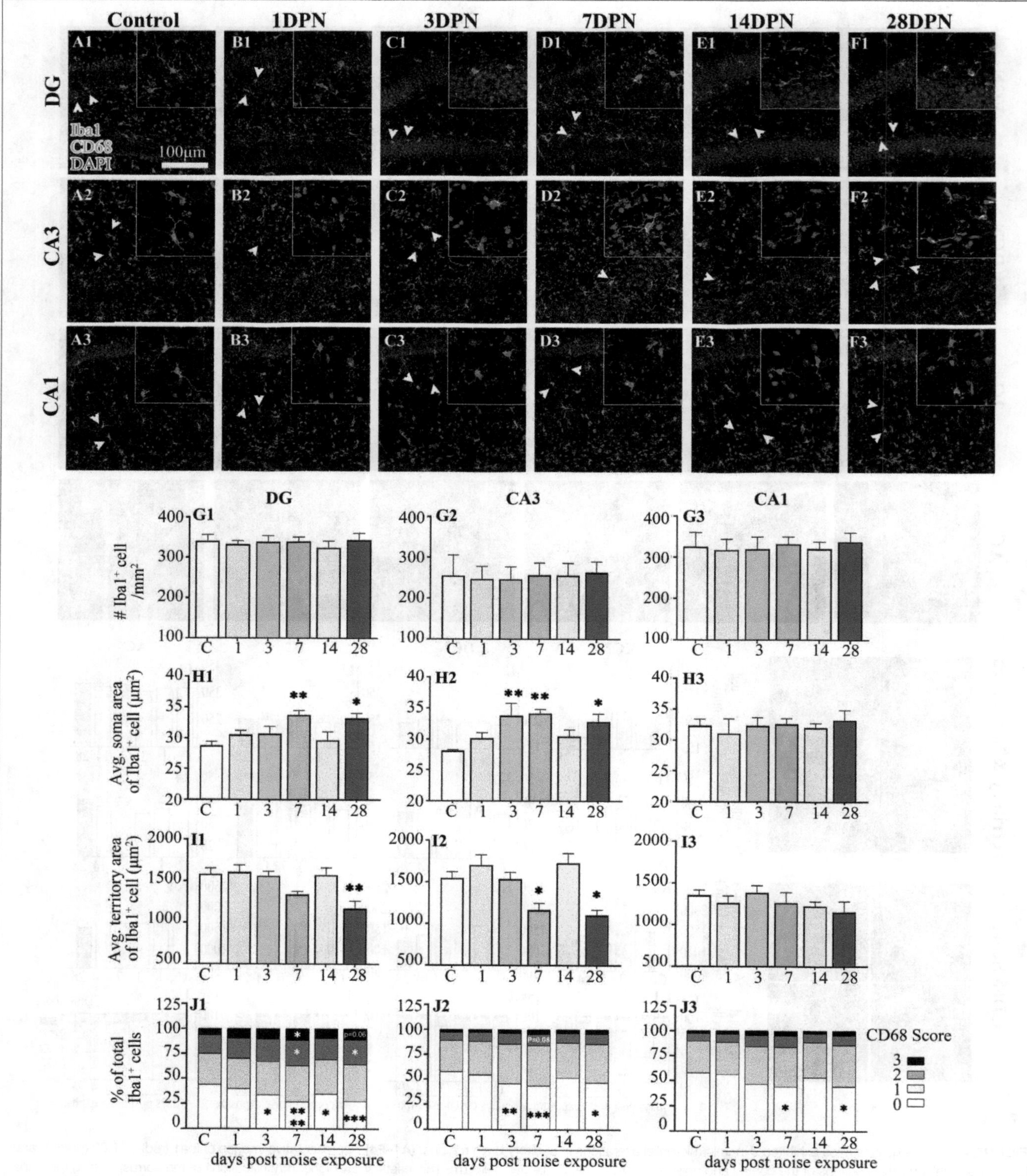

FIGURE 5 | Noise-exposed mice exhibited dynamic microglial alterations in the hippocampus. **(A1–F3)** Representative images of Iba1 (red)-, CD68 (green)-, and DAPI (blue)-stained brain sections of control and noise-exposed mice. Scale bar: 100 μm. The insets show higher magnifications of the corresponding microglia signified by arrowheads. **(G1–J3)** Quantification of the impact of NE on each individual parameter of microglia in the DG, CA3, and CA1. The values are presented as the mean ± SEM of 3–6 mice per group. $*p < 0.05$, $**p < 0.01$, $***p < 0.001$, $****p < 0.0001$ in *post hoc* comparisons between the noise-exposed group and the control group following one-way ANOVA.

(Kleim and Jones, 2008). Microglia play a fundamental role in activity-dependent neuroplasticity. It is well established that microglia can quickly adapt to their environment and modify their functions with a broad spectrum of activation states (Li and Barres, 2018). For instance, these cells can respond to light deprivation and reexposure by changing their morphology and modulating their interactions with neuronal circuits, notably regulating processes that include adult hippocampal neurogenesis and actively contributing to the experience-dependent modification or elimination of a specific subset of synapses in the brain (Tremblay et al., 2010).

In line with previous reports on long-term microglial activation in the cochlear nucleus following inner ear damage that reduced neural output from the cochlea (Campos Torres et al., 1999; Baizer et al., 2015), the present study demonstrated microglial activation in the auditory ROIs of NIHL mice at 28 days after the cessation of NE. Considering the "use-it-or-lose-it" principle of neuroplasticity (Syka, 2002; Kleim and Jones, 2008) and the microglial contribution to neuroplasticity (Wake et al., 2013; Valero et al., 2016), it is plausible to assume that microglial activation represents auditory circuit remodeling following acquired hearing loss (auditory deprivation).

Consistent with previously published data from laboratory experiments (Zhuang et al., 2020), the present study demonstrated a significant effect of NE on the functional phenotypes of microglia in the hippocampal DG and CA3 region but not in the CA1 region. The discrepancy in the outcome after NE between subregions could at least be partially explained by a report indicating that the DG-CA3 subregion is extremely sensitive to changes in information input and plays a key role in auditory information processing while the CA1 subregion is highly resistant to changes in sensory input (Holden et al., 2012). Mounting evidence demonstrates that microglia, the well-known key facilitators of neuronal plasticity, can sense and respond to neuronal activity in a variety of contexts (Umpierre and Wu, 2021). The microglial status is subtly altered by local neuronal activity (Ronzano et al., 2021). As the hippocampus is generally believed to be involved in auditory perception (Moxon et al., 1999; Kraus and Canlon, 2012), it is reasonable to hypothesize that abnormal local neuronal activity caused by a disturbance of auditory input is a major contributor to hippocampal microglial overactivity in mice with acquired peripheral HL.

Microglia are well-known major sources of proinflammatory cytokines and the principal target cells of cytokines (Hanisch, 2002). Chronically activated microglia secrete excessive pro-inflammatory cytokines, which can further induce microglial responses toward a dysregulated phenotype (Voet et al., 2019). Microglial-derived cytokine signals are assumed to propagate through the brain by volume transmission (i.e., diffuse through cerebral spinal fluid, nerve bundles, and perivascular space) and wiring (i.e., through neuronal projections and gap junctions) (Vitkovic et al., 2000; Almeida-Suhett et al., 2017). The hippocampus and the auditory regions make reciprocal connections with each other (Kraus and Canlon, 2012), which would enable the diffusion of cytokines produced by chronically activated microglia in the auditory region to the hippocampus through wiring and/or cerebral spinal fluid. Thus, it cannot be excluded that chronically activated microglia in the auditory region might represent one contributor to the microglial status transition in the hippocampus. However, this hypothesis remains highly speculative in the absence of convincing evidence. Hearing loss (threshold sensitivity loss) from extensive loud noise may occur immediately. The deafening effect of NE includes reversible and irreversible components. After exposure that is intense enough to produce permanent effects, hearing thresholds recover exponentially with increasing post exposure time and reach a steady state within 2~3 weeks (Kujawa and Liberman, 2006). Thus, the significant threshold shift measured at 20 days post exposure represents the magnitude of permanent hearing loss induced by NE in the present study. Moreover, it undoubtedly implies an even greater continuous hearing loss across the 20 days post noise. Intriguingly, although changes in microglia similar to those observed at 28DPN were observed as early as 3DPN, almost no signs of microglial abnormalities were observed at 14DPN in ROIs except the VCN. A similar near-perfect correspondence was seen in hippocampal neurogenesis. These observations provide further evidence for the causal role of permanent HL in microglial dysfunction and hippocampal neurogenesis decline observed long after NE (Zhuang et al., 2020), and they suggest that factors other than HL might serve as a major contributor to the overall alterations that occurred earlier after NE.

Beyond the well-known direct deleterious effects on the auditory system (i.e., hearing loss), exposure to intense noise has previously been shown to acutely activate the stress response (Samson et al., 2007; Frank et al., 2015, 2019; Hahad et al., 2019; Hayes et al., 2019), which has increasingly been linked to both microglial activity (Frank et al., 2019) and adult hippocampal neurogenesis in recent years (Surget and Belzung, 2021). The significantly higher serum corticosterone observed in noise-exposed mice at 0 HPN (i.e., immediately after NE) compared with the control demonstrates a transient stress response induced by noise in the present study.

A recent study has shown that microglia express a diverse array of receptors, which also allows them to respond to stress hormones derived from peripheral and central sources (Frank et al., 2019). Emerging evidence indicates that the activation of microglia by stress results in profound morphological and functional changes that could disrupt neuronal function, impair neurogenesis, and alter cognitive and emotional behavior (Kreisel et al., 2014; Delpech et al., 2015; Frank et al., 2019; Sanguino-Gomez et al., 2021). Furthermore, studies have demonstrated that there are cortisol receptors throughout the hippocampus (Korz and Frey, 2003) and showed that the proliferation of granule cell precursors, and ultimately the production of new granule cells, is dependent on the levels of circulating adrenal steroids (McEwen, 1999). Stressful experiences, which are known to elevate circulating levels of glucocorticoids, inhibit the proliferation of granule cell precursors (Tanapat et al., 1998; McEwen, 1999; Surget and Belzung, 2021) and the survival of newborn neurons (Thomas et al., 2007). Based on these findings and our data, we speculate that the transient stress response caused by NE in our study may have been associated with mediating the functional response of microglia in each target brain region at the early stage after NE (within 1 week);

however, most of the target brain regions showed no abnormal microglia phenotype at 14DPN, suggesting that the transient stress response is insufficient to explain the reappearance of microglia phenotypic abnormalities and aberrant hippocampal neurogenesis in the long term after NE (28DPN) and thus further highlights the major contribution of permanent hearing loss to the prolonged phenotype change of microglia and hippocampal neurogenesis.

In summary, this study observed the effects of acute high-intensity NE on the stress response, hearing threshold, hippocampal neurogenesis, and functional phenotypes of hippocampal and central auditory system microglia. Our results illustrated early but transient and late but progressive microglial activation and hippocampal neurogenesis impairment, an early but transient increase in serum corticosterone, and a permanent moderate-to-severe degree of hearing loss in noise-exposed mice. These findings indicate for the first time that both the stress response and HL are potential contributors to the time-dependent alterations of microglia and hippocampal neurogenesis, which both consist of an early but transient change and a late but enduring change following NE. The noise-induced stress response may be involved with early but transient alterations, while noise-induced permanent HL is more likely to be responsible for late but enduring changes, i.e., microglial dysfunction and hippocampal neurogenesis disturbances that are associated with many neurological diseases (including cognitive impairment and dementia). The microglial overactivation observed in the auditory ROIs may have represented neuronal circuit remodeling closely associated with the acquired peripheral hearing loss caused by high-intensity NE, although it also suggested that the acquired peripheral hearing loss disturbance of auditory input caused by NE induced hippocampal microglia dysfunction and neurogenesis decline. Therefore, we can suggest some reasonable hypotheses based on the available data. Given the pervasiveness of noise in modern life (from commercial, industrial and recreational sources, etc.) and the insidious and progressive nature of neurodegenerative disorders, our observations further highlight that raising awareness of the adverse health impact of noise represents a promising and cost-effective strategy to prevent or delay the onset of dementia.

AUTHOR CONTRIBUTIONS

LL and GT designed the experiment and supervised the project. CY, DX, RL, CF, and YW managed the mouse cohorts. HL, SS, SZ, and QL conducted the noise exposure and ABR measurements. QL, XY, and CW conducted the sample preparation for the histological study and ELISA. QL, HL, and XY performed the histological procedures and data collection. HZ, HL, and CW conducted the data analysis. QL, HZ, YX, and LL were involved in the data interpretation. QL and LL contributed to the manuscript writing. All authors contributed to the article and approved the submitted version.

REFERENCES

Ajami, B., Bennett, J. L., Krieger, C., Tetzlaff, W., and Rossi, F. M. V. (2007). Local self-renewal can sustain CNS microglia maintenance and function throughout adult life. *Nat. Neurosci.* 10, 1538–1543. doi: 10.1038/nn2014

Allen Institute for Brain Science (2008). *The Allen Mouse Brain Atlas* Available online at: https://mouse.brain-map.org/static/atlas (accessed February 11, 2019).

Almeida-Suhett, C. P., Graham, A., Chen, Y., and Deuster, P. (2017). Behavioral changes in male mice fed a high-fat diet are associated with IL-1beta expression in specific brain regions. *Physiol. Behav.* 169, 130–140. doi: 10.1016/j.physbeh.2016.11.016

Angelova, D. M., and Brown, D. R. (2019). Microglia and the aging brain: are senescent microglia the key to neurodegeneration? *J. Neurochem.* 151, 676–688. doi: 10.1111/jnc.14860

Baik, S. H., Kang, S., Lee, W., Choi, H., Chung, S., Kim, J.-I., et al. (2019). A Breakdown in Metabolic Reprogramming Causes Microglia Dysfunction in Alzheimer's Disease. *Cell Metab.* 30, 493–507.e6. doi: 10.1016/j.cmet.2019.06.005

Baizer, J. S., Wong, K. M., Manohar, S., Hayes, S. H., Ding, D., Dingman, R., et al. (2015). Effects of acoustic trauma on the auditory system of the rat: the role of microglia. *Neuroscience* 303, 299–311. doi: 10.1016/j.neuroscience.2015.07.004

Basner, M., Babisch, W., Davis, A., Brink, M., Clark, C., Janssen, S., et al. (2014). Auditory and non-auditory effects of noise on health. *Lancet* 383, 1325–1332. doi: 10.1016/S0140-6736(13)61613-X

Bazargan-Hejazi, S., Dehghan, K., Edwards, C., Mohammadi, N., Attar, S., Sahraian, M. A., et al. (2020). The health burden of non-communicable neurological disorders in the USA between 1990 and 2017. *Brain Commun.* 2:fcaa097. doi: 10.1093/braincomms/fcaa097

Benziger, C. P., Roth, G. A., and Moran, A. E. (2016). The Global Burden of Disease Study and the Preventable Burden of NCD. *Glob. Heart* 11, 393–397. doi: 10.1016/j.gheart.2016.10.024

Braak, H., and Braak, E. (1997). Frequency of stages of Alzheimer-related lesions in different age categories. *Neurobiol. Aging* 18, 351–357. doi: 10.1016/s0197-4580(97)00056-0

Campos Torres, A., Vidal, P. P., and de Waele, C. (1999). Evidence for a microglial reaction within the vestibular and cochlear nuclei following inner ear lesion in the rat. *Neuroscience* 92, 1475–1490. doi: 10.1016/s0306-4522(99)00078-0

Cheng, L., Wang, S. H., Huang, Y., and Liao, X. M. (2016). The hippocampus may be more susceptible to environmental noise than the auditory cortex. *Hear. Res.* 333, 93–97. doi: 10.1016/j.heares.2016.01.001

Chepesiuk, R. (2005). Decibel hell: the effects of living in a noisy world. *Environ. Health Perspect.* 113, A34–A41. doi: 10.1289/ehp.113-a34

Chugh, D., and Ekdahl, C. T. (2016). Interactions Between Microglia and Newly Formed Hippocampal Neurons in Physiological and Seizure-Induced Inflammatory Environment. *Brain Plast.* 1, 215–221. doi: 10.3233/BPL-150014

Collaborators, G. B. D. N. (2019). Global, regional, and national burden of neurological disorders, 1990-2016: a systematic analysis for the Global Burden of Disease Study 2016. *Lancet Neurol.* 18, 459–480. doi: 10.1016/S1474-4422(18)30499-X

Cui, B., Wu, M., She, X., and Liu, H. (2012). Impulse noise exposure in rats causes cognitive deficits and changes in hippocampal neurotransmitter signaling and tau phosphorylation. *Brain Res.* 1427, 35–43. doi: 10.1016/j.brainres.2011.08.035

Davalos, D., Grutzendler, J., Yang, G., Kim, J. V., Zuo, Y., Jung, S., et al. (2005). ATP mediates rapid microglial response to local brain injury in vivo. *Nat. Neurosci.* 8, 752–758. doi: 10.1038/nn1472

De Lucia, C., Rinchon, A., Olmos-Alonso, A., Riecken, K., Fehse, B., Boche, D., et al. (2016). Microglia regulate hippocampal neurogenesis during chronic neurodegeneration. *Brain Behav. Immun.* 55, 179–190. doi: 10.1016/j.bbi.2015.11.001

Delpech, J. C., Madore, C., Nadjar, A., Joffre, C., Wohleb, E. S., and Laye, S. (2015). Microglia in neuronal plasticity: influence of stress. *Neuropharmacology* 96, 19–28. doi: 10.1016/j.neuropharm.2014.12.034

Disouky, A., and Lazarov, O. (2021). Adult hippocampal neurogenesis in Alzheimer's disease. *Prog. Mol. Biol. Transl. Sci.* 177, 137–156. doi: 10.1016/bs.pmbts.2020.09.002

Feder, K., Marro, L., McNamee, J., and Michaud, D. (2019). Prevalence of loud leisure noise activities among a representative sample of Canadians aged 6-79 years. *J. Acoust. Soc. Am.* 146:3934. doi: 10.1121/1.5132949

Femminella, G. D., Ninan, S., Atkinson, R., Fan, Z., Brooks, D. J., and Edison, P. (2016). Does Microglial Activation Influence Hippocampal Volume and Neuronal Function in Alzheimer's Disease and Parkinson's Disease Dementia? *J. Alzheimers Dis.* 51, 1275–1289. doi: 10.3233/JAD-150827

Fernandez-Mendivil, C., Luengo, E., Trigo-Alonso, P., Garcia-Magro, N., Negredo, P., and Lopez, M. G. (2021). Protective role of microglial HO-1 blockade in aging: implication of iron metabolism. *Redox Biol.* 38:101789. doi: 10.1016/j.redox.2020.101789

Frank, M. G., Fonken, L. K., Watkins, L. R., and Maier, S. F. (2019). Microglia: neuroimmune-sensors of stress. *Semin. Cell Dev. Biol.* 94, 176–185. doi: 10.1016/j.semcdb.2019.01.001

Frank, M. G., Watkins, L. R., and Maier, S. F. (2015). The permissive role of glucocorticoids in neuroinflammatory priming: mechanisms and insights. *Curr. Opin. Endocrinol. Diabetes Obes.* 22, 300–305. doi: 10.1097/med.0000000000000168

Gebara, E., Udry, F., Sultan, S., and Toni, N. (2015). Taurine increases hippocampal neurogenesis in aging mice. *Stem Cell Res.* 14, 369–379. doi: 10.1016/j.scr.2015.04.001

Gemma, C., and Bachstetter, A. D. (2013). The role of microglia in adult hippocampal neurogenesis. *Front. Cell. Neurosci.* 7:229. doi: 10.3389/fncel.2013.00229

Goines, L., and Hagler, L. (2007). Noise pollution: a modem plague. *South. Med. J.* 100, 287–294. doi: 10.1097/smj.0b013e3180318be5

GoodSmith, D., Chen, X., Wang, C., Kim, S. H., Song, H., Burgalossi, A., et al. (2017). Spatial Representations of Granule Cells and Mossy Cells of the Dentate Gyrus. *Neuron* 93, 677–690e675. doi: 10.1016/j.neuron.2016.12.026

Gopal, K. V., Mills, L. E., Phillips, B. S., and Nandy, R. (2019). Risk Assessment of Recreational Noise-Induced Hearing Loss from Exposure through a Personal Audio System-iPod Touch. *J. Am. Acad. Audiol.* 30, 619–633. doi: 10.3766/jaaa.17140

Hahad, O., Prochaska, J. H., Daiber, A., and Muenzel, T. (2019). Environmental Noise-Induced Effects on Stress Hormones, Oxidative Stress, and Vascular Dysfunction: key Factors in the Relationship between Cerebrocardiovascular and Psychological Disorders. *Oxid. Med. Cell. Longev.* 2019:4623109. doi: 10.1155/2019/4623109

Hanisch, U. K. (2002). Microglia as a source and target of cytokines. *Glia* 40, 140–155. doi: 10.1002/glia.10161

Hansen, D. V., Hanson, J. E., and Sheng, M. (2018). Microglia in Alzheimer's disease. *J. Cell Biol.* 217, 459–472. doi: 10.1083/jcb.201709069

Hayes, S. H., Manohar, S., Majumdar, A., Allman, B. L., and Salvi, R. (2019). Noise-induced hearing loss alters hippocampal glucocorticoid receptor expression in rats. *Hear. Res.* 379, 43–51. doi: 10.1016/j.heares.2019.04.013

Holden, H. M., Hoebel, C., Loftis, K., and Gilbert, P. E. (2012). Spatial pattern separation in cognitively normal young and older adults. *Hippocampus* 22, 1826–1832. doi: 10.1002/hipo.22017

Hong, S., Beja-Glasser, V. F., Nfonoyim, B. M., Frouin, A., Li, S., Ramakrishnan, S., et al. (2016). Complement and microglia mediate early synapse loss in Alzheimer mouse models. *Science* 352, 712–716. doi: 10.1126/science.aad8373

Imam, L., and Hannan, S. A. (2017). Noise-induced hearing loss: a modern epidemic? *Br. J. Hosp. Med.* 78, 286–290. doi: 10.12968/hmed.2017.78.5.286

Jeschke, M., Happel, M. F. K., Tziridis, K., Krauss, P., Schilling, A., Schulze, H., et al. (2020). Acute and Long-Term Circuit-Level Effects in the Auditory Cortex After Sound Trauma. *Front. Neurosci.* 14:598406. doi: 10.3389/fnins.2020.598406

Kempermann, G., Song, H., and Gage, F. H. (2015). Neurogenesis in the Adult Hippocampus. *Cold Spring Harb. Perspect. Biol.* 7:a018812. doi: 10.1101/cshperspect.a018812

Kleim, J. A., and Jones, T. A. (2008). Principles of experience-dependent neural plasticity: implications for rehabilitation after brain damage. *J. Speech Lang. Hear. Res.* 51, S225–S239. doi: 10.1044/1092-4388(2008/018)

Kohman, R. A., and Rhodes, J. S. (2013). Neurogenesis, inflammation and behavior. *Brain Behav. Immun.* 27, 22–32. doi: 10.1016/j.bbi.2012.09.003

Korz, V., and Frey, J. U. (2003). Stress-related modulation of hippocampal long-term potentiation in rats: involvement of adrenal steroid receptors. *J. Neurosci.* 23, 7281–7287.

Kraus, K. S., and Canlon, B. (2012). Neuronal connectivity and interactions between the auditory and limbic systems. Effects of noise and tinnitus. *Hear. Res.* 288, 34–46. doi: 10.1016/j.heares.2012.02.009

Kraus, K. S., Mitra, S., Jimenez, Z., Hinduja, S., Ding, D., Jiang, H., et al. (2010). Noise trauma impairs neurogenesis in the rat hippocampus. *Neuroscience* 167, 1216–1226. doi: 10.1016/j.neuroscience.2010.02.071

Kreisel, T., Frank, M. G., Licht, T., Reshef, R., Ben-Menachem-Zidon, O., Baratta, M. V., et al. (2014). Dynamic microglial alterations underlie stress-induced depressive-like behavior and suppressed neurogenesis. *Mol. Psychiatry* 19, 699–709. doi: 10.1038/mp.2013.155

Kujawa, S. G., and Liberman, M. C. (2006). Acceleration of age-related hearing loss by early noise exposure: evidence of a misspent youth. *J. Neurosci.* 26, 2115–2123. doi: 10.1523/JNEUROSCI.4985-05.2006

Lagace, D. C., Donovan, M. H., DeCarolis, N. A., Farnbauch, L. A., Malhotra, S., Berton, O., et al. (2010). Adult hippocampal neurogenesis is functionally important for stress-induced social avoidance. *Proc. Natl. Acad. Sci. U. S. A.* 107, 4436–4441. doi: 10.1073/pnas.0910072107

Lazarov, O., and Hollands, C. (2016). Hippocampal neurogenesis: learning to remember. *Prog. Neurobiol.* 138–140, 1–18. doi: 10.1016/j.pneurobio.2015.12.006

Le, T. N., Straatman, L. V., Lea, J., and Westerberg, B. (2017). Current insights in noise-induced hearing loss: a literature review of the underlying mechanism, pathophysiology, asymmetry, and management options. *J. Otolaryngol. Head Neck Surg.* 46:41. doi: 10.1186/s40463-017-0219-x

Li, Q., and Barres, B. A. (2018). Microglia and macrophages in brain homeostasis and disease. *Nat. Rev. Immunol.* 18, 225–242. doi: 10.1038/nri.2017.125

Lin, F. R., Metter, E. J., O'Brien, R. J., Resnick, S. M., Zonderman, A. B., and Ferrucci, L. (2011). Hearing loss and incident dementia. *Arch. Neurol.* 68, 214–220. doi: 10.1001/archneurol.2010.362

Liu, L., Shen, P., He, T., Chang, Y., Shi, L., Tao, S., et al. (2016a). Noise induced hearing loss impairs spatial learning/memory and hippocampal neurogenesis in mice. *Sci. Rep.* 6:20374. doi: 10.1038/srep20374

Liu, L., Wang, F., Lu, H., Cao, S., Du, Z., Wang, Y., et al. (2016b). Effects of Noise Exposure on Systemic and Tissue-Level Markers of Glucose Homeostasis and Insulin Resistance in Male Mice. *Environ. Health Perspect.* 124, 1390–1398. doi: 10.1289/EHP162

Liu, L., Xuan, C., Shen, P., He, T., Chang, Y., Shi, L., et al. (2018). Hippocampal Mechanisms Underlying Impairment in Spatial Learning Long After Establishment of Noise-Induced Hearing Loss in CBA Mice. *Front. Syst. Neurosci.* 12:35. doi: 10.3389/fnsys.2018.00035

Livingston, G., Huntley, J., Sommerlad, A., Ames, D., Ballard, C., Banerjee, S., et al. (2020). Dementia prevention, intervention, and care: 2020 report of the Lancet Commission. *Lancet* 396, 413–446. doi: 10.1016/s0140-6736(20)30367-6

Livingston, G., Sommerlad, A., Orgeta, V., Costafreda, S. G., Huntley, J., Ames, D., et al. (2017). Dementia prevention, intervention, and care. *Lancet* 390, 2673–2734. doi: 10.1016/S0140-6736(17)31363-6

Loughrey, D. G., Kelly, M. E., Kelley, G. A., Brennan, S., and Lawlor, B. A. (2018). Association of Age-Related Hearing Loss With Cognitive Function, Cognitive Impairment, and Dementia: a Systematic Review and Meta-analysis. *JAMA Otolaryngol. Head Neck Surg.* 144, 115–126. doi: 10.1001/jamaoto.2017.2513

McEwen, B. S. (1999). Stress and hippocampal plasticity. *Annu. Rev. Neurosci.* 22, 105–122. doi: 10.1146/annurev.neuro.22.1.105

Meinke, D. K., Finan, D. S., Flamme, G. A., Murphy, W. J., Stewart, M., Lankford, J. E., et al. (2017). Prevention of Noise-Induced Hearing Loss from Recreational Firearms. *Semin. Hear.* 38, 267–281. doi: 10.1055/s-0037-1606323

Mosser, C. A., Baptista, S., Arnoux, I., and Audinat, E. (2017). Microglia in CNS development: shaping the brain for the future. *Prog. Neurobiol.* 149–150, 1–20. doi: 10.1016/j.pneurobio.2017.01.002

Moxon, K. A., Gerhardt, G. A., Bickford, P. C., Austin, K., Rose, G. M., Woodward, D. J., et al. (1999). Multiple single units and population responses during inhibitory gating of hippocampal auditory response in freely-moving rats. *Brain Res.* 825, 75–85. doi: 10.1016/s0006-8993(99)01187-7

Mu, Y., and Gage, F. H. (2011). Adult hippocampal neurogenesis and its role in Alzheimer's disease. *Mol. Neurodegener.* 6:85. doi: 10.1186/1750-1326-6-85

Nelson, D. I., Nelson, R. Y., Concha-Barrientos, M., and Fingerhut, M. (2005). The global burden of occupational noise-induced hearing loss. *Am. J. Ind. Med.* 48, 446–458. doi: 10.1002/ajim.20223

Nimmerjahn, A., Kirchhoff, F., and Helmchen, F. (2005). Resting microglial cells are highly dynamic surveillants of brain parenchyma in vivo. *Science* 308, 1314–1318. doi: 10.1126/science.1110647

Nixon, G. K., Sarant, J. Z., and Tomlin, D. (2019). Peripheral and central hearing impairment and their relationship with cognition: a review. *Int. J. Audiol.* 58, 541–552. doi: 10.1080/14992027.2019.1591644

No authors listed (1990). Noise and hearing loss. National Institutes of Health Consensus Development Conference. *Conn. Med.* 54, 385–391.

Olah, M., Biber, K., Vinet, J., and Boddeke, H. W. (2011). Microglia phenotype diversity. *CNS Neurol. Disord. Drug Targets* 10, 108–118. doi: 10.2174/187152711794488575

Orgeta, V., Mukadam, N., Sommerlad, A., and Livingston, G. (2019). The Lancet Commission on Dementia Prevention, Intervention, and Care: a call for action. *Ir. J. Psychol. Med.* 36, 85–88. doi: 10.1017/ipm.2018.4

Rabinowitz, P. M. (2000). Noise-induced hearing loss. *Am. Fam. Physician* 61, 2759–2760.

Rodriguez-Iglesias, N., Sierra, A., and Valero, J. (2019). Rewiring of Memory Circuits: connecting Adult Newborn Neurons With the Help of Microglia. *Front. Cell Dev. Biol.* 7:24. doi: 10.3389/fcell.2019.00024

Ronzano, R., Roux, T., Thetiot, M., Aigrot, M. S., Richard, L., Lejeune, F. X., et al. (2021). Microglia-neuron interaction at nodes of Ranvier depends on neuronal activity through potassium release and contributes to remyelination. *Nat. Commun.* 12:5219. doi: 10.1038/s41467-021-25486-7

Ryan, A. F., Kujawa, S. G., Hammill, T., Le Prell, C., and Kil, J. (2016). Temporary and Permanent Noise-induced Threshold Shifts: a Review of Basic and Clinical Observations. *Otol. Neurotol.* 37, e271–e275. doi: 10.1097/MAO.0000000000001071

Sahay, A., Scobie, K. N., Hill, A. S., O'Carroll, C. M., Kheirbek, M. A., Burghardt, N. S., et al. (2011). Increasing adult hippocampal neurogenesis is sufficient to improve pattern separation. *Nature* 472, 466–470. doi: 10.1038/nature09817

Sale, A., Berardi, N., and Maffei, L. (2014). Environment and brain plasticity: towards an endogenous pharmacotherapy. *Physiol. Rev.* 94, 189–234. doi: 10.1152/physrev.00036.2012

Salter, M. W., and Stevens, B. (2017). Microglia emerge as central players in brain disease. *Nat. Med.* 23, 1018–1027. doi: 10.1038/nm.4397

Samson, J., Sheeladevi, R., Ravindran, R., and Senthilvelan, M. (2007). Stress response in rat brain after different durations of noise exposure. *Neurosci. Res.* 57, 143–147. doi: 10.1016/j.neures.2006.09.019

Sanguino-Gomez, J., Buurstede, J. C., Abiega, O., Fitzsimons, C. P., Lucassen, P. J., Eggen, B. J. L., et al. (2021). An emerging role for microglia in stress-effects on memory. *Eur. J. Neurosci.* doi: 10.1111/ejn.15188 [Epub Online ahead of print].

Sarlus, H., and Heneka, M. T. (2017). Microglia in Alzheimer's disease. *J. Clin. Invest.* 127, 3240–3249. doi: 10.1172/jci90606

Sato, K. (2015). Effects of Microglia on Neurogenesis. *Glia* 63, 1394–1405. doi: 10.1002/glia.22858

Sierra, A., Encinas, J. M., Deudero, J. J., Chancey, J. H., Enikolopov, G., Overstreet-Wadiche, L. S., et al. (2010). Microglia shape adult hippocampal neurogenesis through apoptosis-coupled phagocytosis. *Cell Stem Cell* 7, 483–495. doi: 10.1016/j.stem.2010.08.014

Spongr, V. P., Flood, D. G., Frisina, R. D., and Salvi, R. J. (1997). Quantitative measures of hair cell loss in CBA and C57BL/6 mice throughout their life spans. *J. Acoust. Soc. Am.* 101, 3546–3553. doi: 10.1121/1.418315

Stansfeld, S. A., and Matheson, M. P. (2003). Noise pollution: non-auditory effects on health. *Br. Med. Bull.* 68, 243–257. doi: 10.1093/bmb/ldg033

Subramaniam, S. R., and Federoff, H. J. (2017). Targeting Microglial Activation States as a Therapeutic Avenue in Parkinson's Disease. *Front. Aging Neurosci.* 9:176. doi: 10.3389/fnagi.2017.00176

Surget, A., and Belzung, C. (2021). Adult hippocampal neurogenesis shapes adaptation and improves stress response: a mechanistic and integrative perspective. *Mol. Psychiatry* doi: 10.1038/s41380-021-01136-8 [Epub Online ahead of print].

Suss, P., and Schlachetzki, J. C. M. (2020). Microglia in Alzheimer's Disease. *Curr. Alzheimer Res.* 17, 29–43. doi: 10.2174/1567205017666200212155234

Syka, J. (2002). Plastic changes in the central auditory system after hearing loss, restoration of function, and during learning. *Physiol. Rev.* 82, 601–636. doi: 10.1152/physrev.00002.2002

Tanapat, P., Galea, L. A., and Gould, E. (1998). Stress inhibits the proliferation of granule cell precursors in the developing dentate gyrus. *Int. J. Dev. Neurosci.* 16, 235–239. doi: 10.1016/s0736-5748(98)00029-x

Tao, S., Liu, L., Shi, L., Li, X., Shen, P., Xun, Q., et al. (2015). Spatial learning and memory deficits in young adult mice exposed to a brief intense noise at postnatal age. *J. Otol.* 10, 21–28. doi: 10.1016/j.joto.2015.07.001

Tejera, D., and Heneka, M. T. (2016). Microglia in Alzheimer's Disease: the Good, the Bad and the Ugly. *Curr. Alzheimer Res.* 13, 370–380. doi: 10.2174/1567205013666151116125012

Thomas, R. M., Hotsenpiller, G., and Peterson, D. A. (2007). Acute psychosocial stress reduces cell survival in adult hippocampal neurogenesis without altering proliferation. *J. Neurosci.* 27, 2734–2743. doi: 10.1523/JNEUROSCI.3849-06.2007

Thomson, R. S., Auduong, P., Miller, A. T., and Gurgel, R. K. (2017). Hearing loss as a risk factor for dementia: a systematic review. *Laryngoscope Investig. Otolaryngol.* 2, 69–79. doi: 10.1002/lio2.65

Tobin, M. K., Musaraca, K., Disouky, A., Shetti, A., Bheri, A., Honer, W. G., et al. (2019). Human Hippocampal Neurogenesis Persists in Aged Adults and Alzheimer's Disease Patients. *Cell Stem Cell* 24, 974–982.e3. doi: 10.1016/j.stem.2019.05.003

Tremblay, M. E., Lowery, R. L., and Majewska, A. K. (2010). Microglial interactions with synapses are modulated by visual experience. *PLoS Biol.* 8:e1000527. doi: 10.1371/journal.pbio.1000527

Uchida, Y., Sugiura, S., Nishita, Y., Saji, N., Sone, M., and Ueda, H. (2019). Age-related hearing loss and cognitive decline - The potential mechanisms linking the two. *Auris Nasus Larynx* 46, 1–9. doi: 10.1016/j.anl.2018.08.010

Umpierre, A. D., and Wu, L. J. (2021). How microglia sense and regulate neuronal activity. *Glia* 69, 1637–1653. doi: 10.1002/glia.23961

Uran, S. L., Caceres, L. G., and Guelman, L. R. (2010). Effects of loud noise on hippocampal and cerebellar-related behaviors. Role of oxidative state. *Brain Res.* 1361, 102–114. doi: 10.1016/j.brainres.2010.09.022

Valero, J., Paris, I., and Sierra, A. (2016). Lifestyle Shapes the Dialogue between Environment, Microglia, and Adult Neurogenesis. *ACS Chem. Neurosci.* 7, 442–453. doi: 10.1021/acschemneuro.6b00009

Vitkovic, L., Konsman, J. P., Bockaert, J., Dantzer, R., Homburger, V., and Jacque, C. (2000). Cytokine signals propagate through the brain. *Mol. Psychiatry* 5, 604–615. doi: 10.1038/sj.mp.4000813

Voet, S., Prinz, M., and van Loo, G. (2019). Microglia in Central Nervous System Inflammation and Multiple Sclerosis Pathology. *Trends Mol. Med.* 25, 112–123. doi: 10.1016/j.molmed.2018.11.005

Wake, H., Moorhouse, A. J., Miyamoto, A., and Nabekura, J. (2013). Microglia: actively surveying and shaping neuronal circuit structure and function. *Trends Neurosci.* 36, 209–217. doi: 10.1016/j.tins.2012.11.007

Xue, J., Guo, H., Gao, Y., Wang, X., Cui, H., Chen, Z., et al. (2019). Altered Directed Functional Connectivity of the Hippocampus in Mild Cognitive Impairment and Alzheimer's Disease: a Resting-State fMRI Study. *Front. Aging Neurosci.* 11:326. doi: 10.3389/fnagi.2019.00326

Young, K., and Morrison, H. (2018). Quantifying Microglia Morphology from Photomicrographs of Immunohistochemistry Prepared Tissue Using ImageJ. *J. Vis. Exp.* 136:57648. doi: 10.3791/57648

Zhao, C., Deng, W., and Gage, F. H. (2008). Mechanisms and functional implications of adult neurogenesis. *Cell* 132, 645–660. doi: 10.1016/j.cell.2008.01.033

Zhuang, H., Yang, J., Huang, Z., Liu, H., Li, X., Zhang, H., et al. (2020). Accelerated age-related decline in hippocampal neurogenesis in mice with noise-induced hearing loss is associated with hippocampal microglial degeneration. *Aging* 12, 19493–19519. doi: 10.18632/aging.103898

18

Correspondence Between Cognitive and Audiological Evaluations Among the Elderly: A Preliminary Report of an Audiological Screening Model of Subjects at Risk of Cognitive Decline with Slight to Moderate Hearing Loss

Alessandro Castiglione[1,2], Mariella Casa[3], Samanta Gallo[2], Flavia Sorrentino[2], Sonila Dhima[2], Dalila Cilia[1], Elisa Lovo[1], Marta Gambin[1], Maela Previato[1], Simone Colombo[1], Ezio Caserta[2], Flavia Gheller[1], Cristina Giacomelli[1], Silvia Montino[1], Federica Limongi[4], Davide Brotto[2], Carlo Gabelli[3], Patrizia Trevisi[1,2], Roberto Bovo[1,2] and Alessandro Martini[1,2]*

[1] Department of Neurosciences, University of Padua, Padua, Italy, [2] Complex Operative Unit of Otolaryngology, Hospital of Padua, Padua, Italy, [3] Regional Center for the Study and Treatment of the Aging Brain, Department of Internal Medicine, Padua, Italy, [4] Institute of Neuroscience, National Research Council, Padua, Italy

***Correspondence:**
Alessandro Castiglione
alessandro.castiglione@unipd.it

Epidemiological studies show increasing prevalence rates of cognitive decline and hearing loss with age, particularly after the age of 65 years. These conditions are reported to be associated, although conclusive evidence of causality and implications is lacking. Nevertheless, audiological and cognitive assessment among elderly people is a key target for comprehensive and multidisciplinary evaluation of the subject's frailty status. To evaluate the use of tools for identifying older adults at risk of hearing loss and cognitive decline and to compare skills and abilities in terms of hearing and cognitive performances between older adults and young subjects, we performed a prospective cross-sectional study using supraliminal auditory tests. The relationship between cognitive assessment results and audiometric results was investigated, and reference ranges for different ages or stages of disease were determined. Patients older than 65 years with different degrees of hearing function were enrolled. Each subject underwent an extensive audiological assessment, including tonal and speech audiometry, Italian Matrix Sentence Test, and speech audiometry with logatomes in quiet. Cognitive function was screened and then verified by experienced clinicians using the Montreal Cognitive Assessment Score, the Geriatric Depression Scale, and further investigations in some. One hundred twenty-three subjects were finally enrolled during 2016–2019: 103 were >65 years of age and 20 were younger participants (as controls). Cognitive functions showed a correlation with the audiological results in post-lingual hearing-impaired patients, in particular in those affected by slight to moderate hearing loss and aged more than 70 years. Audiological testing can thus be useful in clinical assessment and identification of patients at risk of cognitive impairment. The study was limited by its sample size (CI 95%; CL 10%), strict dependence on language, and hearing threshold. Further investigations should be conducted to confirm the reported results and to verify similar screening models.

Keywords: cognitive decline, hearing loss, Italian Matrix Sentence Test, logatomes, signal-to-noise ratio, slope, speech in noise, screening

INTRODUCTION

Aging is epidemiologically associated with increasing prevalence rates of hearing loss and cognitive decline (Lin et al., 2011a,b; Peracino and Pecorelli, 2016). This association has been widely reported in the literature since a study by Herbst and Humphrey (1980). Even if the rational implications are debated in the literature and a causal relationship remains far from being proven, the audiological and cognitive assessment among elderly still remains a key component of a comprehensive and multidisciplinary approach to determining potential frailty (Panza et al., 2015).

Interest in this topic (Thomson et al., 2017) has grown in the last decade mainly due to demographic and sociocultural changes (Homans et al., 2017; Limongi et al., 2017: Livingston et al., 2017; Rooth, 2017); difficulties in treating neurodegenerative disorders, which has led to increased research into modifiable risk factors (Kostoff et al., 2017; Vos et al., 2017); the potential effects of peripheral hearing loss (Lin et al., 2011b; Lin et al., 2013; Wayne and Johnsrude, 2015; Deal et al., 2017); and rehabilitative as well as economical roles of digital devices (such as hearing aids, cochlear implants, over-the-counter amplification products) (Jorgensen and Messersmith, 2015; Cosetti et al., 2016; Nguyen et al., 2017). Additionally, the growing use of new tests and technologies has globally promoted reassessment of cognitive functions (Shen et al., 2016). The clinical distinction between central and peripheral hearing loss facilitates estimation of different contribution rates (Parham and Kost, 2017), even if, in practice, it is very difficult to quantify the relative portions, especially among older adults. In fact, there are different types of hearing impairment, as well as different types of cognitive decline, and these can be differently correlated or respond differently to treatments.

Defining the specific role of audiology in this context is important, and it is necessary to assess, design tests, and determine range limits in aging populations. To this end, the signal-to-noise ratio (SNR) can be used to define different auditory conditions and it is a good candidate for evaluating the contribution of auditory status to high cognitive functions (Panza et al., 2015; Costa et al., 2016; Livingston et al., 2017; Parham and Kost, 2017; Thomson et al., 2017; Jayakody et al., 2018). The Italian Matrix Sentence Test allows adaptive examination and results in noise (Puglisi et al., 2015). In addition, in selected cases, use of logatomes can elucidate auditory functioning in attention and working memory (Muhler et al., 2009; Moradi et al., 2014; Schubotz et al., 2016).

Thus, we performed a prospective study with cross-sectional measurements to evaluate the use of those tools for identifying older adults affected by hearing impairment and at risk of cognitive decline. In addition, the study aims to contribute in establishing age-appropriate reference intervals of specific tools in different hearing and cognitive impairments.

MATERIALS AND METHODS

One hundred sixty-six subjects were screened for inclusion criteria in this study between 2016 and 2019: adults older than 65 years and native Italian speakers with or without hearing loss or cognitive decline were enrolled as cases. The control group consisted of 20 young students (10 females) (median age 21, range 18–42 years) with normal hearing. Younger adults were also included to normalize reference ranges for different ages and to estimate the statistical power, also by comparing with literature on the same topic.

Exclusion criteria were lack of cooperation, life-threatening diseases, psychotropic therapies, history of disabling cardiovascular diseases, ictus or other potential life-threatening conditions, myocardial infarction, transient ischemic attacks or stroke, familiarity of neurodegenerative processes, or in advanced stages of disease. Patients with a history or family history of neurodegenerative diseases were excluded to avoid the contribution of early-onset diseases, which typically have a genetic etiology (Giau et al., 2019). Additionally, adults with hearing aids or cochlear implants were also excluded to avoid interference of digital devices with the acoustic properties of the auditory stimuli, which could significantly modify the SNR (Gallo and Castiglione, 2019). Patients with hearing impairment of genetic origin and those with severe to profound hearing losses were also excluded. These exclusion criteria were comparable to those of previous reports of investigations of mild cognitive impairment (MCI) among the Italian population to yield homogeneous and comparable data for cutoff settings (Bovo et al., 2007; Conti et al., 2015; Santangelo et al., 2015).

Audiological Assessment

An audiological evaluation was carried out by clinicians and technicians with proven experience in the management of hearing loss. Testing included otoscopy, tonal and speech audiometry in quiet, using disyllabic words, the Italian Matrix Sentence Test (OLSA test), with an adaptive SNR (in dB) at which subjects can recognize 50% of the speech material in noise of 65 dB sound pressure level (SPL) in an open set with a frontal speaker (0 degrees) at 1 m distance and the slope in dB/% for speech discrimination in noise. The audiometric tests were randomly administered in a soundproof booth using the

Noah and Otosuite software with standardized Italian language acoustic materials provided by Otometrics (a division of Natus in Taasrup, Denmark) and HörTech (Oldenburg, Germany).

The following data were obtained in a quiet environment: (1) The pure tone average (PTA) value at 0.5, 1, 2, and 4 kHz, in dB HL (PTA dB HL); (2) the signal/speech recognition threshold (SRT), in dB SPL, at which subjects could identify 50% of disyllabic words; (3) speech audiometry with logatomes. The latter were phonetic units without meaning, which can have the following consonant–vowel construction: CVC, VCVC, CVCV. In the Italian language, these structures can be assimilated to form pseudo-words or words non-words and, in general, presented in the following form: VCV or VCVV. Each list used in the present study consisted of 10 randomly selected logatomes. The choice to use this type of speech audiometry aims to minimize the mnemonic effort of the subjects: the speech intelligibility tends to differ between logatomes and words because they are not supported by semantic and long-term memory (Pisoni, 1996; Chan and Alain, 2018). The average of the intrasubject differences has been estimated between 5 and 20% (in favor of words) of recognized signals, even in the best hearing conditions. To identify different groups and carry out statistical analysis, the difference (hereinafter Log. Diff.) between the maximum intelligibility score, in%, for familiar words and the maximum intelligibility score, in%, for logatomes (i.d. maximum speech score with words – maximum speech score with logatomes) was calculated, and the cutoff was arbitrarily set to 10%, as suggested by a previous report (Moradi et al., 2014) to identify subjects potentially out of reference ranges. This allowed correlation among the Log. Diff. and attention or working memory, particularly if this was difficult among older adults (Santangelo et al., 2015). As mentioned before, the difference in percentage of identification of logatomes and words can be set within 10%, at the maximum comfortable level of acoustic signal in dB SPL for normal-hearing adults without cognitive decline. Thus, the maximum speech discrimination score for disyllabic words in a quiet environment is very close to that for logatomes in quiet, independent of differences in intensity levels. Therefore, the difference in a quiet environment should be less than 10%, even at different dB levels (Moradi et al., 2014).

The OLSA test (HörTech) is a versatile examination that is essentially structured into 20 randomized lists of five-word sentences (Houben et al., 2014), semantically unpredictable and administered after a training session to minimize the learning curve. The test can be useful in evaluating a wide range of conditions and treatments: congenital hearing loss, presbycusis, neuropathies, and auditory rehabilitation with hearing aids or cochlear implants. The test yields three main measurements: (1) the SNR, in dB, at which the subject recognizes 50% of the presented words, even if in different sentences (SNR-SRT); (2) the slope of the discrimination function at SRT (Slope) in percentage (%/dB); and (3) the intelligibility percentage score, in terms of estimated accuracy in understanding whole sentences. The global test in itself is an automated version of the synthetic sentence test, termed the synthetic sentences identification test (SSI) (King-Smith and Rose, 1997; Kaernbach, 2001; Buss et al., 2009; MacPherson and Akeroyd, 2014; Kollmeier, 2015). The novelty and the strength of the test are the speech noise material, with features inspired by ICRA noise, and its simplicity in performing adaptive exams (Dreschler et al., 2001; Wagener et al., 2006; Meister et al., 2013; Akeroyd et al., 2015). Reviewing reference ranges and standard deviations for the Italian language of the OLSA test, published by Puglisi et al. (2015), allowed determination of different levels to identify at-risk patients. The cutoff of the SNR dB (SRT) among the elderly was set to - 0.4 dB based on a reference mean level of −6.7 plus 9 standard deviations (3 SDs include 100% of samples divided by age). Thus, older adults are 6–12 SDs away from normal hearing and hearing in a younger population; the slope cutoff was set to 9.4% (reference level of 13.3% minus 3 SDs) (Puglisi et al., 2015). Audiological tests were conducted blinded to the cognitive status.

Cognitive Assessment

Subjects participated in a screening phase. Cognitive function was screened using the Montreal Cognitive Assessment (MoCA, adjusted for education) score: the presence of mild cognitive dysfunction was suspected when the final score was less than 26. Further clinical investigations were carried out by specialists in the management of dementia and cognitive decline (neuropsychologists and geriatricians). In addition, previous clinical data, including neuroimaging, and history available on digital archives were reviewed by medical doctors for definitive assessment. The evaluation was extended in selected cases to confirm screening results, and it included the forward and backward digit span test, drawing tests (clock, cube, house, pentagons), the trail-making test, the digit symbol substitution test, and the Direct Assessment of Functional Status (DAFS) for measuring Alzheimer's disease severity (Zanetti et al., 1998). The DAFS also helped in defining preservations of daily activities. The Geriatric Depression Scale (GDS) (30 items, long form) was used to screen depressive symptoms.

Mild cognitive decline was confirmed when daily activities were preserved, and cognitive decline was defined when these were compromised based on the diagnostic criteria reported in the literature and the DSM-V. Nevertheless, prior to further investigations and final diagnosis, patients were considered as only being at risk of, or likely to have MCI, because the screening model should be not considered diagnostic.

Participants with good cognitive performance and some degree of hearing loss (if any) in few frequencies, but without disabling hearing impairment, were defined healthy: this group was named the "healthy aging."

The cutoff MoCA score for risk of cognitive impairment has been varied (26, 24, 22) to verify differences in specificity and sensitivity (Davis et al., 2015). In addition, for further analysis, the scores for attention and working memory were set to 4.8 (<5) in the digit span test and MoCA (Moradi et al., 2014; Santangelo et al., 2015), whereas the long-term memory score was set to 2.80 (<3). These scores are the approximate normal/average reference values, reduced by 2 SDs (Moradi et al., 2014; Conti et al., 2015; Davis et al., 2015; Santangelo et al., 2015; Castiglione et al., 2016; Kujawski et al., 2018; Siciliano et al., 2019). Subjects with clinical indications were selected for hearing aid prescription, cochlear implantation surgery, or further cognitive investigations.

Statistical Analysis

Statistical analysis was performed through Microsoft Office Excel 2016 (Redmond, WA, United States) with data analysis plug-ins and MedCalc (Ostend, Belgium). The following tests were used: Student's *t*-test, Mann–Whitney test for independent samples (unpaired), Fisher's exact test and relative risk in 2 × 2 tables, analysis of variance (ANOVA), coefficient of Pearson correlation, and multiple regression analysis. Results were considered significant when $p < 0.01$.

Ethical Issues

This study was carried out in accordance with the recommendations of national and international guidelines. All subjects gave written informed consent in accordance with the Declaration of Helsinki. The protocol was approved by the local ethical committee of the University Hospital of Padua. The research was funded by the University of Padua, the Azienda Ospedaliera di Padova, Cochlear Italia Srl, and Amplifon SpA, as part of the main project PRIHTA-IDECO 2013, approved by the local ethics committee in 2016 (n° AO0379-0059267-CE3361/AO/14).

RESULTS

One hundred sixty-six subjects were included in this study between 2016 and 2019, at the clinic of Otorhinolaryngology of the University Hospital of Padua, as part of the PRIHTA-IDECO 2013 project. Forty-three subjects were excluded because of the degree of hearing loss: severe to profound hearing-impaired patients had a speech recognition score below 50%. The other 123 subjects were then divided into two groups: the cases included 103 subjects (51 females) older than 65 years (median age 71, range 65–93 years). The control group consisted of 20 young students with normal hearing (10 females, median age 21, range 18–42 years). Hearing loss among the cases was classified according to the criteria of the World Health Organization. Among the cases were identified 17 (16.50%) subjects with normal hearing, 21 (20.40%) with slight loss of hearing, and 65 (63.10%) with mild to moderate hearing loss, of which four were with characteristics very close to severe losses. There is also a correlation between hearing loss and age and cognitive decline, so that subjects with better hearing and better cognitive performance are grouped in the age group between 65 and 70 years.

A summary of the characteristics of the cases and controls is given in **Table 1**. Distributions by PTA dB HL, age, and MoCA scores are reported in **Table 2**. No differences were found between the left and the right ear, even if the right ear showed slight advantages in discrimination probably due to interhemispheric dominance ($p > 0.05$). The control group allowed normal range adjustment for testing among the elderly and confirmed the feasibility of the test in different audiological and cognitive conditions.

As expected, significant differences were found between cases and controls in all variables, except for sex. Significant differences were also shown between patients with signs of MCI and those with normal cognitive function in terms of PTA, speech in noise, and the slope of psychometric functions. However, in the present study, GDS results are not significant. Among cases, two subgroups were defined: the healthy aging subgroup with a MoCA score > 26, adjusted for education, without signs of decline in cognitive tests or neuroradiological findings, and the MCI subgroup, identified as individuals at risk of MCI through the MoCA test (**Table 3**), and defined by cognitive scores < 26 adjusted for education (Conti et al., 2015). To give comparable results, *t*-tests and Mann–Whitney tests are reported, as many variables can be considered non-parametric, even when values appear parametric; nevertheless, there were no differences between the groups for either test at $\alpha = 0.01$ (**Table 3**).

Comparison of the three groups revealed significant differences, with increasing *p*-value from CONTROLS to MCI patients. ANOVA revealed significant differences among these two groups ($p < 0.001$), and the results are reported in **Figure 1**.

The study of correlation revealed a moderate to strong coefficient between SNR and MoCA scores. Other correlations and multiple regression analysis are shown in **Table 4**. Age showed the highest negative correlation with cognitive results, but it should be noticed that groups were arbitrarily divided by age and that the MoCA scores were adjusted for years of education. Thus, in higher age groups, the MoCA score could be adjusted for age because after 78 years, participants were unlikely to have been attending educational and recreative programs during childhood, as compared to the new 65-year-old subjects of coming decades (Kujawski et al., 2018). Nevertheless, it should be noticed that the SNR showed the highest negative correlation among the audiological testing results and that the multiple regression analysis reached an R^2 of 0.477. These results suggested a strong correlation with cognitive impairment particularly when the variables were considered together. It could be hypothesized that the cognitive results and the audiological tests, when considered together, can explain approximately 50% of the final score (and its variance) obtained for each subject.

In **Tables 5**, **6**, we show the different sensitivity and specificity values for identifying different levels of cognitive impairment. The associated receiver operating characteristic (ROC) curves are illustrated in **Supplementary Figure S1**. The ROC curves show the predictive results of the screening model at various cutoff values. Different ROC curves are shown to compare sensitivity and specificity of different variables for identifying patients with cognitive decline, as represented by a MoCA score < 26 and subsequent confirmed diagnosis of MCI. The SNR reaches highest rates of sensitivity and specificity (**Supplementary Figure S1**). This curve allows intuitive prediction of the sensitivity and specificity of a test for any value obtainable from the test; various tests are also compared to assess which one has the best chance of identifying true positives and true negatives. The audiological evaluation is comparable to those attributed to the MoCA test. Age had suitable characteristics but a lower specificity. These data can only be considered preliminary as a possible screening model that can promote a multidisciplinary approach because the patient often does not know the origin of his own difficulty and may therefore seek help from various specialists. Given that this

TABLE 1 | Major clinical findings in the control group (young adults with normal hearing) and older adults (>65 years, with normal to moderate hearing impairment).

			Controls: 20 (10 F)			P value	Cases: 103 (51 F)		
			Mean	Median	SD	t-test	Mean	Median	SD
		Age (years)	23.20	21	6.22	*<0.001*	72.62	71	7.03
Hearing		PTA dB HL	8.87	10	4.33	***<0.001***	32.77	33.75	15.26
		SRT	13.50	15	5.20	***<0.001***	36.41	35	15.49
		SNR	−6.88	−6.75	0.96	***<0.001***	1.42	−0.3	6.71
		Slope in Noise	15.03	16	4.53	***<0.001***	10.76	10	4.18
		Intelligibility in noise (% of S.I.)	55.48	56	2.9	***<0.001***	50.13	52	7.73
		Logatomes (difference in%)	3.00	2.5	3.35	***<0.001***	11.31	10	12.43
Cognition	MoCA	Tot. MoCA (score)	29.70	30	0.66	***<0.001***	25.15	26	3.89
		Attention and Working Memory	5.80	6	0.41	***<0.001***	4.83	5.00	1.56
		Long-term memory	4.35	4.00	0.67	***<0.001***	2.61	3.00	1.80

F, females; MoCA, Montreal Cognitive Assessment; S.I., Intelligibility (%) of sentences and words in noise around the SNR value; SNR, signal-to-noise ratio; SRT, speech/signal recognition threshold; SD, standard deviation. Bolded values indicate significant results.

TABLE 2 | Age distribution of hearing and cognitive results.

Age (years)	*18–45 (age in years)*	*65–69 (age in years)*	*70–79 (age in years)*	*>79 (age in years)*
n°(of cases)	**20**	**39**	**44**	**20**
MoCA (score)	29.7	27.41	25.15	20.75
Slope (%)	17.3	12.8	10.65	6.95
SNR (dB)	−7	−1.5	1.75	7.89
Intelligibility in Noise (%)	57.9	53	51.25	41.65
PTA (0.5-1-2-4-kHz)	8.62	26.82	33.15	43.5
SRT (%)	9	30.9	36.02	48
Log. Diff. (%)	3	5.5	11.53	22.12
GDS (score)	n.a.	5.48	5.09	5.05
Long Term Memory (score)	4.5	3.8	2.6	2
Attention (score)	5.8	5.8	5.2	3.5
Log Intelligibility (%)	97	77.14	80.6	57.5
MCI (n° of Cases)	0	6	21	17

MoCA, Montreal Cognitive Assessment score (mean); Slope, percentage (mean); SNR, signal-to-noise ratio in dB (mean); S.I., sentence intelligibility in noise, percentage of correct sentences and words (mean); PTA, pure tone average at 500, 1,000, 2,000, and 4,000 Hz (mean in dB HL); SRT, speech/signal recognition threshold, mean in dB SPL of thresholds required to recognize 50% of words in quiet; Log. Diff., difference in% between words intelligibility and logatomes intelligibility (mean); GDS, Geriatric Depression Scale (long form); Memory (long-term), mean of cognitive tests; attention, mean of cognitive tests; MCI, mild cognitive impairment (number of diagnosis for each group); n.a., not applicable. Bolded values indicate significant results.

is proposed as a screening model, high sensitivity is crucial, but subsequent diagnostic confirmation is required.

As mentioned before, the cases were subsequently divided into two subgroups to compare auditory and cognitive functions. In 59 cases, participants were healthy, with good cognitive performance and some degree of hearing loss (if any), but without disabling hearing impairment; this group was named the healthy aging. In contrast, 44 participants were classified as at risk of MCI, showing signs of cognitive impairment. Further cognitive test results and neuroimaging (when possible or indicated) were used to confirm the MoCA results indicative of MCI. Eight of these 44 patients (18.18%) were affected by early-stage vascular cognitive impairment with suggestive neuroradiological findings, 22 (38%) showed memory impairment in multiple domains on cognitive tests, and 14 (38%) were initially classified as having an uncertain or borderline diagnosis (**Table 3**) because of inconclusive diagnostic results or incongruent findings. Eight of the 44 patients (18.18%) were subsequently correctly reevaluated, and MCI in multiple non-amnestic domains was confirmed (**Supplementary Table S1**). The remaining four patients were designated as patients with MCI affecting multiple amnestic domains. Thus, 63.64% (28 of 44) of the screened populations were defined as having amnestic multiple domain MCI, agreeing with reports in the literature. Among the healthy aging group, 9 (of 59) subjects were reevaluated because of inconclusive results probably related to transient anxiety or low attention in performing the test or because they were too fatigued to complete the investigations. Therefore, finally, 23 (of 103) patients required reinterpretation and reanalysis of results.

The relative risk and two-tailed Fisher's exact test for different clinical settings and cutoff values are presented in 2 × 2 tables in **Supplementary Material (Supplementary Table S1)**.

DISCUSSION

In this preliminary study, we found a significant correlation between cognitive scores and SNR, slope, and logatome intelligibility. Even if the MoCA tests should be considered purely indicative and not diagnostic, the results were verified by clinicians experienced in the management of neurodegenerative processes affecting high cognitive functions. To verify the feasibility of a screening model involving audiological tests, the MoCA score was chosen as representative of real-life cognition. Audiological tests were conducted blinded to the cognitive status, and the results were found to correlate statistically significantly. Using these quantitative and semiquantitative parameters, auditory functioning could be assessed, and the risk

TABLE 3 | Comparisons between the healthy aging group and subjects with or at risk of mild cognitive impairment (MCI).

			103 Cases (51 F)						
			At risk of MCI						
			59 Cases (37 F)				44 Cases (14 F)		
			Healthy aging				MCI* (screened by MoCA)		
			Mean	**Median**	**SD**	**p-value**	**Mean**	**Median**	**SD**
		Age	69.34	68	5.61	***<0.001***	76.95	78	6.44
Hearing		PTA dB HL	27.53	23.75	18.41	***<0.001***	49.52	41.25	19.61
		SRT	25.23	25	10.89	***<0.001***	47.30	45	17.75
		SNR dB (SRT)	−0.83	−3.0	6.07	***<0.001***	4.56	2.9	6.49
		Slope in Noise	12.43	12	3.84	***<0.001***	8.67	8	3.98
		Intelligibility in noise	52.65	54	6.26	***<0.001***	46.51	48.5	8.81
		Logatomes (difference in%)	6.16	0	9.97	***<0.001***	18.78	15	13.23
Cognition	MoCA	Tot. MoCA (score)	27.74	28	1.29	***<0.001***	21.67	22	3.54
		Attention and Working Memory	5.70	6	0.57	***<0.001***	3.44	4	1.59
		Long-term memory	3.3	4	1.48	***=0.001***	1.47	1	1.68
	GDS		5.22	4	3.39	***N.S. (p = 0.8)***	5.28	4	4.34

**F, females; MCI, mild cognitive impairment as determined by Montreal Cognitive Assessment (MoCA) scores and confirmed with subsequent investigations by specialists; PTA dB HL, The average of pure tone audiometry around the most important frequencies for speech understanding, that is, 500, 1,000, 2,000, and 4,000 Hz. The p-values are obtained by Student's t-test and the Mann–Whitney test in case of non-parametric variables; GDS, 30-item geriatric depression scale; N.S., not significant; SD, standard deviation. Bolded values indicate significant results.*

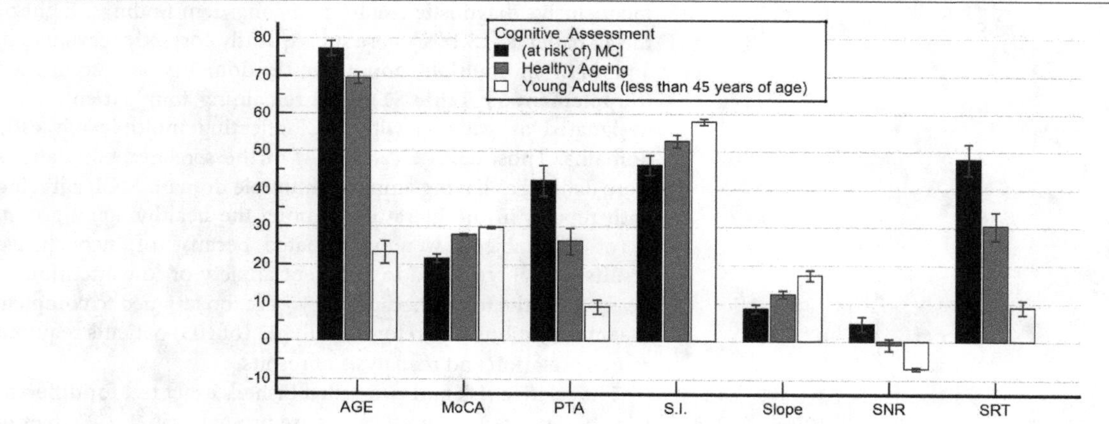

FIGURE 1 | Significant differences among the healthy aging group and the at-risk mild cognitive impairment (MCI) group. This graph shows an analysis of variance for parametric and non-parametric variables. All comparisons were significant; thus, the groups identified through the Montreal Cognitive Assessment (MoCA) test (healthy aging and at risk of MCI) were in fact distinct. They also differed significantly in terms of their audiological profile, although they were not differentiated on the basis of their hearing ability. Healthy aging individuals were also statistically distinct from younger subjects. This suggests cognitive and auditory difficulty/fatigability that physiologically accompanies advancing years. These data, already reported in the literature, were not documented by audiometric comparisons that allow determination of whether loss is paraphysiological. In this way, a healthy aging subject is clearly defined with certain audiometric characteristics: (1) the ability to recognize a signal with a signal-to-noise ratio (SNR) < 0; (2) the pure tone audiometry of less than 30 dB HL; (3) an SRT at rest of less than or equal to 30 dB SPL; (4) a difference between max% words in quiet and logatomes of less than 10; and (5) a slope of psychometric function of greater than 10%. S.I., speech intelligibility in noise. See also **Tables 1–4**.

for cognitive decline can be suspected for further investigations in selected patients. In addition, it is possible to define a reference area or zone, delineated by all of these measures, including individuals with similar characteristics (**Figure 2**). In other words, patients at risk of developing cognitive decline can suffer from a reduced ability to cope with living in a noisy world (auditory frailty). This disadvantage points to the type of rehabilitative action that might reduce the risk of cognitive decline or frailty. The tests might define different contributions to cognitive fatigue by peripheral and central hearing losses, at different ages, thus reflecting a more realistic pattern for longitudinal studies. Even if all tests require cortical efficient functioning, it can be hypothesized that tonal audiometry is one of the simplest tests that a patient can actively perform,

TABLE 4 | Regression analysis and coefficient of correlation of the Montreal Cognitive Assessment (MoCA) score with audiological results.

	Age	*Slope*	*SNR*	*S.I.*	*PTA*	*SRT*	*Log. Diff.*
Coeff. Corr.	−0.670	0.521	−0.544	0.563	−0.469	−0.472	−0.442
R^2	0.449	0.272	0.296	0.317	0.220	0.223	0.195
p_{value}	<0.001	<0.001	<0.001	<0.001	<0.001	<0.001	<0.001
Multiple Regression (Dependent Y MoCA)							
R^2 adjusted	**Multiple corr. coeff.**	**F-ratio**			***P*-value**		
0.477	0.716	14.287			**<0.0001**		

PTA, pure tone average; S.I., sentence intelligibility in noise; SNR, signal-to-noise ratio; SRT, speech/signal recognition threshold; Log. Diff., different discrimination percentages between logatomes and words. Bolded values indicate significant results.

TABLE 5 | Sensitivity and specificity of different audiological results for identifying cognitive impairment.

	MCI				
	TP	**FP**	**TN**	**FN**	**tot**
SNR ≥ -0.4 dB	36	18	41	8	103
Slope ≤ 9.4%	26	9	50	18	103
Logatomes ≥ 10%	38	20	39	6	103
	SNR ≥ -0.4 dB	**≤ 9.4%**	**Log. Diff. ≥ 10%**		
Sens.	0.818	0.743	0.864		
Spec.	0.695	0.735	0.661		

MCI, mild cognitive impairment; Spec, specificity; Sens, sensitivity; SNR, signal-to-noise ratio; tot, total; TP, true positive; FP, false positive; TN, true negative; FN, false negative.

TABLE 6 | Combining Log.Diff.-Slope-SNR (passing two or three criteria for the screening model) increases sensitivity and specificity of audiological screening.

	MCI < 26				
	TP	**FP**	**TN**	**FN**	**tot**
	35	15	44	9	103
	SNR ≥ -0,4 dB AND/OR Slope ≤ 9.4% AND/OR Logatomes Diff. ≥ 10%			***CI 95%***	
Sens.	0.795			0.647–0.902	
Spec.	0.746			0.616–0.850	

Logatomes Diff., the difference in terms of percentage of recognized words/logatomes among the maximum achievable scores in speech audiometry in quiet and the maximum achievable score in logatome audiometry in a quiet environment; MCI, mild cognitive impairment; SNR, signal-to-noise ratio; Sens, sensitivity; Spec, specificity, tot, total; TP, true positive; FP, false positive; TN, true negative; FN, false negative.

and, consequently, it entails poor perceptual involvement of the central neuronal stations. Conversely, progressive involvement of cortical structures is more evident in speech discrimination and in sentence discrimination in noise.

Due to the correlation between hearing loss, aging, and cognitive decline, the results also reflect a pattern of involution, thus the screening model is more congruent for patients with slight to moderate hearing loss among 65–75 years of age (**Table 1**). These results could suggest different contributions of peripheral and central hearing loss to global cognitive functions during aging, and it should suggest range limits for treatments to restore hearing function with hearing aids or cochlear implants.

In the last decade, there has been a great deal of interest in and discussion about the relationship between cognitive decline and hearing loss (Lin et al., 2013; Bernabei et al., 2014; Wayne and Johnsrude, 2015; Hewitt, 2017; Rutherford et al., 2018; Stern and Hilly, 2018; Uchida et al., 2018). Studies on the aging brain have shown that cognitive functions tend to (para-)physiologically decline with advancing years (Ciorba et al., 2011; Ding et al., 2016). In addition, 14.3% of the population over 65 years of age is affected by central auditory processing disorders (CAPD). Older individuals with CAPD seem to be more likely to suffer from dementia than those who are not affected (Martini et al., 2014; Fortunato et al., 2016). The decline can be highlighted in circumstances requiring greater cognitive effort and stressful conditions, such as speech discrimination of words or logatomes in noise or in quiet (Martini et al., 1988; Strauss et al., 2015; Gobara et al., 2016; Taitelbaum-Swead and Fostick, 2016; Bae et al., 2018). Competitive stimuli should be the most sensitive for detecting cognitive efforts or difficulties among elderly people (Pronk et al., 2013). The SNR is a well-known semiquantitative, a parameter, which is useful in the audiological assessment of various conditions of clinical interest, although its role in evaluating cognitive functions is less clear (Pronk et al., 2013; Helfer, 2015; Meister, 2017).

Young subjects have better discrimination than individuals older than 65 years. Furthermore, the use of logatomes can help identify patients with preserved long-term and semantic memory, even though they are at risk of cognitive decline because of impairments in attention and working memory. When semantic content is lacking, speech discrimination requires additional cognitive effort, and subjects with better working memory capacity demonstrate superior performance in the identification of the speech signals (Kim and Oh, 2013). This has been confirmed by neuroimaging studies that show the involvement of both the prefrontal and auditory cortex for the correct identification of ambiguous phonemes (Moradi et al., 2014). In addition, confusion matrices among logatomes (AFA/ATA/ASA, AGIA) can detect some types of cognitive

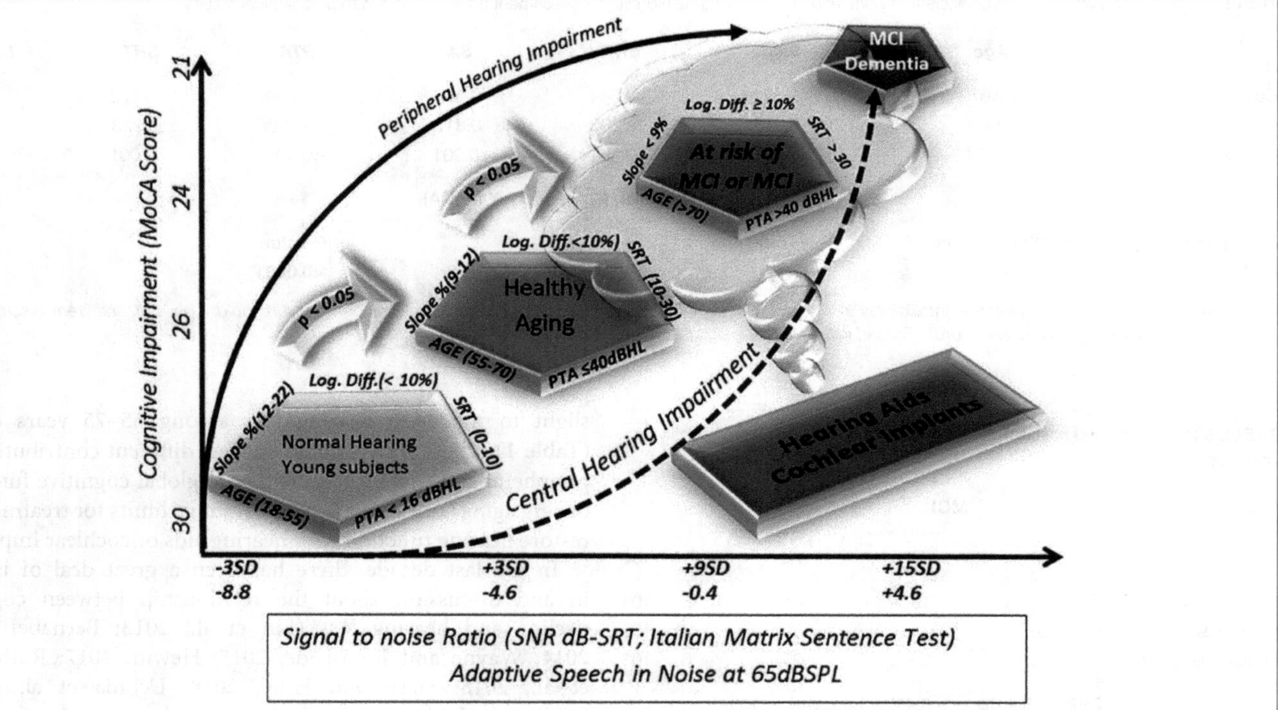

FIGURE 2 | Schematic representation of cognitive decline as defined by different audiological tests. The diagrams summarize the present study. On the *y*-axis, the results of the Montreal Cognitive Assessment (MoCA) score are shown as the average result of the groups shown in the figure as pentagons (ideally defined by five variables, four audiological parameters plus age). On the *x*-axis, there are reference levels for the signal-to-noise ratio (SNR) available in the literature, such as a test for matrices with speech in noise sentences. The test was recently chosen for diffusion in clinical practice in Europe for its easy automatic execution and because it yields easily comparable values regardless of age and language. Starting from the available and official reference levels, and moving in steps of 3 standard deviations, so as to include 100% of the study population, it was possible to identify four different populations, which will by definition be statistically significantly different. The groups used in this study fall exactly within those theoretical values: young subjects, elderly but healthy subjects, and elderly subjects suffering from mild cognitive decline either because they were diagnosed or because they are rated using cognitive tests, and finally, at the opposite extreme, patients suffering from dementia who were so severely affected that they were not able to complete the tests.

disorders among children (Sundstrom et al., 2018), although their role in the audiological and cognitive assessment among older adults is not as clear (Chen and Cowan, 2009). Even if hearing-impaired patients show some disadvantages in speech recognition, the intrasubject differences in identifying words and pseudo-words should be in the 5–20% range (10% ± 2 standard deviation) at the maximum comfortable level of stimulation in dB SPL (Carrat and Carrat, 1992; Apoux et al., 2001; Moradi et al., 2014; Schubotz et al., 2016). Speech audiometry with logatomes might allow identification of those patients who fall outside of this range (**Tables 5, 6**).

Even if it is not routinely performed, such extensive audiological assessment, including SNR, slope of functions, and logatomes, after 55 years of age might help in identifying patients at risk of cognitive decline prior to 65 years of age in the general population.

Nonetheless, due to the limitations of the present study, this report should be considered a tentative preliminary model of auditory screening in the elderly, which must be confirmed in further studies. To the best of our knowledge, reported results and cutoffs should be considered only among older adults with post-lingual mild to moderate hearing loss, and results are more consistent for people between 65 and 75 years of age. These subjects could take advantages from auditory rehabilitation through hearing aids for moderate hearing losses and cochlear implant for severe to profound hearing losses. Unfortunately, patients with severe to profound hearing loss presented limitations in performing all tests, therefore they required specific settings for subsequent investigations, and they were not comparable to elderly patients with better conditions. Consequently, specific populations, such as severe to profound hearing-impaired patients or subjects with cochlear implants and/or hearing aids, require different range references. Furthermore, protocol testing could be time-consuming especially in untrained centers, or among impaired elderly, thus the screening model might be unsustainable in routine or clinical practice. In addition, the fatigue of older adults might be a bias in the final assessment.

CONCLUSION

In conclusion, our study highlights that, in the elderly, audiological assessment by means of SNR, slope of functions, and logatomes might help in further characterization of selected patients because of their correlation with age, high cognitive functions, and hearing loss. These tests might be helpful not only in the detection of hearing loss but also in early identification of the impairment of high cognitive functions. We also suggest that a stricter relation between audiological and neuropsychological assessment of selected patients should be established, and rehabilitation might benefit from such a comprehensive multidisciplinary approach.

Furthermore, our findings indicate that specific audiological results are representative of cognitive functions during aging, following an irregular progression, in part because they can be assimilated into cognitive tests and involve instructions, training, attention, time, accuracy, and cooperation. A mixed contribution of peripheral and central hearing impairment is involved in real life; nevertheless, these impairments contribute differentially during different stages of life. Irrespective of the causative explanation, hearing impairment presents disadvantages at any stage of life and can affect cognition as well as quality of life, increasing the frailty of subjects. Cognitive assessments should be accompanied by auditory testing.

It is important to remark limitations of the present research, thus there are no conclusive evidences on this topic and further investigations are required.

AUTHOR CONTRIBUTIONS

AC supervised the all tests, collected the data, performed the statistical analysis, wrote the main part of the manuscript, and designed the figures and tables. MC helped in the audiological and cognitive assessment, collected the clinical data, and conducted the cognitive tests. SG and MG conducted the literature review, planned part of the work, and wrote part of the manuscript. EL, DC, FS, FG, EC, SG, SC, MP, and SD performed the audiological tests and collected the data. RB, PT, DB, FL, and CGa provided supervision and consultancy on clinical, audiological, and neuroimaging findings. SM and CGi assessed cognitive-communication deficits. AM is the principal investigator of the PRIHTA-IDECO 2013 project and supervised all of the steps of the research.

ACKNOWLEDGMENTS

We would like to thank all participants, colleagues, and technicians who helped in gathering the information presented in this manuscript. We are particularly grateful to the nurses, the students, and the residents who provided support for the research activities. We also thank Cochlear Italia Srl and Amplifon SpA for technical and logistic assistance. The Italian matrix sentence test was provided by MED-EL Italia and GN Hearing Srl (Natus Medical Srl).

SUPPLEMENTARY MATERIAL

FIGURE S1 | Different receiver operating characteristic curves are shown, to compare sensitivity and specificity of different variables for identifying patients with cognitive decline, as represented by a Montreal Cognitive Assessment (MoCA) score < 26.

TABLE S1 | Twenty-three patients with uncertain results were analyzed through the Fisher Exact Test to estimate the identification rate and relative risk of impairment in attention and working memory using logatomes.

REFERENCES

Akeroyd, M. A., Arlinger, S., Bentler, R. A., Boothroyd, A., Dillier, N., Dreschler, W. A., et al. (2015). International collegium of rehabilitative audiology (ICRA) recommendations for the construction of multilingual speech tests. ICRA working group on multilingual speech tests. *Int. J. Audiol.* 54(Suppl. 2), 17–22. doi: 10.3109/14992027.2015.1030513

Apoux, F., Crouzet, O., and Lorenzi, C. (2001). Temporal envelope expansion of speech in noise for normal-hearing and hearing-impaired listeners: effects on identification performance and response times. *Hear. Res.* 153, 123–131. doi: 10.1016/s0378-5955(00)00265-3

Bae, S., Lee, S., Lee, S., Jung, S., Makino, K., Park, H., et al. (2018). The role of social frailty in explaining the association between hearing problems and mild cognitive impairment in older adults. *Arch. Gerontol. Geriatr.* 78, 45–50. doi: 10.1016/j.archger.2018.05.025

Bernabei, R., Bonuccelli, U., Maggi, S., Marengoni, A., Martini, A., Memo, M., et al. (2014). Hearing loss and cognitive decline in older adults: questions and answers. *Aging Clin. Exp. Res.* 26, 567–573. doi: 10.1007/s40520-014-0266-3

Bovo, R., Ortore, R., Ciorba, A., Berto, A., and Martini, A. (2007). Bilateral sudden profound hearing loss and vertigo as a unique manifestation of bilateral symmetric inferior pontine infarctions. *Ann. Otol. Rhinol. Laryngol.* 116, 407–410. doi: 10.1177/000348940711600603

Buss, E., Hall, J. W., and Grose, J. H. (2009). Psychometric functions for pure tone intensity discrimination: slope differences in school-aged children and adults. *J. Acoust. Soc. Am.* 125, 1050–1058. doi: 10.1121/1.3050273

Carrat, R., and Carrat, X. (1992). [Vocal audiometry: the "phonatome" recognition test. Principle, technique, initial results]. *Rev. Laryngol. Otol Rhinol.* 113, 347–353.

Castiglione, A., Benatti, A., Velardita, C., Favaro, D., Padoan, E., Severi, D., et al. (2016). Aging, cognitive decline and hearing loss: effects of auditory rehabilitation and training with hearing aids and cochlear implants on cognitive function and depression among older adults. *Audiol. Neurootol.* 21(Suppl. 1), 21–28. doi: 10.1159/000448350

Chan, T. M. V., and Alain, C. (2018). Listening back in time: does attention to memory facilitate word-in-noise identification? *Atten. Percept. Psychophys.* 81, 253–269. doi: 10.3758/s13414-018-1586-8

Chen, Z., and Cowan, N. (2009). How verbal memory loads consume attention. *Mem. Cognit.* 37, 829–836. doi: 10.3758/MC.37.6.829

Ciorba, A., Benatti, A., Bianchini, C., Aimoni, C., Volpato, S., Bovo, R., et al. (2011). High frequency hearing loss in the elderly: effect of age and noise exposure in an Italian group. *J. Laryngol. Otol.* 125, 776–780. doi: 10.1017/S0022215111001101

Conti, S., Bonazzi, S., Laiacona, M., Masina, M., and Coralli, M. V. (2015). Montreal cognitive assessment (MoCA)-Italian version: regression based norms and equivalent scores. *Neurol. Sci.* 36, 209–214. doi: 10.1007/s10072-014-1921-3

Cosetti, M. K., Pinkston, J. B., Flores, J. M., Friedmann, D. R., Jones, C. B., Roland, J. T., et al. (2016). Neurocognitive testing and cochlear implantation: insights into performance in older adults. *Clin. Interv. Aging* 11, 603–613. doi: 10.2147/CIA.S100255

Costa, M., Lepore, F., Prevost, F., and Guillemot, J. P. (2016). Effects of aging on peripheral and central auditory processing in rats. *Eur. J. Neurosci.* 44, 2084–2094. doi: 10.1111/ejn.13302

Davis, D. H., Creavin, S. T., Yip, J. L., Noel-Storr, A. H., Brayne, C., and Cullum, S. (2015). Montreal Cognitive Assessment for the diagnosis of Alzheimer's disease and other dementias. *Cochrane Database Syst. Rev.* 10:CD010775. doi: 10.1002/14651858.CD010775.pub2

Deal, J. A., Betz, J., Yaffe, K., Harris, T., Purchase-Helzner, E., Satterfield, S., et al. (2017). Hearing impairment and incident dementia and cognitive decline in older adults: the health ABC study. *J. Gerontol. A Biol. Sci. Med. Sci.* 72, 703–709. doi: 10.1093/gerona/glw069

Ding, X. Q., Maudsley, A. A., Sabati, M., Sheriff, S., Schmitz, B., Schutze, M., et al. (2016). Physiological neuronal decline in healthy aging human brain - An in vivo study with MRI and short echo-time whole-brain (1)H MR spectroscopic imaging. *Neuroimage* 137, 45–51. doi: 10.1016/j.neuroimage.2016.05.014

Dreschler, W. A., Verschuure, H., Ludvigsen, C., and Westermann, S. (2001). ICRA noises: artificial noise signals with speech-like spectral and temporal properties for hearing instrument assessment. International collegium for rehabilitative audiology. *Audiology* 40, 148–157. doi: 10.3109/00206090109073110

Fortunato, S., Forli, F., Guglielmi, V., De Corso, E., Paludetti, G., Berrettini, S., et al. (2016). A review of new insights on the association between hearing loss and cognitive decline in ageing. *Acta Otorhinolaryngol. Ital.* 36, 155–166. doi: 10.14639/0392-100X-993

Gallo, S., and Castiglione, A. (2019). The signal to noise ratio assessment in cochlear implanted patients through the Italian Matrix Sentence Test (Oldenburg Test). *Hearing Balance Commun.* 17, 145–148. doi: 10.1080/21695717.2019.1603949

Giau, V. V., Senanarong, V., Bagyinszky, E., An, S. S. A., and Kim, S. (2019). Analysis of 50 neurodegenerative genes in clinically diagnosed early-onset alzheimer's disease. *Int. J. Mol. Sci.* 20:E1514. doi: 10.3390/ijms20061514

Gobara, A., Yamada, Y., and Miura, K. (2016). Crossmodal modulation of spatial localization by mimetic words. *Iperception* 7:2041669516684244.

Helfer, K. S. (2015). Competing speech perception in middle age. *Am. J. Audiol.* 24, 80–83. doi: 10.1044/2015_AJA-14-0056

Herbst, K. G., and Humphrey, C. (1980). Hearing impairment and mental state in the elderly living at home. *Br. Med. J.* 281, 903–905. doi: 10.1136/bmj.281.6245.903

Hewitt, D. (2017). Age-related hearing loss and cognitive decline: you haven't heard the half of it. *Front. Aging Neurosci.* 9:112. doi: 10.3389/fnagi.2017.00112

Homans, N. C., Metselaar, R. M., Dingemanse, J. G., Van Der Schroeff, M. P., Brocaar, M. P., Wieringa, M. H., et al. (2017). Prevalence of age-related hearing loss, including sex differences, in older adults in a large cohort study. *Laryngoscope* 127, 725–730. doi: 10.1002/lary.26150

Houben, R., Koopman, J., Luts, H., Wagener, K. C., Van Wieringen, A., Verschuure, H., et al. (2014). Development of a Dutch matrix sentence test to assess speech intelligibility in noise. *Int. J. Audiol.* 53, 760–763. doi: 10.3109/14992027.2014.920111

Jayakody, D. M. P., Friedland, P. L., Martins, R. N., and Sohrabi, H. R. (2018). Impact of aging on the auditory system and related cognitive functions: a narrative review. *Front. Neurosci.* 12:125. doi: 10.3389/fnins.2018.00125

Jorgensen, L. E., and Messersmith, J. J. (2015). Impact of aging and cognition on hearing assistive technology use. *Semin. Hear.* 36, 162–174. doi: 10.1055/s-0035-1555119

Kaernbach, C. (2001). Slope bias of psychometric functions derived from adaptive data. *Percept. Psychophys.* 63, 1389–1398. doi: 10.3758/bf03194550

Kim, B. J., and Oh, S. H. (2013). Age-related changes in cognition and speech perception. *Korean J. Audiol.* 17, 54–58. doi: 10.7874/kja.2013.17.2.54

King-Smith, P. E., and Rose, D. (1997). Principles of an adaptive method for measuring the slope of the psychometric function. *Vis. Res.* 37, 1595–1604. doi: 10.1016/s0042-6989(96)00310-0

Kollmeier, B. (2015). Overcoming language barriers: matrix sentence tests with closed speech corpora. *Int. J. Audiol.* 54, 1–2. doi: 10.3109/14992027.2015.1074295

Kostoff, R. N., Zhang, Y., Ma, J., Porter, A. L., and Buchtel, H. A. (2017). *Prevention and Reversal of Alzheimer's Disease.* Atlanta: Georgia Institute of Technology.

Kujawski, S., Kujawska, A., Gajos, M., Topka, W., Perkowski, R., Androsiuk-Perkowska, J., et al. (2018). Cognitive functioning in older people. Results of the first wave of cognition of older people, education, recreational activities, nutrition, comorbidities, functional capacity studies (COPERNICUS). *Front. Aging Neurosci.* 10:421. doi: 10.3389/fnagi.2018.00421

Limongi, F., Siviero, P., Noale, M., Gesmundo, A., Crepaldi, G., Maggi, S., et al. (2017). Prevalence and conversion to dementia of Mild Cognitive Impairment in an elderly Italian population. *Aging Clin. Exp. Res.* 29, 361–370. doi: 10.1007/s40520-017-0748-1

Lin, F. R., Metter, E. J., O'Brien, R. J., Resnick, S. M., Zonderman, A. B., and Ferrucci, L. (2011a). Hearing loss and incident dementia. *Arch. Neurol.* 68, 214–220. doi: 10.1001/archneurol.2010.362

Lin, F. R., Thorpe, R., Gordon-Salant, S., and Ferrucci, L. (2011b). Hearing loss prevalence and risk factors among older adults in the United States. *J. Gerontol. A Biol. Sci. Med. Sci.* 66, 582–590. doi: 10.1093/gerona/glr002

Lin, F. R., Yaffe, K., Xia, J., Xue, Q. L., Harris, T. B., Purchase-Helzner, E., et al. (2013). Hearing loss and cognitive decline in older adults. *JAMA Intern. Med.* 173, 293–299. doi: 10.1001/jamainternmed.2013.1868

Livingston, G., Sommerlad, A., Orgeta, V., Costafreda, S. G., Huntley, J., Ames, D., et al. (2017). Dementia prevention, intervention, and care. *Lancet* 390, 2673–2734. doi: 10.1016/S0140-6736(17)31363-6

MacPherson, A., and Akeroyd, M. A. (2014). Variations in the slope of the psychometric functions for speech intelligibility: a systematic survey. *Trends Hear.* 18:2331216514537722. doi: 10.1177/2331216514537722

Martini, A., Bovo, R., Agnoletto, M., Da Col, M., Drusian, A., Liddeo, M., et al. (1988). Dichotic performance in elderly Italians with Italian stop consonant-vowel stimuli. *Audiology* 27, 1–7. doi: 10.3109/00206098809081568

Martini, A., Castiglione, A., Bovo, R., Vallesi, A., and Gabelli, C. (2014). Aging, cognitive load, dementia and hearing loss. *Audiol. Neurootol.* 19(Suppl. 1), 2–5. doi: 10.1159/000371593

Meister, H. (2017). Speech audiometry, speech perception and cognitive functions. German version. *HNO* 65, 189–194. doi: 10.1007/s00106-016-0229-4

Meister, H., Schreitmuller, S., Grugel, L., Beutner, D., Walger, M., and Meister, I. (2013). Examining speech perception in noise and cognitive functions in the elderly. *Am. J. Audiol.* 22, 310–312. doi: 10.1044/1059-0889(2012/12-0067)

Moradi, S., Lidestam, B., Hallgren, M., and Ronnberg, J. (2014). Gated auditory speech perception in elderly hearing aid users and elderly normal-hearing individuals: effects of hearing impairment and cognitive capacity. *Trends Hear.* 18:2331216514545406. doi: 10.1177/2331216514545406

Muhler, R., Ziese, M., and Rostalski, D. (2009). Development of a speaker discrimination test for cochlear implant users based on the oldenburg logatome corpus. *ORL J. Otorhinolaryngol. Relat. Spec.* 71, 14–20. doi: 10.1159/000165170

Nguyen, M. F., Bonnefoy, M., Adrait, A., Gueugnon, M., Petitot, C., Collet, L., et al. (2017). Efficacy of hearing aids on the cognitive status of patients with alzheimer's disease and hearing loss: a multicenter controlled randomized trial. *J. Alzheimers Dis.* 58, 123–137. doi: 10.3233/JAD-160793

Panza, F., Solfrizzi, V., and Logroscino, G. (2015). Age-related hearing impairment-a risk factor and frailty marker for dementia and AD. *Nat. Rev. Neurol.* 11, 166–175. doi: 10.1038/nrneurol.2015.12

Parham, K., and Kost, K. M. (2017). Presbycusis-peripheral and central. *Ear Nose Throat J.* 96, 462–463. doi: 10.1177/014556131709601206

Peracino, A., and Pecorelli, S. (2016). The epidemiology of cognitive impairment in the aging population: implications for hearing loss. *Audiol. Neurootol.* 21(Suppl. 1), 3–9. doi: 10.1159/000448346

Pisoni, D. B. (1996). Word Identification in Noise. *Lang. Cogn. Process.* 11, 681–687.

Pronk, M., Deeg, D. J., Festen, J. M., Twisk, J. W., Smits, C., Comijs, H. C., et al. (2013). Decline in older persons' ability to recognize speech in noise: the influence of demographic, health-related, environmental, and cognitive factors. *Ear Hear.* 34, 722–732. doi: 10.1097/AUD.0b013e3182994eee

Puglisi, G. E., Warzybok, A., Hochmuth, S., Visentin, C., Astolfi, A., Prodi, N., et al. (2015). An Italian matrix sentence test for the evaluation of speech intelligibility in noise. *Int J. Audiol.* 54(Suppl. 2), 44–50. doi: 10.3109/14992027.2015.1061709

Rooth, M. A. (2017). The prevalence and impact of vision and hearing loss in the elderly. *N. C. Med. J.* 78, 118–120. doi: 10.18043/ncm.78.2.118

Rutherford, B. R., Brewster, K., Golub, J. S., Kim, A. H., and Roose, S. P. (2018). Sensation and psychiatry: linking age-related hearing loss to late-life depression and cognitive decline. *Am. J. Psychiatry* 175, 215–224. doi: 10.1176/appi.ajp.2017.17040423

Santangelo, G., Siciliano, M., Pedone, R., Vitale, C., Falco, F., Bisogno, R., et al. (2015). Normative data for the montreal cognitive assessment in an Italian population sample. *Neurol. Sci.* 36, 585–591. doi: 10.1007/s10072-014-1995-y

Schubotz, W., Brand, T., Kollmeier, B., and Ewert, S. D. (2016). The influence of high-frequency envelope information on low-frequency vowel identification in noise. *PLoS One* 11:e0145610. doi: 10.1371/journal.pone.0145610

Shen, J., Anderson, M. C., Arehart, K. H., and Souza, P. E. (2016). Using cognitive screening tests in audiology. *Am. J. Audiol.* 25, 319–331. doi: 10.1044/2016_AJA-16-0032

Siciliano, M., Chiorri, C., Passaniti, C., Sant'elia, V., Trojano, L., and Santangelo, G. (2019). Comparison of alternate and original forms of the Montreal Cognitive Assessment (MoCA): an Italian normative study. *Neurol. Sci.* 40, 691–702. doi: 10.1007/s10072-019-3700-7

Stern, D., and Hilly, O. (2018). [The relationship between hearing loss and cognitive decline in the elderly and the efficiency of hearing rehabilitation in preventing cognitive decline]. *Harefuah* 157, 374–377.

Strauss, A., Henry, M. J., Scharinger, M., and Obleser, J. (2015). Alpha phase determines successful lexical decision in noise. *J. Neurosci.* 35, 3256–3262. doi: 10.1523/JNEUROSCI.3357-14.2015

Sundstrom, S., Lofkvist, U., Lyxell, B., and Samuelsson, C. (2018). Prosodic and segmental aspects of nonword repetition in 4- to 6-year-old children who are deaf and hard of hearing compared to controls with normal hearing. *Clin. Linguist. Phon.* 32, 950–971. doi: 10.1080/02699206.2018.1469671

Taitelbaum-Swead, R., and Fostick, L. (2016). The effect of age and type of noise on speech perception under conditions of changing context and noise levels. *Folia Phoniatr. Logop.* 68, 16–21. doi: 10.1159/000444749

Thomson, R. S., Auduong, P., Miller, A. T., and Gurgel, R. K. (2017). Hearing loss as a risk factor for dementia: a systematic review. *Laryngoscope Investig. Otolaryngol.* 2, 69–79. doi: 10.1002/lio2.65

Uchida, Y., Sugiura, S., Nishita, Y., Saji, N., Sone, M., and Ueda, H. (2018). Age-related hearing loss and cognitive decline - The potential mechanisms linking the two. *Auris Nasus Larynx* 46, 1–9. doi: 10.1016/j.anl.2018.08.010

Vos, S. J. B., Van Boxtel, M. P. J., Schiepers, O. J. G., Deckers, K., De Vugt, M., Carriere, I., et al. (2017). Modifiable risk factors for prevention of dementia in midlife, late life and the oldest-old: validation of the LIBRA Index. *J. Alzheimers Dis.* 58, 537–547. doi: 10.3233/JAD-161208

Wagener, K. C., Brand, T., and Kollmeier, B. (2006). The role of silent intervals for sentence intelligibility in fluctuating noise in hearing-impaired listeners. *Int. J. Audiol.* 45, 26–33. doi: 10.1080/14992020500243851

Wayne, R. V., and Johnsrude, I. S. (2015). A review of causal mechanisms underlying the link between age-related hearing loss and cognitive decline. *Ageing Res. Rev.* 23, 154–166. doi: 10.1016/j.arr.2015.06.002

Zanetti, O., Frisoni, G. B., Rozzini, L., Bianchetti, A., and Trabucchi, M. (1998). Validity of direct assessment of functional status as a tool for measuring Alzheimer's disease severity. *Age Ageing* 27, 615–622. doi: 10.1093/ageing/27.5.615

19

Hearing Loss and Cognition Among Older Adults in a Han Chinese Cohort

Fuxin Ren[1†], Jianfen Luo[2,3†], Wen Ma[4], Qian Xin[5], Lei Xu[2,3], Zhaomin Fan[2,3], Yu Ai[2,3], Bin Zhao[1], Fei Gao[1] and Haibo Wang[2,3*]*

[1] Shandong Medical Imaging Research Institute, Shandong University, Jinan, China, [2] Department of Otolaryngology-Head and Neck Surgery, Shandong Provincial ENT Hospital, Shandong University, Jinan, China, [3] Shandong Provincial Key Laboratory of Otology, Jinan, China, [4] Department of Otolaryngology, Jinan Central Hospital, Shandong University, Jinan, China, [5] The Second Hospital of Shandong University, Jinan, China

***Correspondence:**
Fei Gao
feigao6262@163.com
Haibo Wang
whboto11@163.com*

† These authors have contributed equally to this work

Presbycusis (PC) is associated with cognitive decline and incident dementia. Speech reception thresholds (SRT) are used to assess speech detection, which points toward a central component of PC. However, to the best of our knowledge, no previous study has reported the relationship between SRT and cognitive function in older adults in a Han Chinese cohort. Therefore, in this study, we investigate the association of hearing loss, indexed using pure tone average (PTA) and SRT, with cognitive function in a Han Chinese cohort using a standardized neurocognitive battery. Subjects (aged ≥60 years) with no history of psychiatric or neurological diseases were recruited. All subjects underwent a battery of neuropsychological and auditory tests. According to the PTA of the better ear, the subjects were further divided into PC and normal PTA (NP) groups. Regression analyses were performed to examine the relationship between cognitive function and hearing loss in the PC and NP groups and all subjects when controlling for age, sex, education level, diabetes, smoking, and hypertension. Cognitive function was significantly associated with PTA and SRT in all subjects. In all subjects, the correlations between non-verbal cognitive scores and SRT were stronger than those between non-verbal cognitive scores and PTA, whereas the correlations between verbal cognitive scores and PTA were stronger than those between verbal cognitive scores and SRT. Moreover, the correlations between PTA or SRT and cognitive function in the PC group were in principle stronger than those in the NP group. Our findings indicate that cognitive function is significantly associated with PTA and SRT in older adults in a Han Chinese cohort. Therefore, SRT could be an important auditory test for exploring cognitive decline in PC and could complement PTA.

Keywords: presbycusis, hearing loss, cognition, older adults, speech reception thresholds

INTRODUCTION

Age-related hearing loss, also known as presbycusis (PC), is among the most common chronic diseases in older adults. The prevalence of PC increases with age, and it has been reported that 30–35% of adults between the ages of 65–75 years and 40–50% of adults over the age of 75 years suffer from PC (Nash et al., 2011). The World Health Organization's World Health Statistics report indicated that the average life expectancy in China has increased significantly in recent years (2018). Age-related hearing loss is becoming a major sensory deficit among older adults in China (Luo et al., 2013). Recently, many audiological studies have suggested that PC is associated with cognitive impairment and incident dementia (Gates and Mills, 2005; Lin, 2011; Lin et al., 2011a,b,c; Jayakody et al., 2018). For instance, one cross-sectional study reported that hearing loss of older American adults is independently associated with lower scores on the symbol digit modalities test (SDMT) (Lin, 2011). In addition, reduced cognitive functioning was associated with age-related hearing loss in older European adults (Quaranta et al., 2014). However, to date, there has been a paucity of studies exploring the association between hearing loss and cognitive function in a Han Chinese cohort.

Presbycusis is usually characterized by progressive hearing loss at high frequencies, which are particularly important for speech recognition. Previous studies have shown that PC represents deteriorated function of both the auditory periphery and the central auditory system (Ouda et al., 2015). Hypofunction of the inner ear is the main reason for the peripheral component of PC (Schuknecht and Gacek, 1993). Moreover, poor speech discrimination and deteriorated temporal sound processing reflect a possible central component of PC (Mazelova et al., 2003). However, research into the association between hearing loss and cognitive function has focused solely on hearing as measured by pure tone thresholds, which assess the function of the auditory periphery. Speech reception thresholds (SRT) are used to assess speech detection, which could reflect a central component of PC. To our knowledge, to date there has been a paucity of studies exploring the relationship between SRT and cognitive function in older adults.

Therefore, in the present study, we investigated the association of hearing loss with cognitive function in a Han Chinese cohort using a standardized neurocognitive battery. Hearing loss was assessed using pure tone thresholds and SRT. We hypothesized that cognitive decline would be associated with both pure tone thresholds and SRT.

MATERIALS AND METHODS

Subjects

The study was approved by the Shandong University institutional review board, and each participant provided informed consent. Subjects aged ≥60 years were recruited from the local community. No one had a history of psychiatric or neurological illness. All subjects were Han Chinese.

Assessment of Auditory Function

First, optimal middle ear conditions were confirmed using tympanometry performed with a GSI Tympstar. Then, the air conduction thresholds were measured through pure tone audiometry at the frequencies from 125, 250, 500, 1000, 2000, 4000, and 8000 Hz using a clinical audiometer (GSI AudioStar Pro). The speech-frequency pure-tone average (PTA) for each side of ears was obtained by calculating the average of hearing thresholds at 500, 1000, 2000, and 4000 Hz in air conduction (1). Hearing loss was defined as PTA >25 decibels hearing level (dB HL) for the better ear (World Health Organization [WHO], 2018), and the subjects were further divided into PC and normal PTA (NP) groups. The exclusion criteria in the study were as follows: (1) asymmetric hearing loss, conductive hearing loss and tinnitus; (2) other causes of sensorineural hearing loss different from PC; (3) previous history of hearing aid use, noise exposure, otologic surgery, head trauma and ototoxic drug therapy.

Speech reception thresholds was performed with a clinical audiometer (GSI AudioStar Pro) and equipped with TDH-50P headphones in quiet conditions. First, according to the value of PTA, an initial sound intensity is groped to ensure that the subject is able to exactly recognize 5 spondee words under this intensity. If the subject cannot recognize, the software will increase the initial sound intensity. The software then automatically controls sound intensity: the sound intensity reduces by 5 dB for every five words played. The test is stopped when the subject is unable to exactly recognize five spondee words. Finally, the number of exact recognized words are counted in the whole descending process, then the software subtracts the number of exact recognized words from initial sound intensity and adds a correction factor (2.5 dB), which is the subject's speech recognition threshold.

Assessment of Cognitive Function

First, the subjects' general cognitive function was tested using the Montreal Cognitive Assessment (MoCA) (Galea and Woodward, 2005; Nasreddine et al., 2005). Then, the subjects' verbal learning and memory, attention, psychomotor speed and executive control were tested using the Auditory Verbal Learning Test (AVLT, Chinese version) (Zhao et al., 2012), the Stroop color word interference test (Savitz and Jansen, 2003), the SDMT (Van Schependom et al., 2014), and the trail-making test (TMT) (Sanchez-Cubillo et al., 2009), respectively. The TMT is made up of two parts. In TMT-A part, the subjects were required to draw lines sequentially connecting 25 encircled numbers, that were distributed on a piece of paper in ascending order (from 1 to 25), as soon as possible. Culturally, most Chinese older adults are less familiar with Arabic numerals than Westerners, therefore, a Chinese version of the TMT-B was applied in our study (Lu et al., 2006; Wei et al., 2018). In TMT-B part, the subjects were required to draw a line alternating between squares and circles while connecting the numbers on a page of the same size in ascending order (from 1 to 25) as soon as possible. Cognitive tests in our study were divided into two categories: verbal tests and non-verbal tests. Verbal tests include MoCA, AVLT and Stroop, which means that verbal communication is required in the test. Non-verbal tests include SDMT, TMT-A, and TMT-B, which means that verbal communication is not required in the test. Finally, the subjects' anxiety and depression status were assessed using the hospital anxiety and depression scale (HADS) (Zigmond and Snaith, 1983). The overall testing time was about 60 min in a fixed order.

Statistical Analysis

The two-tailed *t*-test was used to assess group differences in continuous variables, and the chi-square test was used to assess group differences in gender-specific, diabetes, smoking and hypertension. Partial correlation analyses were used to explore the correlations between cognitive function and PTA or SRT in the PC and NP groups and all subjects, controlling for age, sex, education level, diabetes, smoking and hypertension. Stepwise Multiple Linear Regression analyses were then performed in the PC group, NP group and all subjects. PTA/SRT, age, sex, education level, diabetes, smoking, and hypertension are independent variables, and cognition measures are dependent variables. *P*-values of less than 0.05 were accepted as significant.

RESULTS

Demographic and Clinical Characteristics

The demographic and clinical characteristics of the study population are listed in **Table 1**. Eighty subjects aged 60–78 years (40 males/40 females, mean age: 65.78 ± 3.96 years) were screened for inclusion in this study. Thirty-five subjects were assigned to the NP group, and forty-five subjects were assigned to the PC group.

Presbycusis and NP groups did not differ significantly in age, sex or education. Compared to the NP group, the patients with

TABLE 1 | Subjects' demographic and clinical data.

Characteristics	All subjects (*n* = 80)	PC group (*n* = 45)	NP group (*n* = 35)	*P*-value PC vs. NP	Cohen's d PC vs. NP
Gender (male/female)	40/40	23/22	17/18	0.822	–
Age (years)	65.78 ± 3.96	66.29 ± 4.37	65.11 ± 3.30	0.190	0.30
Education (years)	11.50 ± 2.61	11.42 ± 2.35	11.60 ± 2.94	0.771	−0.07
Diabetes (yes/no)	7/73	4/41	3/32	0.960	–
Smoking (yes/no)	21/59	12/33	9/26	0.923	–
Hypertension(yes/no)	39/41	22/23	17/18	0.978	–
Anxiety	3.26 ± 2.40	3.38 ± 2.59	3.11 ± 2.15	0.629	0.11
Depression	3.38 ± 2.83	3.62 ± 3.43	3.06 ± 1.78	0.344	0.20
PTA (dB/HL)	25.97 ± 13.92	35.97 ± 10.18	13.11 ± 3.67	**<0.001**	**2.98**
SRT (dB/HL)	25.93 ± 13.99	35.43 ± 11.16	13.70 ± 4.49	**<0.001**	**2.48**
MoCA	25.68 ± 2.23	25.24 ± 2.79	26.23 ± 0.97	**0.032**	**−0.51**
AVLT	56.63 ± 8.63	55.58 ± 7.90	57.97 ± 9.44	0.232	−0.27
Stroop (s)	131.50 ± 16.20	135.13 ± 16.66	126.83 ± 14.52	**0.022**	**0.53**
SDMT	39.50 ± 15.12	34.71 ± 12.81	45.66 ± 15.80	**0.001**	**−0.76**
TMT-A (s)	48.86 ± 16.91	52.60 ± 16.89	44.06 ± 15.91	**0.024**	**0.53**
TMT-B (s)	140.48 ± 83.65	150.44 ± 85.40	127.66 ± 80.75	0.229	0.27

The data are presented as means ± standard deviations. Values in bold are statistically significant. Cohen's d is an effect size used to indicate the standardized difference between two means. PTA, pure tone average; SRT, speech reception threshold; PC, presbycusis; NP, normal PTA; MoCA, montreal cognitive assessment; AVLT, auditory verbal learning test; SDMT, symbol digit modalities test; TMT, trail-making test; levels of anxiety and depression were assessed according to the hospital anxiety and depression scale (HADS).

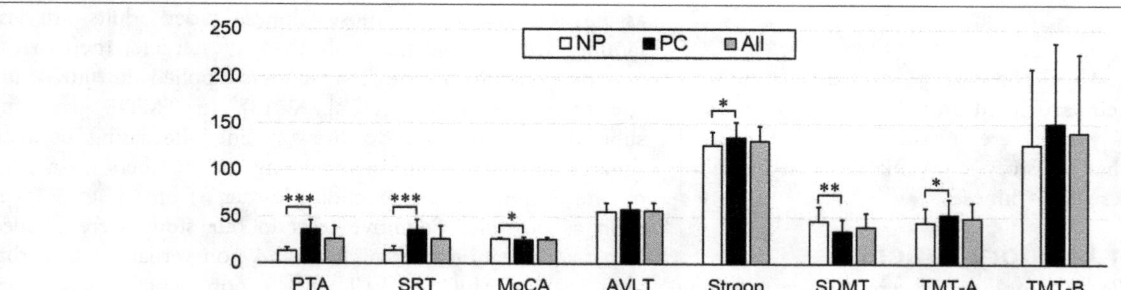

FIGURE 1 | Differences in the neuropsychological and auditory tests between the Normal PTA (NP) group and Presbycusis (PC) group. Compared to the NP group, the patients with PC performed worse on the MoCA, Stroop, SDMT, and TMT-A tests ($p < 0.05$). The PTA and SRT were significantly higher in the patients with PC than in the NP group ($p < 0.001$). Statistical significance was set as *$p < 0.05$, **$p < 0.01$, and ***$p < 0.001$.

PC performed worse on the MoCA, Stroop, SDMT, and TMT-A tests ($p < 0.05$) (**Table 1** and **Figure 1**). The correlations between cognitive outcomes in all subjects, NP and PC group were shown in **Supplementary Table S1**. The PTA and SRT were significantly higher in the patients with PC than in the NP group (PTA, $p < 0.001$; SRT, $p < 0.001$) (**Table 1** and **Figure 1**). All subjects had a type A curve on tympanometry, which indicate normal middle ear function. The hearing thresholds of the left and right ears of all subjects are shown in **Figure 2**. Partial correlation analyses (controlling for age, sex, education level, diabetes, smoking and hypertension) revealed that SRT was positively correlated with PAT in all subjects ($r = 0.945$, $p < 0.001$), in the NP group ($r = 0.472$, $p = 0.013$) and in the PC group ($r = 0.897$, $p < 0.001$), as seen in **Supplementary Figure S1**.

Correlations Between Hearing Loss and Cognitive Function (Table 2)

In all subjects, Pearson correlation analyses revealed that PTA (**Figure 3**) was positively correlated with Stroop ($r = 0.311$, $p = 0.008$), TMT-A ($r = 0.414$, $p < 0.001$), and TMT-B ($r = 0.271$, $p = 0.021$) and negatively correlated with the MoCA ($r = -0.323$, $p = 0.006$), AVLT ($r = -0.262$, $p = 0.026$), and SDMT ($r = -0.489$, $p < 0.001$). SRT (**Figure 4**) was positively correlated with Stroop ($r = 0.298$, $p = 0.011$), TMT-A ($r = 0.427$, $p < 0.001$), and TMT-B ($r = 0.318$, $p = 0.007$), and negatively correlated with the MoCA ($r = -0.297$, $p = 0.011$), AVLT ($r = -0.246$, $p = 0.037$), and SDMT ($r = -0.497$, $p < 0.001$).

In the NP group, Pearson correlation analyses revealed that PTA (**Figure 5**) was positively correlated with Stroop ($r = 0.401$,

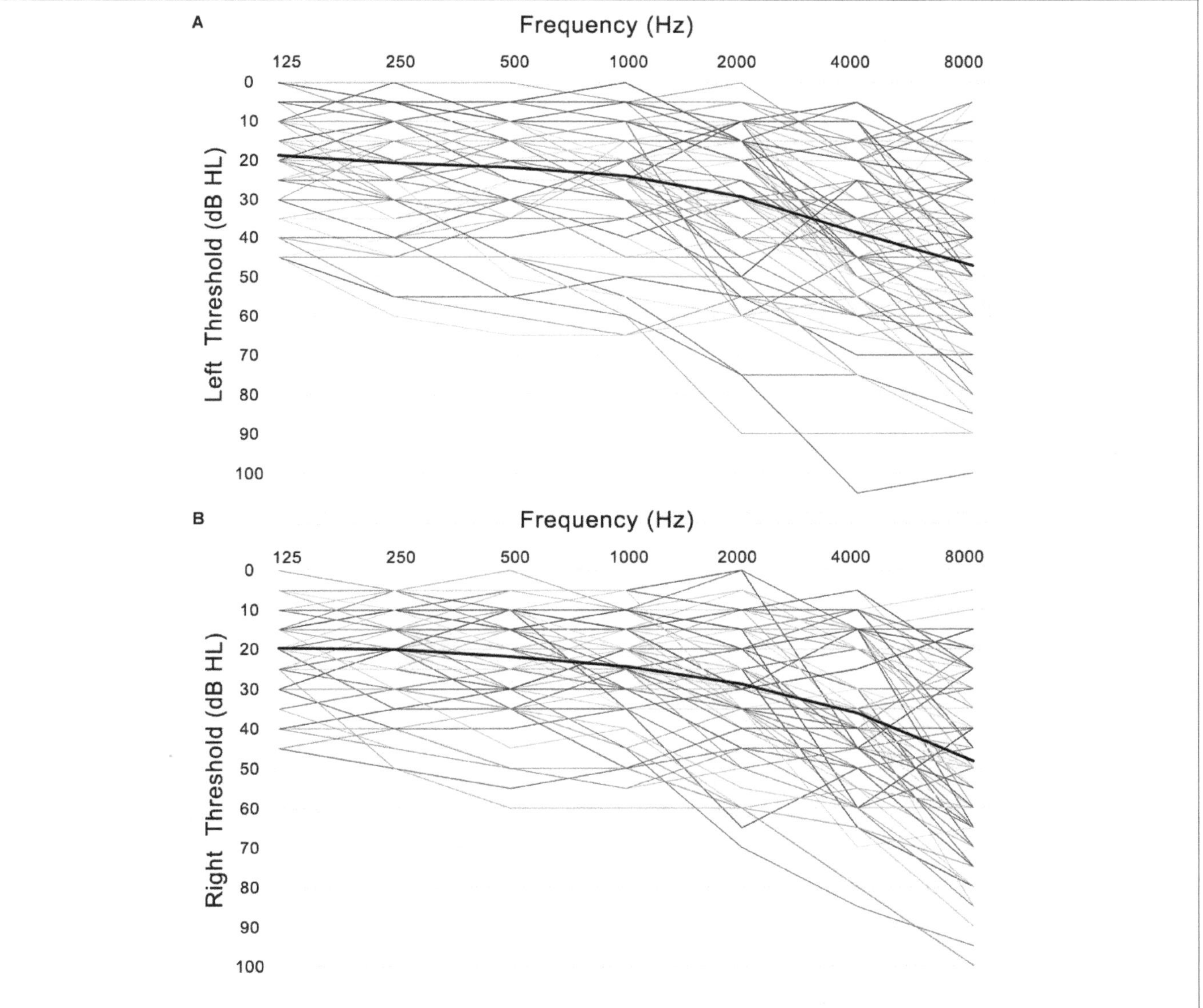

FIGURE 2 | Left **(A)** and right **(B)** ear pure-tone thresholds (dB HL) are plotted for each subject's left and right ear as a function of frequency (Hz) with the mean thresholds across participants and ears (black line).

TABLE 2 | Correlations between audiological (PTA/SRT) and cognitive outcomes (verbal/non-verbal tests).

		Verbal tests			Non-verbal tests		
		MoCA	**AVLT**	**Stroop**	**SDMT**	**TMT-A**	**TMT-B**
All subjects							
PTA	**r**	**−0.323**	**−0.262**	**0.311**	**−0.489**	**0.414**	**0.271**
	p	**0.006**	**0.026**	**0.008**	**<0.001**	**<0.001**	**0.021**
SRT	**r**	**−0.297**	**−0.246**	**0.298**	**−0.497**	**0.427**	**0.318**
	p	**0.011**	**0.037**	**0.011**	**<0.001**	**<0.001**	**0.007**
PC group							
PTA	**r**	**−0.376**	**−0.536**	0.205	**−0.532**	**0.572**	**0.494**
	p	**0.022**	**<0.001**	0.223	**<0.001**	**<0.001**	**0.002**
SRT	**r**	**−0.373**	**−0.574**	0.245	**−0.594**	**0.652**	**0.528**
	p	**0.023**	**<0.001**	0.143	**<0.001**	**<0.001**	**<0.001**
NP group							
PTA	**r**	0.245	−0.379	**0.401**	**−0.430**	0.318	0.091
	p	0.219	0.051	**0.038**	**0.025**	0.106	0.652
SRT	**r**	**0.457**	−0.276	0.297	−0.336	0.175	0.291
	p	**0.017**	0.164	0.132	0.087	0.383	0.141

Partial correlation analyses were used and controlled for age, sex, education level, diabetes, smoking, and hypertension. Bold values indicates a statistically significant difference with a p-value less than 0.05. PTA, pure tone average; SRT, speech reception threshold; PC, presbycusis; NP, normal PTA; MoCA, montreal cognitive assessment; AVLT, auditory verbal learning test; SDMT, symbol digit modalities test; TMT, trail-making test.

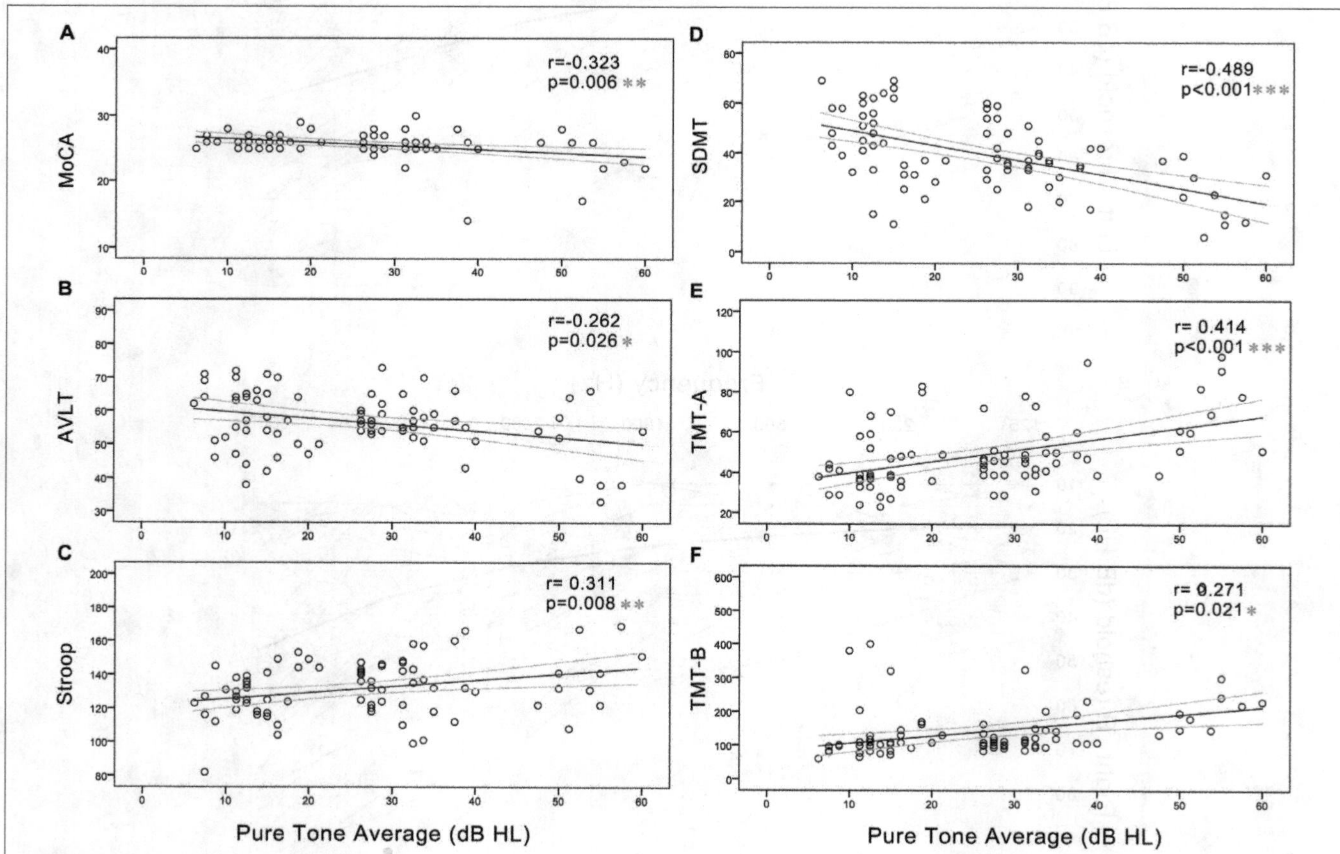

FIGURE 3 | Scatter plots displaying the correlations between PTA and cognitive function in all subjects. Partial correlation analyses (controlling for age, sex, education level, diabetes, smoking, and hypertension) revealed that PTA was positively correlated with **(C)** Stroop ($r = 0.311$, $p = 0.008$), **(E)** TMT-A ($r = 0.414$, $p < 0.001$), and **(F)** TMT-B ($r = 0.271$, $p = 0.021$) and negatively correlated with the **(A)** MoCA ($r = -0.323$, $p = 0.006$), **(B)** AVLT ($r = -0.262$, $p = 0.026$), and **(D)** SDMT ($r = -0.489$, $p < 0.001$). Gray curves: 95% confidence interval of the line of best fit.

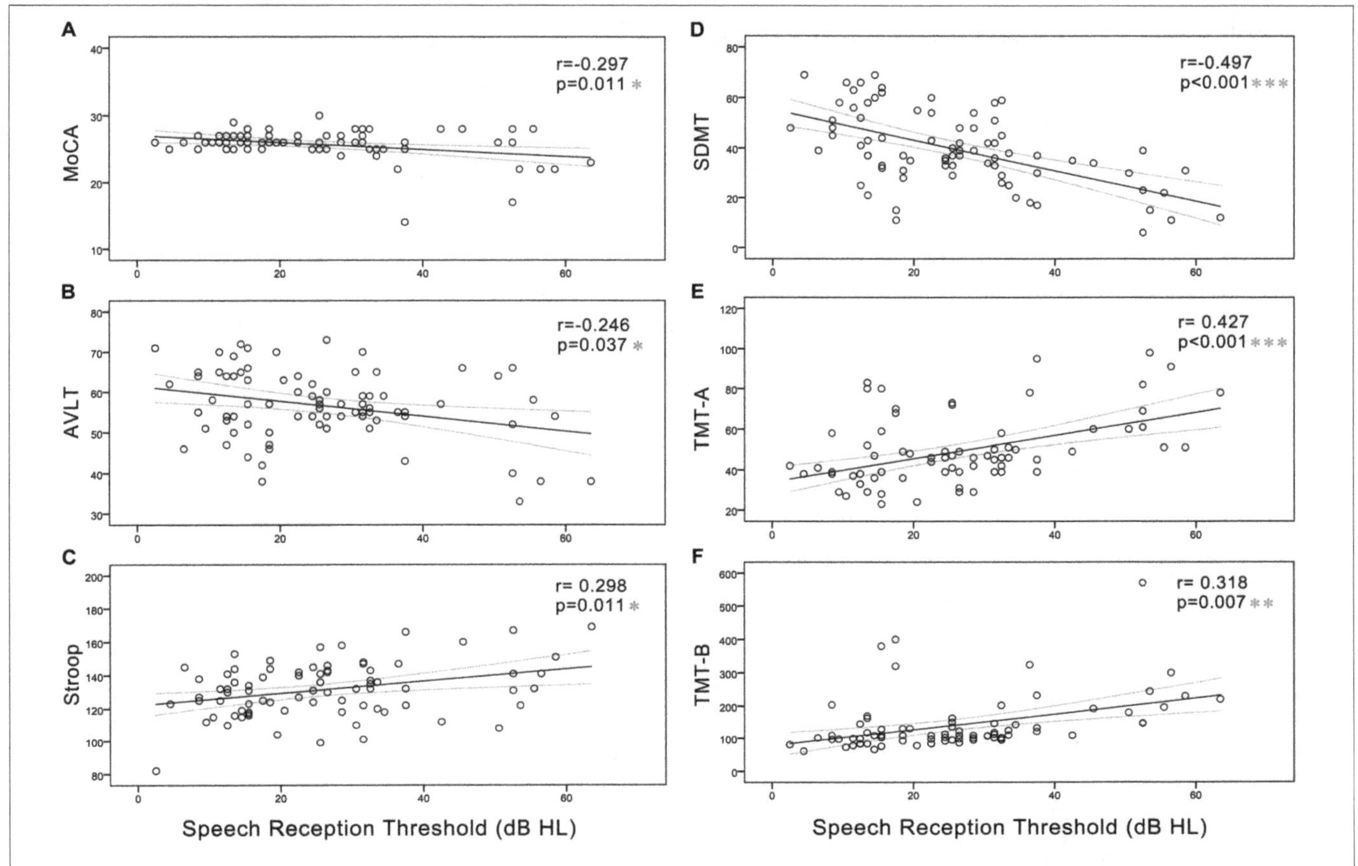

FIGURE 4 | Scatter plots displaying the correlations between SRT and cognitive function in all subjects. Partial correlation analyses (controlling for age, sex, education level, diabetes, smoking, and hypertension) revealed that SRT was positively correlated with **(C)** Stroop ($r = 0.298$, $p = 0.011$), **(E)** TMT-A ($r = 0.427$, $p < 0.001$), and **(F)** TMT-B ($r = 0.318$, $p = 0.007$) and negatively correlated with the **(A)** MoCA ($r = -0.297$, $p = 0.011$), **(B)** AVLT ($r = -0.246$, $p = 0.037$), and **(D)** SDMT ($r = -0.497$, $p < 0.001$). Gray curves: 95% confidence interval of the line of best fit.

$p = 0.038$) and negatively correlated with SDMT ($r = -0.430$, $p = 0.025$). SRT (**Figure 6**) was negatively correlated with SDMT ($r = -0.361, p = 0.033$).

In the PC group, Pearson correlation analyses revealed that PTA (**Figure 5**) was positively correlated with TMT-A ($r = 0.572$, $p < 0.001$), TMT-B ($r = 0.494$, $p < 0.001$), and negatively correlated with MoCA ($r = -0.376, p = 0.022$), AVLT ($r = -0.536$, $p < 0.001$), and SDMT ($r = -0.532, p < 0.001$). SRT (**Figure 6**) was positively correlated with TMT-A ($r = 0.585, p < 0.001$) and TMT-B ($r = 0.602$, $p < 0.001$) and negatively correlated with MoCA ($r = -0.300$, $p = 0.046$), AVLT ($r = -0.408$, $p = 0.005$), and SDMT ($r = -0.622, p < 0.001$).

Regression Analyses Between Hearing Loss and Cognitive Function (Table 3)

Stepwise Multiple Linear Regression Models were established in all subjects. However, some regression models in NP group and PC group could not be established, so were marked as N/A, presumably because of the small sample size of NP group and PC group.

In all subjects, PTA was found to be significant predictors of MoCA ($\beta = -0.050$, $R^2 = 0.345$, $p = 0.001$), AVLT ($\beta = -0.186$, $R^2 = 0.143$, $p = 0.005$), Stroop ($\beta = 0.348$, $R^2 = 0.219$, $p = 0.004$), SDMT ($\beta = -0.532$, $R^2 = 0.322$, $p < 0.001$), TMT-A ($\beta = 0.561$, $R^2 = 0.203$, $p < 0.001$), and TMT-B ($\beta = 1.611$, $R^2 = 0.220$, $p = 0.013$). SRT was found to be significant predictors of MoCA ($\beta = -0.047, R^2 = 0.336, p = 0.002$), AVLT ($\beta = -0.180, R^2 = 0.138$, $p = 0.007$), Stroop ($\beta = 0.324$, $R^2 = 0.206$, $p = 0.007$), SDMT ($\beta = -0.612$, $R^2 = 0.312$, $p < 0.001$), TMT-A ($\beta = 0.571$, $R^2 = 0.213$, $p < 0.001$), and TMT-B ($\beta = 1.851$, $R^2 = 0.219$, $p = 0.005$).

In the PC group, PTA was found to be significant predictors of MoCA ($\beta = -0.096, R^2 = 0.414, p = 0.004$), AVLT ($\beta = -0.362$, $R^2 = 0.343, p < 0.001$), SDMT ($\beta = -0.617, R^2 = 0.459, p < 0.001$), TMT-A ($\beta = 0.988, R^2 = 0.382, p < 0.001$), and TMT-B ($\beta = 4.029$, $R^2 = 0.364, p = 0.040$). SRT was found to be significant predictors of MoCA ($\beta = -0.085, R^2 = 0.434, p = 0.005$), AVLT ($\beta = -0.311$, $R^2 = 0.347, p = 0.001$), SDMT ($\beta = -0.607, R^2 = 0.507, p < 0.001$), TMT-A ($\beta = 0.870, R^2 = 0.505, p < 0.001$), and TMT-B ($\beta = 4.606$, $R^2 = 0.362, p < 0.001$).

In the NP group, PTA was found to be significant predictors of Stroop ($\beta = 1.557, R^2 = 0.129, p = 0.019$) and SDMT ($\beta = -1.687$, $R^2 = 0.128, p = 0.020$). SRT was found to be significant predictors of SDMT ($\beta = -1.268, R^2 = 0.104, p = 0.033$).

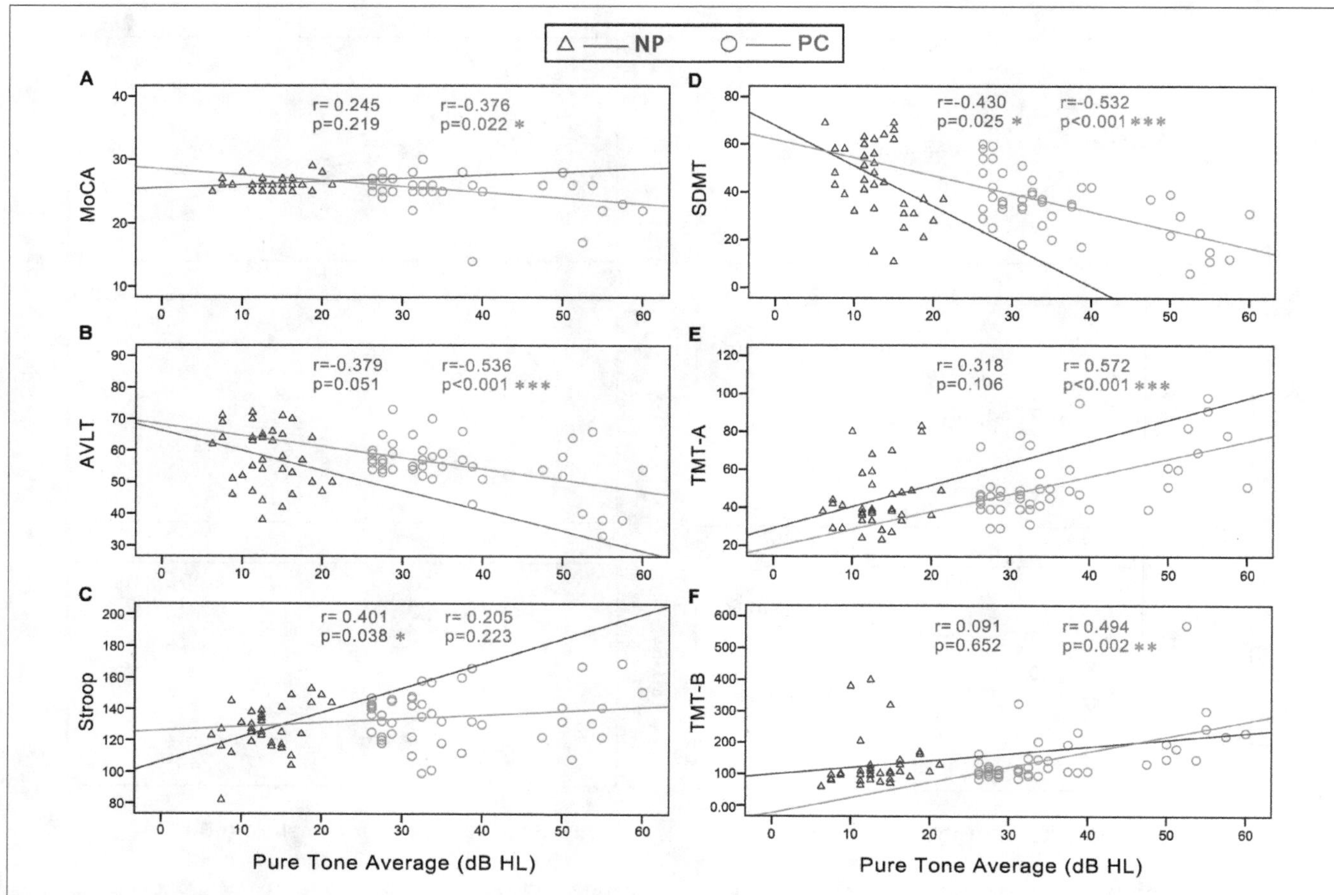

FIGURE 5 | Scatter plots displaying the correlations between PTA and cognitive function in the Normal PTA (NP) group and Presbycusis (PC) group. In the NP group, partial correlation analyses (controlling for age, sex, education level, diabetes, smoking, and hypertension) revealed that PTA was positively correlated with **(C)** Stroop ($r = 0.401$, $p = 0.038$) and negatively correlated with **(D)** SDMT ($r = -0.430$, $p = 0.025$). In the PC group, partial correlation analyses revealed that PTA was positively correlated with **(E)** TMT-A ($r = 0.572$, $p < 0.001$), and **(F)** TMT-B ($r = 0.494$, $p < 0.001$), and negatively correlated with **(A)** MoCA ($r = -0.376$, $p = 0.022$), **(B)** AVLT ($r = -0.536$, $p < 0.001$), and **(D)** SDMT ($r = -0.532$, $p < 0.001$).

DISCUSSION

The results for older adults in a Han Chinese cohort showed that cognitive function was significantly associated with PTA and SRT. In all subjects, the correlations between non-verbal cognitive scores and SRT were stronger than those between non-verbal cognitive scores and PTA, whereas, the correlations between verbal cognitive scores and PTA were stronger than those between verbal cognitive scores and SRT. Moreover, the correlations between PTA or SRT and cognitive function in the PC group were in principle stronger than those in the NP group. Additionally, there was no significant correlation between SRT and cognitive function in the NP group. To the best of our knowledge, this is the first study to elucidate the relationship between SRT and cognitive function in older adults in a Han Chinese cohort.

Previous studies of older American and Australian adults have reported significant relationships between peripheral hearing loss and global cognitive status (Lin et al., 2011a; Gopinath et al., 2012), executive function (Lin, 2011) and psychomotor speed (Lin et al., 2011a). Consistent with these findings, our study indicated, among older adults in a Han Chinese cohort, peripheral hearing, indexed by the four-frequency PTA in the better hearing ear, was significantly related to global cognitive status (MoCA) and multiple domains of cognitive performance, such as psychomotor speed (SDMT), executive function (TMT-A and TMT-B), attention (Stroop) and verbal learning and memory (AVLT). Our results were robust in analyses that accounted for confounders such as age, sex and education level. The strong connection between hearing loss and cognitive decline has been explained by a hypothesis of cognitive resource depletion in older adults (Wayne and Johnsrude, 2015). The hypothesis suggests that hearing loss can lead to increased cognitive resources for understanding acoustically degraded speech. In one functional magnetic resonance imaging study, patients with PC showed greater blood oxygen level-dependent activation responses to acoustic stimuli in the temporal lobes, demonstrating compensatory recruitment of the cortical regions involved in cognitive functions (Ouda et al., 2015). Furthermore, our results demonstrated that the correlations between multiple

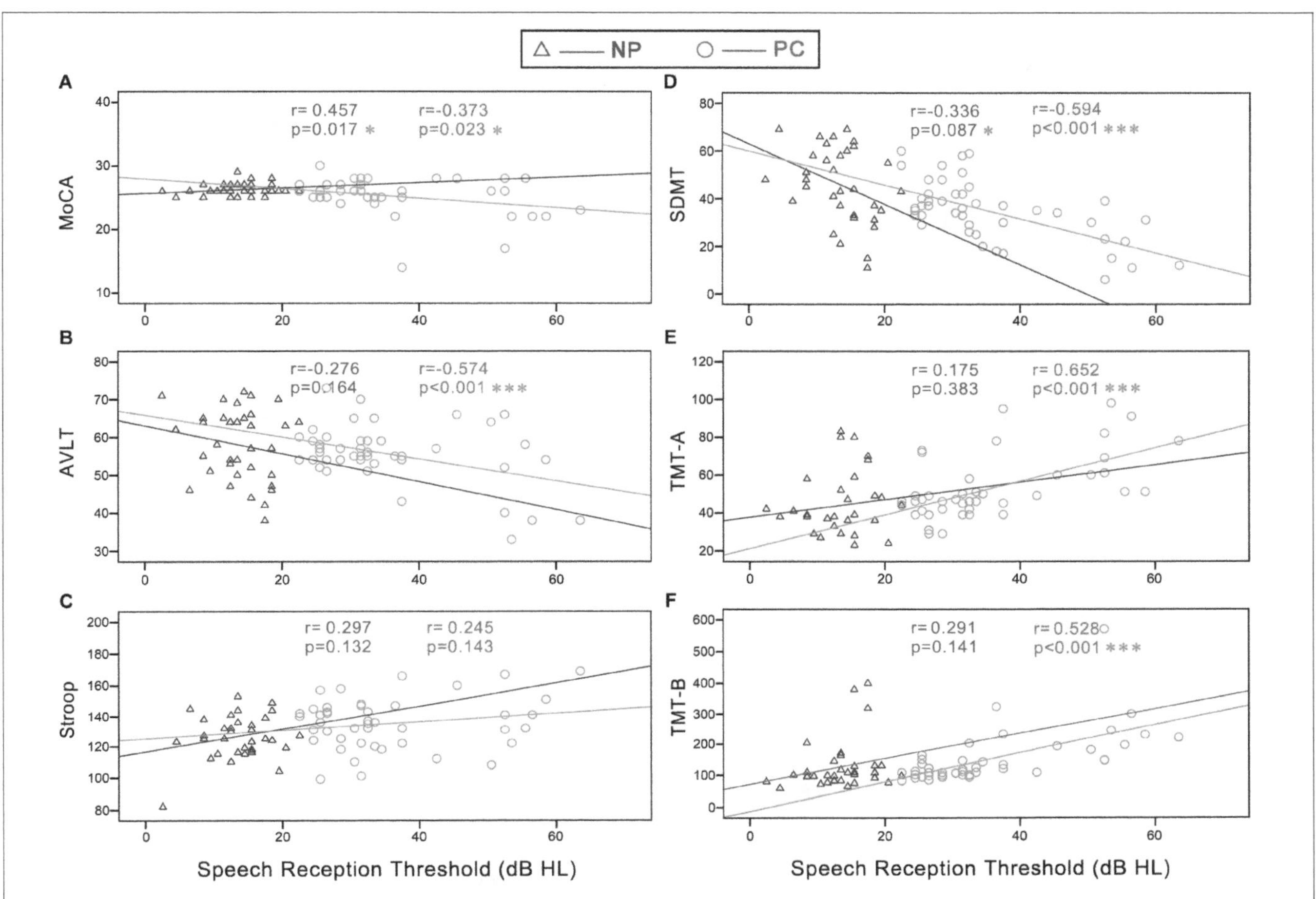

FIGURE 6 | Scatter plots displaying the correlations between SRT and cognitive function in the Normal PTA (NP) group and Presbycusis (PC) group. In the NP group, partial correlation analyses (controlling for age, sex, education level, diabetes, smoking, and hypertension) revealed that SRT was negatively correlated with **(D)** SDMT ($r = -0.361$, $p = 0.033$). In the PC group, Pearson correlation analyses revealed that SRT was positively correlated with **(E)** TMT-A ($r = 0.585$, $p < 0.001$) and **(F)** TMT-B ($r = 0.602$, $p < 0.001$) and negatively correlated with **(A)** MoCA ($r = -0.300$, $p = 0.046$), **(B)** AVLT ($r = -0.408$, $p = 0.005$) and **(D)** SDMT ($r = -0.622$, $p < 0.001$). There were no correlation between SRT and Stroop **(C)** in the NP or PC group.

domains of cognitive performance (e.g., SDMT and TMT) and hearing loss were stronger than those between global cognitive status (e.g., the MoCA) and hearing loss. Tests of multiple domains of cognitive performance are more challenging than the MoCA. Hearing loss could result in a smaller pool of cognitive resources being available for complex cognitive processes, such as psychomotor speed and executive control (Kahneman, 1973).

Pure tone average is considered to be a measure of the auditory periphery because the detection of pure tones relies on cochlear transduction and neuronal afferents to brainstem nuclei, without requiring significant higher auditory cortical processing (Pickles, 1988). It has long been accepted that PC has two components: one that represents aging of the auditory periphery, particularly the inner ear, and another related to aging of the central auditory system. Therefore, in terms of the association between hearing loss and cognitive function, we should take into account the state of both the peripheral hearing and the central auditory system. SRT is used to assess speech detection, and the SRT findings point to a central component of PC. In our study, cognitive function was significantly associated with SRT among older adults. Moreover, in all subjects, the correlations between non-verbal cognitive scores and SRT were stronger than those between non-verbal cognitive scores and PTA, whereas, the correlations between verbal cognitive scores and PTA were stronger than those between verbal cognitive scores and SRT. Therefore, our findings indicated that SRT could be an important auditory test for exploring cognitive decline in PC and could complement PTA. In addition, degraded verbal communication associated with hearing loss may confound cognitive testing. Therefore, non-verbal tests, such as the SDMT and TMT, which do not rely heavily on the presentation of verbal information, were also used in our study; furthermore, mild–moderate hearing loss minimally impairs face-to-face communication in quiet environments, particularly in the setting of testing by experienced examiners (Gordon-Salant, 2005).

Only one study has reported the relationship between SRT and cognitive function in older people (Nkyekyer et al., 2019). In that study, several cognitive domains were associated with SRT, but

TABLE 3 | Stepwise multiple linear regression models (cognitive measures as dependent variables).

Cognitive	Model I(PTA et al.* as independent variables)				Model II(SRT et al.* as independent variables)			
measures	β (95% CI)	R^2	t	p	β (95% CI)	R^2	t	p
All subjects								
MoCA	−0.050 (−0.079 − −0.021)	0.345	−3.393	0.001	−0.047 (−0.076 − −0.018)	0.336	−3.212	0.002
AVLT	−0.186 (−0.315 − −0.057)	0.143	−2.878	0.005	−0.180 (−0.308 − −0.052)	0.138	−2.792	0.007
Stroop SDMT	0.348 (0.117–0.578)	0.219	2.998	0.004	0.324 (0.091 − 0.557)	0.206	2.771	0.007
	−0.532 (−0.742 − −0.322)	0.322	−5.054	< 0.001	−0.612 (−0.813 − −0.411)	0.312	−6.067	< 0.001
TMT-A	0.561 (0.318 − 0.804)	0.203	4.599	< 0.001	0.571 (0.330 − 0.811)	0.213	4.728	< 0.001
TMT-B	1.611 (0.351 − 2.871)	0.220	2.545	0.013	1.851 (0.589 − 3.113)	0.219	2.920	0.005
PC group								
MoCA	−0.096 (−0.160 − −0.033)	0.414	−3.048	0.004	−0.085 (−0.144 − −0.027)	0.434	−2.936	0.005
AVLT	−0.362 (−0.554 − −0.171)	0.343	−3.816	< 0.001	−0.311 (−0.489 − −0.132)	0.347	−3.509	0.001
Stroop SDMT	N/A	N/A	0.919	0.364	N/A	N/A	1.423	0.162
	−0.617 (−0.917 − −0.317)	0.459	−4.154	< 0.001	−0.607 (−0.892 − −0.322)	0.507	−4.303	< 0.001
TMT-A	0.988 (0.588 − 1.388)	0.382	4.999	< 0.001	0.870 (0.529 − 1.210)	0.505	5.160	< 0.001
TMT-B	4.029 (0.260 − 10.341)	0.364	2.122	0.040	4.606 (2.726 − 6.485)	0.362	4.942	< 0.001
NP group								
MoCA	N/A	N/A	0.924	0.392	N/A	N/A	1.489	0.146
AVLT	N/A	N/A	1.098	0.280	N/A	N/A	0.874	0.389
Stroop SDMT	1.557 (0.268 − 2.847)	0.129	2.458	0.019	N/A	N/A	N/A	N/A
	−1.687 (−3.090 − −0.283)	0.128	−2.445	0.020	−1.268 (−2.430 − −0.106)	0.104	−2.221	0.033
TMT-A	N/A	N/A	N/A	N/A	N/A	N/A	N/A	N/A
TMT-B	N/A	N/A	N/A	N/A	N/A	N/A	N/A	N/A

* *Other independent variables include age, sex, education level, diabetes, smoking, and hypertension. PTA, pure tone average; SRT, speech reception threshold; PC, presbycusis; NP, normal PTA; MoCA, montreal cognitive assessment; AVLT, auditory verbal learning test; SDMT, symbol digit modalities test; TMT, trail-making test; levels of anxiety and depression were assessed according to the hospital anxiety and depression scale (HADS); N/A, not available (regression model could not be established).*

only the Stroop measure was associated with PTA. In our study, the sample size is larger than that study, and subjects were further divided into presbycusis and normal PTA groups. Moreover, a Han Chinese cohort and a different set of cognition measures were assessed in our study, and we controlled age, sex, education level and other risk factors for cognitive decline in investigating the correlations between cognition and PTA/SRT.

Despite a growing body of literature documenting significant relationships between peripheral hearing and cognition (Gordon-Salant and Fitzgibbons, 1997; Pichora-Fuller and Singh, 2006; Akeroyd, 2008; Lin, 2011; Grassi and Borella, 2013), a few studies have reported negative results (Gates et al., 2002; Idrizbegovic et al., 2011). For example, one study reported no relationship between peripheral hearing and changes in global mental status over 4 years, after adjusting for covariates (Lin et al., 2004). To determine the extent to which the inclusion of many subjects with NP diffused the effects of peripheral hearing loss on measures of cognition, we repeated our correlation analyses within the NP and PC groups. The correlations between PTA or SRT and cognitive function in the PC group were stronger than those in the NP group. Additionally, there was no significant correlation between SRT and cognitive function in the NP group. This suggests that the significant relationship found between hearing and cognition was mainly driven by the older adults with PC. Therefore, some negative results may be attributed to the inclusion of a sample of older adults with NP.

There are several limitations to the present study. First, as this was a cross-sectional study, although correlations between cognitive impairment and hearing loss were found in older adults, the causation is still unknown. Second, the sample size in the study was relatively small. Third, PTA was only measured at four frequencies in the better ear, and it is likely that many subjects would have had high-frequency sensorineural hearing loss that was not captured in our study due to the limited range of frequencies tested.

CONCLUSION

Our findings indicate that cognitive function is significantly associated with PTA and SRT in older adults in a Han Chinese cohort. Moreover, the correlations between PTA or SRT and cognitive function in the PC group were in principle stronger than those in the NP group. Based on these findings, we argue that SRT could be an important auditory test for exploring cognitive decline in PC and could complement PTA.

AUTHOR CONTRIBUTIONS

FG and HW designed the experiments. FR, JL, WM, and LX carried out the experiments. ZF, YA, and BZ analyzed the experimental results. FG and QX assisted. FR and JL wrote the manuscript.

FUNDING

This work was supported by grants from The National Natural Science Foundation of China (Nos. 81601479 and 81670932); The National 973 Basic Research Program of China (No. 2014CB541703); Shandong Provincial Key Research and Development Program of China (No. 2016GSF201090); The Taishan Scholars Project (No. tsqn201812147); Shandong Provincial Natural Science Foundation of China (Nos. ZR2016QZ007 and 2017CXGC1213); Shandong Provincial Medical and Healthy Technology Development Program of China (No. 2017WS610).

REFERENCES

Akeroyd, M. A. (2008). Are individual differences in speech reception related to individual differences in cognitive ability? A survey of twenty experimental studies with normal and hearing-impaired adults. *Int. J. Audiol.* 47(Suppl. 2), S53–S71. doi: 10.1080/14992020802301142

Galea, M., and Woodward, M. (2005). Mini-mental state examination (MMSE). *Aust. J. Physiother.* 51:198. doi: 10.1016/s0004-9514(05)70034-9

Gates, G. A., Beiser, A., Rees, T. S., D'agostino, R. B., and Wolf, P. A. (2002). Central auditory dysfunction may precede the onset of clinical dementia in people with probable Alzheimer's disease. *J. Am. Geriatr. Soc.* 50, 482–488. doi: 10.1046/j.1532-5415.2002.50114.x

Gates, G. A., and Mills, J. H. (2005). Presbycusis. *Lancet* 366, 1111–1120. doi: 10.1016/s0140-6736(05)67423-5

Gopinath, B., Schneider, J., McMahon, C. M., Teber, E., Leeder, S. R., and Mitchell, P. (2012). Severity of age-related hearing loss is associated with impaired activities of daily living. *Age Ageing* 41, 195–200. doi: 10.1093/ageing/afr155

Gordon-Salant, S. (2005). Hearing loss and aging: new research findings and clinical implications. *J. Rehabil. Res. Dev.* 42(4 Suppl. 2), 9–24.

Gordon-Salant, S., and Fitzgibbons, P. J. (1997). Selected cognitive factors and speech recognition performance among young and elderly listeners. *J. Speech Lang. Hear. Res.* 40, 423–431. doi: 10.1044/jslhr.4002.423

Grassi, M., and Borella, E. (2013). The role of auditory abilities in basic mechanisms of cognition in older adults. *Front. Aging Neurosci.* 5:59. doi: 10.3389/fnagi.2013.00059

Idrizbegovic, E., Hederstierna, C., Dahlquist, M., Kampfe Nordstrom, C., Jelic, V., and Rosenhall, U. (2011). Central auditory function in early Alzheimer's disease and in mild cognitive impairment. *Age Ageing* 40, 249–254. doi: 10.1093/ageing/afq168

Jayakody, D. M., Friedland, P. L., Martins, R. N., and Sohrabi, H. R. (2018). Impact of aging on the auditory system and related cognitive functions: a narrative review. *Front. Neurosci.* 12:125. doi: 10.3389/fnins.2018.00125

Kahneman, D. (1973). *Attention and Effort*. Princeton, NJ: Citeseer.

Lin, F. R. (2011). Hearing loss and cognition among older adults in the United States. *J. Gerontol. A Biol. Sci. Med. Sci.* 66, 1131–1136. doi: 10.1093/gerona/glr115

Lin, F. R., Ferrucci, L., Metter, E. J., An, Y., Zonderman, A. B., and Resnick, S. M. (2011a). Hearing loss and cognition in the baltimore longitudinal study of aging. *Neuropsychology* 25, 763–770. doi: 10.1037/a0024238

Lin, F. R., Metter, E. J., O'Brien, R. J., Resnick, S. M., Zonderman, A. B., and Ferrucci, L. (2011b). Hearing loss and incident dementia. *Arch. Neurol.* 68, 214–220. doi: 10.1001/archneurol.2010.362

Lin, F. R., Thorpe, R., Gordon-Salant, S., and Ferrucci, L. (2011c). Hearing loss prevalence and risk factors among older adults in the United States. *J. Gerontol. A Biol. Sci. Med. Sci.* 66, 582–590. doi: 10.1093/gerona/glr002

Lin, M. Y., Gutierrez, P. R., Stone, K. L., Yaffe, K., Ensrud, K. E., Fink, H. A., et al. (2004). Vision impairment and combined vision and hearing impairment predict cognitive and functional decline in older women. *J. Am. Geriatr. Soc.* 52, 1996–2002. doi: 10.1111/j.1532-5415.2004.52554.x

Lu, J., Guo, Q. H., and Hong, Z. (2006). Trail making test used by Chinese elderly patients with mild cognitive impairment and mild Alzheimer dementia. *Chinese J. Clin. Psychol.* 14, 118–121.

Luo, H., Yang, T., Jin, X., Pang, X., Li, J., Chai, Y., et al. (2013). Association of GRM7 variants with different phenotype patterns of age-related hearing impairment in an elderly male han chinese population. *PLoS One* 8:e77153. doi: 10.1371/journal.pone.0077153

Mazelova, J., Popelar, J., and Syka, J. (2003). Auditory function in presbycusis: peripheral vs. central changes. *Exp. Gerontol.* 38, 87–94. doi: 10.1016/s0531-5565(02)00155-9

Nash, S. D., Cruickshanks, K. J., Klein, R., Klein, B. E., Nieto, F. J., Huang, G. H., et al. (2011). The prevalence of hearing impairment and associated risk factors: the beaver dam offspring study. *Arch. Otolaryngol. Head Neck Surg.* 137, 432–439. doi: 10.1001/archoto.2011.15

Nasreddine, Z. S., Phillips, N. A., Bedirian, V., Charbonneau, S., Whitehead, V., Collin, I., et al. (2005). The montreal cognitive assessment, MoCA: a brief screening tool for mild cognitive impairment. *J. Am. Geriatr. Soc.* 53, 695–699. doi: 10.1111/j.1532-5415.2005.53221.x

Nkyekyer, J., Meyer, D., Pipingas, A., and Reed, N. S. (2019). The cognitive and psychosocial effects of auditory training and hearing aids in adults with hearing loss. *Clin. Interv. Aging* 14, 123–135. doi: 10.2147/CIA.S183905

Ouda, L., Profant, O., and Syka, J. (2015). Age-related changes in the central auditory system. *Cell Tissue Res.* 361, 337–358. doi: 10.1007/s00441-014-2107-2

Pichora-Fuller, M. K., and Singh, G. (2006). Effects of age on auditory and cognitive processing: implications for hearing aid fitting and audiologic rehabilitation. *Trends Amplif.* 10, 29–59. doi: 10.1177/108471380601000103

Pickles, J. O. (1988). *An Introduction to the Physiology of Hearing*. London: Academic press.

Quaranta, N., Coppola, F., Casulli, M., Barulli, M. R., Panza, F., Tortelli, R., et al. (2014). The prevalence of peripheral and central hearing impairment and its relation to cognition in older adults. *Audiol. Neurootol.* 19(Suppl. 1), 10–14. doi: 10.1159/000371597

Sanchez-Cubillo, I., Perianez, J., Adrover-Roig, D., Rodriguez-Sanchez, J., Rios-Lago, M., Tirapu, J., et al. (2009). Construct validity of the trail making test: role of task-switching, working memory, inhibition/interference control, and visuomotor abilities. *J. Int. Neuropsychol. Soc.* 15, 438–450. doi: 10.1017/S1355617709090626

Savitz, J. B., and Jansen, P. (2003). The stroop color-word interference test as an indicator of ADHD in poor readers. *J. Genet. Psychol.* 164, 319–333. doi: 10.1080/00221320309597986

Schuknecht, H. F., and Gacek, M. R. (1993). Cochlear pathology in presbycusis. *Ann. Otol. Rhinol. Laryngol.* 102, 1–16. doi: 10.1177/00034894931020s101

Van Schependom, J., D'hooghe, M., Cleynhens, K., D'hooge, M., Haelewyck, M., De Keyser, J., et al. (2014). The symbol D igit M odalities T est as sentinel test for cognitive impairment in multiple sclerosis. *Eur. J. Neurol.* 21:1219-e72. doi: 10.1111/ene.12463

Wayne, R. V., and Johnsrude, I. S. (2015). A review of causal mechanisms underlying the link between age-related hearing loss and cognitive decline. *Ageing Res. Rev.* 23(Pt B), 154–166. doi: 10.1016/j.arr.2015.06.002

Wei, M., Shi, J., Li, T., Ni, J., Zhang, X., Li, Y., et al. (2018). Diagnostic accuracy of the chinese version of the trail-making test for screening cognitive impairment. *J. Am. Geriatr. Soc.* 66, 92–99. doi: 10.1111/jgs.15135

World Health Organization [WHO] (2018). *World Health Statistics*. Geneva: World Health Organization.

Zhao, Q., Lv, Y., Zhou, Y., Hong, Z., and Guo, Q. (2012). Short-term delayed recall of auditory verbal learning test is equivalent to long-term delayed recall for identifying amnestic mild cognitive impairment. *PLoS One* 7:e51157. doi: 10.1371/journal.pone.0051157

Zigmond, A. S., and Snaith, R. P. (1983). The hospital anxiety and depression scale. *Acta Psychiatr. Scand.* 67, 361–370.

20

Detection of BDNF-Related Proteins in Human Perilymph in Patients with Hearing Loss

Ines de Vries[1†], Heike Schmitt[1,2†], Thomas Lenarz[1,2], Nils Prenzler[1], Sameer Alvi[3], Hinrich Staecker[3], Martin Durisin[1†] and Athanasia Warnecke[1,2†]*

[1] Department of Otolaryngology, Hannover Medical School, Hanover, Germany, [2] Cluster of Excellence Hearing4all, German Research Foundation, Hannover Medical School, Hanover, Germany, [3] Department of Otolaryngology, Head and Neck Surgery, University of Kansas School of Medicine, Kansas City, MO, United States

***Correspondence:**
Athanasia Warnecke
warnecke.athanasia@mh-hannover.de

† These authors have contributed equally to this work

The outcome of cochlear implantation depends on multiple variables including the underlying health of the cochlea. Brain derived neurotrophic factor (BDNF) has been shown to support spiral ganglion neurons and to improve implant function in animal models. Whether endogenous BDNF or BDNF-regulated proteins can be used as biomarkers to predict cochlear health and implant outcome has not been investigated yet. Gene expression of BDNF and downstream signaling molecules were identified in tissue of human cochleae obtained from normal hearing patients (n = 3) during skull base surgeries. Based on the gene expression data, bioinformatic analysis was utilized to predict the regulation of proteins by BDNF. The presence of proteins corresponding to these genes was investigated in perilymph (n = 41) obtained from hearing-impaired patients (n = 38) during cochlear implantation or skull base surgery for removal of vestibular schwannoma by nanoscale liquid chromatography coupled to tandem mass spectrometry (nano LC-MS/MS). Analyzed by mass spectrometry were 41 perilymph samples despite three patients undergoing bilateral cochlear implantation. These particular BDNF regulated proteins were not detectable in any of the perilymph samples. Subsequently, targeted analysis of the perilymph proteome data with Ingenuity Pathway Analysis (IPA) identified further proteins in human perilymph that could be regulated by BDNF. These BDNF regulated proteins were correlated to the presence of residual hearing (RH) prior to implantation and to the performance data with the cochlear implant after 1 year. There was overall a decreased level of expression of BDNF-regulated proteins in profoundly hearing-impaired patients compared to patients with some RH. Phospholipid transfer protein was positively correlated to the preoperative hearing level of the patients. Our data show that combination of gene expression arrays and bioinformatic analysis can aid in the prediction of downstream signaling proteins related to the BDNF pathway. Proteomic analysis of perilymph may help to identify the presence or absence of these molecules in the diseased organ. The impact of such prediction algorithms on diagnosis and treatment needs to be established in further studies.

Keywords: inner ear, perilymph, BDNF, neurotrophin, bioinformatic analysis, proteomics, diagnostics, cochlear implant

INTRODUCTION

One of the challenges in cochlear implantation is to understand the wide variability in performance amongst users. Candidates with similar history and implanted with the same device can demonstrate outcomes on both ends of the spectrum (Carlson et al., 2012). A plethora of factors may contribute to the variance in speech perception including age, duration of deafness, genetics, surgical technique and device characteristics, neuronal survival, electrode position, or central processing abilities (Carlson et al., 2012; Causon et al., 2015; Kral et al., 2016; Shearer et al., 2017). Since human temporal bone studies have recently shown a link between spiral ganglion population and cochlear implant outcomes (Seyyedi et al., 2014), one of the research targets is to maintain the viable population of spiral ganglion neurons for stimulation. Objective measures of cochlear function also suggest that a healthier neuronal population may result in better speech outcomes (Kim et al., 2010). This raises the possibility of modulating spiral ganglion function and health through drug delivery to the inner ear in conjunction with cochlear implantation.

Neurotrophins are the most promising candidates to support the auditory nerve by increasing neuronal survival. Within the murine inner ear, BDNF and NT-3 seem to regulate the connection of hair cells and neurons (Pirvola et al., 1992, 1997; Flores-Otero and Davis, 2011) and to support the survival and synaptic integrity of the auditory nerve (Mellado Lagarde et al., 2013). Damage to the organ of Corti is thought to result in loss of neurotrophin production and secondary degeneration of the spiral ganglion (Lawner et al., 1997; Staecker and Garnham, 2010). In a number of animal models, the delivery of various growth factors to the cochlea has resulted in increased preservation of neurons, re-growth of peripheral processes, and reduction of the threshold of electrical stimulation, suggesting that combining delivery of neurotrophins or neurotrophin mimetics may improve cochlear implant function (Evans et al., 2009; Wan et al., 2014; Budenz et al., 2015; Ramekers et al., 2015; Wise et al., 2016; Pfingst et al., 2017). Pathway analysis suggests that alterations in neurotrophin signaling should result in a broad range of physiologic changes in the cochlea. BDNF in particular appears to play an important role in both the peripheral and central auditory system (Singer et al., 2014). Despite the vast number of preclinical data concerning BDNF and cochlear health, nothing is known hitherto for the human auditory system. Interestingly, prior evaluations to the proteome of human perilymph (Schmitt et al., 2017) did not detect endogenous BDNF. The raw data of all detected proteins in perilymph by mass spectrometry in detail can be perused in the supplementary material of this prior study (Schmitt et al., 2017).

In order to determine whether BDNF and its regulated proteins are expressed in the adult human cochlea, we performed gene array analysis on human cochlear tissue. The results obtained from gene expression analysis were correlated with the previous reported proteome data of human perilymph samples (Schmitt et al., 2017). Based on the neurotrophin hypothesis, we assumed that patients without any RH would demonstrate altered neurotrophin signaling when compared to patients with RH and this would be reflected on the individual proteomic profiles of the perilymph. To evaluate this, we correlated the presence of BDNF-regulated proteins to preoperative hearing levels and postoperative cochlear implant performance data of the patients.

Abbreviations: BDNF, brain derived neurotrophic factor; CDC42, cell division control protein 42 homolog; CID, collision-induced dissociation; CSF, cerebrospinal fluid; GFAP, glial fibrillary acidic protein; GOA, gene ontology annotations; HSP 90, heat shock protein 90; HTA, human transcriptome array; ID, inner diameter; IPA, Ingenuity Pathway Analysis; IRB, Institutional Review Board; LTQ, linear trap quadrupole; NCAM1, neural cell adhesion molecule 1; NELL2, neural tissue-specific epidermal growth factor-like repeat domain-containing protein; LFQ, label free quantification; NH, no hearing; NT-3, neurotrophin 3; p75NTR, p75 neurotrophin receptor; PI3K, phosphoinositide 3-kinase; PTA, pure tone average; RAS, rat sarcoma; RH, residual hearing; TdT, terminal deoxynucleotidyltransferase; Trk, receptor tyrosine kinase.

MATERIALS AND METHODS

Perilymph and Cochlear Tissue Sampling

Collection of human cochlear tissue for gene array analysis was approved by the University of Kansas School of Medicine Institutional Review Board. Cochleae from three patients with normal hearing were obtained during a transcochlear approach to the posterior fossa for removal of meningioma and analyzed for growth factor gene expression.

Human perilymph was collected with a modified micro glass capillary during inner ear surgeries from 38 patients including three patients undergoing a bilateral cochlear implantation (37 perilymph samples during cochlear implantations and 4 during vestibular schwannoma surgeries) as already described in our previous study (Schmitt et al., 2017). The present study is an extension of a previous study (Schmitt et al., 2017). The data were analyzed with regard to pre-implantation hearing thresholds and cochlear implantation outcome. Patients aged 9 months up to 80 years with different etiologies for sensorineural hearing loss (e.g., Menière's disease, connatal cytomegalovirus infection, large vestibular aqueduct, CHARGE syndrome, meningitis, and auditory neuropathy) were included in this study. In addition, included patients were implanted with different cochlear implant devices and electrode arrays. A short version of the demographic data of the 38 patients undergoing cochlear implantation with perilymph sampling is depicted in **Table 1**. Detailed information about the individual patients is presented in the supporting information (**Supplementary Table S1**). The perilymph samples were obtained by puncturing of the round window membrane directly before the insertion of a cochlear implant electrode array. Protocols for collection of specimens were approved by the Ethics Committee of Hannover Medical School for perilymph by cochlear implantation (approval no. 1883-2013) and for perilymph during translabyrinthal vestibular schwannoma surgeries (approval no. 2403-2014).

Written informed consent was obtained from every patient included in this study.

Genomic Evaluation

Tissue of the cochleae from three patients with normal hearing, undergoing a transcochlear approach to the posterior fossa

TABLE 1 | Demographic data of the 41 patients undergoing CI surgery with perilymph sampling.

Demographic data	Age (mean in years)	n* (%)
Patients	44.4	41 (100)
Male	44.3	23 (56.1)
Female	44.7	18 (43.9)
No hearing (NH)	36.5	27 (65.9)
Residual hearing (RH)	59.8	14 (34.1)
Children (0–18 years)	2.7	12 (29.3)
Adults (19–80)	61.7	29 (70.7)

**Bilateral samples of patients (n = 3) counted as two individual patients.*

for removal of meningioma were analyzed for growth factor gene expression. The lateral wall, basilar membrane and a portion of the modiolus were removed with an alligator forceps and immediately placed in RNAlater (Qiagen, cat #76104). Total RNA was extracted with Trizol reagent (Thermo Fisher Scientific, cat #15596018) and purified by centrifuging with phase lock heavy gel (Tiagen, cat # WMS-2302830). RNA was analyzed using the Agilent RNA6000 Pico kit in an Agilent Bioanalyzer 2100 to identify RNA degradation if present. Using an Affymetrix GeneChip WT Pico labeling kit, 50 ng of total RNA was TdT end labeled with biotin and hybridized on an Affymetrix HTA 2.0 array. After washing and staining, the chip was read with an Affymetrix GeneChip Scanner 3000 7G using a single scan with default normalization. Expression of genes present at 2 logs over baseline was evaluated. Data (genomic and proteomic) were uploaded into IPA software (Qiagen Bioinformatics) and evaluated based on the effects of varying expression of BDNF. Some proteins were subjected to classification by GOA using *UniProt* (UniProt Consortium, 2015).

Proteomic Analysis

In a prior study, intraoperative perilymph sampling method and analysis by an in depth shot gun proteomics approach were established allowing the analysis of hundreds of proteins simultaneously in very small sample sizes in a microliters range (Schmitt et al., 2017). Perilymph samples were prepared for LC-MS/MS analysis by alkylation and separated using sodium dodecyl sulfate polyacrylamide gel electrophoresis as previously described (Schmitt et al., 2017). Peptide samples were separated with a nano-flow ultra-high pressure liquid chromatography system (RSLC, Thermo Fisher Scientific) equipped with a trapping column (3 μm C18 particle, 2 cm length, 75 μm ID, Acclaim PepMap, Thermo Fisher Scientific) and a 50 cm long separation column (2 μm C18 particle, 75 μm ID, Acclaim PepMap, Thermo Fisher Scientific). The RSLC system was coupled online via a Nano Spray Flex Ion Source II (Thermo Fisher Scientific) to an LTQ-Orbitrap Velos mass spectrometer. Metal-coated fused-silica emitters (SilicaTip, 10 μm i.d., New Objectives) and a voltage of 1.3 kV were used for the electrospray. Overview scans were acquired at a resolution of 60 k in a mass range of m/z 300–1600 in the orbitrap analyzer and stored in profile mode. The top 10 most intensive ions of charges two or three and a minimum intensity of 2000 counts were selected for CID fragmentation with a normalized collision energy of 38.0, an activation time of 10 ms and an activation Q of 0.250 in the LTQ. Fragment ion mass spectra were recorded in the LTQ at normal scan rate and stored as centroid m/z value and intensity pairs. Active exclusion was activated so that ions fragmented once were excluded from further fragmentation for 70 s within a mass window of 10 ppm of the specific m/z value. The relative protein quantification was performed by LFQ and was determined as LFQ intensity (Schmitt et al., 2017, 2018).

Additionally, proteins were subjected to classification by GOA using *UniProt* (UniProt Consortium, 2015). The Gene Ontology (GO) classification allows a mapping of the proteins into the categories *molecular function*, *biological process*, and *cellular compartment*. Proteins were described using a standardized vocabulary of the *UniProt* Knowledgebase by uploading the UniProt IDs of the proteins to the *UniProt* website http:/www.uniprot.org.

Audiology: Classification of Patients by Audiogram Data

Before surgery and perilymph sampling, pure tone audiometry was performed using a calibrated audiometer according to DIN EN 60318 to detect the acoustic hearing threshold. The test method follows DIN ISO 8253 with headphones for air conduction and headset for bone conduction in both ears. The PTA was analyzed for the frequency region of 500, 1000, and 2000 Hz. This classification was used for a direct correlation of the hearing loss of patients with LFQ intensity of detected proteins.

For the classification of severity of hearing loss in decibels (dB) and percent hearing impairment, a previously described method was used (Shearer et al., 1993). Therefore, the PTA was calculated for the frequency region of 500, 1000, 2000, and 3000 Hz. To obtain an ear-specific level, 25 dB was subtracted from this PTA and multiplied by the factor 1.5. This method includes a broader range of frequency values and allows a more precise classification of severity of hearing loss, especially in our cochlear implant patients with severe hearing loss in the low frequency area. The preoperative audiograms were used to assign patients to one of the two groups:

No hearing: PTA threshold of 91 dB or higher, 100% hearing impairment, $n = 27$ ears.

Residual hearing: PTA threshold of less than 91 dB, some RH, $n = 14$ ears.

Additionally, the postoperative hearing performance with a cochlear implant 1 year after implantation of the 38 patients with perilymph sampling was analyzed. Therefore, data of three audiologic tests (HSM sentence test in quiet and in noise at 10 dB, Freiburg monosyllable word test) 1 year after implantation were included. From the 29 adult patients, the majority of the patients participated in the three tests: HSM sentence test in quiet ($n = 15$), HSM sentence test in noise 10 dB ($n = 20$), Freiburg monosyllable word test ($n = 22$). For children, these types of tests were not applicable.

Statistical Analysis

Mass spectrometric raw data were processed using Max Quant software (version 1.4) and human entries of Swissprot/UniProt database. The threshold for protein identification was set to 0.01 on peptide and protein level.

Data were evaluated with multiple correlation analysis, or generation of heat maps and analysis with Fisher's exact test (Graph Pad Prism V 7). Significance was set at $p < 0.05$.

RESULTS

BDNF and TrkB Are Expressed in the Normal Hearing Human Cochlea

There is only very limited data on neurotrophin signaling in the adult human cochlea. Expression of BDNF mRNA and associated signaling molecules were determined by evaluating cochlear cDNA libraries from patients with normal hearing undergoing surgical removal of rare meningiomas anterior to the brainstem via a transcochlear approach. In these surgeries, hearing was sacrificed to gain better access to the tumor and thus also to the normal hearing cochlea.

Both BDNF and the TrkB receptor were expressed in all three specimens. The array did not differentiate between transcript variants. The low affinity p75NTR was also detectable in all three specimens. To determine the biologically significant pathways regulated by BDNF in the cochlea, we determined which components of neurotrophin signaling were present at a high level in the normal inner ear. As depicted in **Figure 1**, there is a high level of expression of the Ras/ERK pathway members and of CREB. These pathways are not only specific to neurotrophin signaling but may provide targets for pharmacological intervention for experimental or therapeutic purposes.

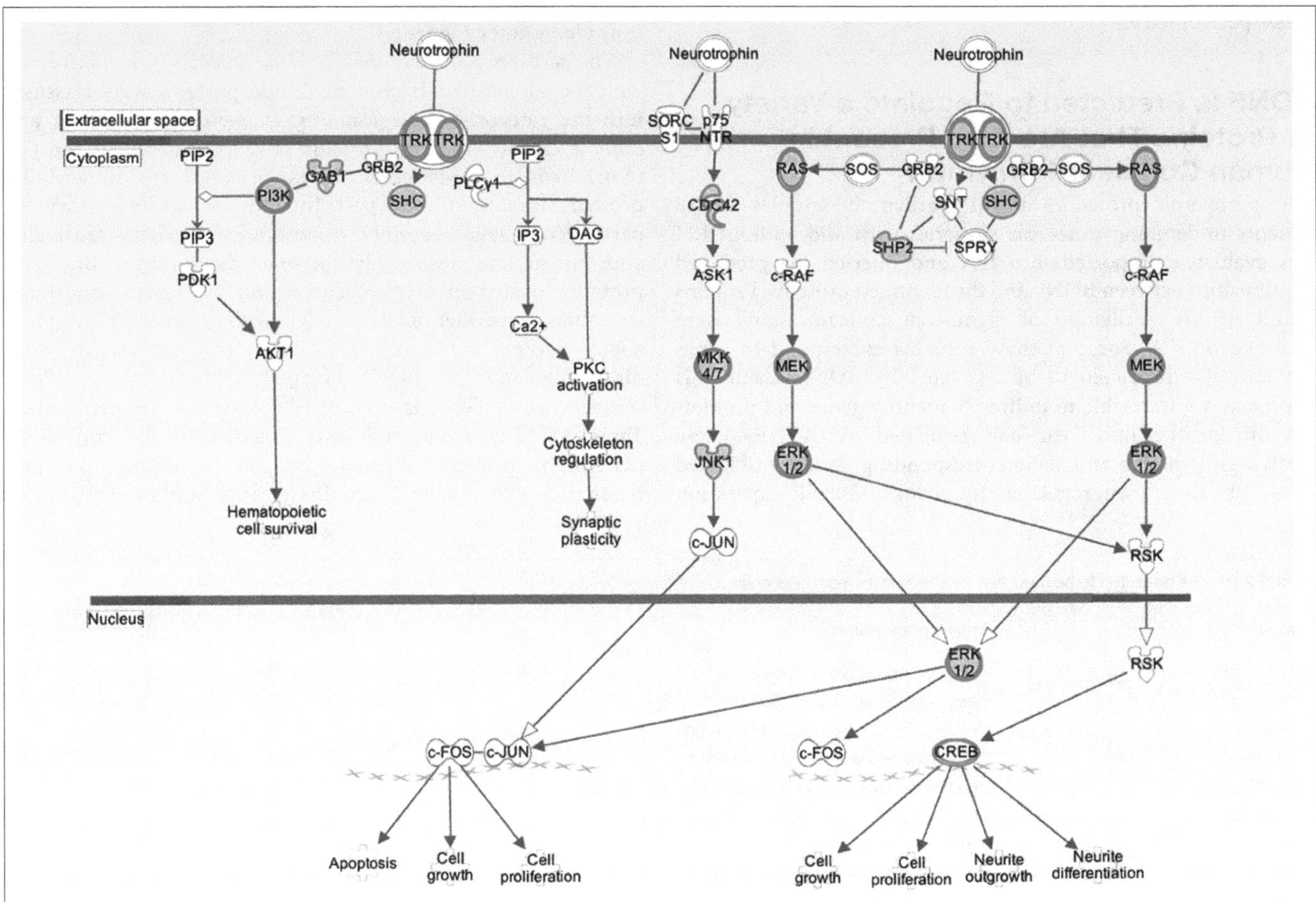

FIGURE 1 | Analysis of human inner ear transcriptome over-layed on a generic human neurotrophin signaling pathway. Purple/gray proteins represent gene products/proteins identified at 10 log folds expression over baseline in the cochlear transcriptome. This suggests that those particular signaling pathways play an active role in the inner ear. Both the high affinity Trk receptor which is found in the spiral ganglion and the low affinity p75NTR which is thought to be in Schwann and glial cells are represented. p75NTR was detectable at 2 log fold expression over baseline expression. The downstream signaling genes were expressed at significantly higher levels.

BDNF Is Predicted to Regulate a Variety of Genes Involved in Neuronal Health in the Human Cochlea

Ingenuity Pathway Analysis software was used to identify pathways related to BDNF signaling that are expressed in all 3 cDNA samples from the normal hearing patients described above at 10-fold higher levels than baseline gene expression levels. In addition, the same software was used to identify the expression of genes in the normal cochlea that are predicted to be regulated by BDNF. A range of proteins, many of which have not been evaluated for their effect on hearing and cochlear biology, have been predicted by the IPA Knowledgebase (**Table 2**). Functions of these genes include microtubule assembly, synaptic vesicle trafficking, protein folding, DNA binding, transcriptional regulation, actin binding, axonogenesis, myelination, ribosomal function, and differentiation. Proteins corresponding to the genes from the cochlear cDNA library (results from mRNA analysis) that were predicted to be regulated by BDNF were not found in the perilymph samples analyzed by mass spectrometry.

BDNF Is Predicted to Regulate a Variety of Proteins That Are Also Present in Human Cochlear Perilymph

The perilymph proteome in 41 perilymph samples of 38 patients undergoing inner ear surgeries with and without RH was evaluated, imported into IPA and queried for predicted relationships between BDNF and the identified proteins. Proteins found in the perilymph at significant concentrations were analyzed by IPA. Some of these proteins correspond to genes that are also predicted to be regulated by BDNF. Using this approach, we were able to indirectly identify genes and proteins relevant to the inner ear and regulated by BDNF. These perilymph proteins and their corresponding genes anticipated to be up and down regulated by reduced BDNF expression and proteins that are predicted to be regulated by reduced BDNF but with no information about the direction of regulation are summarized in **Table 3**. The proteins in **Table 3** are ranked by the occurrence of the protein in perilymph samples of the patients within the three subgroups (downregulated, upregulated, with no information about regulation). Proteins were not detected in every perilymph sample. Proteins listed above in the subgroups have less abundance in the samples of the patients, meaning the proteins are detected in a low number of samples. However, the proteins at the bottom of the subgroup lists are detected in many samples of our patient cohort. Depicted in **Supplementary Figure S1** are the proteins detected in % of the patients. In conclusion, these 41 proteins of the 878 previously determined proteins present in perilymph (Schmitt et al., 2017) were identified in the IPA Knowledgebase as being regulated by BDNF (**Table 3**). There was a wide range of expression profile for the different proteins in different patients with some proteins being expressed in only a few of patients and others being found in every patient, depicted in the supporting information (**Supplementary Figure S1**).

For a more detailed view, GOA analysis was performed with the 41 perilymph proteins. These proteins were classified into the categories *biological process*, *molecular function*, and *cellular component*. The proteins were considered in the GO terms *cellular components*. Most proteins are intracellular proteins located in cell part (mainly intracellular organelle parts), organelle (mainly membrane-bounded organelle), and membrane (especially plasma membrane). But also proteins located in extracellular region part like extracellular exosomes were identified. A table with detailed information about proteins detected in >80% of patients or with direct regulation by BDNF mapped to the category *cellular components* by GOA is exemplarily shown in **Supplementary Table S2**. The main *molecular function* of the considered perilymph proteins depicts besides molecular function regulation and catalytic activity clearly binding with focus

TABLE 2 | Genes predicted to be regulated by BDNF in the normal cochlea.

Symbol	Entrez gene name	Location
ATAT1	Alpha tubulin acetyltransferase 1	Cytoplasm
BDNF	Brain derived neurotrophic factor	Extracellular space
C5orf34	Chromosome 5 open reading frame 34	Other
CADPS2	Calcium dependent secretion activator 2	Plasma membrane
DNAJC21	DnaJ heat shock protein family (Hsp40) member C21	Other
HIST1H2AL	Histone cluster 1H2A family member I	Nucleus
ITIH3	Inter-alpha-trypsin inhibitor heavy chain 3	Extracellular space
MALAT1	Metastasis associated lung adenocarcinoma transcript 1 (non-protein coding)	Nucleus
MYH8	Myosin heavy chain 8	Cytoplasm
OMG	Oligodendrocyte myelin glycoprotein	Plasma membrane
PRSS12	Protease, serine 12	Extracellular space
RPL35A	Ribosomal protein L35a	Cytoplasm
SEMA3E	Semaphorin 3E	Extracellular space
SLC16A7	Solute carrier family 16 member 7	Plasma membrane
TMEM45A	Transmembrane protein 45A	Plasma membrane

TABLE 3 | Perilymph proteins and corresponding abbreviations (gene names) and Uniprot IDs anticipated to be up and down regulated and with no information about regulation by simulation that cochlear BDNF is reduced.

Downregulated	**Symbol**	**Uniprot ID**
Neurexin-1 beta	*NRXN1*	F8WB18
Cell division control protein 42 homolog	*CDC42*	P60953
Ubiquitin carboxyl-terminal hydrolase isozyme L1	*UCHL1*	D6RE83
Myelin proteolipid protein	*PLP1*	P60201
Myelin basic protein	*MBP*	E9PMR5
Ryanodine receptor 3	*RYR3*	Q15413
14-3-3 protein gamma	*YWHAG*	P61981
Ryanodine receptor 2	*RYR2*	H7BY35
Osteopontin	*SPP1*	P10451
Protein kinase C-binding protein NELL2	*NELL2*	F8VVB6
Heat shock protein HSP 90-alpha	*HSP90AA1*	P07900
Neural cell adhesion molecule 1	*NCAM1*	Q92823
Glial fibrillary acidic protein	*GFAP*	P14136
Upregulated		
Tripeptidyl-peptidase 1	*TPP1*	O14773
Laminin subunit gamma-1	*LAMC1*	P11047
Dihydropyrimidinase-related protein 2	*DPYSL2*	Q16555
Reelin	*RELN*	P78509
Ferritin light chain	*FTL*	P02792
Plexin-B2	*PLXNB2*	O15031
Agrin	*AGRN*	O00468
Annexin A5	*ANXA5*	P08758
Filamin-B	*FLNB*	O75369
Ribonuclease inhibitor	*RNH1*	P13489
Filamin-A	*FLNA*	Q5HY54
78 kDa glucose-regulated protein	*HSPA5*	P11021
Neutrophil gelatinase-associated lipocalin	*LCN2*	P80188
Annexin A2	*ANXA2*	P07355
Phospholipid transfer protein	*PLTP*	P55058
Vimentin	*VIM*	P08670
No information about regulation		
Gamma-secretase C-terminal fragment 59 (Amyloid beta A4 protein)	*APP*	E9PG40
Carboxypeptidase E	*CPE*	P16870
Chromogranin-A	*CHGA*	P10645
Glutamine synthetase	*GLUL*	P15104
Inter-alpha-trypsin inhibitor heavy chain H3	*ITIH3*	Q06033
Vasorin	*VASN*	Q6EMK4
Protein S100-A9	*S100A9*	P06702
Fibrinogen beta chain	*FGB*	P02675
Plasminogen	*PLG*	P00747
Actin, cytoplasmic 1	*ACTB*	P60709
Apolipoprotein E	*APOE*	P02649
Alpha-2-macroglobulin	*A2M*	P01023

on protein and ion binding. The perilymph proteins are involved in manifold *biological processes* with focus on biological regulation. Many proteins are also participated in cellular, developmental and metabolic processes as well as in cellular component regulation, response to stimulus and localization.

Severity of Hearing Loss Correlates to Overall Lower Expression of Perilymph Proteins Predicted to Be Regulated by BDNF

Using IPA software, we identified proteins detected in perilymph with direct or indirect regulation by BDNF and we grouped these regulated perilymph proteins by expected change in expression level when BDNF is decreased. The IPA Knowledgebase predicted that 13 proteins would be down regulated and 16 proteins would be up regulated when BDNF expression diminished (**Table 3**). No predictive information on up or down regulation could be found for the 12 remaining proteins (**Table 3**). Patients were divided into two groups, patients with and without RH based on a cutoff of 90 dB PTA, and correlated to the three groups of proteins regulated by BDNF. These results are shown as a heat map depicting the presence and concentration of the various proteins in patients with and without RH (**Figure 2**). Patients with no preoperative RH had significantly lower levels of the proteins predicted to be down regulated when BDNF decreases (**Figure 2**; left side; $p = 0.007$; Fisher's exact test). For proteins that are predicted to be up regulated, there was also a significant difference between the groups (**Figure 2**; middle; $p = 0.02$; Fisher's exact test). For proteins determined to be regulated by BDNF expression but without predictable change direction, there was no statistically significant difference between RH and non-hearing patients (**Figure 2**; right side).

Preoperative Hearing Loss Correlates to Decreased Perilymph Expression of Phospholipid Transfer Protein

The proteins listed in **Table 3** were correlated to the preoperative hearing level and postoperative performance data with the cochlear implant 1 year after implantation. Comparison of protein levels (LFQ intensity) to the patients' preoperative PTA showed a slightly significant correlation between preoperative PTA and level of phospholipid transfer protein (PLTP) (Pearson $r = -0.3658$; $p = 0.0187$) shown in **Figure 3**. Correlation of the other proteins to the PTA was not significant. PLTP was detectable in the perilymph of the majority of the patients (36/41).

Additionally, the correlation of the relative PLTP concentration (LFQ intensity) in perilymph at the time point during surgery to postoperative hearing performance 1 year after hearing restoration with a cochlear implant was analyzed. Data of audiologic tests (HSM sentence test in quiet and in noise 10 dB, Freiburg monosyllable word test) 1 year after implantation were used for a correlation analysis. Data of the majority of the patients, children excluded, were analyzed: HSM sentence test in quiet ($n = 15$), HSM sentence test in noise 10 dB ($n = 20$), Freiburg monosyllable word test ($n = 22$). There might be a trend toward better understanding in patients with higher PLTP levels in perilymph is shown in **Figure 4**. For confirming these hypotheses further studies are required.

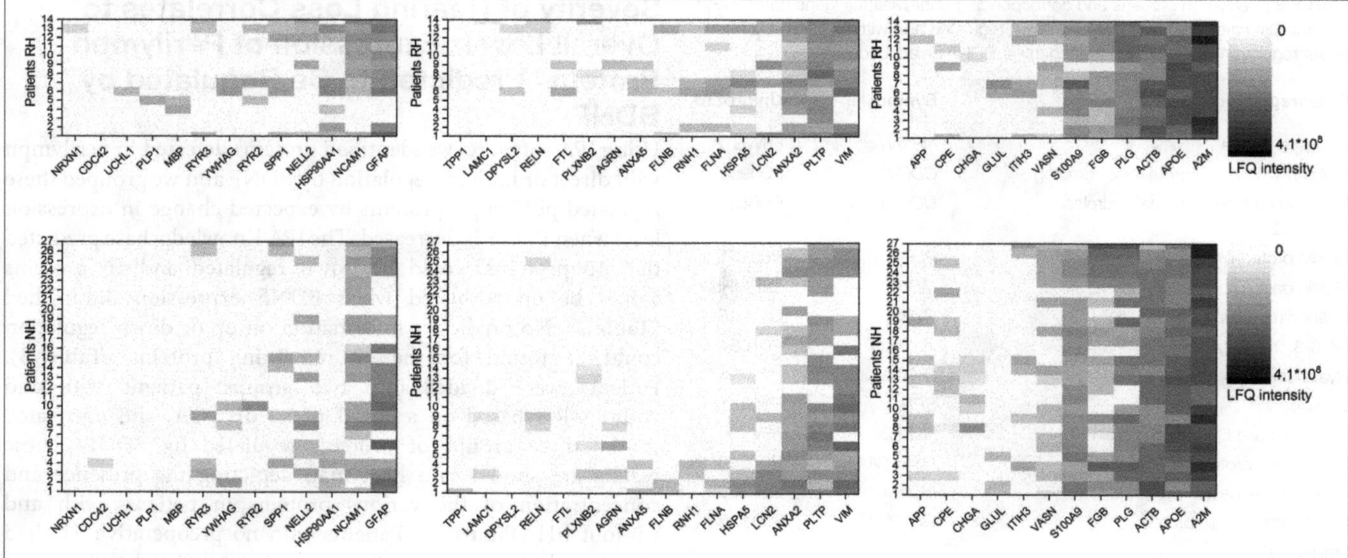

FIGURE 2 | Heat map of proteins predicted to be regulated by BDNF. Shown are proteins anticipated to be downregulated with decrease in BDNF for patients with (RH) and without (NH) residual hearing on the left. Proteins anticipated to be upregulated with decrease in BDNF for patients with (RH) and without (NH) residual hearing in the middle and proteins with no information about the regulation with decrease in BDNF for patients with (RH) and without (NH) residual hearing on the right. Protein values of patients with RH are shown in the upper row, data of patients NH in the lower row. The concentration of the individual proteins was analyzed by label free quantification (LFQ) in human perilymph samples and an increase is shown with deeper shades of violet.

DISCUSSION

The integrity of the spiral ganglion is thought to play a key role in cochlear implant function. Since the studies of Spoendlin demonstrated that aminoglycoside injury of the peripheral auditory system in cats resulted in a secondary degeneration of the spiral ganglion (Spoendlin, 1975), there has been significant interest in understanding the mechanisms that maintain spiral ganglion integrity and function. In humans, the process of spiral ganglion degeneration appears to occur at a different rate than in animal models. There clearly are variations in spiral ganglion populations that occur with different disease processes (Otte et al., 1978). The relationship between spiral ganglion integrity and cochlear implant outcomes in humans has been more difficult to establish. Initial temporal bone studies did not show a clear relationship between spiral ganglion counts and implant outcomes (Fayad et al., 1991). More recent studies with larger numbers, however, do show a relationship between speech outcomes and the quantity of spiral ganglion neurons (Seyyedi et al., 2014). To assess the functionality of the remaining spiral ganglion neurons, animal studies have been used to correlate changes in the electrically evoked compound actual potential of guinea pigs with intact or impaired spiral ganglion neurons (Pfingst et al., 2015b). This potentially correlates to measurable changes in patients undergoing cochlear implantation since an abnormal growth function of the electrically evoked compound action has been correlated to poor cochlear implant speech outcomes (Kim et al., 2010).

An important question that arises is whether neurotrophic factors can influence neuronal survival in humans treated with cochlear implants. Amongst the most studied candidates are the neurotrophins. The function of BDNF in the adult rodent auditory system was recently reviewed (Singer et al., 2014). Diverse studies mainly using knockout and conditional knockout mice suggest that BDNF is initially expressed in auditory hair cells. During maturation of hearing, the pattern of BDNF expression changes to inner phalangeal cells, pillar cells (the cells surrounding the inner hair cell) and spiral ganglion cells

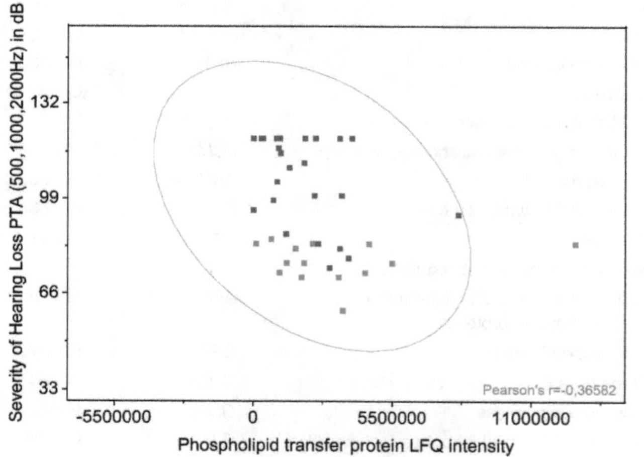

FIGURE 3 | Comparison of PLTP protein levels to the patients' preoperative pure tone average (PTA). Shown is a significant correlation between preoperative PTA (500, 1000, and 2000 Hz) and presence of PLTP. The protein levels were analyzed by label free quantification (LFQ intensity) in human perilymph samples.

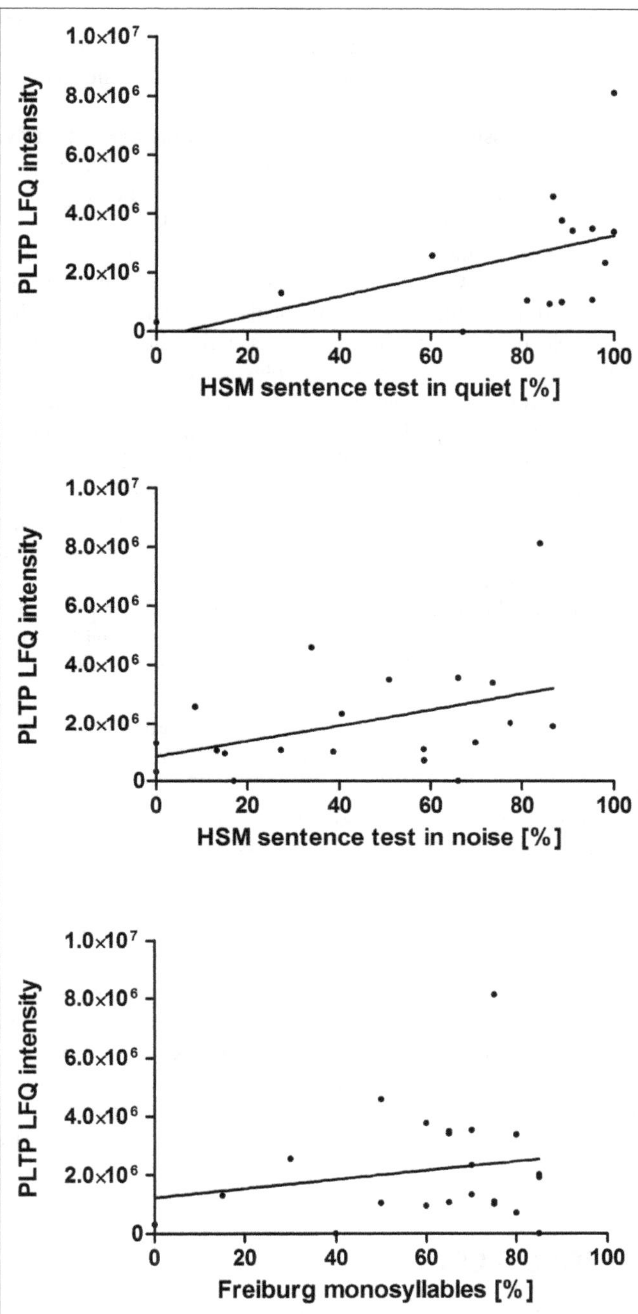

FIGURE 4 | Correlation of the PLTP protein levels to the patients' postoperative hearing performance. Audiologic test data of 29 adult patients of the 41 patients with perilymph sampling 1 year after cochlear implantation are depicted as speech understanding in %. The HSM sentence test in quiet (n = 15) is shown on the top, the HSM sentence test in noise at 10 dB (n = 20) in the middle and the Freiburg monosyllable word test (n = 22) at the bottom. The protein levels were analyzed by label free quantification (LFQ intensity) in human perilymph samples.

(Fritzsch et al., 2004; Kersigo and Fritzsch, 2015; Johnson Chacko et al., 2017). One of the key roles of BDNF in the adult auditory system may include maintenance of ribbon synapse integrity (Zuccotti et al., 2012; Singer et al., 2014). The role of BDNF in the human adult auditory system is less defined. A number of studies have looked at the expression of neurotrophin and their receptors in normal adult human cochlear tissue from cochleae harvested during acoustic neuroma surgery. The TrkB receptor was found to be expressed in the spiral ganglion neurons and in nerve fibers underneath outer hair cells (Liu et al., 2011). BDNF expression was not detectable by immunohistochemistry (Liu et al., 2011). A recent *in situ* hybridization study in adult human inner ear tissue, however, has found BDNF mRNA in auditory hair cells and supporting cells (Johnson Chacko et al., 2017). Expression of the low affinity p75NTR was demonstrated in Schwann cells and glial cells but not in spiral ganglion neurons (Liu et al., 2012). Currently, no human data exists demonstrating what changes in neurotrophin signaling occur as a result of hearing loss. The signaling pathways of BDNF are well understood. Consequently, a potential method of evaluating BDNF effects in the human inner ear is to look at the downstream effects of BDNF signaling.

In the central nervous system, there are clear links to a variety of neurodegenerative pathologies and decreased levels of BDNF expression (Lu et al., 2013). Besides direct degeneration of the tissues producing BDNF, the expression of BDNF can be modulated by inflammatory mediators which may be present as a consequence of cochlear implantation (Calabrese et al., 2014). Additionally, as shown in many studies, BDNF can autoregulate its expression (Zheng et al., 2012). Animal studies have shown that implant function can be improved after cochlear damage by either co-infusing BDNF or inducing production of BDNF through gene therapy (Staecker and Garnham, 2010; Budenz et al., 2012). A key factor in translating these finding into human studies is to identify patients with insufficient endogenous BDNF production or signaling. In addition to electrophysiological measures (Pfingst et al., 2015a), direct or indirect indicators of neurotrophin function in perilymph may be detectable. Unlike in CSF (Calderon-Garciduenas et al., 2016; Li et al., 2016; Martin-de-Pablos et al., 2018), direct detection of BDNF by mass spectrometry have not been demonstrated in perilymph yet (Schmitt et al., 2017).

In the herein presented study, analysis of gene expression in three normal human patients showed the presence of BDNF, TrkB and the p75NTR in the cochlea, supplementing information gained from prior immunohistochemical studies. We compared these data with analysis of proteins in the perilymph of patients undergoing cochlear implantation, therefore having hearing loss, and analyzed their relationship to BDNF signaling. Based on profiling, we show that expression of signaling cascades downstream from neurotrophic tyrosine kinase receptors and the low affinity p75NTR are active in the normal cochlea (**Figure 1**). There is active expression of PI3K, CDC42, and RAS (**Figure 1**) resulting in activation of pathways that maintain cell survival, growth, and neuritogenesis (Sandhya et al., 2013). Using IPA software, we identified a subgroup of the 878 expressed perilymph proteins, identified, and described in a previous study (Schmitt et al., 2017), that may be regulated by BDNF (**Table 3**). The 41 proteins identified based on their relationship to BDNF signaling may be related to the hearing level of the patients since different protein levels between the two patients groups were analyzed (patients with RH and patients with profound hearing loss).

For the proteins that are predicted to be down regulated if BDNF is reduced, patients with no RH prior to implantation expressed lower or absent levels of these proteins. For this group of proteins, ryanodine receptors 2 and 3, and HSP 90 are hair cell specific, so their reduction could be a reflection of loss of hair cells rather than changes in BDNF signaling (Lim et al., 1996; Mammano et al., 2007). Within this group, NELL2 is a spiral ganglion marker (Nelson et al., 2002). GFAP is a marker for spiral ganglion glial cells and supporting cells (Rio et al., 2002) and NCAM1 is associated with the spiral ganglion (Terkelsen et al., 1989). Individually, these proteins did not correlate to preoperative hearing levels. A potential explanation of this is found in the adult rodent data. If BDNF really is only expressed in the higher frequency region of the adult cochlea as suggested by Zuccotti et al. (2012), then our RH and non-hearing patients may not have a significant difference in BDNF expression since most patients undergoing implantation have RH only at lower frequencies. A larger cohort of patients with variable hearing loss will be needed to further refine these outcomes. Interestingly, among these proteins osteopontin is a marker for vestibular hair cells and may also be expressed in lower levels in the marginal cells and in the spiral ganglion (Sakagami, 2000). This protein has a decreased expression in patients without RH, suggesting that there may also be differences in balance function that can be assayed through this approach.

For the proteins that were predicted to be upregulated when BDNF is reduced, filamin A and B are actin binding proteins which can be found in hair cell stereocilia (Ramakrishnan et al., 2012). Plexins are members of a family of transmembrane proteins that control axonal growth and have been demonstrated in the developing spiral ganglion (Lu et al., 2011). Annexin A5 has been described as being present in high concentration in hair cell stereocilia (Krey et al., 2016). Within this group, the patients with profound hearing loss expressed a significantly reduced proteome, when considering proteins regulated by BDNF (**Figure 2**). Again, this may reflect the overall degeneration of the organ of Corti rather than a BDNF regulatory effect. Within this subgroup, however, phospholipid transfer protein showed a statistically significant correlation to preoperative PTA. This protein is generally identified with lipid metabolism but has been identified in the developing inner ear as expressed in cells of a non-hair cell lineage during development (Scheffer et al., 2015). By GOA the molecular, function of this protein is characterized by lipid transporter activity (including phospholipids and ceramides like diacylglycerol, phosphatidic acid, sphingomyelin, phosphatidylcholine, phosphatidylglycerol, cerebroside, and phosphatidyl ethanolamine). Additionally, this protein is involved in different biological processes like ceramide transport, flagellated sperm motility, high-density lipoprotein particle remodeling, lipid metabolic process, lipid transport, phospholipid transport, positive regulation of cholesterol efflux, and vitamin E biosynthetic process. Interestingly, a link between PLTP and the amyloid precursor protein (APP) was discussed suggesting that a deficiency of these proteins accelerates memory dysfunction in mouse models. Additionally, PLTP might play an important role in autophagy modulation (Tong et al., 2015). Its function in the adult inner ear is not defined yet.

When discussing the results obtained from the present study, several limitations need to be considered. The population of the patients included into our analysis is highly heterogenous with different anatomic and molecular pathologies. This can certainly add to the variability in the perilymph proteome that we showed in this study and in prior studies (Schmitt et al., 2017, 2018). In addition, different cochlear implant devices with various electrode arrays have been used for the treatment of the hearing loss, adding more variables to be considered when analyzing the hearing performance with the device. Finally, the low number of patients included and the vast number of proteins identified in the perilymph are limiting the statistical power of the study. The influence of age and gender on gene and protein expression needs also consideration. Thus, future studies need to concentrate on a higher number of homogenous groups of patients.

Despite the limitations, evaluation of the perilymph proteome offers a novel approach for the indirect evaluation of a wide range of biological effects within the cochlea of patients undergoing cochlear implantation. Animal studies have demonstrated that BDNF supplementation can enhance spiral ganglion survival (Evans et al., 2009; Wan et al., 2014; Budenz et al., 2015; Ramekers et al., 2015; Wise et al., 2016; Pfingst et al., 2017). Despite temporal bone pathology and physiological evidence that spiral ganglion survival is variable between disease processes and affects cochlear implant outcomes, we have a very incomplete understanding of the diseased human inner ear. Cochlear "health" is hypothesized to have a significant impact on cochlear implant outcomes (Pfingst et al., 2015b, 2017). The human perilymph proteome in implant patients consists of greater than 800 individual proteins. By focusing on proteins that are regulated by BDNF, we can analyze subgroups that may reflect changes in BDNF signaling or even allow the identification of markers that may reflect BDNF signaling or demonstrate degeneration of hair cells and supporting cells within the organ of Corti.

CONCLUSION

We have demonstrated that BDNF is expressed in cochlear tissue in normal hearing individuals. Patients with profound hearing loss have less BDNF-regulated proteins in their perilymph when compared to patients with some RH. In addition, the expression level of PLTP correlated not only to preoperative hearing but also tend to improved outcome with cochlear implants in individual patients. This initial study identifies a group of proteins that may potentially serve as markers for inner ear health as it relates to cochlear implantation. In order to use this tool for the identification of biomarkers or for the reliable prediction of cochlear implant outcome, large applied studies need to be performed.

AUTHOR CONTRIBUTIONS

IdV acquired and analyzed the data, and wrote the first draft of the manuscript. HS processed and analyzed the perilymph, and wrote the manuscript. TL designed the study, provided financial support, and approved the manuscript. NP collected the perilymph, provided and analyzed the human data, and approved the manuscript. SA performed the bioinformatics analysis of the data, and approved the manuscript. HS designed the study, performed the bioinformatics analysis of the data, and wrote the manuscript. MD collected the perilymph, provided and analyzed the human data, approved the manuscript, and provided financial support. AW designed the study, collected the perilymph, analyzed the data, and wrote the manuscript.

REFERENCES

Budenz, C. L., Pfingst, B. E., and Raphael, Y. (2012). The use of neurotrophin therapy in the inner ear to augment cochlear implantation outcomes. *Anat. Rec.* 295, 1896–1908. doi: 10.1002/ar.22586

Budenz, C. L., Wong, H. T., Swiderski, D. L., Shibata, S. B., Pfingst, B. E., and Raphael, Y. (2015). Differential effects of AAV.BDNF and AAV.Ntf3 in the deafened adult guinea pig ear. *Sci. Rep.* 5:8619. doi: 10.1038/srep08619

Calabrese, F., Rossetti, A. C., Racagni, G., Gass, P., Riva, M. A., and Molteni, R. (2014). Brain-derived neurotrophic factor: a bridge between inflammation and neuroplasticity. *Front. Cell Neurosci.* 8:430. doi: 10.3389/fncel.2014.00430

Calderon-Garciduenas, L., Avila-Ramirez, J., Calderon-Garciduenas, A., Gonzalez-Heredia, T., Acuna-Ayala, H., Chao, C. K., et al. (2016). Cerebrospinal fluid biomarkers in highly exposed pm2.5 urbanites: the risk of alzheimer's and parkinson's diseases in young mexico city residents. *J. Alzh. Dis.* 54, 597–613. doi: 10.3233/JAD-160472

Carlson, M. L., Driscoll, C. L., Gifford, R. H., and McMenomey, S. O. (2012). Cochlear implantation: current and future device options. *Otolaryngol. Clin. North. Am.* 45, 221–248. doi: 10.1016/j.otc.2011.09.002

Causon, A., Verschuur, C., and Newman, T. A. (2015). A Retrospective analysis of the contribution of reported factors in cochlear implantation on hearing preservation outcomes. *Otol. Neurotol.* 36, 1137–1145. doi: 10.1097/MAO.0000000000000753

Evans, A. J., Thompson, B. C., Wallace, G. G., Millard, R., O'Leary, S. J., Clark, G. M., et al. (2009). Promoting neurite outgrowth from spiral ganglion neuron explants using polypyrrole/BDNF-coated electrodes. *J. Biomed. Mater. Res. A* 91, 241–250. doi: 10.1002/jbm.a.32228

Fayad, J., Linthicum, F. H. Jr., Otto, S. R., Galey, F. R., and House, W. F. (1991). Cochlear implants: histopathologic findings related to performance in 16 human temporal bones. *Ann. Otol. Rhinol. Laryngol.* 100, 807–811. doi: 10.1177/000348949110001004

Flores-Otero, J., and Davis, R. L. (2011). Synaptic proteins are tonotopically graded in postnatal and adult type I and type II spiral ganglion neurons. *J. Comp. Neurol.* 519, 1455–1475. doi: 10.1002/cne.22576

Fritzsch, B., Tessarollo, L., Coppola, E., and Reichardt, L. F. (2004). Neurotrophins in the ear: their roles in sensory neuron survival and fiber guidance. *Prog. Brain Res.* 146, 265–278. doi: 10.1016/S0079-6123(03)46017-2

Johnson Chacko, L., Blumer, M. J. F., Pechriggl, E., Rask-Andersen, H., Dietl, W., Haim, A., et al. (2017). Role of BDNF and neurotrophic receptors in human inner ear development. *Cell Tissue Res.* 370, 347–363. doi: 10.1007/s00441-017-2686-9

Kersigo, J., and Fritzsch, B. (2015). Inner ear hair cells deteriorate in mice engineered to have no or diminished innervation. *Front. Aging Neurosci.* 7:33. doi: 10.3389/fnagi.2015.00033

Kim, J. R., Abbas, P. J., Brown, C. J., Etler, C. P., O'Brien, S., and Kim, L. S. (2010). The relationship between electrically evoked compound action potential and speech perception: a study in cochlear implant users with short electrode array. *Otol. Neurotol.* 31, 1041–1048. doi: 10.1097/MAO.0b013e3181ec1d92

Kral, A., Kronenberger, W. G., Pisoni, D. B., and O'Donoghue, G. M. (2016). Neurocognitive factors in sensory restoration of early deafness: a connectome model. *Lancet Neurol.* 15, 610–621. doi: 10.1016/S1474-4422(16)00034-X

Krey, J. F., Drummond, M., Foster, S., Porsov, E., Vijayakumar, S., Choi, D., et al. (2016). Annexin A5 is the most abundant membrane-associated protein in stereocilia but is dispensable for hair-bundle development and function. *Sci. Rep.* 6:27221. doi: 10.1038/srep27221

Lawner, B. E., Harding, G. W., and Bohne, B. A. (1997). Time course of nerve-fiber regeneration in the noise-damaged *mammalian* cochlea. *Int. J. Dev. Neurosci.* 15, 601–617. doi: 10.1016/S0736-5748(96)00115-3

Li, W., Li, X., Xin, X., Kan, P. C., and Yan, Y. (2016). MicroRNA-613 regulates the expression of brain-derived neurotrophic factor in alzheimer's disease. *Biosci. Trends* 10, 372–377. doi: 10.5582/bst.2016.01127

Lim, H. H., Miller, J. M., Dolan, D. F., Raphael, Y., and Altschuler, R. A. (1996). "Noise-induced expression of heat shock proteins in the cochlea," in *Scientific Basis of NoiseInduced Hearing Loss*, eds A. Axelsson, H. Borchgrevink, R. P. Hamernik, P.-A. Hellstrom, and R. J. Salvi (New York,NY: Thieme Medical Publishers), 43–49.

Liu, W., Glueckert, R., Kinnefors, A., Schrott-Fischer, A., Bitsche, M., and Rask-Andersen, H. (2012). Distribution of P75 neurotrophin receptor in adult human cochlea-an immunohistochemical study. *Cell Tissue Res.* 348, 407–415. doi: 10.1007/s00441-012-1395-7

Liu, W., Kinnefors, A., Bostrom, M., and Rask-Andersen, H. (2011). Expression of TrkB and BDNF in human cochlea-an immunohistochemical study. *Cell Tissue Res.* 345, 213–221. doi: 10.1007/s00441-011-1209-1203

Lu, B., Nagappan, G., Guan, X., Nathan, P. J., and Wren, P. (2013). BDNF-based synaptic repair as a disease-modifying strategy for neurodegenerative diseases. *Nat. Rev. Neurosci.* 14, 401–416. doi: 10.1038/nrn3505

Lu, C. C., Appler, J. M., Houseman, E. A., and Goodrich, L. V. (2011). Developmental profiling of spiral ganglion neurons reveals insights into auditory circuit assembly. *J. Neurosci.* 31, 10903–10918. doi: 10.1523/JNEUROSCI.2358-11.2011

Mammano, F., Bortolozzi, M., Ortolano, S., and Anselmi, F. (2007). Ca2+ signaling in the inner ear. *Physiology* 22, 131–144. doi: 10.1152/physiol.00040.2006

Martin-de-Pablos, A., Cordoba-Fernandez, A., and Fernandez-Espejo, E. (2018). Analysis of neurotrophic and antioxidant factors related to midbrain dopamine neuronal loss and brain inflammation in the cerebrospinal fluid of the elderly. *Exp. Gerontol.* 110, 54–60. doi: 10.1016/j.exger.2018.05.009

Mellado Lagarde, M. M., Cox, B. C., Fang, J., Taylor, R., Forge, A., and Zuo, J. (2013). Selective ablation of pillar and deiters' cells severely affects cochlear postnatal development and hearing in mice. *J. Neurosci.* 33, 1564–1576. doi: 10.1523/JNEUROSCI.3088-12.2013

Nelson, B. R., Matsuhashi, S., and Lefcort, F. (2002). Restricted neural epidermal growth factor-like like 2 (NELL2) expression during muscle and neuronal differentiation. *Mech. Dev.* 119(Suppl. 1), S11–S19. doi: 10.1016/S0925-4773(03)00084-4

Otte, J., Schunknecht, H. F., and Kerr, A. G. (1978). Ganglion cell populations in normal and pathological human cochleae. implications for cochlear implantation. *Laryngoscope* 88(8 Pt 1), 1231–1246. doi: 10.1288/00005537-197808000-00004

Pfingst, B. E., Colesa, D. J., Swiderski, D. L., Hughes, A. P., Strahl, S. B., Sinan, M., et al. (2017). Neurotrophin gene therapy in deafened ears with cochlear implants: long-term effects on nerve survival and functional measures. *J. Assoc. Res. Otolaryngol.* 18, 731–750. doi: 10.1007/s10162-017-0633-9

Pfingst, B. E., Hughes, A. P., Colesa, D. J., Watts, M. M., Strahl, S. B., and Raphael, Y. (2015a). Insertion trauma and recovery of function after cochlear implantation: Evidence from objective functional measures. *Hear. Res.* 330(Pt A), 98–105. doi: 10.1016/j.heares.2015.07.010

Pfingst, B. E., Zhou, N., Colesa, D. J., Watts, M. M., Strahl, S. B., Garadat, S. N., et al. (2015b). Importance of cochlear health for implant function. *Hear. Res.* 322, 77–88. doi: 10.1016/j.heares.2014.09.009

Pirvola, U., Hallbook, F., Xing-Qun, L., Virkkala, J., Saarma, M., and Ylikoski, J. (1997). Expression of neurotrophins and Trk receptors in the developing, adult, and regenerating avian cochlea. *J. Neurobiol.* 33, 1019–1033. doi: 10.1002/(SICI)1097-4695(199712)33:7<1019::AID-NEU11>3.0.CO;2-A

Pirvola, U., Ylikoski, J., Palgi, J., Lehtonen, E., Arumae, U., and Saarma, M. (1992). Brain-derived neurotrophic factor and neurotrophin 3 mRNAs in the peripheral target fields of developing inner ear ganglia. *Proc. Natl. Acad. Sci. U.S.A.* 89, 9915–9919. doi: 10.1073/pnas.89.20.9915

Ramakrishnan, N. A., Drescher, M. J., Khan, K. M., Hatfield, J. S., and Drescher, D. G. (2012). HCN1 and HCN2 proteins are expressed in cochlear hair cells: HCN1 can form a ternary complex with protocadherin 15 CD3 and F-actin-binding filamin A or can interact with HCN2. *J. Biol. Chem.* 287, 37628–37646. doi: 10.1074/jbc.M112.375832

Ramekers, D., Versnel, H., Strahl, S. B., Klis, S. F., and Grolman, W. (2015). Temporary neurotrophin treatment prevents deafness-induced auditory nerve degeneration and preserves function. *J. Neurosci.* 35, 12331–12345. doi: 10.1523/JNEUROSCI.0096-15.2015

Rio, C., Dikkes, P., Liberman, M. C., and Corfas, G. (2002). Glial fibrillary acidic protein expression and promoter activity in the inner ear of developing and adult mice. *J. Comp. Neurol.* 442, 156–162. doi: 10.1002/cne.10085

Sakagami, M. (2000). Role of osteopontin in the rodent inner ear as revealed by in situ hybridization. *Med. Electron. Microsci.* 33, 3–10. doi: 10.1007/s007950000001

Sandhya, V. K., Raju, R., Verma, R., Advani, J., Sharma, R., Radhakrishnan, A., et al. (2013). A network map of BDNF/TRKB and BDNF/p75NTR signaling system. *J. Cell Commun. Signal.* 7, 301–307. doi: 10.1007/s12079-013-0200-z

Scheffer, D. I., Shen, J., Corey, D. P., and Chen, Z. Y. (2015). Gene expression by mouse inner ear hair cells during development. *J. Neurosci.* 35, 6366–6380. doi: 10.1523/JNEUROSCI.5126-14.2015

Schmitt, H., Roemer, A., Zeilinger, C., Salcher, R., Durisin, M., Staecker, H., et al. (2018). Heat shock proteins in human perilymph: implications for cochlear implantation. *Otol. Neurotol.* 39, 37–44. doi: 10.1097/MAO.0000000000001625

Schmitt, H. A., Pich, A., Schroder, A., Scheper, V., Lilli, G., Reuter, G., et al. (2017). Proteome analysis of human perilymph using an intraoperative sampling method. *J. Proteome Res.* 16, 1911–1923. doi: 10.1021/acs.jproteome.6b00986

Seyyedi, M., Viana, L. M., and Nadol, J. B. Jr. (2014). Within-subject comparison of word recognition and spiral ganglion cell count in bilateral cochlear implant recipients. *Otol. Neurotol.* 35, 1446–1450. doi: 10.1097/MAO.0000000000000443

Shearer, A. E., Eppsteiner, R. W., Frees, K., Tejani, V., Sloan-Heggen, C. M., Brown, C., et al. (2017).). Genetic variants in the peripheral auditory system significantly affect adult cochlear implant performance. *Hear. Res.* 348, 138–142. doi: 10.1016/j.heares.2017.02.008

Shearer, A. E., Hildebrand, M. S., and Smith, R. J. H. (1993). *Hereditary Hearing Loss and Deafness Overview*. Seattle, WA: University of Washington.

Singer, W., Panford-Walsh, R., and Knipper, M. (2014). The function of BDNF in the adult auditory system. *Neuropharmacology* 76(Pt C), 719–728. doi: 10.1016/j.neuropharm.2013.05.008

Spoendlin, H. (1975). Retrograde degeneration of the cochlear nerve. *Acta Otolaryngol.* 79, 266–275. doi: 10.3109/00016487509124683

Staecker, H., and Garnham, C. (2010). Neurotrophin therapy and cochlear implantation: translating animal models to human therapy. *Exp. Neurol.* 226, 1–5. doi: 10.1016/j.expneurol.2010.07.012

Terkelsen, O. B., Bock, E., and Mollgard, K. (1989). NCAM and Thy-1 in special sense organs of the developing mouse. *Anat. Embryol.* 179, 311–318. doi: 10.1007/BF00305057

Tong, Y., Sun, Y., Tian, X., Zhou, T., Wang, H., Zhang, T., et al. (2015). Phospholipid transfer protein (PLTP) deficiency accelerates memory dysfunction through altering amyloid precursor protein (APP) processing in a mouse model of Alzheimer's disease. *Hum. Mol. Genet.* 24, 5388–5403. doi: 10.1093/hmg/ddv262

UniProt Consortium (2015). UniProt: a hub for protein information. *Nucleic Acids Res.* 43, D204–D212. doi: 10.1093/nar/gku989

Wan, G., Gomez-Casati, M. E., Gigliello, A. R., Liberman, M. C., and Corfas, G. (2014). Neurotrophin-3 regulates ribbon synapse density in the cochlea and induces synapse regeneration after acoustic trauma. *eLife* 3:e03564. doi: 10.7554/eLife.03564

Wise, A. K., Tan, J., Wang, Y., Caruso, F., and Shepherd, R. K. (2016). Improved auditory nerve survival with nanoengineered supraparticles for neurotrophin delivery into the deafened cochlea. *PLoS One* 11:e0164867. doi: 10.1371/journal.pone.0164867

Zheng, F., Zhou, X., Moon, C., and Wang, H. (2012). Regulation of brain-derived neurotrophic factor expression in neurons. *Int. J. Physiol. Pathophysiol. Pharmacol.* 4, 188–200.

Zuccotti, A., Kuhn, S., Johnson, S. L., Franz, C., Singer, W., Hecker, D., et al. (2012). Lack of brain-derived neurotrophic factor hampers inner hair cell synapse physiology, but protects against noise-induced hearing loss. *J. Neurosci.* 32, 8545–8553. doi: 10.1523/JNEUROSCI.1247-12.2012

Permissions

All chapters in this book were first published by Frontiers; hereby published with permission under the Creative Commons Attribution License or equivalent. Every chapter published in this book has been scrutinized by our experts. Their significance has been extensively debated. The topics covered herein carry significant findings which will fuel the growth of the discipline. They may even be implemented as practical applications or may be referred to as a beginning point for another development.

The contributors of this book come from diverse backgrounds, making this book a truly international effort. This book will bring forth new frontiers with its revolutionizing research information and detailed analysis of the nascent developments around the world.

We would like to thank all the contributing authors for lending their expertise to make the book truly unique. They have played a crucial role in the development of this book. Without their invaluable contributions this book wouldn't have been possible. They have made vital efforts to compile up to date information on the varied aspects of this subject to make this book a valuable addition to the collection of many professionals and students.

This book was conceptualized with the vision of imparting up-to-date information and advanced data in this field. To ensure the same, a matchless editorial board was set up. Every individual on the board went through rigorous rounds of assessment to prove their worth. After which they invested a large part of their time researching and compiling the most relevant data for our readers.

The editorial board has been involved in producing this book since its inception. They have spent rigorous hours researching and exploring the diverse topics which have resulted in the successful publishing of this book. They have passed on their knowledge of decades through this book. To expedite this challenging task, the publisher supported the team at every step. A small team of assistant editors was also appointed to further simplify the editing procedure and attain best results for the readers.

Apart from the editorial board, the designing team has also invested a significant amount of their time in understanding the subject and creating the most relevant covers. They scrutinized every image to scout for the most suitable representation of the subject and create an appropriate cover for the book.

The publishing team has been an ardent support to the editorial, designing and production team. Their endless efforts to recruit the best for this project, has resulted in the accomplishment of this book. They are a veteran in the field of academics and their pool of knowledge is as vast as their experience in printing. Their expertise and guidance has proved useful at every step. Their uncompromising quality standards have made this book an exceptional effort. Their encouragement from time to time has been an inspiration for everyone.

The publisher and the editorial board hope that this book will prove to be a valuable piece of knowledge for researchers, students, practitioners and scholars across the globe.

List of Contributors

Yi Xu, Huiying Guo, Hui Cao, Jing Zhang and Dong Yang
Department of Otorhinolaryngology, Tianjin Medical University General Hospital, Tianjin, China

Yan Li
Department of Anesthesiology, Tianjin Jizhou People's Hospital, Tianjin, China

Dandan Guo and Xin Zhang
Department of Neurology, Tianjin Medical University General Hospital, Tianjin, China

Xin Li
Department of Otorhinolaryngology, Beijing Tsinghua Changgung Hospital, School of Clinical Medicine, Tsinghua University, Beijing, China

Jun Tu, Jinghua Wang and Xianjia Ning
Department of Neurology, Tianjin Medical University General Hospital, Tianjin, China
Laboratory of Epidemiology, Tianjin Neurological Institute, Tianjin, China
Key Laboratory of Post-Neuroinjury Neuro-Repair and Regeneration in Central Nervous System, Tianjin Neurological Institute, Ministry of Education and Tianjin City, Tianjin, China

Xuexin Tian, Yimeng Liu and Jieqing Cai
Department of Otolaryngology Head & Neck Surgery, Zhujiang Hospital, Southern Medical University, Guangzhou, China

Zengzhi Guo and Fei Chen
Department of Electrical and Electronic Engineering, Southern University of Science and Technology, Shenzhen, China

Jie Tang
Department of Otolaryngology Head & Neck Surgery, Zhujiang Hospital, Southern Medical University, Guangzhou, China
Department of Physiology, School of Basic Medical Sciences, Southern Medical University, Guangzhou, China
Hearing Research Center, Southern Medical University, Guangzhou, China
Key Laboratory of Mental Health of the Ministry of Education, Southern Medical University, Guangzhou, China

Yan Zhao
Department of Physiology, School of Basic Medical Sciences, Southern Medical University, Guangzhou, China

Wenlu Pan
Department of Physiology, School of Basic Medical Sciences, Southern Medical University, Guangzhou, China
Functional Nucleic Acid Basic and Clinical Research Center, Department of Physiology, School of Basic Medical Sciences, Changsha Medical College, Changsha, China

Jing Pan and Hongzheng Zhang
Department of Otolaryngology Head and Neck Surgery, Zhujiang Hospital, Southern Medical University, Guangzhou, China
Hearing Research Center, Southern Medical University, Guangzhou, China

Qixuan Wang, Minfei Qian and Hao Wu
Department of Otolaryngology-Head and Neck Surgery, Ninth People's Hospital, Shanghai Jiao Tong University School of Medicine, Shanghai, China
Ear Institute, Shanghai Jiao Tong University School of Medicine, Shanghai, China
Shanghai Key Laboratory of Translational Medicine on Ear and Nose Diseases, Shanghai, China

Lu Yang and Yingying Hong
Department of Otolaryngology-Head and Neck Surgery, Ninth People's Hospital, Shanghai Jiao Tong University School of Medicine, Shanghai, China
Hearing and Speech Center, Ninth People's Hospital, Shanghai Jiao Tong University School of Medicine, Shanghai, China

Zhiwu Huang
Department of Otolaryngology-Head and Neck Surgery, Ninth People's Hospital, Shanghai Jiao Tong University School of Medicine, Shanghai, China
Ear Institute, Shanghai Jiao Tong University School of Medicine, Shanghai, China
Shanghai Key Laboratory of Translational Medicine on Ear and Nose Diseases, Shanghai, China
Hearing and Speech Center, Ninth People's Hospital, Shanghai Jiao Tong University School of Medicine, Shanghai, China

Xueling Wang
Department of Otolaryngology-Head and Neck Surgery, Ninth People's Hospital, Shanghai Jiao Tong University School of Medicine, Shanghai, China
Ear Institute, Shanghai Jiao Tong University School of Medicine, Shanghai, China
Shanghai Key Laboratory of Translational Medicine on Ear and Nose Diseases, Shanghai, China
Biobank, Ninth People's Hospital, Shanghai Jiao Tong University School of Medicine, Shanghai, China

Bo Liu and Shuo Wang
Beijing Institute of Otolaryngology, Otolaryngology-Head and Neck Surgery, Beijing Tongren Hospital, Capital Medical University, Beijing, China

Xinxing Fu
Beijing Institute of Otolaryngology, Otolaryngology-Head and Neck Surgery, Beijing Tongren Hospital, Capital Medical University, Beijing, China
Medical School, The University of Western Australia, Crawley, WA, Australia
Ear Science Institute Australia, Subiaco, WA, Australia

Robert H. Eikelboom
Medical School, The University of Western Australia, Crawley, WA, Australia
Ear Science Institute Australia, Subiaco, WA, Australia
Department of Speech Language Pathology and Audiology, University of Pretoria, Pretoria, South Africa

Dona M. P. Jayakody
Medical School, The University of Western Australia, Crawley, WA, Australia
Ear Science Institute Australia, Subiaco, WA, Australia
WA Centre for Health and Ageing, The University of Western Australia, Crawley, WA, Australia

Juanjuan Gao, Junyan Chen, Jia Xu, Sichao Liang and Haijin Yi
Department of Otolaryngology, Head and Neck Surgery, Beijing Tsinghua Changgung Hospital, School of Clinical Medicine, Tsinghua University, Beijing, China

Tongxiang Diao, Xin Ma and Lisheng Yu
Department of Otolaryngology, Head and Neck Surgery, People's Hospital, Peking University, Beijing, China

Junbo Zhang
Department of Otolaryngology, Head and Neck Surgery, Peking University First Hospital, Beijing, China

Maoli Duan
Department of Clinical Science, Intervention and Technology, Karolinska Institute, Stockholm, Sweden
Department of Otolaryngology, Head and Neck Surgery & Audiology and Neurotology, Karolinska University Hospital, Karolinska Institute, Stockholm, Sweden

Lena L. N. Wong
Faculty of Education, The University of Hong Kong, Pokfulam, Hong Kong SAR, China

Qi Gao
Department of Electrical and Electronic Engineering, Southern University of Science and Technology, Shenzhen, China
Faculty of Education, The University of Hong Kong, Pokfulam, Hong Kong SAR, China

Yuyang Wang, Chaogang Wei, Tianyu Xin and Yuhe Liu
Department of Otolaryngology, Head and Neck Surgery, Peking University First Hospital, Beijing, China

Lili Liu and Xinlin Hou
Department of Pediatrics, Peking University First Hospital, Beijing, China

Ying Zhang and Qiang He
Department of Otolaryngology, Head and Neck Surgery, The Second Hospital of Hebei Medical University, Shijiazhuang, China

Yan-Xin Chen, Xin-Ran Xu, Shuo Huang, Rui-Rui Guan, Xiao-Yan Hou, Jia-Qiang Sun and Jing-Wu Sun
Department of Otolaryngology-Head and Neck Surgery, The First Affiliated Hospital of USTC, Division of Life Sciences and Medicine, University of Science and Technology of China, Hefei, China

Xiao-Tao Guo
Department of Otolaryngology-Head and Neck Surgery, The First Affiliated Hospital of USTC, Division of Life Sciences and Medicine, University of Science and Technology of China, Hefei, China
CAS Key Laboratory of Brain Function and Diseases, School of Life Sciences, University of Science and Technology of China, Hefei, China

Pingping Guo
Department of Medical Ultrasound, Affiliated Tumor Hospital of Guangxi Medical University, Nanning, China

Siyuan Lang, Muliang Jiang and Zisan Zeng
Department of Radiology, First Affiliated Hospital of Guangxi Medical University, Nanning, China

Yifeng Wang
Institute of Brain and Psychological Sciences, Sichuan Normal University, Chengdu, China

Zuguang Wen
Department of Radiology, Seventh Affiliated Hospital of Sun Yat-sen University, Shenzhen, China

Yikang Liu
Department of Otorhinolaryngology Head and Neck Surgery, First Affiliated Hospital of Guangxi Medical University, Nanning, China

Bihong T. Chen
Department of Diagnostic Radiology, City of Hope National Medical Center, Duarte, CA, United States

Tingzhi Deng, Xiaoya Liu, Jia Mi, Chunhua Yang, Cuifang Yao and Geng Tian
Precision Medicine Research Center, School of Pharmacy, Binzhou Medical University, Yantai, China

Xicheng Song
Department of Otorhinolaryngology-Head and Neck Surgery, Yantai Yuhuangding Hospital, Qingdao University, Yantai, China

Jingjing Li
Precision Medicine Research Center, School of Pharmacy, Binzhou Medical University, Yantai, China
Department of Otorhinolaryngology-Head and Neck Surgery, Yantai Yuhuangding Hospital, Qingdao University, Yantai, China
Second Clinical Medical College, Binzhou Medical University, Yantai, China

Jian Liu
Department of Plastic Surgery, Shandong Provincial Qianfoshan Hospital, The First Affiliated Hospital of Shandong First Medical University, Jinan, China

Fuyi Xu
Precision Medicine Research Center, School of Pharmacy, Binzhou Medical University, Yantai, China
Department of Genetics, Genomics and Informatics, The University of Tennessee Health Science Center, Memphis, TN, United States

Lu Lu
Department of Genetics, Genomics and Informatics, The University of Tennessee Health Science Center, Memphis, TN, United States

Jonas Bergquist
Precision Medicine Research Center, School of Pharmacy, Binzhou Medical University, Yantai, China
Department of Chemistry – BMC, Analytical Chemistry and Neurochemistry, Uppsala University, Uppsala, Sweden

Helen Wang
Department of Medical Biochemistry and Microbiology, BMC, Uppsala University, Uppsala, Sweden

Qing Yin Zheng
Department of Otolaryngology-Head and Neck Surgery, Case Western Reserve University, Cleveland, OH, United States

Susanna S. Kwok, Xuan-Mai T. Nguyen and Diana D. Wu
Carle Illinois College of Medicine, University of Illinois Urbana-Champaign, Urbana, IL, United States

Raksha A. Mudar
Department of Speech and Hearing Sciences, University of Illinois Urbana-Champaign, Urbana, IL, United States

Daniel A. Llano
Carle Illinois College of Medicine, University of Illinois Urbana-Champaign, Urbana, IL, United States
Department of Speech and Hearing Sciences, University of Illinois Urbana-Champaign, Urbana, IL, United States
Department of Molecular and Integrative Physiology, University of Illinois Urbana-Champaign, Urbana, IL, United States
Beckman Institute for Advanced Science and Technology, University of Illinois Urbana-Champaign, Urbana, IL, United States
Carle Neuroscience Institute, Carle Foundation Hospital, Urbana, IL, United States

Rui Guo, Yang Li, Jiao Liu, Shusheng Gong and Ke Liu
Department of Otolaryngology Head and Neck Surgery, Beijing Friendship Hospital, Capital Medical University, Beijing, China

Jing Liu, Xinyi Huang and Jiping Zhang
Key Laboratory of Brain Functional Genomics, Ministry of Education, NYU–ECNU Institute of Brain and Cognitive Science at NYU Shanghai, School of Life Sciences, East China Normal University, Shanghai, China

Junbo Wang, Jiahao Liu, Yiqing Zheng and Maojin Liang
Department of Otolaryngology, Sun Yat-sen Memorial Hospital, Guangzhou, China

Kaiyin Lai and Suiping Wang
South China Normal University, Guangzhou, China

Qi Zhang
School of Foreign Languages, Shenzhen University, Shenzhen, China

Qian Li, Hong Li and Haiqing Liu
School of Life Science and Technology, Southeast University, Nanjing, China

Xiuting Yao, Conghui Wang, Chenxi Yang, Hong Zhuang, Yu Xiao, Rui Liu, Sinuo Shen, Shaoyang Zhou, Chenge Fu, Yifan Wang and Lijie Liu
Medical College, Southeast University, Nanjing, China

Dan Xu
School of Public Health, Southeast University, Nanjing, China

Gaojun Teng
Jiangsu Key Laboratory of Molecular Imaging and Functional Imaging, Department of Radiology, Medical School, Zhongda Hospital, Southeast University, Nanjing, China

Alessandro Castiglione, Patrizia Trevisi, Roberto Bovo and Alessandro Martini
Department of Neurosciences, University of Padua, Padua, Italy
Complex Operative Unit of Otolaryngology, Hospital of Padua, Padua, Italy

Dalila Cilia, Elisa Lovo, Marta Gambin, Maela Previato, Simone Colombo, Flavia Gheller, Cristina Giacomelli and Silvia Montino
Department of Neurosciences, University of Padua, Padua, Italy

Samanta Gallo, Flavia Sorrentino, Sonila Dhima, Ezio Caserta and Davide Brotto
Complex Operative Unit of Otolaryngology, Hospital of Padua, Padua, Italy

Mariella Casa and Carlo Gabelli
Regional Center for the Study and Treatment of the Aging Brain, Department of Internal Medicine, Padua, Italy

Federica Limongi
Institute of Neuroscience, National Research Council, Padua, Italy

Fuxin Ren, Bin Zhao and Fei Gao
Shandong Medical Imaging Research Institute, Shandong University, Jinan, China

Jianfen Luo, Lei Xu, Zhaomin Fan, Yu Ai and Haibo Wang
Department of Otolaryngology-Head and Neck Surgery, Shandong Provincial ENT Hospital, Shandong University, Jinan, China
Shandong Provincial Key Laboratory of Otology, Jinan, China

Wen Ma
Department of Otolaryngology, Jinan Central Hospital, Shandong University, Jinan, China

Qian Xin
The Second Hospital of Shandong University, Jinan, China

Ines de Vries, Nils Prenzler and Martin Durisin
Department of Otolaryngology, Hannover Medical School, Hanover, Germany

Heike Schmitt, Thomas Lenarz and Athanasia Warnecke
Department of Otolaryngology, Hannover Medical School, Hanover, Germany
Cluster of Excellence Hearing4all, German Research Foundation, Hannover Medical School, Hanover, Germany

Sameer Alvi and Hinrich Staecker
Department of Otolaryngology, Head and Neck Surgery, University of Kansas School of Medicine, Kansas City, MO, United States

Index

Printed in the USA
CPSIA information can be obtained
at www.ICGtesting.com
JSHW051400091023
49903JS00006B/219